Antiepileptic Drugs
Combination Therapy and Interactions

This book reviews the use of antiepileptic drugs focussing on the interactions between these drugs, and between antiepileptics and other drugs. These interactions can be beneficial or can cause harm. The aim of this book is to increase awareness of the possible impact of combination pharmacotherapies. Pharmacokinetic and pharmacodynamic interactions are discussed supported by clinical and experimental data. The book consists of five parts covering the general concepts and advantages of combination therapies, the principles of drug interactions, the mechanisms of interactions, drug interactions in specific populations or in patients with co-morbid health conditions, concluding with a look at the future directions for this field of research. The book will be of interest to all who prescribe antiepileptics to epileptic and non-epileptic patients, including epileptologists, neurologists, neuropediatricians, psychiatrists and general practitioners.

Antiepileptic Drugs

Combination Therapy and Interactions

Edited by

Jerzy Majkowski
The Foundation of Epileptology, Warsaw

Blaise F. D. Bourgeois
Harvard Medical School, USA

Philip N. Patsalos
Institute of Neurology, UK

and

Richard H. Mattson
Yale University School of Medicine, USA

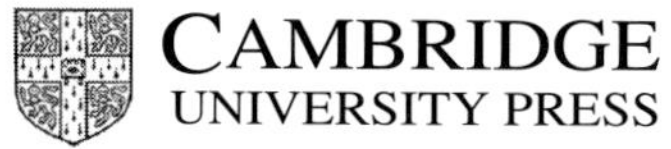

CAMBRIDGE
UNIVERSITY PRESS

PUBLISHED BY THE PRESS SYNDICATE OF THE UNIVERSITY OF CAMBRIDGE
The Pitt Building, Trumpington Street, Cambridge, United Kingdom

CAMBRIDGE UNIVERSITY PRESS
The Edinburgh Building, Cambridge CB2 2RU, UK
40 West 20th Street, New York, NY 10011-4211, USA
477 Williamstown Road, Port Melbourne, VIC 3207, Australia
Ruiz de Alarcón 13, 28014 Madrid, Spain
Dock House, The Waterfront, Cape Town 8001, South Africa

http://www.cambridge.org

First published 2005

Printed in the United Kingdom at the University Press, Cambridge

Typeface: Minion 10.5/14 pt   System: QuarkXpress®

A catalog record for this book is available from the British Library

ISBN-10 0 521 82 219 X
ISBN-13 978 0 521 82 219 0

The publisher has used its best endeavors to ensure that the URLs
for external websites referred to in this book are correct and
active at the time of going to press. However, the publisher has
no responsibility for the websites and can make no guarantee
that a site will remain live or that the content is or will
remain appropriate.

Every effort has been made in preparing this book to provide accurate and
up-to-date information that is in accord with accepted standards and practice at the
time of publication. Nevertheless, the authors, editors and publisher can make no
warranties that the information contained herein is totally free from error, not least
because clinical standards are constantly changing through research and regulation.
The authors, editors and publisher therefore disclaim all liability for direct or
consequential damages resulting from the use of material contained in this book.
Readers are strongly advised to pay careful attention to information provided by the
manufacturer of any drugs or equipment that they plan to use.

Contents

List of contributors

Professor Albert P. Aldencamp
Department of Neurology, University
Hospital of Maastricht, PO Box 21, NL 2100
AB, Heeze, The Netherlands

Professor Blaise F. D. Bourgeois
Children's Hospital – HU2, Harvard Medical
School, 300 Longwood Avenue, Boston,
MA 02115, USA

Dr Catherine Chiron
Hospital Necker-Enfants Malades, 149 Rue
de Sevres, Paris 75015, France

Dr Massimo Cincotta
Unit of Neurology, Santa Maria Nuova
Hospital, Florence, Italy

Dr James C. Cloyd
College of Pharmacy, University of
Minnesota, Room 7101, Weaver Densford
Hall, 308 Harvard St SE, Minneapolis,
MN 55455 0353, USA

Dr Jeannine M. Conway
College of Pharmacy, University of
Minnesota, 7-170 WDH, 308 Harvard St SE,
Minneapolis, MN 55455, USA

Professor Stanislaw J. Czuczwar
Department of Pathophysiology, Medical
Academy, Jaczewskiego 8, 820-090 Lublin,
Poland

Dr Mark de Krom
Department of Neurology, University
Hospital of Maastricht, PO Box 21, NL 2100
AB, Heeze, The Netherlands

Professor Olivier Dulac
Hospital Necker-Enfants Malades, 149 Rue
de Sevres, Paris 75015, France

Professor Carlos A. Fontes Ribeiro
Department of Pharmacology,
Faculty of Medicine, 3000 Coimbra,
Portugal

Professor Jacqueline French
Department of Neurology, 3 West Gates,
Hospital of the University of Pennsylvania,
3400 Spruce St, PA 19104, USA

Professor Walter Fröscher
Department of Neurology and Epileptology,
Die Weissenau (Department of Psychiatry I),
University of Ulm, D-88214 Ravensburg,
Germany

Dr Michael R. Johnson
Division of Neurosciences and Psychological
Medicine, Imperial College London,
Charing Cross Hospital, London,
W6 8RP, UK

Dr Daniel M. Jonker
Epilepsy Institute of the Netherlands (SEIN),
Achterweg 5, NL 21 03 SW,
Heemstede, The Netherlands

Dr Irene Kotsopoulos
Department of Neurology, University
Hospital of Maastricht, PO Box 21,
NL 2100 AB, Heeze, The Netherlands

Professor Rene Levy
Department of Pharmaceutics, School of
Pharmacy, University of Washington,
Health Sciences Center H-Wing, Suite 272,
Seattle, WA 98195, USA

Professor Fernando H. Lopes da Silva
Epilepsy Institute of the Netherlands
(SEIN), Achterweg 5, NL 21 03 SW,
Heemstede, The Netherlands

Professor Jerzy Majkowski
Diagnostic and Therapeutic Center for
Epilepsy, Foundation of Epileptology, ul
Wiertnicza 122, 02-952 Warsaw, Poland

Dr Emma Mason
Department of Pharmacology, Therapeutics
and Toxicology, Wales College of Medicine,
Cardiff University, Heath Park, Cardiff,
CF14 4XN, UK

Professor Richard H. Mattson
Department of Neurology, Yale University
701 LC1, 33 Cedar Street, New Haven,
CT 06510, USA

Dr Theodor W. May
Biochemisches Labor der Gesellschaft für
Epilepsieforchung, Maraweg 13, D-33617
Bielefeld, Germany

Dr Andrea Messori
Unit of Pharmacy, Careggi Hospital,
Florence, Italy

Dr Marco Mula
Amadeo Avogadro University,
C.so Mazzini, 18 28100 Novara, Italy

Professor Philip N. Patsalos
Pharmacology and Therapeutic Unit,
Department of Clinical and Experimental
Epilepsy, Institute of Neurology, Queen
Square, London, WC1N 3BG; The National
Society for Epilepsy, Chalfont St Peter, UK

Professor Emilio Perucca
Clinical Pharmacology Unit, University of
Pavia, Piazza Botta 10, I 27100 Pavia, Italy

Dr John R. Pollard
Department of Neurology, 3 West Gates,
Hospital of the University of Pennsylvania,
3400 Spruce St, PA 19104, USA

Dr Bernhard Rambeck
Biochemisches Labor der Gesellschaft für
Epilepsieforschung, Maraweg 13, D-33617
Bielefeld, Germany

Dr Elizabeth Rey
Hôpital Saint Vincent de Paul, Paris, France

Professor Philip A. Routledge
Department of Pharmacology, Therapeutics
and Toxicology, Wales College of Medicine,
Cardiff University, Heath Park, Cardiff,
CF14 4XN, UK

Professor Matti Sillanpää
Department of Public Health, 20014 Turku
University, Turku, Finland

Professor Edoardo Spina
Department of Clinical and Experimental
Medicine and Pharmacology, University of
Messina, Policlinico Universitario, Via
Consolare Valeria, 98125 Messina, Italy

Professor Michael R. Trimble
The National Hospital for Neurology and
Neurosurgery, Institute of Neurology,
Queen Square, London, WC1N 3BG, UK

Dr Jan Vermeulen
Epilepsy centre SEIN, Heemstede,
The Netherlands

Dr Rob A. Voskuyl
LACDR, Division of Pharmacology,
Gorlaeus Laboratories, Postbus 9502,
2300 RA, Leiden, The Netherlands

Dr Matthew C. Walker
Pharmacology and Therapeutic Unit,
Department of Clinical and Experimental
Epilepsy, Institute of Neurology,
Queen Square, London, WC1N 3BG, UK

Dr Mark S. Yerby
North Pacific Epilepsy Research, 2455 NW
Marshall St, Ste 14, Portland, OR 97201,
USA

Dr Gaetano Zaccara
Department of Neurology, Ospedale S.M.
Nuova, Piazza S.M. Nuova 1, 50124
Florence, Italy

Foreword

It is my special pleasure to introduce this book about the principles on which to base combination antiepileptic drug (AED) therapy and its related problems.

As reviewed in the excellent opening chapter by Mason and Routledge, therapeutic strategies involving the combination of different drugs are currently used to treat hypertension, infectious diseases and cancer in an attempt to enhance efficacy, reduce unwanted side effects and decrease the of probability of developing resistance. However, their disadvantages may exceed their benefits. First of all, drug toxicity may actually be increased by combination therapy as a result of negative pharmacodynamic interactions and the increased probability of idiosyncratic reactions. Secondly, the management of combination therapy is complicated by pharmacokinetic interactions. Thirdly, the risks of non-compliance and medication error are significantly greater with a multiple drug regimen.

How these general concepts apply to pharmacological antiepileptic therapy is dealt with by the most authoritative specialists in the first three parts of the book, which give considerable space to pharmacokinetic and pharmacodynamic interactions, while the fourth part develops these questions further with special regard to the patients' age, associated health problem (neurological or general), and sexual life (contraception, pregnancy, etc.). The reader is thus guided in understanding the rationale for combining AEDs, and made aware of the caveats that need to be taken into account.

In an ideal situation, we should consider AED combinations in such a way as to ensure that each pharmacological ingredient targets a specific epileptogenic mechanism. Unfortunately, our current understanding of the basic mechanisms of epileptogenesis and drug activity is still too limited to make such rational polypharmacy feasible. However, the favourable effects of some combinations based on traditional or newly developed AEDs (or both) is documented in the literature and here critically reviewed. This information is relevant and important when choosing the drug combinations to be prescribed to patients failing to respond to single drug regimens on the basis of exploiting the potential synergies of different drugs.

It is worth noting that the availability of newly developed AEDs has made multiple drug regimens increasingly frequent in clinical practice because, until the efficacy and tolerability of a given new drug are fully understood it would be inappropriate (and in many instances illegal) to use it as a first choice monotherapy. A good knowledge of the advances and drawbacks of combination therapy is essential for the everyday use of new AEDs.

Appropriate attention is given to the pharmacogenetic aspects underlying the variables that may influence AED responses and interaction profiles, such as metabolism, pharmacokinetics and pharmacodynamics, and there is a critical discussion of the usefulness and pitfalls of genetic screening. Pharmacogenetics and pharmacogenomics are currently seen as speculative perspectives, but it is worth bearing in mind that it is already possible to characterize individuals on the basis of the polymorphisms of genes encoding drug metabolic enzymes, even though the relevance of this approach to the clinical use of combination therapy has not yet been assessed.

This book will stimulate new thoughts and ideas, and I am sure that all of its readers will learn something even about what at first glance may seem familiar subjects. For instance, although I was of course aware that most drug formulations contain multiple ingredients, it had not occurred to me that this makes the very concept of monotherapy rather relative as the active principle may make up as little as 8% of a tablet's weight, with the rest consisting of coating and binding agents, fillers, dyes, preservatives, and solubilising and disintegrating ingredients which, however rarely, may give rise to dose-related or idiosyncratic reactions in susceptible subjects.

In summary, this book will provide readers an updated account of the state of the art and an appraisal of the exciting perspectives of an important aspect of pharmacological antiepileptic therapy. The editors (Jerzy Majkowski, Blaise Bourgeois, Philip Patsalos and Richard Mattson) wrote some of the critical chapters themselves, but also gathered a highly authoritative group of other scientists in order to cover the field comprehensively. In thanking them for this, I wish the book the success it deserves.

Giuliano Avanzini
President of the International League Against Epilepsy

Foreword

Drug interactions may be regarded as a stimulating challenge by the pharmacologist but by the physician responsible for management of the patient, interactions are often considered cumbersome and a vexing factor complicating treatment. Drug interactions are particularly common in the treatment of patients with epilepsy. Although monotherapy has been the favoured treatment strategy for the last 25 years or so, up to 50% may not achieve satisfactory seizure control while on the first drug they have been prescribed. A high proportion of these patients will eventually end up taking a combination of different antiepileptic drugs. Until now, the selection of drug combinations has more often been the result of chance or the physician's individual preferences rather than being rational or evidence-based. Given the long duration of epilepsy treatment, most patients will frequently be prescribed drugs for other conditions too. Conventional antiepileptic drugs have been among the most prone to pharmacokinetic interactions, and pharmacodynamic interactions occur whenever two drugs are used together. For all these reasons, the topic of combination therapy and drug interactions is of great importance and up-to-date knowledge is an essential basis for a rational approach to the pharmacological treatment of people with epilepsy.

The editors of the current book on *Antiepileptic drugs: combination therapy and interactions* have managed to gather an international group of experts to cover these and related issues in a comprehensive volume. The reader is provided the relevant general background, along with in-depth coverage of pharmacokinetic and pharmacodynamic interactions as well as interactions in specific patient populations. It is made clear that while pharmacokinetic interactions in most cases are negative, recent advances in our understanding of drug metabolism enable us to predict and avoid adverse interactions. Drug level monitoring can help us manage those interactions that cannot be avoided. Pharmacodynamic interactions are not always adverse. Some are advantageous, improving the therapeutic index, and could be exploited to the benefit of our patients. This volume, which should be of interest to all physicians engaged in the treatment of patients with epilepsy, shows how far we have advanced from the level where interactions could be regarded as just an unwieldy factor complicating pharmacotherapy. Instead, the data provided will hopefully serve as a platform for more rational and effective therapeutic strategies in the future for epilepsy patients in need of combination therapy.

Torbjörn Tomson
Chairman, Commission on Therapeutic Strategies,
International League Against Epilepsy

Acknowledgements

This book has arisen as a result of the activities of the International League Against Epilepsy's (ILAE) Sub-commission of Polytherapy and Drug Interactions of the Commission on Therapeutic Strategies. Under the auspices of the Sub-commission, three international pre-congress symposia/satellite symposia were organised during the 1st European Congress of Epileptology, Oporto, Portugal, 1994; the 3rd European Congress of Epileptology, Warsaw, Poland, 1998; and the XIV Conference on Epilepsy, Warsaw, Poland, 2000. These symposia brought together internationally recognised experts in the field of antiepileptic drug interactions and it is these experts that have contributed the chapters that constitute this book. The activities of the Sub-commission of Polytherapy and Drug Interactions and thus this book would not have been possible without the generous financial support of the ILAE, Polish Society of Epileptology, Abbott, Aventis, GlaxoSmithKline, Hoechst Marion Roussel, Novartis, Ortho (Johnson and Johnson) and Pfizer.

J. Majkowski, B.F.D. Bourgeois, P.N. Patsalos and R.H. Mattson

Part I

Introduction

Combination therapy of diseases: general concepts

Emma Mason and Philip A. Routledge

Department of Pharmacology, Therapeutics and Toxicology, Wales College of Medicine, Cardiff University, Cardiff, UK

> Many drugs are excellent when mingled and many are fatal
>
> Homer 950 EC

Historical aspects

Combination therapy has been used since therapeutics was first practiced. The physician or *asu* of Mesopotamia in 1700 BC used combinations of several plants, minerals and animal products in concoctions, salves and fomentations (Lyons and Petrucelli, 1987). We know little of the efficacy or toxicity of these combined medications. However, the Babylonian code of Hammurabi states that a doctor who causes the death of a patient or loss of an eye should lose his hands. It would not have been surprising if such stringent punishments encouraged the use of a large number of non-toxic (and possibly non-efficacious) medicines. At least this would have ensured that the physician could continue to be able to mix his own preparations.

Since many early drugs were of plant origin, the use of single herbal preparations containing many potentially active ingredients resulted in combination therapy, albeit often unknowingly. Thus cannabis, advocated by the Red Emperor (Shen Nung) around 2800 BC contains around 30 cannabinoid compounds, and debate still rages today as to whether cannabis has greater therapeutic efficacy than single cannabinoid therapy (e.g. with delta-9 tetrahydrocannabinol) in certain medical conditions. Traditional Chinese medicines continue to be used regularly by up to half the population of China (Encyclopaedia Britannica, 1999), and contain several constituents prescribed in individualized doses in a *bespoke* fashion. The patient takes these ingredients home and boils them in a soup, before consuming the broth.

In 1753, the Scottish physician and sailor, James Lind described one of the first controlled trials of drug therapy in history, which he had performed 6 years earlier. He administered a combination treatment for scurvy containing nutmeg, garlic mustard seed, *rad. raphan*, balsam of Peru and gum myrrh to two sailors for 6 days.

It is not surprising that the sailors who improved most were not these two individuals, but two others given another 'combination therapy' – two oranges and a lemon (Lind, 1753)!

The deliberate combination of medicines continued to be practiced right through into the nineteenth and twentieth centuries, although not embraced by all physicians.

William Withey Gull (1816–1890) particularly condemned prescriptions containing multiple drugs. He was a passionate advocate of the scientific basis of medicine and stated that '*The road to a clinic goes through the pathologic museum and not through the apothecary's shop*'. Drug combinations were often contained in medicines, the contents of which were kept secret from the patient. Dr Pierce's Pleasant Purgative Pills were said to combine the active principles of several unspecified vegetable compounds which 'in some inexplicable manner, gradually changed certain morbid conditions of the system, and established a healthy condition instead' (Pierce, 1891). Dr Pierce did not patent his proprietary medicines as 'cure-alls', but others did patent theirs, since there was little or no government regulation of ingredients or need to verify claims of therapeutic efficacy. It was not until 1938, a year after 105 people died due to an elixir of sulfonamide made up of 70% diethylene glycol that the US government legislation was introduced to ensure labeling of all ingredients and prevention of false claims of efficacy (Routledge, 1998a).

The issue of toxicity of ingredients, which still occurs today (Stephens, 1998) is a reminder that most formulations of medicines contain several ingredients, some of which may rarely cause either dose-related (Type A) or idiosyncratic (Type B) toxicity in certain susceptible individuals. Thus, the active principle may constitute as little as 8% of the weight of a typical tablet, and the remainder may include coating and binding agents, fillers, dyes, preservatives, solubilizing and disintegrating agents (Freestone, 1969). To this extent, combination therapy with several compounds occurs when only one medicine is prescribed, although the other ingredients are inactive in most individuals. However, changes to the formulation may affect bioavailability, and were responsible for an outbreak of phenytoin (diphenylhydantoin) toxicity in Australia when lactose was substituted for calcium sulfate as an excipient (Tyrer *et al.*, 1970).

A scientific basis for the value of combination therapy was established in the 1940s. Waksman had discovered streptomycin as the first compound to be effective in the treatment of tuberculosis (Waksman, 1949). Indeed the efficacy of streptomycin in tuberculosis was the subject of the first published randomized controlled trial in medicine (Medical Research Council (MRC), 1948). It was soon realized that streptomycin monotherapy required the use of large doses, which could cause significant toxicity. The emergence of streptomycin resistance was also soon recognized, and combination therapy was seen to be a possible answer to this serious problem. Thus a trial of para-aminosalicylic acid and streptomycin in pulmonary tuberculosis

Table 1.1 Principles for the development of chemotherapeutic regimens in oncology

1   Each single agent should have activity against the disease
2   The agents should have different mechanisms of action
3   The agents should have non-overlapping toxicity profiles
4   The regimen should combine cell cycle specific and cell cycle non-specific agents

found a reduction in streptomycin resistance from 67% in the streptomycin-only group to 10% in those treated with both agents concomitantly (MRC, 1950).

It soon became clear that similar principles applied to the treatment of malignant cells as to slow-growing pathogenic bacteria such as *Mycobacterium tuberculosis*. This led not only to the use of combination chemotherapy of cancer according to specific principles shown in Table 1.1 (Muggia and Von Hoff, 1997). The first three of these principles are generally applicable to combination therapy in other condi-tion, although some exceptions will be highlighted in this chapter. Before discussing the possible advantages and disadvantages of combination therapy, it is important to define and discuss two terms that have been used in this context, sometimes interchangeably.

Polypharmacy

The term polypharmacy has been in use in medicine for around 40 years. One of the first occasions on which it was used was in the context of multiple drug admin-istration versus hypnosis for surgical patients (Bartlett, 1966). This early paper did not make any suggestion that polypharmacy was a bad practice, but a subsequent review of polypharmacy in America highlighted the potential problems that polypharmacy could produce (Hudson, 1968). Indiscriminate polypharmacy has been identified as a major medical problem in some developing countries and a challenge for the World Health Organisation's action program on essential drugs (Hogerzeil *et al.*, 1993).

The strict definition of the word in *The New Shorter Oxford Dictionary* (1993) is '*the use of several drugs or medicines together in the treatment of disease*'. However this initially rather non-judgemental definition is immediately qualified with the rider '*frequently with the suggestion of indiscriminate, unscientific or excessive pre-scription*'. Other authors have assumed that the administration of an excessive number of drugs is implicit in the definition (*Online Medical Dictionary*, 1997). This has led to the use of the term rational polypharmacy to distinguish the appropriate use of drug combinations from indiscriminate use of several medi-cines concurrently (Kalviainen *et al.*, 1993; Reus, 1993; Wolkowitz, 1993). Thus polypharmacy tends to be a pejorative term for excessive irrational drug use, although the drugs may be being used for a range of medical conditions rather than for a single disease.

Polytherapy

The first record of the use of this term listed on *Medline* was just over 20 years ago (1978) in the context of epilepsy management (Deisenhammer and Sommer, 1978). Since then it has been used predominantly in this therapeutic area, and largely by German, Italian, Spanish and French authors. It has not entered general use in the UK, where combination therapy is generally the preferred term for use of more than one drug for the same condition. The definition in the *Online Medical Dictionary* is '*A therapy that uses more than one drug*'. It thus differs from polypharmacy in that it normally refers to the use of drugs for the same medical condition rather than for a group of existing medical conditions. In the following discussion, we will treat the term polytherapy as synonymous with combination therapy, a term that is more widely accepted across the spectrum of therapeutics and throughout Europe and the USA.

Epidemiology of combination therapy

Although, around 10% of the general population take more than one prescribed medicine, the incidence of combination therapy is even greater in the elderly, in females and in those who have had recent hospital admission (Nobili *et al.*, 1997; Teng Liaw, 1997). Stewart and Cooper reviewed a number of studies and concluded that patients aged over 65 years use on average 2–6 prescribed medications and 1–3.4 non-prescribed medications (Stewart and Cooper, 1994).

The effects of multiple drug administration on the incidence of adverse drug reactions were first studied by May and co-workers in 10 518 patients hospitalized on a general medical service during a 5-year period (May *et al.*, 1977). Their data suggested a disproportionately increased risk of adverse drug reactions for patients, the more drugs they were receiving. A significant proportion of these adverse drug reactions were due to adverse interactions between two or more co-prescribed agents.

In a case-control study by Hamilton and co-workers (who over the 3-year period 1993–1995 studied more than 157 000 patients in the USA) the drug combination most often associated with hospital admission was angiotensin converting enzyme (ACE) inhibitors co-prescribed with potassium replacement therapy. Combinations with inhibitors of drug metabolism (particularly macrolide antibiotics such as erythromycin) formed the next most frequent group of agents associated with increased hospitalization (Hamilton *et al.*, 1998).

Advantages of combination therapy

Efficacy can be enhanced by combination therapy

One of the first indications that the use of more than one agent could be more effective than the use of either agent as monotherapy was in the treatment of severe infections (e.g. bacterial endocarditis) with combinations of penicillin and an aminoglycoside (Wilson *et al.*, 1978). It later became clear that this *synergism* was achieved by a dual action on bacterial growth. Penicillins inhibited cell wall synthesis while the aminoglycoside inhibited protein synthesis. Synergism was also demonstrated between loop diuretics and thiazides, since each acted at a different site on the nephron to reduce sodium and water reabsorption. This combination (e.g. frusemide and metolazone) is still used to produce diuresis in resistant congestive cardiac failure. Thus combination therapy normally involves the use of two or more drugs with different mechanism of action, and therefore normally from different drug classes.

The effects of some drug combinations are merely additive rather than synergistic. Nevertheless, the combination produces more efficacy than the use of each single agent alone and this can be of therapeutic benefit. Patients may now leave hospital after acute myocardial infarction on a beta-blocker, ACE inhibitor, antiplatelet agent (e.g. aspirin) and lipid lowering agent (e.g. statin), all having been shown individually to provide secondary preventive benefit in this situation. In heart failure, ACE inhibitors, beta-blockers and spironolactone have been shown to reduce mortality when added to standard therapy. Ischemic heart disease, heart failure and hypertension are heterogeneous diseases with multiple mechanisms contributing to their pathogenesis. It is therefore not surprising that more than one mechanism of action (and therefore more than one drug) may be needed to treat the underlying problems. In addition, several of these chronic diseases result in multiple end-organ damage and several drugs may be needed to treat the multiple pathologies associated with them.

Monotherapy is effective in only around 50% of hypertensive patients, but efficacy can be increased to around 80% with the judicious use of combination therapy (Mancia *et al.*, 1996). The need for combination therapy is also demonstrated by the hypertension optimal treatment (HOT) study. Depending on the target blood pressure, up to 74% of patients needed more than one drug to achieve the required blood pressure (Hansson *et al.*, 1998; Opie, 1998). It is also interesting to note that in this study, patients randomized to acetylsalicylic acid had significantly reduced rates of major cardiovascular events. Thus combined antihypertensive and antiplatelet therapy is valuable, even though these drugs are producing their beneficial effects in completely different ways.

Anticonvulsant drugs are also thought to have a range of different mechanisms of action, but that the same principles should also apply. Even with carefully instituted and monitored monotherapy, only 70–80% of patients will achieve satisfactory control of their epilepsy (Jallon, 1997) so that combination therapy may be an option that should be considered.

Combination therapy may help to reduce the incidence and/or severity of adverse drug reactions

Dose-related (Type A) adverse drug reactions are thought to make up around 75% of all adverse drug reactions (Routledge, 1998b). Combinations of medicines with different spectra of adverse drug reactions may therefore allow reduction of dose of each compound to levels that are less likely to produce clinically relevant toxicity. This principle (i.e. that the agents should have non-overlapping toxicity) is one of the underlying reasons for the general use of combination chemotherapy in cancer (Muggia and Von Hoff, 1997). In the case of tuberculosis, the use of triple and quadruple antituberculous chemotherapy has allowed some potentially toxic agents (e.g. ethambutol and pyrazinamide) to be used at lower and therefore safer doses than previously. This approach has also allowed shorter treatment courses, thus reducing duration of exposure to risk of toxicity. In hypertension combinations of low doses of two agents from different classes have been shown to provide additional antihypertensive efficacy, thereby minimizing the likelihood of dose-dependent adverse effects.

Combination therapy can prevent the development of resistance

The experience of treatment of tuberculosis indicated that combination therapy might help to prevent the emergence of resistant bacteria. Chambers and Sande (1996) have elegantly argued that if spontaneous mutation were the major mechanism by which bacteria acquired antibiotic resistance, combination chemotherapy should be effective. They illustrate their argument with the example of a micro-organism that has a frequency of development of resistance to one drug of 10^{-7} and to a second drug of 10^{-6}. In this case, the probability of independent mutation of resistance to both drugs in a single cell would be the product of the two frequencies (i.e. 10^{-13}) making the likelihood of development of resistance extremely small. Such arguments clearly apply to other situations such as oncology where the development of resistance can otherwise limit drug efficacy. They are less relevant to the treatment of other diseases.

Disadvantages of combination therapy

The evidence for the benefits of combined therapy is often poor

At the beginning of the last century, therapeutics was based more on the experience of others, rather than on firm evidence. Thus Wilson was able to state that although many remedies had been tried and were still in favor for the treatment of epilepsy, the only ones that have any effect are the bromides of potassium, sodium and ammonium. It is interesting to note that 'the best results seem to follow the administration of all three in a combined dose' (Wilson, 1912).

In diabetes, the benefits of combination therapy with a biguanide (e.g. metformin) and sulfonylurea (e.g. glibenclamide), in patients with Type 2 (non-insulin-dependent) diabetes who are inadequately controlled with either agent alone, have been claimed for 40 years. The mechanism of action of these two drug classes is different. Biguanides such as metformin (which first became available in Europe in 1957), work by increasing the action of insulin in peripheral tissues and reducing hepatic glucose output due to inhibition of gluconeogenesis. Sulfonylureas act primarily by potentiating glucose-stimulated insulin release from functioning pancreatic islet beta-cells (O'Meara *et al.*, 1990), although studies of insulin secretion at the same plasma glucose concentrations before and during long-term sulfonylurea therapy have shown increased beta-cell sensitivity to glucose and continuously augmented insulin secretion (Gerich, 1989). However, the evidence for combined therapy sulfonylurea/biguanide was relatively sparse for many years, and rested largely on a single non-randomized observational trial of 108 sulfonylurea failures (Clarke and Duncan, 1965). It was only 30 years later that controlled trials confirmed the benefits of this combination of agents (Hermann *et al.*, 1994; DeFronzo, 1995).

In his article on rational polypharmacy in epilepsy, Richens points out that few randomized placebo-controlled studies have been undertaken to compare the relative merits of monotherapy and combination therapy with respect to seizure control (Richens, 1995). Evidence-based medicine should play an important role in the therapeutics of epilepsy, as it has increasingly done in other areas of disease management.

Toxicity may be greater with combination therapy than monotherapy

One of the principles of combination therapy in cancer is that the agents should have non-overlapping toxicity. Clearly this is not always possible, even in oncology, since many anti-cancer drugs share similar toxicity profiles (e.g. myelotoxicity). It may also be difficult to achieve in other therapeutic areas.

It is possible that combination therapy is a risk factor in the production of sudden unexpected death in epilepsy, although the use of more than one drug may just reflect the severe unstable nature of the epilepsy in such individuals (Nilsson *et al.*, 2001). It is also possible that combination therapy is associated with greater risk of anticonvulsant embryopathy in infants exposed to anticonvulsant drugs in utero, (control frequency 8.5%, monotherapy 20.6%, combination therapy 28.0%) so that the risks from each agent in this situation may be additive (Holmes *et al.*, 2001).

Non-steroidal anti-inflammatory drugs (NSAIDs) used in the treatment of arthritis can increase the risk of peptic ulcer by around four-fold in patients aged

65 years or older (Griffin *et al.*, 1991). Corticosteroids are also used in some patients with arthritis, particularly rheumatoid arthritis. Piper and colleagues, using the same design and patient database as Griffin, showed that the estimated relative risk for the development of peptic ulcer disease among current users of oral corticosteroids (but not NSAIDs) was 1.1 (i.e. a 10% increase in risk). However, patients concurrently receiving corticosteroids and NSAIDs had a risk for peptic ulcer disease that was 15 times greater than that of non-users of either drug (Piper *et al.*, 1991).

Similarly, compared with non-users of either drug, the relative risk of hemorrhagic peptic ulcer disease among current users of both anticoagulants and NSAIDs was 12.7 (95% confidence interval, 6.3–25.7)(Shorr *et al.*, 1993). However, the prevalence of NSAID use among anticoagulant users was 13.5%, the same as in those who were not using anticoagulants. Thus toxicity of drug combinations may sometimes be synergistic and be greater than the sum of the risks of toxicity of either agent used alone.

Enhanced toxicity of drug combinations may sometimes be due to pharmacokinetic interaction. Herpes Zoster infections are not uncommon in immunocompromised patients, and anti-viral agents may be required. Unfortunately 19 people with cancer and Herpes Zoster died in Japan in 1993 because of fluoro-pyrimidine toxicity, caused by the inhibition of 5-fluorouracil metabolism by the metabolite of a new anti-viral agent, sorivudine. Sixteen of the deaths occurred after the drug had been licensed, illustrating that not all drug interactions may be recognized before marketing and widespread exposure to the offending combination of agents occurs (Watabe, 1996).

In 1997, Mibefradil (Posicor) was marketed in the USA and Europe for the treatment of hypertension and angina as an exciting new molecule that selectively blocked T-calcium channels (Frishman, 1997). It was already known before marketing that mibefradil inhibited the metabolism of three potentially toxic agents, astemizole, cisapride and terfenadine. Soon further clinically significant interactions with cyclosporin and tricyclic antidepressants were being reported. It was known that mibefradil could inhibit the action of cytochrome P450 3A4 and thus reduce the clearance of other drugs that were metabolized by this enzyme. In December 1997, because of seven reports of statin-induced rhabdomyolysis in patients receiving simvastatin and mibefradil, lovastatin and simvastatin were added to the list of those that should never be co-administered with mibefradil. This was of particular importance, since hypertension and hypercholesterolemia are important and often co-existing risk factors for ischemic heart disease.

Finally, as a result of the number of serious interactions, the manufacturers announced the withdrawal of mibefradil from the market in 1998; almost exactly a year after the drug had been given marketing approval (Po and Zhang, 1998). Recently Wandel and co-workers have used a human intestinal cancer-derived cell which expresses P-glycoprotein to show that mibefradil is not only a substrate for

P-glycoprotein, but may well be a potent inhibitor of this efflux pump mechanism (Wandel *et al.*, 2000). Thus its combined effects on CYP3A and P-glycoprotein could explain the magnitude of the effect of its interactions with other drugs. Thus the clinical significance of potential interactions may not be fully realized until after marketing.

Combination therapy may be associated with increased risk of non-compliance (non-concordance)

Compliance with therapy is an essential prerequisite of obtaining the benefits of the drugs. The use of combination therapy means that the patient has to take more tablets, unless the drugs have been formulated in a combined preparation. If two drugs are being used in combination, the dose of each should be adjusted to achieve optimal benefit. Thus, patient compliance is essential, yet more difficult to achieve. If patients perceive that they are being overmedicated, they self-report that their compliance falls (Fincke *et al.*, 1998). Polypharmacy may thus result in poor compliance, which may itself result in failure of therapy. This mechanism has been reported to be a problem in individuals with epilepsy (Lambie *et al.*, 1981), and an important factor precipitating admission to hospital for seizure (Lambie *et al.*, 1986).

To obviate the problem of multiple medication use, many fixed-dose drug combinations are marketed. The use of such combinations is advantageous only if the ratio of the fixed doses corresponds to the needs of the individual patient. In the USA, a fixed-dose combination of drugs is considered a 'new drug' and as such must be approved by the Food and Drug Administration (FDA) before it can be marketed, even though the individual drugs are available for concurrent use. To be approved, certain conditions must be met. Either the two drugs must act to achieve a better therapeutic response than either drug alone (e.g. many antihypertensive drug combinations); or one drug must act to reduce the incidence of adverse effects caused by the other (e.g. a diuretic that promotes the urinary excretion of K^+ combined with a K^+-sparing diuretic) (Nies and Spielberg, 1996).

Combination therapy may be associated with an increased risk of medication error

Misuse of medications is a major cause of morbidity and mortality. Patients' medication bottles and their reported use of medications were compared with physicians' records of outpatients in Boston, Massachusetts. Discrepancies were present in 239 patients (76%). The 545 discrepancies in these patients were the result of patients taking medications that were not recorded ($n = 278$ [51%]); patients not taking a recorded medication ($n = 158$ [29%]) and differences in dosage ($n = 109$ [20%]). Older age and polypharmacy were the most significant correlates of discrepancy (Bedell *et al.*, 2000).

Conclusions

Combination therapy is an essential therapeutic tool, although one that can all too often be misused, to the detriment of the patient. The efficacy of many treatment schedules can be enhanced by combination therapy, and this approach may help to reduce the incidence and/or severity of adverse drug reactions. In cancer and anti-infective chemotherapy, combination therapy can prevent or at least delay the development of resistance.

However there is often a dearth of robust evidence for the benefits of certain drug combinations. Increased toxicity, sometimes as a result of direct interaction, is also a possibility. Finally combination therapy may be associated with an increased risk of non-compliance (non-concordance). A good working knowledge of the pharmacology of the drugs prescribed, and the potential for interaction is an important part of obtaining the benefits of combination therapy and minimizing toxicity. In addition, the risk of medication error in patients on multiple medicines means that physicians should check medication lists with patients carefully. Since patients are major stakeholders in the prescribing process, they should be encouraged to engage in a 'prescribing partnership'. They can help in the monitoring of therapy by alerting physicians, pharmacists and other healthcare professionals to problems that occur, especially when new drugs are introduced or doses of existing agents are changed (Seymour and Routledge, 1998).

REFERENCES

Bartlett EE. Polypharmacy versus hypnosis in surgical patients. *Pac Med Surg* 1966; **74**: 109–112.

Bedell SE, Jabbour S, Goldberg R, *et al*. Discrepancies in the use of medications: their extent and predictors in an outpatient practice. *Arch Intern Med* 2000; **160**: 2129–2134.

Chambers HF, Sande MA. Antimicrobial agents: general considerations. In *Goodman and Oilman's The Pharmacological basis of Therapeutics*, 9th edn. USA: McGraw Hill, 1996.

DeFronzo RA, Goodman A and the Multicenter Metformin Study Group. Efficacy of metformin in patients with non-insulin-dependent diabetes mellitus. *New Engl J Med* 1995; **335**: 541–549.

Deisenhammer E, Sommer R. Blood level of antiepileptic drugs and therapeutic effect in mono- and polytherapy. *Nervenarzt* 1978; **49**: 674–677.

Duncan LJ, Clarke BF, Munro JF. The treatment of diabetes mellitus with oral hypoglycaemic drugs. *Curr Med Drug* 1965; **5**: 23–32.

Encyclopaedia Britannica on CD ROM, Multimedia Edition. 1999.

Fincke BG, Miller DR, Spiro A III. The interaction of patient perception of overmedication with drug compliance and side effects. *J Gen Intern Med* 1998; **13**: 182–185.

Freestone DS. Formulation and therapeutic efficacy of drugs used in clinical trials. *Lancet* 1969; **2**: 98–99.

Frishman WH. Mibefradil: A new selective T-channel calcium antagonist for hypertension and angina pectoris. *J. Cardiovasc Pharmacol Ther* 1997; **2**: 321–330.

Gerich JE. Oral hypoglycaemic agents. *New Engl J Med* 1989; **321**: 1231–1235.

Griffin MR, Piper JM, Daugherty JR, *et al.* Nonsteroidal anti-inflammatory drug use and increased risk for peptic ulcer disease in elderly persons. *Ann Intern Med* 1991; **114**: 257–263.

Hamilton RA, Briceland LL, Andritz MH. Frequency of hospitalization after exposure to known drug–drug interactions in a Medicaid population. *Pharmacotherapy* 1998; **18**: 1112–1120.

Hansson L, Zanchetti A, Carruthers SG, *et al.* Effects of intensive blood-pressure lowering and low-dose aspirin in patients with hypertension: principal results of the Hypertension Optimal Treatment randomised trial. *Lancet* 1998; **351**: 1755–1762.

Hermann LS, Schersten B, Bitzen PO, *et al.* Therapeutic comparison of metformin and sulfonylurea, alone and in various combinations. *Diabetes Care* 1994; **17**: 1100–1109.

Hogerzeil HV, Bimo, Ross-Degnan D, Laing RO, *et al.* Field tests for rational drug use in twelve developing countries. *Lancet* 1993; **342**: 1408–1410.

Holmes LB, Harvey EA, Coull BA, *et al.* The teratogenicity of anticonvulsant drugs. *New Engl J Med* 2001; **344**: 1132–1138.

Hudson RP. Polypharmacy in twentieth century America. *Clin Pharmacol Ther* 1968; **9**: 2–10.

Jallon P. Monotherapy and polytherapy use of anti-epileptic drugs. Development of views. *Rev Neurol (Paris)* 1997; **153**(Suppl. 1): 829–833.

Kalviainen R, Keranen T, Riekkinen Sr PJ. Place of newer antiepileptic drugs in the treatment of epilepsy. *Drugs* 1993; **46**: 1009–1024.

Lambie DG, Johnson RH, Stanaway L. Prescribing patterns for epilepsy. *New Zeal Med J* 1981; **93**: 15–19.

Lambie DG, Stanaway L, Johnson RH. Factors which influence the effectiveness of treatment of epilepsy. *Aust NZ J Med* 1986; **16**: 779–784.

Lind J. *A Treatise of the Scurvy*. In three parts. Containing an inquiry into the nature, causes and cure, of that disease; together with a critical and chronological view of what has been published on the subject. Edinburgh: Printed by Sands, Murray and Cochran for A. Kincaid and A. Donaldson, 1753.

Lyons AS, Petrucelli RJ. *Medicine: An Illustrated History*. New York: Harry N Abrams, Inc., 1987.

Mancia G, *et al.* Guidelines for the treatment of hypertension: a commentary. *Curr Ther Res* 1996; **57**: 3–15.

Materson BJ, Reda DJ, Cushman WC. Department of Veterans Affairs single-drug therapy of hypertension study. Revised figures and new data. Department of Veterans Affairs Cooperative Study Group on Antihypertensive Agents. *Am J Hypertens* 1995; **8**: 189–192.

May FE, Fuller S, Stewart RB. Drug use and adverse drug reactions prior to and during hospitalization. *J Amer Pharm Assoc* 1977; **17**: 560–563.

Medical Research Council. Streptomycin treatment of pulmonary tuberculosis: a Medical Research Council investigation. *Br Med J* 1948; **2**: 769–782.

Treatment of pulmonary tuberculosis with streptomycin and para-aminosalicilic acid. *Br Med J* 1950; **2**: 1073–1083.

Muggia FM, Von Hoff DD. Malignant diseases. In *Avery's Drug Treatment*, 4th edn. T. M. Speight, N. H. G. Holford, eds. Auckland: Adis International, 1997.

Nies AS, Spielberg SP. Principles of therapeutics. In *Goodman and Oilman's The Pharmacological Basis of Therapeutics*, 9th edn. USA: McGraw Hill, 1996.

Nilsson L, Bergman U, Diwan V, *et al.* Antiepileptic drug therapy and its management in sudden unexpected death in epilepsy: a case-control study. *Epilepsia* 2001; **42**: 667–673.

Nobili A, Tettamanti M, Frattura L, *et al.* Drug use by the elderly in Italy. *Ann Pharmacother* 1997; **31**: 416–422.

O'Meara NM, Shapiro ET, van Cauter E, *et al.* Effect of glyburide on b-cell responsiveness to glucose in non-insulin-dependent diabetes mellitus. *Am J Med* 1990; **89**(Suppl. 2A): 11S–16S.

Online Medical Dictionary. http://www.medic8.com/MedicalDictionary.htm

Opie LH. Principles of combination therapy for hypertension. What we learn from HOT and other studies – a personal point of view. *Cardiovasc Drug Ther* 1998; **12**: 425–429.

Pellock JM. Antiepileptic drug therapy in the United States: a review of clinical studies and unmet needs. *Neurology* 1995; **45**: 817–824.

Pierce RV. *The Peoples Common Sense Medical Adviser in Plain English or Medicine Simplified*, 26th edn. Buffalo, NY: World's Dispensary Printing Office and Bindery, 1891.

Piper JM, Ray WA, Daugherty JR, *et al.* Corticosteroid use and peptic ulcer disease: role of nonsteroidal anti-inflammatory drugs. *Ann Intern Med* 1991; **114**: 735–740.

Po AL, Zhang WY. What lessons can be learnt from withdrawal of mibefradil from the market? *Lancet* 1998; **351**: 1829–1830.

Reus VI. Rational polypharmacy in the treatment of mood disorders. *Ann Clin Psychiatry* 1993; **5**: 91–100.

Richens A. Rational polypharmacy. *Seizure* 1995; **4**: 211–214.

Routledge P. 150 years of pharmacovigilance. *Lancet* 1998a; **351**: 1200–1201.

Routledge P. In *Detection of New Adverse Reactions*, 4th edn. M. D. B. Stephens, J. C. C. Talbot, P. A. Routledge, eds. London: Macmillan Reference Ltd., 1998b.

Seymour RM, Routledge PA. Important drug–drug interactions in the elderly. *Drug Ageing* 1998; **6**: 485–494.

Shorr RI, Ray WA, Daugherty JR, *et al.* Concurrent use of nonsteroidal anti-inflammatory drugs and oral anticoagulants places elderly persons at high risk for hemorrhagic peptic ulcer disease. *Arch Intern Med* 1993; **153**(14): 1665–1670.

Stephens M. In *Detection of New Adverse Reactions*, 4th edn. M. D. B. Stephens, J. C. C. Talbot, P. A. Routledge, eds. London: Macmillan Reference Ltd., 1998.

Stewart RB, Cooper JW. Polypharmacy in the aged. Practical solutions. *Drug Aging* 1994; **4**: 449–461.

Teng Liaw ST. Drug interactions among the elderly. *Aust Fam Phys* 1997; **26**: 355–357.

The New Shorter Oxford Dictionary. L. Brown, ed. Oxford: Oxford University Press, 2001.

Tyrer JH, Eadie MJ, Sutherland JM, *et al.* Outbreak of anticonvulsant intoxication in an Australian city. *Br Med J* 1970; **4**: 271–273.

Waksman SA (ed.). *Streptomycin: Nature, and Practical Applications.* Baltimore: The Williams & Wilkins Co., 1949.

Wandel C, Kim RB, Guengerich FP, *et al.* Mibefradil is a P-glycoprotein substrate and a potent inhibitor of both P-glycoprotein and CYP3A in vitro. *Drug Metab Dispos* 2000; **28**: 895–898.

Watabe T. Strategic proposals for predicting drug–drug interactions during new drug development: based on sixteen deaths caused by interactions of the new antiviral sorivudine with 5-fluorouracil prodrugs. *J Toxicol Sci* 1996; **21**: 299–300.

Wilson A. Diseases of the brain and nervous system. In *The Modern Physician.* London: Caxton Publishing Company, 1912.

Wilson WR, Geraci IE, Wilkowske CJ, *et al.* Short-term intramuscular therapy with procaine penicillin plus streptomycin for infective endocarditis due to *viridans* streptococci. *Circulation* 1978; **57**: 1158–1161.

Wolkowitz OM. Rational polypharmacy in schizophrenia. *Ann Clin Psychiat* 1993; **5**: 79–90.

2

Combination therapy with antiepileptic drugs: potential advantages and problems

Richard H. Mattson

Department of Neurology, Yale University, New Haven, CT, USA

Rationale for combination therapy

Antiepileptic drug (AED) treatment of epilepsy to prevent or minimize recurrent epileptic seizures begins with the use of a single agent as monotherapy. The primary reason why two or more drugs are used together is the failure of monotherapy to control the seizures. Depending on the type of seizures and epilepsy syndrome, control may be complete or very poor. In adult-onset seizures control varies between 35% and 60% for partial seizures and 10% and 20% higher for tonic–clonic seizures after 1-year follow-up (Mattson *et al.*, 1985, 1992, 1996; Richens *et al.*, 1994; Heller *et al.*, 1995; Kwan and Brodie, 2000). The long-term response is less favorable for some patients because breakthrough seizures occur over time although others enter remission (Richens *et al.*, 1994; Heller *et al.*, 1995). Seizures associated with idiopathic generalized epilepsies are usually more easily controlled.

When seizures continue despite increasing doses of the initial AED to the maximum that can be tolerated, a second drug is usually added to the first in an effort to achieve better control. In those patients with particularly refractory seizures/epilepsy, three and even four AEDs are occasionally employed. The overall indications for and selection of combined therapy as well as the associated problems encountered are issues of importance.

When initial monotherapy fails to provide adequate seizure control despite being optimally given, an alternative AED is added and, when possible, is titrated up gradually. Dose increases are made as tolerated and as needed to obtain control. The intent is to taper the first AED to again achieve monotherapy. If addition of a second drug fails, another is recommended as an alternate until it is clear that control cannot be achieved with use of a single agent. In actual practice it is common for the second AED to be added without tapering of the first. At times, the patient may be unwilling to change the medical regimen if complete or significantly improved control has been achieved with a combination of two or more AEDs for fear of a recurrent seizure with all the attendant medical and social complications.

Background

The use of combination therapy for management of medical or psychiatric problems extends far back, even before the time when pharmacodynamically active products became available. When Locock and later others used bromides for treatment of seizures, they often combined multiple agents, although only bromides ultimately proved effective. Turner (1907) stated 'perhaps the drug most frequently used as a substitute for, or as an adjuvant to, the bromides is *borax* (sodium biborate)'. Others included belladonna, zinc salts and opium. Similarly, when Hauptmann (1912) first introduced phenobarbital (PB), it was often used in combination with the bromides. This pattern has persisted with virtually every new AED introduced. The addition was usually made to improve seizure control. After the introduction of phenytoin (PHT), Yahr and colleagues (1953) reported that PHT was more successful than PB but the combination produced the best control of seizures in patients not controlled by either alone. Indeed, a product became available from Parke-Davis known as phelantin that contained 100 mg of dilantin and 32 mg of PB. New onset patients could be put on the combination without ever trying monotherapy. The lack of dosing flexibility together with studies by Reynolds and co-workers (1981) as well as Schmidt (1983) in the early 1980s emphasized that monotherapy was as effective as polytherapy in the majority of patients and was associated with fewer adverse effects. A shift to the use of monotherapy followed and has remained the accepted principle to the present time.

Potential advantages of combination therapy

It is assumed that combined AEDs work to increase efficacy (Table 2.1) either by an additive and/or synergistic effect or by achieving infra-additive adverse effects (Bourgeois and Dodson, 1988; Chapter 9, this book) allowing a higher dose to be administered. Unfortunately, more often such combinations add adverse effects at the same time and fail to improve the overall outcome or success.

Table 2.1 Advantages for combinations of AEDs

Broader spectrum
Additive efficacy
Complementary mechanisms
Decreased adverse effects
Counteracting adverse effects

Different seizure types

Combination therapy is clearly indicated when two or more seizure types exist that fail to respond to any one agent. For example, until the introduction of valproate (VPA) with its broad spectrum of action it was necessary to combine both an anti-absence drug, ethosuximide, with another AED effective against tonic–clonic seizures, such as PB or PHT, for patients with generalized idiopathic epilepsy having both seizure types. With the introduction of new AEDs since the 1990s, many of which have broad-spectrum efficacy, the need for such combination therapy is less frequent.

Different antiepileptic mechanisms

The concept of rational polytherapy is based on the realization that most AEDs have different mechanisms and act, at least in part if not primarily, at one site to produce an anti-seizure effect. PHT, for example, has well defined effects at the sodium channel to block high-frequency discharge of action potentials. PB has an action at the gamma amino butyric acid (GABA)-A receptor enhancing chloride flux. This effect increases hyperpolarization leading to inhibition of neuronal depolarization. This concept of combining complementary mechanisms is 'rational' and, as noted below, is one of the most commonly used. Similar principles would favor other combinations such as PHT or other AEDs active at the sodium channel (carbamazepine, CBZ; lamotrigine, LTG) with GABA-active drugs such as barbiturates, vigabatrin (VGB) or tiagabine (TGB). Combinations might also include drugs whose mechanism is unclear or unknown (VPA; levetiracetam, LEV), or multiple (topiramate, TPM; felbamate, FBM). By this reasoning it would not be rational to combine AEDs with similar mechanism such as PHT with CBZ or oxcarbazepine (OXC) with CBZ. However, some evidence (below) suggests these latter combinations may be effective. As with all combinations, the actual evidence favoring 'rational' polytherapy is lacking and the concept remains theoretical.

Additive efficacy/infra-additive adverse effects

A third reason for combined AED therapy is to achieve infra-additive adverse effects and equal or better efficacy. By selecting AEDs with *different* adverse effect profiles, it might be expected that efficacy would be additive while adverse effects would remain tolerable. For example, dose-related adverse effects of CBZ often first appear as dizziness or visual dysfunction (blurring or diplopia) whereas PB causes sedation and cognitive compromise as doses increase. In theory, giving modest doses of both drugs should provide additive efficacy while keeping the AED levels sufficiently low to remain under the threshold for tolerability problems. In contrast, monotherapy doses increased to achieve comparable efficacy would usually double the adverse effects. Other combinations can be readily considered using this logic.

Counteracting adverse effects

A fourth potential advantage of combination therapy is to add efficacy at the same time using AEDs with *counteracting* adverse effects. For example, combining TPM with VPA would utilize a drug causing weight loss with one causing weight gain. The help in ameliorating tremor by TPM would also decrease this side effect of VPA.

Pharmacoeconomic benefits

Although combination therapy usually adds to the cost of drugs, it can be theorized that a combination of PB with low doses of any other AED would be less expensive than high doses of any other drug even in monotherapy due to the very low cost of PB. Another potentially less costly combination is the use of low dose VPA with LTG. The relatively less costly VPA markedly inhibits LTG clearance, making it possible to give a half or less of LTG, the more expensive drug, and achieve comparable LTG blood levels to what would be obtained if giving double the dose as monotherapy.

Evidence of benefits of combination therapy versus monotherapy

Although many theoretical advantages can be proposed for combination therapy as noted above, it must be emphasized that there is no evidence to prove a benefit. That is not to say there is no benefit. It only emphasizes that there is a need for evidence. The only prospective, randomized, double-blind comparison between monotherapy and combination AED treatment was been carried out and published by Deckers and colleagues (2001). They compared CBZ monotherapy to VPA combined with CBZ in patients with new onset epilepsy. Doses were selected to reflect comparable 'drug loads' and were intended to be low. Adverse effects were the primary outcome. No significant difference was found for adverse effects (or control) although withdrawals showed a trend favoring combination therapy. Unfortunately, the number of patients entered (130) was too small to detect possible clinically meaningful differences. Although this design using new onset epilepsy patients is of interest, it is not the setting in which combination therapy is commonly employed. It might be a concept to consider when initiating therapy despite the many reasons to avoid combinations as noted below.

In fact, combination therapy is almost always selected when monotherapy has failed to control seizures in a more refractory population. No prospective efficacy studies have been conducted comparing monotherapy to combinations of AEDs in patients not controlled on monotherapy when titrated to maximally tolerated doses.

The typical clinical trial design for licensing of a new AED adds an investigational AED to a regimen of one or more drugs that failed monotherapy. All approved new

AEDs have demonstrated improved control by some efficacy outcome measure. However, compared to the placebo control groups, the add-on investigational group has always been associated with more adverse effects. In addition, the designs do not increase doses of pre-study medication in the placebo group to an amount producing comparable amounts of adverse effects. If improved efficacy could still be detected in such a setting, it would be strong evidence for greater effect for combination therapy.

A prospective combination trial was attempted in the original Veterans Administration (VA) study comparing CBZ, PB, PHT and primidone (PRM). Patients failing acceptable control on monotherapy despite maximally tolerated doses on initial or a second alternate drug were randomized to a two-drug combination. Unfortunately only 89 patients entered this protocol and had a 1-year follow-up. Nine of the patients (11%) were fully controlled. Although this is a small number, it provided evidence of increased efficacy. However, a quantitative measure of adverse effects (Cramer, 1983) showed scores higher than the monotherapy groups, suggesting better control came at least in part at the cost of more side effects.

In an often cited abstract Hakkarainen (1980) reported the results of a group of 100 patients randomized to either CBZ or PHT. After a year of treatment one half were controlled. Those failing were crossed to the other drug for the next year and another 17% came under control. Those still not controlled were placed on the combination and another 15% achieved remission. This work was never published in full text to allow scrutiny of the methods and results. A limitation of interpreting studies such as those above to show efficacy of combination therapy is the fact that some spontaneous remission occurs in epilepsy and inclusion of a parallel group maintained on monotherapy would be needed to demonstrate a true difference.

Evidence that AED combinations are more effective than monotherapy also can be inferred from the repeated observations that testing of new AEDs for regulatory approval is carried out by showing efficacy of an added drug compared to placebo as add-on to failed treatment with one or more drugs. However, such trials inevitably show more adverse effects of some type than the placebo group. Other observations suggesting added efficacy of AED combinations are common in epilepsy monitoring units. In an effort to record events on CCTV/EEG, AEDs are commonly reduced sequentially. The occurrence of attacks after one or more drugs is removed and another continues to be administered implies the drug removed was contributing to seizure control.

Potential problems with combined AEDs

Problems with combination AED therapy are given in Table 2.2.

Table 2.2 Problems with combination AED therapy

Increased adverse effects
Pharmacokinetic interactions
New active metabolites
Choice of combination
Method of initiation/discontinuation

Additive adverse effects

Add-on trials for licensing of all the new AEDs have demonstrated a statistically significant improvement in the percentage of patients achieving a 50% or greater reduction in seizures compared to placebo. Although this seems to provide clear evidence of better control with use of combined agents, virtually all trials reveal more adverse effects in the arm with an add-on drug than in the placebo arm. It is likely that drug combinations with similar adverse effects of central nervous system type are more likely to become poorly tolerated. For example, adding LTG to CBZ in clinical trials caused dizziness in 38% of patients, an additive adverse effect common to both AEDs, whereas when studied as monotherapy only 8% reported dizziness. The increased side effects may be difficult to attribute to any of a combination of drugs.

In addition to increased additive or supra-additive adverse effects from pharmacodynamic mechanisms, CBZ and LTG in combination were found to have similar dose-related central nervous system (CNS) side effects and often caused dizziness, ataxia, and visual complaints when used together. Similarly LTG and VPA often increase tremor well above what is seen in monotherapy.

Pharmacokinetic interactions

All the older AEDs (CBZ, PB, PRM, PHT, VPA) are associated with potentially clinically important interactions when used in combination (Perucca *et al.*, 2002). VPA inhibits PB, PRM and CBZ epoxide metabolism leading to increased blood levels with associated side effects. VPA also inhibits the clearance of LTG at times, leading to rapid elevation of LTG levels and increased risk of a hypersensitivity reaction. PB, PRM and PHT induce the clearance of CBZ and VPA such that the elimination half-life of these drugs is approximately half of what is found when the drugs are given as monotherapy. Unless more frequent dosing is given (with increased chance of non-compliance), or extended release formulations are used, peak and trough effects can lead to swings from side effects to insufficient control. Similar effects result when these inducing drugs are combined with some of the newer AEDs (LTG; TPM; zonisamide, ZNS). These problems are sufficient that the text, *Antiepileptic Drugs* (Levy *et al.*, 2002), devotes a chapter to this topic for each of the AEDs.

Active metabolites

Combinations of AEDs may produce pharmacodynamically active metabolites not present in clinically relevant concentrations when drugs are used as monotherapy. These include the conversion of PRM to PB in much greater proportion when co-administered with PHT. The consequence is that giving PRM in such a combination essentially means the PRM is little more than a more costly pro-drug for PB. CBZ is metabolized into the 10–11 epoxide (CBZ-E), a pharmacodynamically active product. The quantities are usually sufficiently low to be of minimal clinical effect when CBZ is used as monotherapy. When PHT is co-administered, the conversion to CBZ-E is enhanced. If VPA is combined with CBZ, inhibition of CBZ-E hydrolase occurs and levels of the CBZ-E may rise to clinically meaningful amounts. These changes may contribute to efficacy and, perhaps more importantly, to side effects.

VPA given in moderate dose is primarily metabolized to the 2-ene derivative in the mitochondria. When used at higher doses, and especially if co-administered with enzyme-inducing drugs such as PB or PHT, significant metabolism occurs in the hepatic CYP 450 system causing omega oxidation and producing putatively hepatotoxic and teratogenic products.

Selection of AED combinations

The principles that are used in selection of an added drug are different mechanisms and/or different adverse effects expectation, with the goal of an overall greater efficacy without a parallel increase in intolerable adverse effects. However, it must be re-emphasized that no clinical data from controlled randomized studies exist to address this theoretical issue. CBZ, LTG, or PHT, sodium channel active drugs having primarily vestibulo-cerebellar dose-related adverse effects, should be an appropriate combination with GABA-active drugs such as VGB or TGB with adverse effects of sedation or cognitive type.

CBZ, LTG, and PHT work at least in part by action at the sodium channel to prevent rapid neuronal firing and seizure spread. VGB or TGB act to increase GABA inhibitory effect and presumably provide different and complementary action. Some support of this concept was reported in the study of Tanganelli and Regestra (1996) in a comparative trial of CBZ or VGB alone or in combination. Although this is a 'rational' combination, it implies that we understand the mechanism by which the AEDs work. CBZ and PHT are both thought to function by preventing rapid firing due to action at the sodium channel. Consequently, combining both drugs should not be useful if the first was maximally given. In fact, however, this 'non-rational' combination has been effective in clinical practice going back to early reports by Troupin and Hakkarainen (Dodrill and Troupin, 1977; Hakkarainen, 1980). Similar experience has shown that the combination of two closely related AEDs, CBZ and OXC may prove more effective that either used alone (Barcs *et al.*, 2000).

Problems with the process of combining AEDs

When a decision is made to add a second or third AED after monotherapy has failed an adequate trial, the decision needs to be made not only what drug should be selected but how the drug should be given. Questions arise concerning initial dose, titration rate and target dose. Clinical responses of achieving seizure control or, more frequently, limitations of tolerability are the main guidelines. Adverse effects may appear as the second (or third) AED is titrated up. It is unclear whether the escalation of the add-on drug should be slowed/reversed or whether the baseline drug dose should be decreased to allow higher doses of the add-on AED. The adverse effects may be attributed erroneously to the add-on AED. For example, sedation was often observed when VPA was combined with PB. Evidence made clear that the side effect often was due to marked elevation of PB levels as a consequence of inhibition of PB metabolism by VPA rather than a direct effect of VPA.

Expense

Combinations of AEDs may double the cost of using monotherapy with a few exceptions mentioned above. In some cases combining an enzyme-inducing drug such as PHT with CBZ or VPA increases the clearance, often requiring a much larger dose to achieve blood levels comparable to those achieved with monotherapy. An even greater expense can be incurred by combining one of these older enzyme-inducing drugs with one of the costlier new AEDs, LTG, OXC, TPM or ZNS.

Summary

The failure of monotherapy to prevent seizures in 20–60% of patients (depending on seizure and epilepsy type) has led to combinations of AEDs to achieve better control. Although persuasive evidence indicates such treatment may improve control, the benefit is usually modest and adverse effects are almost always increased for both pharmacokinetic and pharmacodynamic reasons. No adequate randomized prospective clinical trials have compared combination of AED treatment with monotherapy in either new onset or refractory epilepsy. The absence of evidence does not mean combination therapy is not helpful, but until such evidence becomes available, treatment decisions unfortunately must be based on Level III and IV evidence.

REFERENCES

Barcs G, Walker EB, Elger CE, *et al.* Oxcarbazepine placebo-controlled, dose-ranging trial in refractory partial epilepsy. *Epilepsia* 2000; **41**: 1597–1607.

Bourgeois BFD, Dodson WE. Antiepileptic and neurotoxic interactions between antiepileptic drugs. In *Antiepileptic Drug Interactions*. W. H. Pitlick, ed. New York: Demos, 1988: 209–219.

Brodie MJ, Yuen AW. Lamotrigine substitution study: evidence for synergism with sodium valproate? 105 study group. *Epilepsy Res* 1997; **26**: 423–432.

Cramer J. A method for quantification for the evaluation of antiepileptic drug therapy. *Neurology* 1983; **33**(Suppl. 1): 26–37.

Deckers CLP, Hekster YA, Keyser A, *et al.* Monotherapy versus polytherapy for epilepsy: a multicenter double-blind randomized study. *Epilepsia* 2001; **42**: 1387–1394.

Dodrill CB, Troupin AS. Psychotropic effects of carbamazepine in epilepsy: a double-blind comparison with phenytoin. *Neurology* 1977; **27**: 1023–1028.

Hakkarainen H. Carbamazepine vs diphenylhydantoin vs their combination in adult epilepsy. *Neurology* 1980; **30**: 354.

Hauptmann A. Luminal bei epilepsie. *Muenchener Medizinsche Wochenschrift* 1912; **57**: 1907–1909.

Heller AJ, Chesterman P, Elwes RDC, *et al.* Phenobarbitone, phenytoin, carbamazepine or sodium valproate for newly diagnosed adult epilepsy: a randomized comparative monotherapy trial. *J Neurol Neurosurg Psychiatr* 1995; **58**: 44–50.

Kwan P, Brodie MJ. Comparison of carbamazepine, phenobarbital, phenytoin and primidone in partial and secondarily generalized tonic–clonic seizures. *New Engl J Med* 1985; **313**: 145–151.

Kwan P, Brodie MJ. Early identification of refractory epilepsy. *New Engl J Med* 2000; **342**: 314–319.

Levy RH, Mattson RH, Meldrum BS, Perucca E (eds.). *Antiepileptic Drugs*, 5th edn. Philadelphia: Lippincott Williams and Wilkins, 2002.

Mattson RH, Cramer JC, Collins JF, *et al.* A comparison of valproate with carbamazepine for the treatment of complex partial seizures and secondarily generalized tonic–clonic seizures in adults. *New Engl J Med* 1992; **327**: 765–771.

Mattson RH, Cramer JC, Collins and the VA Cooperative Epilepsy Study Group. Prognosis for complete control of complex partial and secondarily generalized tonic–clonic seizures. *Neurology* 1996; **47**: 68–76.

Perucca E, Levy RH. Combination therapy and drug interactions. In *Antiepileptic Drugs*, 5th edn. R. H. Levy, R. H. Mattson, B. S. Meldrum, E. Perucca, eds. Philadelphia: Lippincott Williams and Wilkins, 2002: 96–102.

Reynolds EH, Shorvon SD. Monotherapy or polytherapy for epilepsy? *Epilepsia* 1981; **22**: 1–10.

Richens A, Davidson DLW, Cartlidge NEF, *et al.*, on behalf of the EPITEG Collaborative Group. A multicentre comparative trial of sodium valproate and carbamazepine in adult onset epilepsy, *J Neurol Neurosurg Psychiatr* 1994; 57: 682–687.

Schmidt D. Reduction of two-drug therapy in intractable epilepsy. *Epilepsia* 1983; **24**: 368–376.

Stephens LJ, Brodie MJ. Seizure freedom with more than one antiepileptic drug. *Seizure* 2002; **11**: 349–351.

Tanganelli P, Regestra G. Vigabatrin vs carbamazepine monotherapy in newly diagnosed focal epilepsy: a randomized response conditional cross-over study. *Epilepsy Res* 1996; **25**: 257–262.

Turner WA. *Epilepsy – The Study of the Idiopathic Disease*. London: McMillan and Co., Limited, 1907: 234–236.

Yahr MD, Sciarra D, Carter S, *et al.* Evaluation of standard anticonvulsant therapy in three hundred nineteen patients. *JAMA* 1953; **150**: 663–667.

3

Pharmacogenetic aspects

Matthew C. Walker[1], Michael R. Johnson[2] and Philip N. Patsalos[1]

[1] Pharmacology and Therapeutic Unit, Department of Clinical and Experimental Epilepsy, Institute of Neurology, Queen Square, London, UK
[2] Division of Neurosciences and Psychological Medicine, Imperial College London, Charing Cross Hospital, London, UK

Introduction

Pharmacogenetics and pharmacogenomics are fields which show how the genetic make-up of an individual can influence drugs effects. In epilepsy it is one part of a number of influences that determine drug responsiveness. Other contributors are age, sex, concomitant medication, other illnesses and cause and type of epilepsy. The cause and type of epilepsy may have a complex interaction with the genetics of drug response, as the genes that contribute to epilepsy can directly affect drug responsiveness (see below), and epilepsy itself may influence genetic expression. The observation that inherited differences can affect drug disposition, adverse effects and responsiveness is not new. The observation that there are slow metabolizers of phenytoin was made in the 1960s (Kutt *et al.*, 1964), and later this was noted to be an inherited familial trait (Vasko *et al.*, 1980; Vermeij *et al.*, 1988).

The human genome project will undoubtedly revolutionize the practice of medicine. The relatively small number of human genes (approximately 30 000–40 000; International Human Genome Sequencing Consortium, 2001) and the growth of rapid sequencing technology has brought the possibility of complete genome screening closer to reality. Variation in these genes, environmental factors, and their joint interactions determine our individual response to drugs. Human genetic variation mostly consists of single nucleotide polymorphisms (SNPs) and small insertion or deletion (INDELS) polymorphisms. Over 1.4 million SNPs were identified in the initial sequencing of the human genome (International SNP Map Working Group, 2001). Most of these lie in non-coding regions of the genome, with fewer (approximately 60 000) identified within exons (coding regions of the genes). Between any two genomes there are an estimated 2.3 million variants and on a population level, up to 10 million variant positions with a frequency of more than 1%. Due to linkage disequilibrium, certain patterns of SNPs within a gene are found within specific populations (Salisbury *et al.*, 2003), which may enable a reduction in the number of SNPs that need to be genotyped in order to screen for the association of variability in a gene with disease and drug response. Although technology has advanced, in many instances tests of the gene product (e.g. enzyme activity) rather than for the gene itself may be cheaper, more reliable and more relevant (see review by Streetman *et al.*, 2000).

Genetic polymorphisms can influence antiepileptic drug (AED) responses and, during polytherapy, their interaction profile by influencing metabolism, central nervous system penetration, pharmacodynamics and adverse events. We will consider the evidence for each of these in turn before reviewing the use and pitfalls of genetic screening.

Metabolism

Lipophilic drugs cannot be easily eliminated from the body, and thus are biotransformed to more hydrophilic compounds that are then easily excreted. This biotransformation involves either modification of functional groups (phase I) or conjugation with hydrophilic moieties (phase II). Both of these systems are under extensive genetic control. Most of our presently available AEDs are metabolized by the cytochrome P450 (CYP) system. The CYP system consists of a number of different enzymes, and the classification of these, adopted in 1996, was into CYP{number}{letter}{number}*{number} groups (Nelson *et al.*, 1996). The first number groups into families which have greater than 40% protein sequence homology, the subsequent letter into subfamilies that have greater than 55% homology, the second number into members of subfamilies that are encoded by a particular gene, and the number following the '*' represents specific alleles of that gene. Four isoenzymes (CYP3A4, CYP2D6, CYP2C9 and CYP1A2) are known to be responsible for the metabolism of 95% of all drugs, and there are extensive pharmacogenetic polymorphisms for each of the enzymes. Three isoenzymes (CYP2C9, CYP2C19 and CYP3A4) are of particular importance in relation to AED metabolism and interactions (Rendic and Di Carlo, 1997). Indeed the two enzymes that have received the most attention have been CYP2C9 and CYP2C19. CYP2C9 is the dominant enzyme in the metabolism of phenytoin, and the two alleles CYP2C9*2 and CYP2C9*3 have impaired enzymatic activity compared to CYP2C9*1 (Aithal *et al.*, 1999); those with either a CYP2C9*2 or CYP2C9*3 allele need a phenytoin dose that is 30% lower than those who have only CYP2C9*1 (van der Weide *et al.*, 2001). Due to impaired enzymatic activity, those patients with a CYP2C9*2 or CYP2C9*3 allele are more likely to experience metabolic interactions during combination therapy with phenytoin and an interacting drug (Meyer, 2000). CYP2C19 is also involved in the metabolism of phenytoin, but to a lesser degree and consequently CYP2C19 polymorphism has less of an effect on phenytoin metabolism and its propensity to interact with concomitant drugs. CYP2C19 is, however, the dominant enzyme in the metabolism of phenobarbitone, and CYP2C19 allelic variation has been associated with decreased metabolism and also an increased propensity for metabolic interactions. Decreased metabolism is especially common in the Japanese population where 8% of patients with epilepsy may be poor phenobarbitone metabolizers (Mamiya *et al.*, 2000) and may be more prone to metabolic interactions.

Like CYP-mediated reactions, glucuronidation processes are susceptible to inhibition and induction.

Phase II metabolism is also subject to genetic variation. Uridine glucuronyl transferases (UGTs) are a family of enzymes that catalyze the process of glucuronidation and comprise two distinct families, UGT1 and UGT2, with eight isoenzymes identified in each family. The UGT1A4 isoenzyme plays an important role in the glucuronidation of lamotrigine (Green *et al.*, 1995), whereas the isoenzyme isoforms catalyzing the glucuronide conjugation of valproic acid have not yet been elucidated. Patients with Gilbert's syndrome (unconjugated hyperbilirubinaemia due to a mutation in a gene coding for UGT) have over 30% lower clearances and higher half-lives for lamotrigine when compared to healthy volunteers (Posner *et al.*, 1989). Certain drug interactions with lamotrigine can be explained by the glucuronidation pathway, such as the reduction of lamotrigine serum concentrations by oral contraceptives (Sabers *et al.*, 2001) and the potential reductions in olanzipine glucuronidation by lamotrigine (Linnet, 2002). Such interactions are likely to be affected by polymorphisms and mutations in the genes coding for UGT, although this remains to be tested.

Genotyping to determine drug metabolism probably has a limited role in epilepsy for two main reasons:

1 for many AEDs, there is not a clear relationship between plasma concentrations and efficacy/adverse events;
2 AEDs are titrated up slowly and concomitant blood level monitoring often gives an accurate idea if patients are slow or fast metabolizers.

This contrasts with the now commonly used screening of children for thiopurine *S*-methyltransferase deficiency before beginning mercaptopurine treatment for acute lymphoblastic leukemia (McLeod and Siva, 2002). In these cases the children are given acute courses of a drug whose efficacy and side-effect profile is closely related to plasma concentrations. An exceptional use for genotyping for drug metabolism may come into use for AEDs which have potential metabolites that are toxic (see below), and geneotyping may prove useful in predicting drug–drug interactions.

Central pharmacokinetics

The point of action for AEDs is the brain, and so AEDs have to be able to cross the blood–brain barrier. Transport proteins regulate the flux of drugs across the blood–brain barrier. Many of these proteins belong to the ATP-binding cassette family of membrane transporters of which P-glycoprotein is the most extensively studied (Lee *et al.*, 2001; Sisodiya, 2003). P-glycoprotein at the blood–brain barrier limits the accumulation of specific drugs in the central nervous system by transporting the drugs out of the brain. The role of such transporters in epilepsy remains uncertain (Sisodiya, 2003). This is partly because there is at present no consensus on which AEDs are transported by these proteins (see, for example Potschka *et al.*, 2001 and Owen *et al.*, 2001). Nevertheless, upregulation of these proteins is associated with drug resistant epilepsy in both humans and animal models (Sisodiya, 2003). Furthermore, a specific SNP in the gene encoding P-glycoprotein, ABCB1, has a strong association with AED resistance (Siddiqui *et al.*, 2003). This SNP is in a non-coding portion of the gene and thus its functional significance is uncertain – it is probable that it is associated with a separate functional SNP in an exon (Siddiqui *et al.*, 2003). This raises a problem with the use of SNPs in order to determine biological function, as they could be associated with SNPs elsewhere in the gene or even on other genes and thus unless a change of function of the gene product is demonstrated, such SNPs should only be used as biological markers as they may not be causal. The use of such markers for drug resistance could be useful for determining early referral for surgery, the spectrum of drug responsiveness or even the use of concomitant blockers of such transporters. In addition, the finding that carbamazepine may inhibit P-glycoprotein, albeit at high concentrations (Weiss *et al.*, 2003), raises the possibility that certain AED interactions could be explained by competitive inhibition of these drug transporters. In such instances, polymorphisms could determine the degree to which such interactions occur.

Pharmacodynamics

There is, at present, scant human evidence that genotype contributes to AED responsiveness, despite considerable evidence that receptor and channel subtypes determine drug pharmacodynamics. Genes that determine the type of epilepsy can influence drug pharmacodynamics by two specific mechanisms. First the epilepsy type and the pathophysiological substrate of the epilepsy could influence drug pharmacodynamics and secondly a genetic mutation could lead to both a channel that is 'responsible' for the epilepsy and also particularly sensitive/resistant to specific drugs. Thus, the first of these influences can be illustrated by the idiopathic generalized epilepsies which are largely genetically determined. Despite the likelihood that there are many genes determining the subtype and expression of these epilepsies, they are characterized by seizures with similar pathophysiological substrates. Thus absence seizures are generated within a recurrent loop between the thalamus and neocortex, and their generation is dependent upon oscillatory behavior mediated by gamma amino butyric acid (GABA)$_A$ receptors, GABA$_B$ receptors, T-type calcium channels and glutamate receptors (Crunelli and Leresche, 2002). One hypothesis is that hyperpolarization of the thalamocortical neurons in the thalamus mediated by GABAergic inhibition leads to activation of T-type calcium currents which open on neuronal depolarization, resulting in repetitive spiking that activates neurons in the neocortex which in turn stimulate the thalamic reticular nucleus leading to GABAergic inhibition of the thalamocortical (relay) neurons, and so the cycle continues (Danober *et al.*, 1998; Huguenard, 1999). The pathophysiological substrates of absence seizures lead to specific pharmaco-dynamic actions that may largely be independent of the genetic defects underlying the generation of such seizures. Within this circuit, clonazepam preferentially inhibits the thalamic reticular neurons, perhaps due to the higher expression of α3-containing GABA$_A$ receptors (Browne *et al.*, 2001). Ethosuximide, a drug whose main action may be on T-type calcium channels, has a specific action on absence seizures. Drugs that increase ambient GABA, such as tiagabine and vigabatrin, and GABA$_B$ receptor agonists can hyperpolarize thalamocortical neurons and so can have a pro-absence effect (Danober *et al.*, 1998). Also certain other drugs such as carbamazepine and phenytoin can worsen absence seizures; the mechanism of this is unknown, but does not seem to be a class effect, as lamotrigine, a drug that also inhibits sodium channels (see below) has an antiabsence effect (Frank *et al.*, 1999).

That genes that determine specific epilepsies could also influence drug responsiveness has been well documented recently. Autosomal dominant frontal lobe epilepsy is an epilepsy that can result from a mutation in the gene for the α4 subunit of the nicotinic receptor. How this mutation results in the epilepsy remains a topic for speculation, but an interesting observation is that this mutation also renders the receptor more sensitive to carbamazepine (Picard *et al.*, 1999), and this tallies with clinical experience as carbamazepine is a very effective treatment in this disorder. A note of caution needs to be raised here: a mutation of a specific channel does not necessarily mean that drugs acting at that channel are more likely to be effective. Thus benign neonatal convulsions result from mutations in KCNQ2 and KCNQ3 potassium channels (these channels make up the M potassium current – a potassium current that is 'switched off' by muscarinic receptor activation; Tatulian *et al.*, 2001). A facile interpretation is that drugs that act at these potassium channels are likely to be most effective in this epilepsy, and such a drug exists; retigabine (Tatulian *et al.*, 2001). Yet one could equally expect drugs that act at muscarinic receptors to be effective, and with further thought, and the realization that epilepsy is a network phenomenon that involves a multitude of receptors and channels, one could predict the efficacy of drugs acting at quite separate targets. In fact this epilepsy responds very well to a range of conventional AEDs. Nevertheless certain genetic defects could prevent the efficacy of certain drugs. An interesting finding is that of a mutation of the γ subunit of the $GABA_A$ receptors underlying absence epilepsy with febrile seizures in a large family (Wallace *et al.*, 2001). This mutation, along with other mutations in the same subunit, possibly results in seizures by decreasing the function of $GABA_A$ receptors containing this subunit (Baulac *et al.*, 2001; Bianchi *et al.*, 2002). Yet this mutation also renders the receptors benzodiazepine insensitive, and thus possibly makes this a benzodiazepine-resistant epilepsy (Wallace *et al.*, 2001).

Genetic differences could also affect the channels to which specific drugs are targeted, and may be independent of those genes that are contributing/determining the epilepsy. Voltage-dependent sodium channels and $GABA_A$ receptors are two of the main targets for presently available AEDs, and the effect of drugs on these targets is subtype dependent. Since drug action is critically dependent on subunit composition, it is easy to appreciate how genetic polymorphisms could have a strong influence on drug effects. We will use these two targets as illustrations of how genetic differences can influence drug effects, and how those genes that determine the epilepsy syndrome could similarly affect drug responsiveness.

Voltage-gated sodium channels are responsible for the rising phase of the action potential in excitable cells and membranes, and are thus critical for action potential generation and propagation (Catterall, 2000). The sodium channel exists in three principle conformational states:

1 at hyperpolarized potentials the channel is in the resting closed state;
2 with depolarization the channels convert to an open state that conducts sodium ions;
3 the channel then enters a closed, non-conducting, inactivated state, this inactivation is removed by hyperpolarization.

In this manner, depolarization results in a transient inward sodium current that rapidly inactivates.

The sodium channel consists of a 260-kDa α subunit that forms the sodium selective pore. This α subunit consists of four homologous domains (I–IV) that each consist of six α-helical transmembrane segments (S1–6). The highly charged S4 segments are responsible for voltage-dependent activation. A 'hinged lid' consisting of the intracellular loop connecting domains III and IV that can only close following voltage-dependent activation provides the mechanism of inactivation (Catterall, 2000).

In the central nervous system, the α subunit is associated with two auxiliary β subunits ($\beta1$ and $\beta2$) that influence the kinetics and voltage dependence of the gating. There are at least 10 different sodium channel isoforms ($Na_v1.1$–1.9 and Na_x). Five of these isoforms are present in the central nervous system – $Na_v1.1$–1.3, $Na_v1.5$ (in the limbic system) and $Na_v1.6$; these isoforms have some functional differences that are of physiological importance. Certain receptor subtypes, such as $Na_v1.6$ are more prone to late openings following a depolarization that can lead to persistent sodium currents that can contribute top burst firing. Sodium channels are additionally modulated by protein phosphorylation, which can affect the peak sodium current, and the speed and voltage dependence of channel inactivation (Catterall, 2000).

Many drugs including certain anesthetics and antiarrhythmics exert their therapeutic effect by preferential binding to the inactivated state of the sodium channel (Catterall, 2000). This has two effects: first to shift the voltage dependence of inactivation towards the resting potential (i.e the channels become inactive at lower membrane potentials), and secondly to delay the return of the channel to the resting, closed conformation following hyperpolarization. Phenytoin, lamotrigine and carbamazepine have a similar mode of action (Lang *et al.*, 1993; Kuo, 1998). All bind in the inner pore of the sodium channel, and their binding is mutually exclusive (Kuo, 1998). There are, however, differences in the fashion in which drugs interact with adjacent amino acids that can partly explain drug specific effects (Ragsdale *et al.*, 1996; Liu *et al.*, 2003); AEDs perhaps have more complex interactions with surrounding amino acids than do local anesthetics (Liu *et al.*, 2003), and will have their effects modified by a greater number of possible polymorphisms. Indeed, mutations of single amino acids affect the binding of individual drugs to different degrees, indicating that these drugs interact in an overlapping, but non-identical, manner with a common receptor site (Ragsdale *et al.*, 1996). Sodium channels from patients with refractory temporal lobe epilepsy may be selectively resistant to carbamazepine (Remy *et al.*, 2003).

There are other drugs such as valproate that inhibit rapid repetitive firing (McLean and Macdonald, 1986), but act at a different site from the site on which carbamazepine, lamotrigine and phenytoin act (Xie *et al.*, 2001). Thus there could be single amino acid substitutions that would affect sodium channel inhibitors (but not necessarily all drugs acting on that channel), and also amino acid substitutions that could result in resistance to specific drugs.

$GABA_A$ receptors are the target for a number of AEDs since alterations in $GABA_A$ receptor-mediated transmission have been implicated in the pathogenesis of epilepsy. $GABA_A$ receptors are mainly expressed post-synaptically in the brain (pre-synaptic $GABA_A$ receptors have been described within the spinal cord). $GABA_A$ receptors are constructed from five of at least 16 subunits, grouped in seven classes: α, β, γ, δ, σ, ε and π (Mehta and Ticku, 1999). This permits a vast number of putative receptor isoforms. The subunit composition determines the specific effects of allosteric modulators of $GABA_A$ receptors, such as neurosteroids, zinc and benzodiazepines (Mehta and Ticku, 1999). Importantly the subunit composition of $GABA_A$ receptors expressed in neurons can change during epileptogenesis, and these changes influence the pharmacodynamic response to drugs (Brooks *et al.*, 1998). $GABA_A$

receptor activation results in the early rapid component of inhibitory transmission. Since GABA$_A$ receptors are permeable to chloride and, less so, bicarbonate, the effects of GABA$_A$ receptor activation on neuronal voltage are dependent on the chloride and bicarbonate concentration gradients across the membrane (Macdonald and Olsen, 1994). In neurons from adult animals, the extracellular chloride concentration is higher than the intracellular concentration resulting in the equilibrium potential of chloride being more negative than the resting potential. Thus GABA$_A$ receptor activation results in an influx of chloride and cellular hyperpolarization. This chloride gradient is maintained by a membrane potassium/chloride co-transporter, KCC2 (Rivera *et al.*, 1999). Absence of this transporter in immature neurons results in a more positive reversal potential for chloride, and thus GABA$_A$ receptor activation in these neurons produces neuronal depolarization (Ben-Ari *et al.*, 1994; Rivera *et al.*, 1999). Under these circumstances GABA$_A$ receptors can mediate excitation rather than inhibition. Thus the expression of KCC2 could influence the response to drugs acting at GABA$_A$ receptors, and importantly the expression of KCC2 can be modified by epileptogenesis. Thus, polymorphisms in genes that do not directly code for the GABA$_A$ receptor could influence the pharmacodynamic response of drugs acting on this receptor.

Benzodiazepines are specific modulators of GABA$_A$ receptors and act at GABA$_A$ receptors that contain an α1, α2, α3 or α5 subunit in combination with a γ subunit (Mehta and Ticku, 1999). Drugs acting at the benzodiazepine site have different affinities for the different α subunit-containing GABA$_A$ receptors, and this specificity can affect pharmacodynamic response (McKernan *et al.*, 2000). This is due perhaps to the varied distribution of these receptors in the brain. Thus the α1 subunit-containing receptors seem to have mainly a sedative effect, and are perhaps responsible for this side effect of benzodiazepines (McKernan *et al.*, 2000). This may also explain why zolpidem, a drug that has great affinity for GABA$_A$ receptors containing the α1 subunit has marked sedative effects and weak anticonvulsant efficacy (Crestani *et al.*, 2000). More selective ligands could thus result in benzodiazepine agonists that have less sedative effect and greater anticonvulsant potential. Importantly, single amino acid substitutions rendering certain subunits insensitive to benzodiazepines can thus radically alter the profile of these drugs. Importantly, a mutation in the γ subunit has been found to underlie a specific epilepsy syndrome in some families, and this mutation renders the GABA$_A$ receptors benzodiazepine insensitive. It is likely that a range of polymorphisms in the GABA$_A$ receptor are likely to underlie the range of clinical responses to these drugs (adverse effects, efficacy, tolerance etc.). Even drugs that are less selective than benzodiazepines (e.g. barbiturates) still show some preference for certain GABA$_A$ receptor subtypes.

The manner by which polymorphisms and receptor expression can affect drug interactions is an unexplored area, but it is easy to speculate that certain pharmacodynamic interactions are receptor subtype dependent. For example, the enhancement of the action of tiagabine (increasing extracellular GABA) on $GABA_A$ receptors by a benzodiazepine would require the presence of benzodiazepine-sensitive $GABA_A$ receptors, and the extent of such an interaction could thus be determined by polymorphisms and mutations in specific receptor subunits.

Adverse events

The spectrum of adverse events may also depend upon receptor and channel polymorphisms, but most of these are likely to be dose related and inconsequential. There is unlikely to be a role for screening for these. There are, however, serious adverse events with AED use that may benefit from pharmacogenetic screening. Pharmacogenetic screening of serious adverse events that result from drug metabolites is potentially a powerful application. Felbamate has three primary metabolites, 2-hydroxy, *p*-hydroxy, and monocarbamate metabolites (Kapetanovic *et al.*, 1998). The monocarbamate metabolite is eventually metabolized to a carboxylic acid (3-carbamoyl-2-phenylpropionic acid), which is the major metabolite of felbamate in humans (Kapetanovic *et al.*, 1998). Metabolism of the monocarbamate metabolite can also result in the formation of a reactive aldehyde, atropaldehyde that could be responsible for aplastic anemia and hepatic damage associated with this drug. Enzymatic defects in the metabolism of the monocarbamate metabolite may result in the overproduction of atropaldehyde, or defects in the conjugation of atropaldehyde with glutathione (and thus detoxification) could lead to its accumulation; screening for these defects could result in identification of those who are susceptible to the serious adverse effects of felbamate, and could result in the wider use of a potentially very effective drug. Many adverse effects such as rash have an immunological basis, and these are frequently associated with human leukocyte antigen (HLA) type, providing a possible method of screening for other idiopathic adverse events. The association with HLA does not always indicate an immunological basis as HLA-determining genes on chromosome 6 can be in linkage disequilibrium with other genes (i.e. the occurrence of a specific HLA type may increase the chance of a specific polymorphism in a neighboring but distinct gene) (see, for example Pirmohamed *et al.*, 2001).

There could also be a place for screening for chronic adverse events. Reduced folate levels have been associated with chronic AED treatment. A possible consequence of this is hyperhomocysteinaemia. Hyperhomocysteinaemia is associated with vascular disease and so a prediction would be that AED therapy, through reducing folate levels, would increase homocysteine levels and result in an increase in cardiovascular disease. This could explain the increased incidence of cardiovascular disease in patients with epilepsy. Such associations have been described, and indeed it has been noted that patients receiving phenytoin and carbamazepine, who are homozygous for the thermolabile genotype of methylenetetrahydrofolate reductase gene (MTHFR), are at significant risk of hyperhomocysteinaemia (Yoo and Hong, 1999). Similarly gum hypertrophy with phenytoin is a problem that may occur in up to 50% of the patients treated with phenytoin. In cats the main metabolite of phenytoin, *p*-hydroxyphenol-5-phenylhydantoin (*p*-HPPH), has been shown to induce gingival overgrowth (Hassell and Page, 1978), and it may be that those who produce higher concentrations of *p*-HPPH (i.e. the fast metabolizers) have a higher incidence of gum hypertrophy. Undoubtedly there are other genetic factors at play that may affect fibroblasts and gingival inflammation (Seymour *et al.*, 1996).

Lastly there may be strong genetic determinants in AED teratogenicity. Defects in detoxification pathways such as epoxide hydrolase, which detoxifies epoxides, have been implicated in increasing the risk of fetal malformations. One of the oxidized products of phenytoin is an arene oxide (epoxide). It has been proposed that these arene oxide metabolites can covalently bind to cell macromolecules, resulting in cell death, hypersensitivity and even birth defects (Spielberg *et al.*, 1981; Strickler *et al.*, 1985). A defect in epoxide hydrolase has been proposed to increase the risk of fetal malformations (Strickler *et al.*, 1985; Buehler *et al.*, 1990). Furthermore developmental homeobox genes may play an important role, as it has been shown that certain mutations result in an increased chance of valproate-associated malformations in mice (Faiella *et al.*, 2000).

The predisposition to the formation of toxic metabolites, and an enhanced susceptibility to the adverse effects of these metabolites will undoubtedly lead to enhanced toxicity with specific drug combinations. Conversely, there may be certain drug combinations that could be protective in that they may reduce the serum concentrations of responsible metabolites. Identification of relevant polymorphisms may help tailor AED therapy and drug combinations in pregnant women.

Misconceptions about the use of genetic tests

We have shown above that genetic polymorphisms may have a profound effect on drug responsiveness and drug interactions. How useful will genetic testing be? The purpose of a diagnostic test is to provide increased certainty of the presence or absence of a disease. Pharmacogenetic tests are performed in an attempt to predict the therapeutic or adverse consequences of a drug in an unexposed individual. As such, they are screening tests not diagnostic tests and whilst screening tests may have health benefits, the harm that can result from inappropriate tests or their inappropriate interpretation is well documented (Sackett, 1991; Grimes and Schulz, 2002). Here we review the utility of genetic testing to predict drug response

Table 3.1 Discriminative value of genetic test (T) for drug outcome (D)

		Disease outcome		
		D+	D−	
Test	T+	19	1000	1019
(T)	T−	1	98 980	98 981
		20	99 980	100 000

The background risk of SJS or TEN with lamotrigine is estimated at 2 in 10 000 (see text). D+: presence; D−: absence of SJS/TEN following 100 000 hypothetical exposures. T refers to a + or − test result.

Sensitivity (probability of T+ in people with D+):   19/20   = 0.95
Specificity (probability of T− in people without D−): 98 980/99 980 = 0.99
PPV (probability of D+ in people with T+):   19/1019   = 0.02
NPV (probability of of D− in people with T−):   98 980/98 981 = 0.99 999

(pharmacogenetics) in the context of the intrinsic epidemiological constraints on genetic tests. We do not consider other important aspects of genetic testing including ethical, legal and social implications (Rothstein and Epps, 2001).

The principles of screening tests are best considered by means of an example. Consider an hypothetical genetic test for predicting the risk of Stevens–Johnson syndrome (SJS) and toxic epidermal necrolysis (TEN) in response to lamotrigine. The precise risk of SJS/TEN following lamotrigine use is unknown. Such data are uncertain because of an inability to control for confounding, low risk and (relatively) small numbers of exposed individuals. Observational studies by prescription event monitoring in general practice, however, suggest an approximate risk of 0.1/1000 patient months of exposure, with most cases occurring in the first 2 months of use (Mackay *et al.*, 1997; Rzany *et al.*, 1999). Suppose we have a genetic test for identifying patients at risk of SJS/TEN with lamotrigine that has sensitivity 95% and specificity 99%. Intuitively one might consider this an 'excellent' test, but how will such a test perform in clinical practice?

The effectiveness of a screening test can be evaluated using a 2×2 table that relates test result to drug outcome. The ability of our hypothetical test to discriminate those at risk of SJS/TEN from those not at risk is illustrated in Table 3.1. Table 3.1 shows how the four indices of a test's validity, sensitivity, specificity and positive and negative predictive value are calculated. For the clinician, who wishes to predict the probability of a patient developing SJS/TEN with lamotrigine, the key index is the positive predictive value (PPV – the probability of the disease given a positive test result). In the example cited (Table 3.1), it can be seen that although

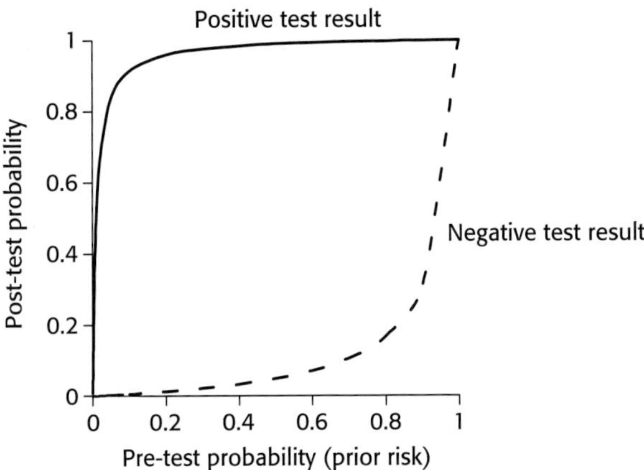

Figure 3.1   Influence of pre-test probability (prior risk) on the probability of a disease after a negative and positive screening test result (test sensitivity is 95% and specificity 99%)

the test has both high sensitivity (95%) and high specificity (99%), the predictive value of a positive test result (PPV) is only 2%. Although the probability of SJS/TEN following a positive test result has risen substantially from 2 in 10 000 to 2 in 100, it remains the case that 98% of patients testing positive will not develop SJS/TEN. This example illustrates how, in low prevalence settings, even good tests may have low predictive value. Thus, for a test with a sensitivity 95% and a specificity 99%, PPV only exceeds 90% when prior risk exceeds 1 in 11 (Figure 3.1). If prior risk is not considered when interpreting the result of the test, a positive result might deny some epilepsy patients the opportunity of an appropriate treatment.

The above discussion illustrates how the probability of a specific drug outcome after a screening test is dependent on prior risk. Knowledge of prior risk is therefore critical for interpreting the result of a screening test. Yet, even for serious adverse drug reactions (ADRs), an accurate estimate of prior risk may not be available. Co-medication, co-morbidity, age, sex, weight, duration of treatment, renal and liver function, under- and over-reporting as well as misdiagnosis all confound the accurate assessment of prior risk. Moreover, in routine clinical practice the dependency of test performance on prior risk is frequently under-appreciated, resulting in badly interpreted test results (Johnson *et al.*, 2001). Without accurate prevalence data, the clinical utility of a predictive genetic test will have to be determined by prospective randomized controlled trial. Yet methodology for the evaluation of new diagnostic techniques remains poorly defined, it is less advanced than that relating to the assessment of new therapies and there are no formal standards for the acceptance of new diagnostic procedures (Knottnerus, 2002).

The predictive value of a pharmacogenetic test can also be viewed from a genetic epidemiological perspective. Whilst some have argued that genetic testing will be widely used to predict a person's probability of developing a disease, others have pointed to limitations based on the low magnitude of relative risk and incomplete penetrance associated with various genotypes in the general population (Holtzman and Marteau, 2000; Vineis *et al.*, 2001). Using simple epidemiological principles, Holtzman and Marteau (2000) demonstrated that under most conditions, common genotypes associated with common human diseases will have little predictive power. We can apply similar principles when considering the potential for pharmacogenetic tests to yield clinically useful predictive value. The PPV of a test for a genetic susceptibility factor (this might denote the alleles that a person possesses at a single gene locus on homologous chromosomes or a complex genomic profile) is a function of the frequency of the genetic factor in the population, its relative risk and the prevalence of the drug outcome (Lilienfeld and Lilienfeld, 1980; Khoury *et al.*, 1985; Holtzman and Marteau, 2000). This can be appreciated if we consider a gene test (or genomic profile) for a drug response (adverse or therapeutic) with a prior risks prevalence of 1 in 100 and 1 in 10 (Table 3.2). Thus the drug response of interest may occur in persons with a specific genotype (G) as well as in persons without that genotype ($1-G$). Individuals without the specific genotype may still experience the drug response of interest due to locus and allelic heterogeneity, environmental variation and/or stochastic factors.

If $r+$ is the risk associated with exposure to genotype, and $r-$ the risk associated with non-exposure, then the relative risk for the drug response conferred by the susceptibility phenotype $(R) = r+/r-$. The prevalence of the drug response (D) will include cases that arise from exposure to the genotype $(G \times r+)$ as well as cases that arise from unrelated mechanisms $((1 - G) \times r-)$. Substituting PPV for $r+$, this can be re-written as:

$$D = G \times \text{PPV} + (1 - G) \times \text{PPV}/R$$

which, solved for

$$\text{PPV} = DR \times 100/G(R - 1) + 1 \quad \text{(expressed as a \%)}$$

The PPV of a test based on a genetic susceptibility factor can now be estimated across a range of D, R and G values. Table 3.2 lists PPV across a range of G and R values for a drug response with a prevalence of 1 in 100 and 1 in 10. For an outcome with prior risk of 1 in 100, it can be seen that only when the frequency of the susceptibility factor is low, and the genotype relative risk is high, will PPV be high. Whilst this 'Mendelian' situation may account for some drug responses, it seems just as likely that genotypes will confer lower relative risk for a specific drug response and thus lower PPV. Where the prevalence of the outcome of interest is lower (as, for example

Table 3.2 PPV of a screening test for a genetic susceptibility factor (genotype) for a drug response (adverse or therapeutic) with a prior risk of 1 in 100 and 1 in 10

Genotype frequency	Genotype relative risk									
	2	5	10	20	50	2	5	10	20	50
	PPV: 1 in 100 (%)					*PPV: 1 in 10 (%)*				
0.001	2.0	5.0	9.9	19.6	47.7	20.0	50.0	99.1		
0.01	2.0	4.8	9.2	16.8	33.6	19.8	48.1	91.7		
0.1	1.8	3.6	5.3	6.9	8.5	18.2	35.7	52.6	69.0	84.7
0.3	1.5	2.3	2.7	3.0	3.2	15.4	22.7	27.0	29.8	31.8

in the risk of SJS/TEN with lamotrigine), then PPV will be even lower. Of course, where the outcome is more prevalent (e.g., 1 in 10 exposures, Table 3.2), then PPV will be higher. In this situation, whilst there may be no point in testing people if the prevalent outcome is a beneficial drug response, there may be value in identifying people without genetic susceptibility to a prevalent harmful response.

What is clear, at the moment however, is that there is a lack of data on which to base predictions regarding the potential utility of pharmacogenetic testing. Epidemiological considerations such as those above highlight that if genetic tests for drug outcomes (therapeutic or adverse) are to become widely used, they will need to be validated, easy to use, unambiguous, and provide a significant improvement over current clinical practice. Physicians are used to working within established risk scenarios, and may not adapt easily to genetically altered benefit–risk trade-offs. Clinical and cost effectiveness of pharmacogenetic tests may need to be established in prospective randomized trials and their use may require new professional standards of testing and test interpretation. The degree to which pharmacogenetic tests become integrated into routine clinical practice will be determined as much by epidemiological constraints as the important legal, ethical, social and commercial aspects of genetic testing.

REFERENCES

Aithal GP, Day CP, Kesteven PJL, *et al.* Association of polymorphisms in the cytochrome P450 CYP2C9 with warfarin dose requirement and risk of bleeding complications. *Lancet* 1999; **353**: 717–719.

Baulac S, Huberfeld G, Gourfinkel-An I, *et al.* First genetic evidence of GABA(A) receptor dysfunction in epilepsy: a mutation in the gamma2-subunit gene. *Nat Genet* 2001; **28**: 46–48.

Ben-Ari Y, Tseeb V, Raggozzino D, *et al.* Gamma-aminobutyric acid (GABA): a fast excitatory transmitter which may regulate the development of hippocampal neurons in early postnatal life. *Prog Brain Res* 1994; **102**: 261–273.

Bianchi MT, Song L, Zhang H, *et al.* Two different mechanisms of disinhibition produced by GABAA receptor mutations linked to epilepsy in humans. *J Neurosci* 2002; **22**: 5321–5327.

Brooks KA, Shumate MD, Jin H, *et al.* Selective changes in single cell GABA(A) receptor subunit expression and function in temporal lobe epilepsy. *Nat Med* 1998; **4**: 1166–1172.

Browne SH, Kang J, Akk G, *et al.* Kinetic and pharmacological properties of GABA$_A$ receptors in single thalamic neurons and GABAA subunit expression. *J Neurophysiol* 2001; **86**: 2312–2322.

Buehler BA, Delimont D, van Waes M, *et al.* Prenatal prediction of risk of the fetal hydantoin syndrome. *New Engl J Med* 1990; **322**: 1567–1572.

Catterall WA. From ionic currents to molecular mechanisms: the structure and function of voltage-gated sodium channels. *Neuron* 2000; **26**: 13–25.

Crestani F, Martin JR, Mohler H, *et al.* Mechanism of action of the hypnotic zolpidem in vivo. *Br J Pharmacol* 2000; **131**: 1251–1254.

Crunelli V, Leresche N. Childhood absence epilepsy: genes, channels, neurons and networks. *Nat Rev Neurosci* 2002; **3**: 371–382.

Danober L, Deransart C, Depaulis A, *et al.* Pathophysiological mechanisms of genetic absence epilepsy in the rat. *Prog Neurobiol* 1998; **55**: 27–57.

Faiella A, Wernig M, Consalez GG, *et al.* A mouse model for valproate teratogenicity: parental effects, homeotic transformations, and altered HOX expression. *Hum Mol Genet* 2000; **9**: 227–236.

Frank LM, Enlow T, Holmes GL, *et al.* Lamictal (lamotrigine) monotherapy for typical absence seizures in children. *Epilepsia* 1999; **40**: 973–979.

Green MD, Bishop WP, Tephley TR. Expressed human UGT1.4 protein catalyzes the formation of quaternary ammonium-linked glucuronides. *Drug Metab Disp* 1995; **23**: 299–302.

Grimes DA, Schulz KF. Uses and abuses of screening tests. *Lancet* 2002; **359**: 881–884.

Hassell TM, Page RC. The major metabolite of phenytoin (Dilantin) induces gingival overgrowth in cats. *J Periodont Res* 1978; **13**: 280–282.

Holtzman NA, Marteau TM. Will genetics revolutionize medicine? *New Engl J Med* 2000; **343**: 141–144.

Huguenard JR. Neuronal circuitry of thalamocortical epilepsy and mechanisms of antiabsence drug action. *Adv Neurol* 1999; **79**: 991–999.

International Human Genome Sequencing Consortium. Initial sequencing and analysis of the human genome. *Nature* 2001; **409**(6822): 860–921.

International SNP Map Working Group. A map of human genome sequence variation containing 1.42 million single nucleotide polymorphisms. *Nature* 2001; **409**: 928–933.

Johnson MR, Good CD, Penny WD, *et al.* Playing the odds in clinical decision making: lessons from berry aneurysms undetected by magnetic resonance angiography. *Br Med J* 2001; **322**: 1347–1349.

Kapetanovic IM, Torchin CD, Thompson CD, *et al.* Potentially reactive cyclic carbamate metabolite of the antiepileptic drug felbamate produced by human liver tissue in vitro. *Drug Metab Dispos* 1998; **26**: 1089–1095.

Khoury MJ, Newill CA, Chase GA. Epidemiological evaluation of screening for risk factors: application to genetic screening. *Am J Public Health* 1985; **75**: 1204–1208.

Knottnerus JA, van Weel C, Muris JWM. Evaluation of diagnostic procedures. *Br Med J* 2002; **324**: 477–480.

Kuo CC. A common anticonvulsant binding site for phenytoin, carbamazepine, and lamotrigine in neuronal Na+ channels. *Mol Pharmacol* 1998; **54**: 712–721.

Kutt H, Wolk M, Scherman R, *et al.* Insufficient parahydroxylation as a cause of diphenylhydantoin toxicity. *Neurology* 1964; **14**: 542–548.

Lang DG, Wang CM, Cooper BR. Lamotrigine, phenytoin and carbamazepine interactions on the sodium current present in N4TG1 mouse neuroblastoma cells. *J Pharmacol Exp Ther* 1993; **266**: 829–835.

Lee G, Dallas S, Hong M, *et al.* Drug transporters in the central nervous system: brain barriers and brain parenchyma considerations. *Pharmacol Rev* 2001; **53**: 569–596.

Lilienfeld AM, Lilienfeld DE. *Foundations of Epidemiology*, 2nd edn. New York: Oxford University Press, 1980.

Linnet K. Glucuronidation of olanzapine by cDNA-expressed human UDP-glucuronosyltransferases and human liver microsomes. *Hum Psychopharmacol* 2002; **17**: 233–238.

Liu G, Yarov-Yarovoy V, Nobbs M, *et al.* Differential interactions of lamotrigine and related drugs with transmembrane segment IVS6 of voltage-gated sodium channels. *Neuropharmacology* 2003; **44**: 413–422.

Macdonald RL, Olsen RW. GABAA receptor channels. *Ann Rev Neurosci* 1994; **17**: 569–602.

Mackay FJ, Wilton LV, Pearce GL, *et al.* Safety of long term lamotrigine in epilepsy. *Epilepsia* 1997; **38**: 881–886.

Mamiya K, Hadama A, Yukawa E, *et al.* CYP2C19 polymorphism effect on phenobarbitone. Pharmacokinetics in Japanese patients with epilepsy: analysis by population pharmacokinetics. *Eur J Clin Pharmacol* 2000; **55**: 821–825.

McKernan RM, Rosahl TW, Reynolds DS, *et al.* Sedative but not anxiolytic properties of benzodiazepines are mediated by the GABA(A) receptor alpha1 subtype. *Nat Neurosci* 2000; **3**: 587–592.

McLean MJ, Macdonald RL. Sodium valproate, but not ethosuximide, produces use- and voltage-dependent limitation of high frequency repetitive firing of action potentials of mouse central neurons in cell culture. *J Pharmacol Exp Ther* 1986; **237**: 1001–1011.

McLeod HL, Siva C. The thiopurine *S*-methyltransferase gene locus – implications for clinical pharmacogenomics. *Pharmacogenomics* 2002; **3**: 89–98.

Mehta AK, Ticku MK. An update on GABA$_A$ receptors. *Brain Res Rev* 1999; **29**: 196–217.

Meyer UA. Pharmacogenetics and adverse drug reactions. *Lancet* 2000; **356**: 1667–1671.

Nelson DR, Koymans L, Kamataki T, *et al.* P450 superfamily: update on new sequences, gene mapping, accession numbers and nomenclature. *Pharmacogenetics* 1996; **6**: 1–42.

Owen A, Pirmohamed M, Tettey JN, *et al.* Carbamazepine is not a substrate for P-glycoprotein. *Br J Clin Pharmacol* 2001; **51**: 345–349.

Picard F, Bertrand S, Steinlein OK, *et al.* Mutated nicotinic receptors responsible for autosomal dominant nocturnal frontal lobe epilepsy are more sensitive to carbamazepine. *Epilepsia* 1999; **40**: 1198–1209.

Pirmohamed M, Lin K, Chadwick D, *et al.* TNFalpha promoter region gene polymorphisms in carbamazepine-hypersensitive patients. *Neurology* 2001; **56**: 890–896.

Posner J, Cohen AF, Land G, *et al.* The pharmacokinetics of lamotrigine (BW430C) in healthy subjects with unconjugated hyperbilirubinaemia (Gilbert's syndrome). *Br J Clin Pharmacol* 1989; **28**: 117–120.

Potschka H, Fedrowitz M, Loscher W. P-glycoprotein and multidrug resistance-associated protein are involved in the regulation of extracellular levels of the major antiepileptic drug carbamazepine in the brain. *Neuroreport* 2001; **12**: 3557–3560.

Ragsdale DS, McPhee JC, Scheuer T, *et al.* Common molecular determinants of local anesthetic, antiarrhythmic, and anticonvulsant block of voltage-gated Na^+ channels. *Proc Natl Acad Sci USA* 1996; **93**: 9270–9275.

Remy S, Gabriel S, Urban BW, *et al.* A novel mechanism underlying drug resistance in chronic epilepsy. *Ann Neurol* 2003; **53**: 469–479.

Rendic S, Di Carlo FJ. Human cytochrome P450 enzymes: a status report summarizing their reactions, substrates, inducers, and inhibitors. *Drug Metab Rev* 1997; **29**: 413–580.

Rivera C, Voipio J, Payne JA, *et al.* The K^+/Cl^- co-transporter KCC2 renders GABA hyperpolarizing during neuronal maturation. *Nature* 1999; **397**: 251–255.

Rothstein MA, Epps PG. Ethical and legal implications of pharmacogenomics. *Nat Rev Genet* 2001; **2**: 228–229.

Rzany B, Correia O, Kelly JP, *et al.* Risk of Stevens–Johnson syndrome and toxic epidermal necrolysis during first weeks of antiepileptic therapy: a case control study. *Lancet* 1999; **353**: 2190–2194.

Sabers A, Buchholt JM, Uldall P, *et al.* Lamotrigine plasma levels reduced by oral contraceptives. *Epilepsy Res* 2001; **47**: 151–154.

Sackett DL. *Clinical Epidemiology: A Basic Science for Clinical Medicine.* Boston: Little Brown, 1991.

Salisbury BA, Pungliya M, Choi JY, *et al.* SNP and haplotype variation in the human genome. *Mutat Res* 2003; **526**: 53–61.

Seymour RA, Thomason JM, Ellis JS. The pathogenesis of drug-induced gingival overgrowth. *J Clin Periodontol* 1996; **23**: 165–175.

Siddiqui A, Kerb R, Weale ME, *et al.* Association of multidrug resistance in epilepsy with a polymorphism in the drug-transporter gene ABCB1. *New Engl J Med* 2003; **348**: 1442–1448.

Sisodiya SM. Mechanisms of antiepileptic drug resistance. *Curr Opin Neurol* 2003; **16**: 197–201.

Spielberg SP, Gordon GB, Blake DA, *et al.* Anticonvulsant toxicity in vitro: possible role of arene oxides. *J Pharmacol Exp Ther* 1981; **217**: 386–389.

Streetman DS, Bertino Jr JS, Nafziger AN. Phenotyping of drug-metabolizing enzymes in adults: a review of in-vivo cytochrome P450 phenotyping probes. *Pharmacogenetics* 2000; **10**: 187–216.

Strickler SM, Dansky LV, Miller MA, *et al.* Genetic predisposition to phenytoin-induced birth defects. *Lancet* 1985; **2**: 746–749.

Tatulian L, Delmas P, Abogadie FC, *et al.* Activation of expressed KCNQ potassium currents and native neuronal M-type potassium currents by the anti-convulsant drug retigabine. *J Neurosci* 2001; **21**(15): 5535–5545.

van der Weide J, Steijns LS, van Weelden MJ, *et al.* The effect of genetic polymorphism of cytochrome P450 CYP2C9 on phenytoin dose requirement. *Pharmacogenetics* 2001; **11**: 287–291.

Vasko MR, Bell RD, Daly DD, *et al.* Inheritance of phenytoin hypometabolism: a kinetic study of one family. *Clin Pharmacol Ther* 1980; **27**: 96–103.

Vermeij P, Ferrari MD, Buruma OJ, *et al.* Inheritance of poor phenytoin parahydroxylation capacity in a Dutch family. *Clin Pharmacol Ther* 1988; **44**: 588–593.

Vineis P, Schulte P, McMichael AJ. Misconceptions about the use of genetic tests in populations. *Lancet* 2001; **357**: 709–712.

Wallace RH, Marini C, Petrou S, *et al.* Mutant GABA(A) receptor gamma2-subunit in childhood absence epilepsy and febrile seizures. *Nat Genet* 2001; **28**: 49–52.

Weiss J, Kerpen CJ, Lindenmaier H, *et al.* Interaction of antiepileptic drugs with human P-glyco-protein in vitro. *J Pharmacol Exp Ther* 2003; **307**: 262–267.

Xie X, Dale TJ, John VH, *et al.* Electrophysiological and pharmacological properties of the human brain type IIA Na$^+$ channel expressed in a stable mammalian cell line. *Pflügers Arch* 2001; **441**: 425–433.

Yoo JH, Hong SB. A common mutation in the methylenetetrahydrofolate reductase gene is a determinant of hyperhomocysteinemia in epileptic patients receiving anticonvulsants. *Metabolism* 1999; **48**: 1047–1051.

Part II

Pharmacokinetic interactions

4

Pharmacokinetic principles and mechanisms of drug interactions

Philip N. Patsalos

Pharmacology and Therapeutics Unit, Department of Clinical and Experimental Epilepsy, Institute of Neurology, London, UK
The National Society for Epilepsy, Chalfont St Peter, UK

Introduction

In recent years, many of the fundamental principles and concepts of pharmacokinetics have emerged from studies with antiepileptic drugs (AEDs). Pharmacokinetics describes how a drug is absorbed, distributed, metabolized, and ultimately excreted from the body. These characteristics will determine not only the ease of clinical use of the drug (e.g. how it is prescribed) and whether or not a patient will comply with its prescription, but also the pharmacokinetics of a drug has a direct impact on a drug's efficacy. During combination therapy with AEDs and indeed with AEDs and other drugs, there is potential for interference in pharmacokinetic processes and these interactions can be of major clinical significance. In this chapter, we review the various pharmacokinetic principles that are important to drug interactions and relate these to the major mechanisms of drug interactions.

Mechanisms of drug interactions

There are two basic types of drug interaction, pharmacokinetic and pharmacodynamic. Pharmacokinetic interactions are associated with changes in drug disposition, which are readily measured in that changes in drug concentrations in plasma occur. These interactions, which in fact can be associated with a change in plasma concentration of either the drug or its metabolite(s) or both, involve a change in the absorption, distribution, or elimination of the affected drug and account for most known interactions (Patsalos and Perucca, 2003a). Pharmacodynamic interactions are also important but are less well recognized and occur between drugs that have similar or opposing pharmacological mechanisms of action. These interactions take place at the cellular level where drugs act, leading to additive, supra-additive, or infra-additive effects in relation to a therapeutic response or drug toxicity. Pharmacodynamic interactions are not associated with any change in the plasma concentration of either drug and are reviewed in detail in Chapter 9.

As pharmacokinetic interactions can occur during any stage of drug disposition (i.e. during absorption, distribution, metabolism, or elimination) these stages are discussed in greater detail below.

Absorption

Absorption is the entry of drug molecules into the systemic circulation via the mucous membranes of the gut or lungs, via the skin, or from the site of an injection. Although drug interactions with AEDs are rare during absorption, such interactions can be important in some cases. For example, when phenytoin is ingested with certain nasogastric feeds, it is thought to bind to constituents of the feeding formulas to form insoluble complexes that cannot be absorbed (Bauer, 1982; Hatton, 1984; Worden *et al.*, 1984). Therefore, phenytoin absorption is impaired. Another example is that of antacids which have been shown to reduce the absorption of some AEDs (e.g. phenytoin, phenobarbitone, carbamazepine, and gabapentin) by decreasing the acidity of the stomach (Patsalos and Perucca, 2003b).

Another, useful, interaction is that with activated charcoal which both impairs drug absorption and adsorbs drug secreted into the intestine. This interaction is exploited clinically to hasten the elimination of phenobarbitone, phenytoin, and carbamazepine in overdose patients (Neuvonen *et al.*, 1978; Neuvonen and Elonen, 1980; Mauro *et al.*, 1987; Weichbrodt and Elliot, 1987).

In recent years, evidence has accumulated that transporters, particularly P-glycoprotein, may play an important role in the gastrointestinal absorption of many drugs (Lin and Yamazaki, 2003), including digoxin (Hoffmeyer *et al.*, 2000) and cyclosporine (Fricker *et al.*, 1996; Lown *et al.*, 1997). Whether P-glycoprotein contributes to the gastrointestinal absorption of AEDs is unknown. As the distribution of P-glycoprotein varies significantly across the gastrointestinal tract, its role and contribution to drug absorption may vary for different drugs (Cox *et al.*, 2002). Furthermore, the expression of P-glycoprotein in many tissues, including the gut, is subject to inhibition and induction by co-administered drugs, and many inhibitors and inducers of the cytochrome P450 (CYP) isoenzyme CYP3A4 may inhibit or induce P-glycoprotein activity (Wacher *et al.*, 1995; Jette *et al.*, 1996; Schuetz *et al.*, 1996; Verschraagen *et al.*, 1999). Therefore, overall, based on these observations, it cannot be excluded that some AED interactions currently ascribed to other mechanisms could in fact be mediated by modulation of P-glycoprotein function at the level of drug absorption or distribution. This possibility needs to be investigated.

Distribution

Distribution is the movement of drug molecules between the various water, lipid, and protein compartments in the body, including the movement of drugs to their sites of action, metabolism, and elimination. Interactions involving the distribution of drugs are difficult to ascertain. For example, during combination therapy with vigabatrin and phenytoin, phenytoin plasma concentrations are reduced by approximately 30%. Although the mechanism of this interaction is unknown, it is thought to involve an effect on phenytoin distribution (Tonini *et al.*, 1992).

Drug distribution is affected by protein binding in the circulation and the primary proteins to which drugs bind are albumin and α-glycoprotein, with albumin being by far the most important in relation to AEDs. Since the non-protein-bound drug concentration is that that is available for distribution in the body in general, and in relation to AEDs for distribution into the brain, and is pharmacologically active, plasma protein binding is important. Therefore, interactions involving competition between two drugs for plasma-protein-binding sites may affect drug distribution. However, these interactions are only important for drugs which are highly protein bound (>90%), and among AEDs, only phenytoin, valproic acid, diazepam, and tiagabine have this characteristic (Perucca, 2001; Table 4.1).

Competition of drugs for albumin binding sites depends on both the affinity and the concentration of the two drugs. Drugs with lower affinity and lower concentration will be displaced. The most commonly occurring plasma-protein-binding displacement interaction involving AEDs is the displacement of phenytoin by valproic acid (Patsalos and Lascelles, 1977a; Perucca *et al.*, 1980). As the free fraction of phenytoin increases, total systemic clearance also increases, leading to a decline in total phenytoin concentration. Unbound (pharmacologically active) drug concentrations are dependent on drug dose and hepatic intrinsic clearance. Therefore, although at steady state a displacement interaction may transiently increase the unbound concentration of phenytoin, the concentration should return to its pre-interaction value, assuming there has not been any alteration in hepatic intrinsic clearance (e.g. due to concurrent inhibition). Thus, although typically this interaction results in a fall in total phenytoin concentration while the concentration of free, pharmacologically active, phenytoin is usually unaltered (Tsanaclis *et al.*, 1984), in some patients a modest rise in free phenytoin concentration may actually be seen, due to a concomitant inhibition of phenytoin metabolism by valproic acid (Patsalos and Lascelles, 1977b). Awareness of this interaction is important for interpretation of plasma drug concentration measurements since in this setting the "therapeutic" range of total plasma phenytoin concentrations is shifted towards lower values and therapeutic and toxic effects will occur at total drug concentrations lower than usual. Patient management may best be guided by monitoring free unbound phenytoin concentrations (Patsalos, 2001, 2002).

Table 4.1 Some pharmacokinetic characteristics the various AEDs

AED	% bound	Undergoes metabolic transformation	Undergoes renal elimination	Elimination half-life $(h)^a$
Carbamazepine	75	Yes	No	16–24
Clobazam	85	Yes	No	10–58
Clonazepam	85	Yes	No	19–40
Diazepam	98	Yes	No	24–48
Ethosuximide	0	Yes	No	40–60
Felbamate	25	Yes	Yes	13–23
Gabapentin	0	No	Yes	5–9
Lamotrigine	56	Yes[d]	No	22–38
Levetiracetam	0	Yes[e]	Yes	6–8
Oxcarbazepine[b]	40	Yes	Yes	5–30
Phenobarbitone	50	Yes	Yes	80–100
Phenytoin[c]	90	Yes	No	7–42
Primidone	25	Yes	Yes	8–12
Tiagabine	98	Yes	No	5–8
Topiramate	15	Yes	Yes	19–25
Valproic acid	90	Yes	No	8–18
Vigabatrin	0	No	Yes	5–7
Zonisamide	60	Yes	Yes	57–68

[a]Values relate to patients co-administered with non-interacting drugs.

[b]Refers to the mono-hydroxy metabolite of oxcarbazepine.

[c]Dose or plasma concentration dependent.

[d]Refers to glucuronide metabolite of lamotrigine.

[e]Metabolism is non-hepatic.

Tolbutamide and phenylbutazone also interact with phenytoin by simultaneously displacing phenytoin from its protein-binding site and inhibiting its metabolism (Tassaneeyakul *et al.*, 1992). Thus, the same precautions described above for valproic acid would also apply.

AEDs that are not protein bound (Table 4.1; ethosuximide, gabapentin, levetiracetam, and vigabatrin) would not be susceptible to protein-binding displacement interactions.

Distribution of AEDs from the blood compartment to the brain is very necessary for a successful therapeutic outcome. There is evidence that the efflux of some AEDs, including carbamazepine, felbamate, lamotrigine, phenobarbitone, and phenytoin, across the blood–brain barrier is mediated by p-glycoprotein (Potschka and Loscher, 2001; Potschka *et al.*, 2001, 2002; Rizzi *et al.*, 2002). Furthermore, p-glycoprotein overexpression in brain tissue may limit the penetration of AEDs to their sites of action and may be a mechanism of pharmacoresistance in epilepsy (Sisodiya, 2003). Therefore, the possibility exists that AEDs may compete for transport across the blood-brain barrier via p-glycoprotein mechanisms.

Metabolism

Metabolism is the most important mechanism of elimination and accounts for the majority of clinically relevant drug interactions with AEDs. By far the most important system for AED metabolism is that involving the CYP system (e.g. carbamazepine, phenobarbitone, phenytoin, tiagabine, topiramate, zonisamide, and felbamate). However, metabolic pathways such as conjugation involving uridine glucuronyl transferases (UGTs) (e.g. lamotrigine and valproic acid) and β-oxidation (e.g. valproic acid) are also important.

CYP enzymes are a major component of the mixed function oxidase system that is located in the smooth endoplasmic reticulum of the cells of almost all tissues. The highest concentrations of CYP enzymes are found in the liver and four of these isoenzymes (CYP3A4, 50%; CYP2D6, 25%; CYP2C9, 15%; CYP1A2, 5%) are known to be responsible for the metabolism of 95% of all drugs (Spatzenegger and Jaeger, 1995). Furthermore, 50–70% of all drugs might be substrates for CYP3A4 and three isoenzymes (CYP3A4, CYP2C9 and CYP2C19) are of particular importance in relation to AED interactions (Rendic and Di Carlo, 1997). CYP3A4 and CYP2C9, which are responsible for the metabolism of carbamazepine and phenytoin respectively, are susceptible to induction and inhibition by many compounds and carbamazepine is capable of inducing its own metabolism (autoinduction) via its action on the CYP3A4 isoenzyme. If two drugs are metabolized by, or act upon, the same isoform of CYP, then drug interactions are more likely. Phenobarbitone, primidone, phenytoin, and carbamazepine are inducers of CYP isoenzymes, whereas valproate is an inhibitor (Mather and Levy, 2000).

The UGT family of enzymes are involved in the catalysis of glucuronidation processes and comprise two distinct families, UGT1 and UGT2. To date eight isoenzymes have been identified in each family. The glucuronidation of lamotrigine is by the UGT1A4 isoenzyme, whereas the isoenzyme isoform catalysing the glucuronide conjugation of valproic acid has not yet been identified (Green *et al.*, 1995). Glucuronidation processes, just like those mediated by CYPs, are susceptible to inhibition and induction.

Of all AEDs, phenytoin has the greatest propensity to interact. Phenytoin binds loosely to CYP isoenzymes and consequently it is easily displaced from its binding sites by other drugs. Consequently, its metabolism is readily inhibited. Furthermore, the fact that the metabolism of phenytoin is saturable makes phenytoin particularly susceptible to problematic interactions. As the metabolism of phenytoin is primarily via the isoenzyme CYP2C9 (responsible for approximately 80% of the metabolism of phenytoin) whilst the isoenzyme CYP2C9 contribution is limited (responsible for the remaining 20%) the clinical significance of an interaction will very much depend on which isoenzyme is involved. Thus, amiodarone, which interacts with CYP2C9, will have a greater effect on the plasma concentration of phenytoin compared with cimetidine, which interacts with CYP2C19.

By far the most important pharmacokinetic interactions with AEDs are those which are related to induction or inhibition of drug metabolism (Anderson, 1998; Patsalos and Perucca, 2003a). Enzyme inhibition is the phenomenon by which a drug or its metabolite(s) blocks the activity of one or more drug-metabolizing enzymes resulting in a decrease in the rate of metabolism of the affected drug. This, in turn, will lead to increased plasma concentrations of the affected drug and, possibly, clinical toxicity. Inhibition is usually competitive in nature and dose dependent, and tends to begin as soon as sufficient concentrations of the inhibitor are achieved, with significant inhibition being often observed within 24 h after addition of the inhibitor (Anderson, 1998). However, the time scale of the maximal pharmacological potentiation consequent to an inhibitory interaction depends on the elimination half-life of the affected drug with potentiation of drug activity occurring more quickly if the drug has a short half-life. As a rule, a new steady-state plasma concentration will be achieved at a time that is equivalent to five half-life values of the affected drug (Figure 4.1). For example, lamotrigine has a half-life

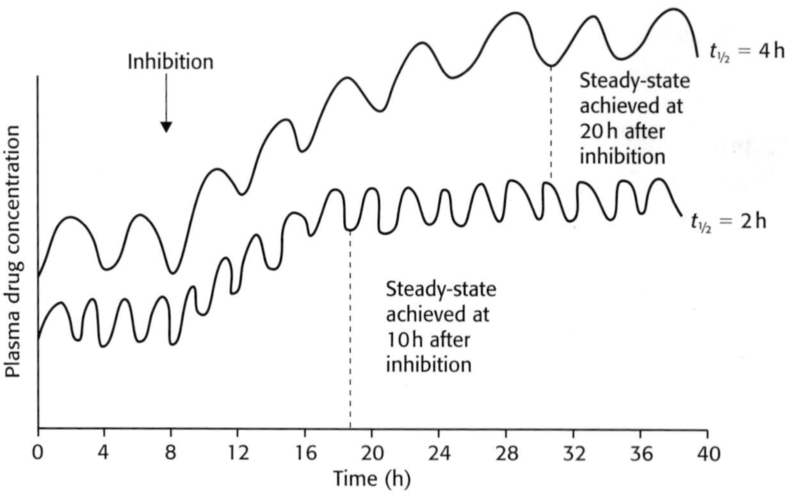

Figure 4.1   A schematic showing how the elapsed time after an inhibitory interaction and maximal pharmacological potentiation is dependent on the elimination half-life ($t_{1/2}$) of a drug. A new steady-state plasma concentration is typically achieved at a time representing five $t_{1/2}$ values

value of approximately 1.5 days, and therefore its maximal pharmacological potentiation occurs 7.5 days later (Table 4.1). In contrast, the maximal pharmacological potentiation of phenobarbitone will occur 20 days later because its half-life is longer (approximately 4 days). If drug interactions result in an increased plasma concentration of a drug or its active metabolite, then the patient may experience toxicity and side effects, in which case it may be necessary to reduce the dose of the affected drug. However, in some patients, an increase in plasma drug concentration may actually enhance the therapeutic response, particularly if the concentration was previously sub-therapeutic. An extended half-life may also mean that the frequency of dosing can be reduced, which may actually help to improve compliance.

Enzyme induction, which is the consequence of an increase in the synthesis of CYP isoenzymes in the liver and in other tissues resulting in an increase in enzyme activity, becomes apparent more slowly than that of inhibition (Perucca *et al.*, 1984; Su *et al.*, 1998). The elevated enzyme activity, in turn, results in an increase in the rate of metabolism of drugs, which are substrates of those isoenzymes, leading to a decrease in plasma concentration of the affected drug. In this setting the pharmacological effect of the drug will be reduced. However, if the affected drug has a pharmacologically active metabolite (e.g. the epoxide of carbamazepine), induction can result in increased metabolite concentration and seizure control may continue to be effective, but the possibility of an increase in drug toxicity is also greater. A further example involves the induction of disopyramide and amiodarone by enzyme-inducing AEDs whereby formation of an active metabolite complicates dosage requirements after induction has occurred (Aitio *et al.*, 1981; Nolan *et al.*, 1990). As enzyme induction requires synthesis of new enzymes, the time course of induction is dependent on the rate of enzyme synthesis and degradation and the time to reach steady-state concentrations of the inducing drug. Thus, the time course of induction is usually dose dependent and gradual (Perucca, 1987; Patsalos *et al.*, 1988).

It should be remembered that both enzyme induction and enzyme inhibition are reversible processes and that upon the removal of an interacting drug, drug dosage re-adjustments will be necessary.

AEDs that are not subject to hepatic metabolism (gabapentin, levetiracetam, and vigabatrin) would not be susceptible to metabolic interactions (Table 4.1).

Elimination

Elimination is the removal of drug molecules from the body by excretion, usually by the kidneys, or by biotransformation/metabolism (primarily CYPs), mainly in the liver. Excretion is important for water-soluble drugs and the water-soluble metabolites of lipid-soluble drugs. Conjugation by UGT isoenzymes usually results in the production of pharmacologically inactive and less lipid-soluble metabolites, which are often excreted in the urine or in the bile. Although drug interactions affecting renal excretion are rare with AEDs, AEDs that undergo extensive renal elimination in unchanged form may be susceptible to interactions affecting the excretion process, particularly when the latter involves active transport mechanisms or when the ionized state of the drug is highly sensitive to changes in urine pH (Bonate *et al.*, 1998). For example, probenecid increases the plasma concentration of penicillin by competing for the same active transport system in the kidneys and consequently reduces the renal excretion of penicillin (Hansten, 1998). Also, agents which cause alkalinization of urine, reduce the reabsorption of phenobarbitone from the renal tubuli and consequently enhance its elimination (Powell *et al.*, 1981). The latter interaction is exploited therapeutically in severe cases of barbiturate intoxication. It should be borne in mind that although vigabatrin, gabapentin, levetiracetam, topiramate and felbamate are renaly excreted, it has not been established whether or not this occurs by active transport systems (Table 4.1). Nevertheless, other drugs that are similarly excreted could potentially interact with these AEDs.

REFERENCES

Aitio ML, Mansury L, Tala E, *et al*. The effects of enzyme induction on the metabolism of disopyramide in man. *Br J Clin Pharmacol* 1981; **11**: 279–285.

Anderson GD. A mechanistic approach to antiepileptic drug interactions. *Ann Pharmacother* 1998; **32**: 554–563.

Bauer LA. Interference of oral phenytoin absorption by continuous nasogastric feeding. *Neurology* 1982; **32**: 570–572.

Bonate PL, Reith K, Weir S. Drug interactions at the renal level. Implications for drug development. *Clin Pharmacokinet* 1998; **34**: 375–404.

Cox DS, Scott KR, Gao H, *et al*. Effect of P-glycoprotein on the pharmacokinetics and tissue distribution of enaminone anticonvulsants: analysis by population and physiological approaches. *J Pharmacol Exp Ther* 2002; **302**: 1096–1104.

Fricker G, Drewe J, Huwyler J, *et al*. Relevance of P-glycoprotein for the enteral absorption of cyclosporine A: in vitro-in vivo correlation. *Br J Pharmacol* 1996; **118**: 1841–1847.

Green MD, Bishop WP, Tephly TR. Expressed human UGT1. 4 protein catalyzes the formation of quaternary ammonium-linked glucuronides. *Drug Metab Disp* 1995; **23**: 299–302.

Hansten PD. Understanding drug interactions. *Sci Med* 1998; January/February: 16–25.

Hatton RC. Dietery interaction with phenytoin. *Clin Pharm* 1984; **3**: 110–111.

Hoffmeyer S, Burk O, von Richter O, *et al*. Functional polymorphisms of the human multidrug resistance gene: multiple sequence variations and correlation of one allele with P-glycoprotein expression and activity in vivo. *Proc Natl Acad Sci USA* 2000; **97**: 3473–3478.

Jette L, Beaulieu E, Leclerc JM, *et al*. Cyclosporin A treatment induces overexpression of P-glycoprotein in the kidney and other tissues. *Am J Physiol* 1996; **270**: F756–F765.

Lin JH, Yamazaki M. Role of P-glycoprotein in pharmacokinetics. *Clin Pharmacokinet* 2003; **42**: 59–98.

Lown KS, Mayo RR, Leichtman AB, *et al.* Role of intestinal P-glycoprotein (mdr1) in interpatient variation in the oral bioavailability of cyclosporin. *Clin Pharmacol Ther* 1997; **62**: 248–260.

Mather GG, Levy RH. Anticonvulsants. In *Metabolic Drug Interactions*, R. H. Levy, K. E. Thummel, W. F. Trager, P. D. Hansten, M. Eichelbaum, eds. Philadelphia, USA: Lippincott Williams & Wilkins, 2000; 217–232.

Mauro LS, Mauro VF, Brown DL, *et al.* Enhancement of phenytoin elimination by multiple-dose activated charcoal. *Ann Emerg Med* 1987; **16**: 1132–1135.

Neuvonen PJ, Elfving SM, Elonen E. Reduction of absorption of digoxin, phenytoin and aspirin by activated charcoal in man. *Eur J Clin Pharmacol* 1978; **13**: 213–218.

Neuvonen PJ, Elonen E. Effect of activated charcoal on absorption and elimination of phenobarbitone, carbamazepine and phenylbutazole in man. *Eur J Clin Pharmacol* 1980; **17**: 51–57.

Nolan PE, Marcus FI, Karol MD, *et al.* Effect of phenytoin on the clinical pharmacokinetics of amiodarone. *J Clin Pharmacol* 1990; **30**: 1112–1119.

Patsalos PN. Therapeutic drug monitoring in epilepsy – principles and concepts. *Epilepsy Monit* 2001; **5**: 1–6.

Patsalos PN. Therapeutic drug monitoring in epilepsy – the established and the new antiepileptic drugs. *Epilepsy Monit* 2002; **6**: 1–8.

Patsalos PN, Lascelles PT. Effect of sodium valproate on plasma protein binding of diphenylhydantoin. *J Neurol Neurosurg Psychiat* 1977a; **40**: 570–574.

Patsalos PN, Lascelles PT. In vitro hydroxylation of diphenylhydantoin and its inhibition by other commonly used anticonvulsants. *Biochem Pharmacol* 1977b; **26**: 1929–1933.

Patsalos PN, Lascelles PT. Clinically important drug interactions in epilepsy: general features and interactions between antiepileptic drugs. *Lancet Neurol* 2003a; **2**: 347–356.

Patsalos PN, Perucca E. Clinically important drug interactions in epilepsy: interactions between antiepileptic drugs and other drugs. *Lancet Neurol* 2003b; **2**: 473–481.

Patsalos PN, Duncan JS, Shorvon SD. Effect of the removal of antiepileptic drugs on antipyrine kinetics in patients taking polytherapy. *Br J Clin Pharmacol* 1988; **26**: 253–259.

Perucca E. Clinical implications of hepatic microsomal enzyme induction by antiepileptic drugs. *Pharmacol Ther* 1987; **33**: 139–144.

Perucca E. The clinical pharmacology and therapeutic use of the new antiepileptic drugs. *Fund Clin Pharmacol* 2001; **15**: 405–417.

Perucca E, Hebdige S, Frigo GM, *et al.* Interaction between phenytoin and valproic acid: plasma protein binding and metabolic effects. *Clin Pharmacol Ther* 1980; **28**: 779–789.

Perucca E, Hedges A, Makki KA, *et al.* A comparative study of the enzyme inducing properties of anticonvulsant drugs in epileptic patients. *Br J Clin Pharmacol* 1984; **18**: 401–110.

Potschka H, Loscher W. Multidrug resistance-associated protein is involved in the regulation of extracellular levels of phenytoin in the brain. *Neuroreport* 2001; **12**: 2387–2389.

Potschka H, Fedrowitz M, Loscher W. P-glycoprotein and multidrug resistance-associated protein are involved in the regulation of extracellular levels of the major antiepileptic drug carbamazepine in the brain. *Neuroreport* 2001; **12**: 3557–3560.

Potschka H, Loscher W. P-Glycoprotein-mediated efflux of phenobarbital, lamotrigine, and felbamate at the blood-brain barrier: evidence from microdialysis experiments in rats. *Neurosci Lett* 2002; **327**: 173–176.

Powell JR, Nelson E, Conrad KA, *et al.* Phenobarbital clearance, elimination with alkaline diuresis, and bioavailability in adults. *Clin Pharmacol Ther* 1981; **29**: 273.

Rendic S, Di Carlo FJ. Human cytochrome P450 enzymes: a status report summarizing their reactions, substrates, inducers, and inhibitors. *Drug Metab Rev* 1997; **29**: 413–580.

Rizzi M, Caccia S, Guiso G, *et al.* Limbic seizures induce P-glycoprotein in rodent brain: functional implications for pharmacoresistance. *J Neurosci* 2002; **22**: 5833–2539.

Schuetz EG, Beck WT, Schuetz JD. Modulators and substrates of P-glycoprotein and cytochrome P4503A coordinately up-regulated these proteins in human carcinoma cells. *Mol Pharmacol* 1996; **49**: 311–318.

Sisodiya SM. Mechanisms of antiepileptic drug resistance. *Curr Opin Neurol* 2003; **16**: 197–201.

Spatzenegger M, Jaeger W. Clinical importance of cytochrome P450 in drug metabolism. *Drug Metab Rev* 1995; **27**: 397–417.

Su T, He W, Gu J, *et al.* Differential xenobiotic induction of CYP2A5 in mouse liver, kidney, lung, and olfactory mucosa. *Drug Metab Dispos* 1998; **26**: 822–824.

Tassaneeyakul W, Veronese ME, Birkett DJ, *et al.* Co-regulation of phenytoin and tolbutamide metabolism in humans. *Br J Clin Pharmacol* 1992; **34**: 494–498.

Tonini M, Gatti G, Manzo L, *et al.* Vigabatrin does not affect the intestinal absorption of phenytoin in rat duodeno-jejunal loops in situ. *Pharmacol Res* 1992; **26**: 201–205.

Tsanaclis LM, Allen J, Perucca E, *et al.* Effect of valproate on free plasma phenytoin concentrations. *Br J Clin Pharmacol* 1984; **18**: 17–20.

Verschraagen M, Koks CHW, Schellens JHM, *et al.* P-glycoprotein system as a determinant of drug interactions: the case of digoxin-verapamil. *Pharmacol Res* 1999; **40**: 301–306.

Wacher VJ, Wu CY, Benet LZ. Overlapping substrate specificities and tissue distribution of cytochrome P4503A and P-glycoprotein: implications for drug delivery and activity in cancer chemotherapy. *Mol Carcinog* 1995; **13**: 129–134.

Weichbrodt GD, Elliot DP. Treatment of phenytoin toxicity with repeated doses of activated charcoal. *Ann Emerg Med* 1987; **16**: 1387–1389.

Worden Jr JP, Wood Jr CA, Workman CH. Phenytoin and nasogastric feedings. *Neurology* 1984; **34**: 132.

5

Predictability of metabolic antiepileptic drug interactions

Edoardo Spina[1], Emilio Perucca[2] and Rene Levy[3]

[1] Section of Pharmacology, Department of Clinical and Experimental Medicine and Pharmacology, University of Messina, Messina, Italy
[2] Clinical Pharmacology Unit, University of Pavia, Pavia, Italy
[3] Department of Pharmaceutics, University of Washington, Seattle, WA, USA

Principles of drug metabolism

Many drugs are lipid soluble, weak organic acids or bases that are not readily eliminated from the body, being reabsorbed into the blood from the glomerular filtrate. Metabolic processes are necessary to convert a drug into one or more metabolites which are chemically different from the parent compound, but generally more polar and water soluble, facilitating their excretion in urine or bile. Although metabolism usually results in inactivation or detoxification, many drug metabolites have pharmacological activity. Metabolites may occasionally be much more active than the parent compound (which then may be designated as a prodrug), they may exert effects similar to or different from those of the parent molecule, or they may be responsible for toxic effects (Perucca and Richens, 1995). When metabolites are active, termination of their action occurs by further biotransformation or by direct excretion of the metabolite in urine or bile.

The chemical reactions involved in the biotransformation of drugs are catalyzed by various enzyme systems and are conventionally divided into phase I (functionalization) and phase II (conjugation) biotransformation reactions, which may occur in series. Phase I reactions involve the addition of a polar functional group (e.g. a hydroxyl group) or the deletion of a non-polar alkyl group (e.g. *N*-demethylation) by oxidation, reduction, or hydrolysis. In phase II or conjugation reactions, the drug or the phase I metabolite are covalently attached to a water-soluble endogenous substrate (e.g. glucuronic acid, acetic acid, sulfate, amino acids or glutathione), usually resulting in an inactive, easily excretable compound.

The liver is usually the main organ responsible for phase I and phase II reactions, but other organs such as the gastrointestinal tract, the kidney, the lungs, the brain, the blood, the skin and the placenta may also contribute to metabolism. In the hepatocyte, phase I oxidative enzymes are located almost exclusively in the smooth endoplasmic reticulum, along with the phase II enzyme, glucuronyltranferase. Other phase II enzymes responsible for conjugation reactions are found predominantly in the cytoplasm.

Major drug-metabolizing enzymes

Knowledge of the main enzyme systems involved in the biotransformation of antiepileptic drugs (AEDs) is essential for understanding the principles and mechanisms of metabolically based drug interactions involving these drugs.

The cytochrome P450 system

The cytochrome P450 (CYP) system constitutes a superfamily of isoenzymes that are responsible for the oxidative metabolism of many endogenous (e.g. steroids, prostaglandins and fatty acids) and exogenous compounds (e.g. many drugs). These isoenzymes are haemoproteins located in the membranes of the smooth endoplasmic reticulum in the liver and in many extrahepatic tissues (Guengerich, 1997a), and they are subdivided into families, subfamilies and isoenzymes according to a nomenclature system based on amino acid sequence homology (Nelson *et al.*, 1996). Each enzyme is designated with the root CYP followed by a first Arabic number indicating the 'family' (>40% sequence identity within family members), a capital letter designating the 'subfamily' (>59% sequence identity within subfamily members), and a second Arabic number representing individual isoenzymes. The major CYP enzymes involved in drug metabolism in humans belong to families 1, 2 and 3, which together represent approximately 70% of the total CYP content in human liver (Shimada *et al.*, 1994). The most important isoforms playing a major role in the biotransformation of therapeutic agents are CYP1A2, CYP2C9, CYP2C19, CYP2D6, CYP2E1 and CYP3A4, and these will be discussed in more detail below. Each CYP isoform is a specific gene product and possesses a characteristic but relatively broad spectrum of substrate specificity. Different CYP isoforms may display overlapping substrate specificities.

There is a large variability in the expression and activity of these isoenzymes, which may lead to interindividual differences in drug exposure. Such a variability results from genetic, pathophysiological and environmental factors, including concomitant administration of other drugs. A number of genes coding for CYP isoforms have variant alleles resulting from mutations, and these mutations can result in enzyme variants with higher, lower or no activity, or in the very absence of the enzyme. The existence of mutated alleles in at least 1% of the population is referred to as genetic polymorphism (Meyer, 1994). The CYP polymorphisms that have the greatest clinical implications are CYP2D6, CYP2C9 and CYP2C19.

In recent years, the major CYP isoenzymes have been characterized at the molecular level and their different substrates, inhibitors and inducers have been identified (Rendic and Di Carlo, 1997). As indicated in Table 5.1, the majority of AEDs are metabolized by CYP enzymes and some may also inhibit or induce, to varying degrees, one or more of these isoforms. The activity of CYP enzymes can be evaluated in vitro and in vivo. In vitro studies provide a screening method for evaluating drug affinities as substrates, inhibitors or inducers. In vivo studies include phenotyping and/or genotyping tests. Phenotyping tests are based upon administration of a single dose of a probe compound to an individual, followed by measurement of urinary or plasma concentrations of the test compound and its major metabolite(s). The ratio of parent drug/metabolite (metabolic ratio, MR) is used as a measure of the activity of the enzyme responsible for the formation of that metabolite. Genotyping is performed by using polymerase chain reaction (PCR)-based assays and restriction fragment length polymorphism (RFLP) analyses and allows detection of allelic variants for the genes coding for the polymorphic enzymes.

CYP1A2

CYP1A2 accounts for approximately 13% of total hepatic CYPs and represents the primary enzyme responsible for the metabolism of many drugs, including phenacetin, paracetamol, tacrine, theophylline, caffeine, clozapine and olanzapine (Miners and McKinnon, 2000). Although CYP1A2 has not been found to play a major role in the metabolism of any AED, it does contribute to a minor extent to carbamazepine metabolism (Patsalos *et al.*, 2002). Phenacetin and theophylline are frequently used as in vitro probes for CYP1A2, and caffeine is also widely used as a marker for CYP1A2 activity in vivo. Though CYP1A2 activity does not seem to be polymorphically distributed, it shows large interindividual variability.

Furafylline and α-naphtoflavone are potent selective inhibitors of CYP1A2 and, therefore, may be used in vitro to evaluate the contribution of this isoform in drug-metabolizing pathways. Fluvoxamine is also a potent, but not selective, inhibitor of CYP1A2. The activity of CYP1A2 is induced by polycyclic aromatic hydrocarbons (including those found in charcoal-broiled foods and cigarette smoke), rifampicin, omeprazole and, possibly, by phenobarbital, phenytoin and carbamazepine (Guengerich, 1997a). Two polymorphisms have been reported which seem to enhance the inducibility of CYP1A2 (Nakajima *et al.*, 1999; Sachse *et al.*, 1999), but the clinical implications of this observation have not been clarified.

CYP2C9 and CYP2C19

The human CYP2C subfamily, which accounts for approximately 20% of total CYPs expressed in human liver, includes at least four members: CYP2C8, CYP2C9, CYP2C18 and CYP2C19 (Rettie *et al.*, 2000). The relative contributions of these

Table 5.1 Substrates, probe drugs, inhibitors and inducers of the major CYP isoforms involved in drug metabolism

Isoenzymes	Substrates	Probe drugs	Inhibitors	Inducers
CYP1A2	Antidepressants: amitryptyline, clomipramine, imipramine, fluvoxamine, mirtazepine Antipsychotics: clozapine, olanzapine, haloperidol Methylxanthines: theophylline, caffeine Miscellaneous: phenacetin, paracetamol, tacrine, tamoxifen, *R*-warfarin	*In vitro* Phenacetin *O*-deethylation Theophylline 8-hydroxylation *In vivo* Caffeine	Furafylline α-naphtoflavone Fluvoxamine Ciprofloxacin Clarithromycin	Cigarette smoke Rifampicin Carbamazepine Barbiturates Phenytoin Charcoal-broiled meat
CYP2C9	AEDs: phenytoin, phenobarbital NSAIDs: diclofenac, ibuprofen, naproxen, piroxicam, celecoxib Miscellaneous: *S*-warfarin, tolbutamide, losartan, torasemide, fluvastatin	*In vitro* Phenytoin *p*-hydroxylation Tolbutamide 4-hydroxylation *S*-w(s)-warfarin hydroxylation *In vivo* Diclofenac, Losartan *S*-warfarin Tolbutamide	Sulfaphenazole Amiodarone Fluconazole Miconazole Valproic acid Fluoxetine Fluvoxamine	Rifampicin Barbiturates Phenytoin Carbamazepine
CYP2C19	AEDs: *S*-mephenytoin, methylphenobarbital, phenytoin, diazepam Antidepressants: amitryptyline, clomipramine, imipramine, citalopram, moclobemide Miscellaneous: omeprazole, propranolol, proguanil, *R*-warfarin	*In vitro* *S*-mephenytoin 4′-hydroxylation *In vivo* *S*-mephenytoin Omeprazole	Omeprazole Ticlopidine Fluvoxamine Felbamate Topiramate (weak)	Rifampicin Barbiturates Phenytoin Carbamazepine
CYP2D6	Antidepressants: amitryptyline, clomipramine, imipramine, desipramine, nortriptyline, fluoxetine, paroxetine, fluvoxamine, citalopram, venlafaxine, mianserine, mirtazepine	*In vitro* Dextrometorphan *O*-demethylation Debrisoquine	Quinidine Propafenone Thioridazine Perphenazine	*No inducer known*

	Antipsychotics: thioridazine, perphenazine, fluphenazine, zuclopenthixol, haloperidol, risperidone, clozapine, olanzapine, chlorpromazine Opioids: codeine, dextromethorphan, tramadol β-blockers: alprenolol, bufuralol, metoprolol, propanolol, timolol, pindolol Antiarrhythmics: encainide, flecainide, propafenone, sparteine Miscellaneous: debrisoquine, phenformin	4-hydroxylation Bufuralol 1′-hydroxylation *In vivo* Debrisoquine Dextrometorphan Sparteine Metoprolol Desipramine	Fluoxetine Paroxetine Haloperidol	
CYP2E1	Ethanol, halotane, dapsone, isoniazid, chlorzoxazone, felbamate, phenobarbital	*In vitro* Chlorzoxazone 6-hydroxylation *In vivo* Chlorzoxazone	Disulfiram	Ethanol Isoniazid
CYP3A4	AEDs: carbamazepine, ethosuximide, tiagabine, zonisamide, some benzodiazepines (e.g. alprazolam, midazolam, triazolam) Antidepressants: amitryptyline, clomipramine, imipramine, sertraline, nefazodone, mirtazepine Antipsychotics: clozapine, risperidone, quetiapine, ziprasidone, haloperidol Calcium antagonists: diltiazem, nifedipine, verapamil, felodipine Miscellaneous: cisapride, terfenadine, astemizole, cyclosporine, tacrolimus, erythromycin, clarithromycin, tamoxifen, amiodarone, quinidine, itraconazole, ketoconazole, indinavir, ritonavir	*In vitro* Midazolam 1′-hydroxylation Erythromycin *N*-demethylation Testosterone 6β-hydroxylation *In vivo* Nifedipine Midazolam Cortisol Dapsone Erythromycin	Ketoconazole Itraconazole Fluconazole Erythromycin Troleandomycin Ritonavir Indinavir Fluvoxamine Grapefruit juice	Carbamazepine Barbiturates Phenytoin Rifampicin St. John's wort Glucocorticoids[a] Oxcarbazepine[a] Topiramate[a] Felbamate[a]

[a] Weaker or tissue-selective inducers.

isoforms to total CYP2C content in human liver are about 60% for 2C9, 35% for 2C8, 4% for 2C18 and 1% for 2C19. Of these isoforms, CYP2C9 and CYP2C19 seem to be the most important for drug metabolism, although CYP2C8 should not be neglected as it contributes to the metabolism of carbamazepine (Kerr *et al.*, 1994). As CYP2C9 and CYP2C19 show a 91% identity in amino acid sequence, many substrates of CYP2C9 are also metabolized, at least in part, by CYP2C19.

CYP2C9 plays an important role in the oxidation of many drugs, including phenytoin, phenobarbital, *S*-warfarin, tolbutamide, losartan, fluvastatin and many non-steroidal anti-inflammatory agents such as diclofenac, ibuprofen and piroxicam (Perucca and Richens, 1995; Guengerich, 1997a). CYP2C9 is polymorphically expressed in humans. To date, three different allelic variants have been identified, that code for enzymes with different catalytic activity (Miners and Birkett, 1998). The frequencies of the defective alleles CYP2C9*2 and CYP2C9*3 vary between 8% and 12% and 3% and 8%, respectively among Whites, but they are somewhat lower in Orientals and black Africans. Subjects carrying two mutated alleles for CYPC9*3 lack almost completely CYP2C9 activity, and, therefore, are unable to metabolize important CYP2C9 substrates such as phenytoin and *S*-warfarin (Brandolese *et al.*, 2001). While sulfaphenazole is the prototypic inhibitor for CYP2C9, other inhibitors include valproic acid, amiodarone, fluconazole and miconazole.

CYP2C19 is involved to a significant extent in the biotransformation of methylphenobarbital, phenytoin, omeprazole, proguanil, citalopram and tricyclic antidepressants (demethylation reactions) (Guengerich, 1997a). However, the prototype substrate for this isoform is the *S*-enantiomer of mephenytoin, which undergoes *p*-hydroxylation at position 4 on its aromatic ring. The exclusive participation of CYP2C19 in this metabolic pathway is the basis for the use of *S*-mephenytoin as an in vitro and in vivo probe for CYP2C19 activity. CYP2C19 also exhibits an important genetic polymorphism. The frequency of the poor metabolizer (PM) phenotype varies from approximately 3% in Whites to 12–25% in many Asian populations, while in black Africans PM frequencies vary between 4% and 7% (Goldstein, 2001). The major defective alleles responsible for the PM phenotype are CYP2C19*2, the most common among Whites and Orientals, and CYP2C19*3, found at a frequency of about 12% among Orientals, but almost absent among Whites. The activity of CYP2C19 may be inhibited by felbamate, omeprazole, ticlopidine, fluvoxamine and, possibly, topiramate.

Inducers of the activity of CYP2C isoforms include barbiturates, phenytoin, carbamazepine and rifampicin.

CYP2D6

Although expressed at low levels (2% of hepatic CYPs) compared with other human CYPs, CYP2D6 plays an important role in the biotransformation of a large number of drugs (Zanger and Eichelbaum, 2000). To date, however, none of the major AEDs has been found to be metabolized to a significant extent by CYP2D6.

Debrisoquine, sparteine, dextromethorphan and desipramine have been validated as probe drugs for CYP2D6. This enzyme exhibits an important genetic polymorphism. PMs lack CYP2D6 activity and represent approximately 3–10% of Whites, but only 1–2% of Orientals (Evans *et al.*, 1980). Among extensive metabolizers (EMs), the catalytic activity varies largely, and a subgroup of subjects with extremely high enzyme activity have been classified as ultrarapid metabolizers (UMs) (Johansson *et al.*, 1993). The CYP2D6 gene is extremely polymorphic with more than 70 allelic variants described so far (Bertilsson *et al.*, 2002). Three major mutated alleles, CYP2D6*3, CYP2D6*4 and CYP2D6*5, account for 90–95% of the PM alleles in Whites, and CYP2D6*4 is the most common allele associated with the PM phenotype in Whites (allele frequency of about 21%). CYP2D6*4 is almost absent in Orientals, which may account for the low incidence of PMs in these populations. On the other hand, the high frequency (up to 50%) of the CYP2D6*10 allele among Orientals, and its absence among Whites, may explain the slightly lower CYP2D6 activity found in Oriental EMs compared to Whites. The frequency of the CYP2D6*5 allele, with deletion of the entire CYP2D6 gene, is about 4–6% and is similar in different ethnic populations. Individuals heterozygous for the defect alleles have lower enzyme activity than homozygous EMs. On the other hand, alleles with duplication or multiduplication of a functional CYP2D6*2 gene are associated with an increased CYP2D6 activity: the frequency of this condition varies from 1–2% in Swedes to up to 7–10% in Spaniards and Southern Italians (Bertilsson, 2002).

Quinidine, fluoxetine, paroxetine and different phenothiazines are potent inhibitors of CYP2D6. In contrast to all other CYPs involved in drug metabolism, CYP2D6 does not appear to be inducible, an important consideration in predicting interactions caused by AEDs.

CYP2E1

CYP2E1, which represents approximately 7% of total human hepatic CYPs, is of greater importance in toxicants' metabolism than in drug metabolism (Raucy and Carpenter, 2000). CYP2E1 is responsible for the metabolism of ethanol, halotane and dapsone, and plays a minor role in the oxidative biotransformation of felbamate and phenobarbital. Chlorzoxazone has been suggested as probe drug for CYP2E1. CYP2E1 activity is inhibited by disulfiram and is induced by ethanol and isoniazid.

CYP3A4

The CYP3A subfamily, which includes the isoforms 3A4, 3A5 and 3A7, is the most abundant in human liver, accounting for approximately 30% of total CYP content.

CYP3A4 is the predominant isoform in adults, is present both in the liver and in the small intestine, and participates in the biotransformation of more than 50% of all eliminated by metabolism drugs (Wrighton and Thummel, 2000). CYP3A4 is the primary enzyme responsible for the metabolism of carbamazepine, ethosuximide, tiagabine and zonisamide, and it is also involved in the biotransformation of felbamate (Perucca and Richens, 1995). Other drugs primarily metabolized by this isoform include immunosuppressants (e.g. cyclosporin and tacrolimus), triazolobenzodiazepines (e.g. alprazolam, midazolam and triazolam), non-sedating antihistamines (e.g. terfenadine and astemizole), calcium antagonists (e.g. diltiazem, verapamil, nifedipine and other dihydropyridines), cholesterol lowering drugs (e.g. simvastatin and lovastatin), antiarrhythmics (e.g. amiodarone and quinidine), and several steroids (e.g. cortisol, ethinylestradiol and levonogestrel). Index reactions for CYP3A4 activity in vitro include midazolam and triazolam 1- and 4-hydroxylation, nifedipine dehydrogenation and testosterone 6β-hydroxylation. Cortisol, nifedipine, erythromycin and midazolam have been used as in vivo probes.

The hepatic and enteric location of CYP3A4 makes it well suited to play a significant role in first-pass (or presystemic) drug metabolism. Furthermore, the considerable overlap in substrate selectivity and tissue localization of CYP3A4 and P-glycoprotein, an intestinal transport protein located in the small bowel, has led to the hypothesis that this transporter and enzyme pair act as a co-ordinated barrier against xenobiotics at the intestinal level (Schuetz *et al.*, 1996). Although CYP3A4 drug-metabolizing activity varies more than 20-fold among individuals, it has a unimodal distribution and does not appear to be subject to genetic polymorphism. Its wide interindividual variability is caused, at least in part, by modulation of CYP3A4 activity by many environmental compounds, including dietary constituents and medications.

Compounds that inhibit CYP3A4 activity include azole antimycotics (e.g. ketoconazole and itraconazole), macrolide antibiotics (e.g. erythromycin and troleandomycin), HIV protease inhibitors (e.g. ritonavir and indinavir), nefazodone and some of the furanocoumarin dimers found in grapefruit juice (Guengerich, 1997b). The hepatic and, possibly, the intestinal CYP3A4 isoforms are induced by glucocorticoids (e.g. dexamethasone), rifampicin, phenobarbital, phenytoin and carbamazepine. Felbamate, oxcarbazepine and topiramate appear to exert a selective inducing effect on CYP3A4 activity, at least in some tissues.

Recent studies indicate that CYP3A5 can account for more than 50% of total CYP3A hepatic and jejunal content in 30% of Whites and 50% of African Americans. This behavior has been associated with the *CYP3A5*1* wild-type allele (Lamba *et al.*, 2002). Such individuals will exhibit more variability in clearance of CYP3A substrates and more variability in drug interactions since CYP3A5 appears less inhibitable than CYP3A4.

Epoxide hydrolases

Epoxide hydrolases (EHs) belong to the group of hydrolytic enzymes which also includes esterases, proteases, dehalogenases and lipases. EHs catalyze a specialized form of hydrolysis, called hydration, where water is added to a compound without causing its cleavage into separate components (Omcienski, 2000). These enzymes hydrate epoxides and arene oxides to dihydrodiol and diol-epoxide metabolites.

Many epoxide intermediates, formed during oxidation of xenobiotics and endogenous substances, are reactive electrophilic species that may act as critical initiators of cellular damage through protein and RNA adduction as well as genetic mutation. Through inactivation of epoxides, EHs are usually implicated in detoxification processes, although in certain instances they may be involved in bio-activation. Five classes of EHs have been described: (a) cholesterol oxide hydrolase; (b) hepoxylin A_3 hydrolase; (c) leukotriene A_4 hydrolase; (d) soluble EH; and (e) microsomal EH.

Microsomal EH catalyzes the *trans*-addition of water to a broad range of epoxides and arene oxides derived from xenobiotics, resulting in the formation of dihydrodiol products. This enzyme exhibits a broad-substrate specificity and plays a role in the metabolism of some AEDs. Phenobarbital, phenytoin and carbamazepine, in particular, are metabolized by CYP isoenzymes to epoxide intermediates, which have been implicated in idiosyncratic adverse drug reactions and teratogenicity. Since these epoxide intermediates can be substrates for microsomal EH, it has been hypothesized that EH enzymatic status may modulate the individual susceptibility to adverse drug reactions (Lindhout, 1992).

Unlike other epoxides, the 10,11-epoxide metabolite of carbamazepine is chemically stable and retains anticonvulsant activity. The clearance of this metabolite is controlled by microsomal EH activity. In vitro and in vivo interaction studies with carbamazepine-10,11-epoxide have indicated that valpromide, valnoctamide and, to a lesser extent, valproic acid are inhibitors of microsomal EH (Kerr *et al.*, 1989; Pisani *et al.*, 1993). Another AED, progabide, has been reported to inhibit microsomal EH both in vivo and in vitro (Kroetz *et al.*, 1993). The activity of microsomal EH may be moderately induced by phenobarbital, phenytoin and carbamazepine.

Uridine diphosphate-glucuronosyltransferases

Uridine diphosphate (UDP)-glucuronosyltransferases (UDPGTs) are a subset of enzymes belonging to the superfamily of UDP-glycosyltransferases (UGTs) (Liston *et al.*, 2001). These enzymes, which catalyze the glucuronidation of a large number of endobiotics and xenobiotics, are located in the endoplasmic reticulum, mainly in the liver, but also in the kidney, intestine, skin, lung, prostate and brain.

Glucuronidation, which is the most common pathway in phase II drug metabolism, involves the transfer of the glucuronyl moiety of uridine diphosphate glucuronic acid (UDPGA) to the substrate, with subsequent release of UDP. While most substrates undergo glucuronide conjugation after phase I reactions, in some cases, i.e. morphine and valproic acid, direct conjugation proceeds without phase I functionalization of the parent compound. In general, glucuronidation leads to formation of water-soluble inactive metabolites, but active and reactive glucuronide metabolites have also been described, as in the case of morphine.

In recent years, at least 33 families within the UGTs superfamily have been identified and classified by a nomenclature similar to that used for the CYP system (Mackenzie *et al.*, 1997). Various UDPGTs have been characterized and assigned to the UGT1 and UGT2 gene families. Among the isoforms of the UGT1 family, UGT1A3 is involved in the *O*-glucuronidation of valproic acid and UGT1A4 has been found to be the major isoform responsible for the *N*-glucuronidation of lamotrigine (Dickins and Chen, 2002) and retigabine (Hiller *et al.*, 1999). Among the isoforms of the UGT2 family, the UGT2B7 variant also appears to contribute to the *O*-glucuronidation of valproic acid (Jin *et al.*, 1993).

In contrast to extensive documentation for CYP-mediated drug interactions, there are fewer data on interactions involving glucuronidation. Any substrate of UGT has the potential to competitively inhibit glucuronidation of other substrates metabolized by the same enzyme. Unlike the CYP system, no specific inhibitors of individual UGT isoforms have been identified. Valproic acid has been reported to inhibit several glucuronidation reactions, while phenobarbital, phenytoin, carbamazepine and, to a lesser extent, oxcarbazepine may act as inducers (Perucca and Richens, 1995; Perucca, 2001). In particular, phenobarbital appears to induce UGT1A1, the major enzyme responsible for the glucuronidation of bilirubin, ethinylestradiol and the opioids buprenorphine, nalorphine and naltrexone (Bock *et al.*, 1999).

Enzyme induction and enzyme inhibition

Drug interactions involving CYP isoforms and other drug-metabolizing enzymes may result from one of two processes, enzyme induction or inhibition.

Enzyme induction

The activity of drug-metabolizing enzymes in the liver and/or extrahepatic tissues may be increased ('induced') by chronic administration of several exogenous agents including drugs, industrial contaminants, dietary or voluctuary substances, as well as by endogenous compounds (Guengerich, 1997b). Although induction involves predominantly CYP isoenzymes, other enzymes including microsomal EH and UGTs may be affected. Morphologically, enzyme induction may be associated with a proliferation of the smooth endoplasmic reticulum and hepatic hypertrophy. From a biological point of view, induction is an adaptive response that protects the cells from toxic xenobiotics by increasing the detoxification activity. Therefore, it is to be expected that induction will result in decreased concentration of an active compound. However, for those agents that are inactive but are biotransformed to active metabolites, enzyme induction may paradoxically increase pharmacological or toxicological activity.

Enzyme induction is the consequence of an increased concentration of the enzyme protein (Lin and Lu, 1998; Thummel *et al.*, 2000). In most cases, this involves an enhanced protein synthesis resulting from an increase in gene transcription, usually mediated by intracellular receptors. However, enzyme induction may also occur by an inducer-mediated decrease in rate of enzyme degradation, mainly through protein stabilization. Each inducer has its own specificity in inducing a given range of drug-metabolizing enzymes, and several mechanisms of induction are often activated by a single agent, but to a different extent. Five main mechanisms of induction have been established to date (Fuhr, 2000). The two best known are the polycyclic aromatic hydrocarbon type and the phenobarbital type of induction.

Induction mediated by the aryl hydrocarbon receptor

Polycyclic aromatic hydrocarbons such as benzo(a)pyrene and 3-methylcholanthrene are environmental contaminants formed by incomplete combustion of organic matter, i.e. cigarette smoke and charcoal-broiled beef. These agents selectively induce CYP1A1 and CYP1A2, but they can also stimulate the activity of other enzymes such as UGTs. The mechanism of this type of induction has been well characterized and involves a sequence of events: initial binding of the inducer to the intracellular aryl hydrocarbon (Ah) receptor, dissociation of heat-shock 90 proteins from the receptor, translocation of the receptor–ligand complex into the nucleus, binding to the Ah receptor nuclear translocator (Arnt), binding of the Ah–Arnt complex to response elements on the CYP1A genes, resulting in increased gene transcription (Sogawa and Fujii-Kuriyama, 1997). In addition to polycyclic aromatic hydrocarbons, certain constituents of cruciferous vegetables, and certain drugs, such as omeprazole and rifampicin, appear to induce CYP1A enzymes by the same mechanism (Fuhr, 2000).

The constitutive androstane receptor and phenobarbital-type induction

Phenobarbital is recognized as the prototype of a class of agents known to induce drug metabolism (Perucca and Richens, 1995). Many other compounds, including phenytoin, primidone, carbamazepine, rifampicin and the oxazaphosphorines cyclophosphamide and ifosfamide have been shown to stimulate drug-metabolizing enzymes with an induction pattern which overlaps, at least in part, with that of barbiturates. Early investigations in liver microsomes from individuals exposed to phenobarbital and in primary cultures of human hepatocytes have documented the ability of phenobarbital to induce CYP enzymes, but the specific isoforms induced could not be identified. More recently, with the improvement in culture techniques and the development of isoform-specific reagents, it has been possible to demonstrate that the cluster of enzymes induced by phenobarbital and related agents appears to include several CYPs such as CYP2C subfamily members, CYP3A4, CYP2B6, possibly CYP1A2, but not CYP2D6 (Fuhr, 2000). In addition, microsomal EH and some UGTs appear to be induced by these agents. Thus, the drugs metabolized by enzymes subject to phenobarbital-type induction include a major fraction of all drugs undergoing biotransformation. Endogenous compounds, such as cortisol, testosterone and vitamin D_3, are also susceptible to induction by phenobarbital and related agents (Perucca, 1978).

Recent evidence suggests that the orphan receptor constitutive androstane receptor (CAR) is the molecular target and mediator of phenobarbital-type induction (Sueyoshi *et al.*, 1999). It should be pointed out that the molecular mechanism of phenobarbital-type induction may show partial overlap with that of the pregnane X receptor (PXR), which mediates CYP3A4 induction by rifampicin and glucocorticoids.

Induction mediated by the PXR

This type of induction, previously called the rifampicin/glucocorticoid-type induction, has as target CYP3A4 enzymes, mainly in the gut. Induction involves the binding of CYP3A4 inducers, including several steroids, rifampicin and phenobarbital, to the human PXR (Fuhr, 2000).

Enzyme induction by ethanol

The ethanol-type induction is probably limited to a single target, CYP2E1. Unlike other types of induction mediated by intracellular 'receptors', ethanol-type induction occurs through protein stabilization mediated by the binding of the inducers to the active site of the enzyme (Gonzalez *et al.*, 1991). Ethanol-type inducers stabilize the enzyme by protecting it from degradation, resulting in accumulation of the enzyme. Inducers of CYP2E1 are often substrates of the same enzyme and include ethanol, isoniazid and many organic solvents such as acetone, benzene and carbon tetrachloride.

Induction caused by peroxisome proliferators

This type of induction is mediated by binding to two peroxisome proliferator-activated receptors (PPARs), PPARα and PPARγ. PPARα controls the transcription of genes encoding for enzymes mediating the metabolism of lipoproteins and fatty acids, while PPARγ is involved in adipogenesis. Typical peroxisome proliferator inducers are members of the classes of fibrates and glitazones (Fuhr, 2000).

Enzyme induction as a cause of drug interactions

Enzyme induction is a slow regulatory process, which is dose and time dependent (Perucca, 1978, 1987; Perucca *et al.*, 1984). In other words, the extent of induction is generally proportional to the dose of the inducing agent and, since the process usually requires synthesis of new enzyme, it occurs with some delay after the exposure to the inducing agent. In practice, the time required for induction depends on the time to reach the steady state of the inducing agent (approximately five elimination half-lives) and the rate of synthesis of the enzyme(s). Similarly, the time course of de-induction is also gradual and depends on the rate of degradation of the enzyme and the time required to eliminate the inducing drug. Either of these two processes could be the rate-limiting step. As far as classical enzyme-inducing AEDs are concerned, induction by phenobarbital is usually manifest after approximately 1 week, with maximal effect occurring after 2–3 weeks following initiation of therapy. De-induction follows a similar time course (Anderson and Graves, 1994; Anderson, 1998). With phenytoin, maximal induction or de-induction occur approximately 1–2 weeks after initiation or removal of therapy respectively (Anderson and Graves, 1994; Anderson, 1998). Carbamazepine is the only AED which significantly induces its own metabolism (autoinduction) and, as a result of this, its plasma clearance more than doubles during the initial weeks of therapy. The time course of carbamazepine autoinduction should be completed within approximately 3–5 weeks (Anderson and Graves, 1994; Anderson, 1998).

Enzyme induction may have a profound impact on the pharmacokinetics of drugs metabolized by the susceptible enzyme(s) (Perucca, 1978). Elevated enzyme concentrations in the eliminating organ(s) generally result in an increase in the rate of metabolism of the affected drug, leading to a decrease in serum drug concentrations and, possibly, decreased clinical efficacy. If the affected drug has an active metabolite, induction can result in increased metabolite concentrations and possibly enhanced toxicity. There are three different situations where enzyme induction plays a role in therapeutic decision-making: addition of a medication when an inducer is already present, addition of an inducer to an existing therapy, and removal of an inducer from chronic therapy. In the first two cases a higher dose of the affected drug will be needed to achieve or maintain clinical efficacy, while a reduction of the dose of the affected drug may be necessary to prevent toxicity after removal of the inducer. The magnitude and timing of these interactions are critical to allow clinicians to adjust dosages in order to maintain therapeutic effects and prevent toxicity.

Enzyme induction represents a common problem in the management of epilepsy. Based on their enzyme-inducing properties, phenobarbital, phenytoin and carbamazepine have been reported to increase the clearance or reduce the therapeutic efficacy of many different compounds including other AEDs (Perucca, 1982;

2001). As a general rule, these compounds will induce the biotransformation of any drug that is primarily metabolized by CYP3A4, CYP2C9, CYP2C19 and, possibly, CYP1A2 (see Table 5.1). The possibility of induction of CYP1A2 by carbamazepine is supported by evidence that this agent increases the metabolic clearance of CYP1A2 substrates such as olanzapine and *R*-warfarin, and increases the percentage of labelled caffeine exhaled as carbon dioxide, a marker of CYP1A2 activity in vivo (Parker *et al.*, 1998). Because the induction profiles of phenobarbital, phenytoin and carbamazepine are not fully overlapping, stimulation of the metabolism of all drugs listed in Table 5.1 may not necessarily be observed with each of these AEDs. Moreover, in some cases enzyme induction and inhibition may occur at the same time, complicating the prediction process. In any case, clinically relevant interactions should be expected when enzyme-inducing agents are co-administered with drugs with a low therapeutic index such as warfarin, oral contraceptives or cyclosporin (Anderson, 1998). When active metabolites are formed, enzyme induction may result in potentiation of therapeutic and/or toxic effects. For example, the enhanced hepatotoxicity of valproic acid in children concurrently treated with enzyme inducers could be explained by accelerated formation of reactive oxidation products (Kondo *et al.*, 1990).

In addition to classical enzyme-inducing AEDs, some newer agents, namely felbamate, oxcarbazepine and topiramate, may produce significant enzyme induction, though the spectrum of enzymes induced by these agents appears to be more restricted. In particular, felbamate may induce the activity of CYP3A4 (Glue *et al.*, 1997), as indicated by a decrease in the plasma concentrations of CYP3A4 substrates such as carbamazepine (Fuerst *et al.*, 1988), ethinylestradiol and gestodene (Saano *et al.*, 1995). Unlike carbamazepine, oxcarbazepine is not subject to autoinduction, but it may selectively induce the specific isoforms of the CYP3A group involved in the metabolism of oral contraceptives (Fattore *et al.*, 1999) and dihydropyridine calcium antagonists (Zaccara *et al.*, 1993). In addition, oxcarbazepine may also induce UGTs, as suggested by a significant acceleration of lamotrigine clearance (May *et al.*, 1999). Topiramate is also a weak inducer of CYP3A4, because at dosages above 200 mg/day it may decrease plasma concentrations of ethinylestradiol by approximately 30% with a risk of failure of contraception (Rosenfeld *et al.*, 1997). At lower dosages, topiramate does not appear to affect the metabolism of steroid contraceptives (Doose *et al.*, 2003), reinforcing the important concept that enzyme induction is a dose-dependent phenomenon. Recent evidence indicates that topiramate, at higher dosages, may induce CYP3A4 by activation of PXA (Nalloni *et al.*, 2003)

Enzyme inhibition

Enzyme inhibition is the most common mechanism underlying drug interactions. A large number of compounds may inhibit the activity of drug-metabolizing enzymes, in particular with CYPs. As a consequence of enzyme inhibition, the rate of metabolism of a particular agent is decreased, resulting in increased plasma drug concentrations and potential enhancement of its pharmacological effects.

The mechanisms of enzyme inhibition include reversible inhibition, slowly reversible inhibition and irreversible inhibition (Lin and Lu, 1998; Thummel *et al.*, 2000). In reversible inhibition, the normal function of the enzyme is restored after the inhibitor has been eliminated from the body. In contrast, the loss of enzyme activity caused by irreversible inhibition persists even after the elimination of the inhibitor, and de novo biosynthesis of new enzyme is the only means by which activity can be restored.

Reversible inhibition

This type of enzyme inhibition is probably the most common and, kinetically, it can be subdivided further into competitive, non-competitive and uncompetitive inhibition (Lin and Lu, 1998). Competitive inhibition involves a mutually exclusive competition between the substrate and the inhibitor for binding to the catalytic site of the enzyme. Competitive inhibitors can be non-substrates with nevertheless high binding affinity: binding of the inhibitor prevents the substrate from binding to the active site of the enzyme and, therefore, the substrate cannot be metabolized. This inhibition can be reversed by increasing the concentration of the substrate. In the case of non-competitive inhibition, the inhibitor binds to another site of the enzyme and the inhibitor does not affect the binding of the substrate, but formation of the enzyme–inhibitor complex results in loss of enzyme activity. Uncompetitive inhibition occurs when the inhibitor does not bind to the enzyme, but to the enzyme–substrate complex, and again formation of the enzyme–substrate–inhibitor complex results in loss of enzyme activity.

Slowly reversible inhibition

Several drugs undergo metabolic activation by CYP enzymes to form inhibitory metabolites. These metabolites can form stable complexes with the prosthetic haem of CYPs, the so-called metabolic intermediate (MI) complexes, so that the CYP isoform is sequestered in a functionally inactive state (Lin and Lu, 1998). While in vitro MI complexation can be reversed, in vivo the MI complex is usually so stable that the CYP involved in the complex is not available for drug metabolism, and the activity can be restored only after synthesis of new enzyme. The effect of this inhibition may, therefore, persist well after the elimination of the interacting drug. Troleandomycin and erythromycin are probably the best-known macrolide antibiotics involved in the formation of MI complexes. These two agents are associated with a clinically significant inhibition of the CYP3A4-mediated metabolism of carbamazepine (Spina *et al.*, 1996). Hydrazine derivatives represent another class of compounds that may form stable complexes with the haem of CYP enzymes. Among these agents, isoniazid may cause a significant inhibition of phenytoin metabolism (Patsalos *et al.*, 2002), probably through MI complexation with CYP enzymes involved in its biotransformation.

Irreversible inhibition

Some drugs are oxidized by CYPs to reactive intermediates that then cause irreversible inactivation of the enzyme (Lin and Lu, 1998). As metabolic activation is required for enzyme inactivation, these agents are classified as mechanism-based inactivators or suicide inhibitors. This inactivation of CYPs may result from irreversible alteration of the haem or protein, or a combination of both. Classical examples of compounds that alkylate the prosthetic haem group and inactivate the enzyme include olefins, acetylenes and dihydropyridines. Chloramphenicol provides perhaps the best example of a drug causing irreversible (suicide) inactivation of CYP through protein modification.

Enzyme inhibition as a cause of drug interactions

Competitive inhibition is typically a rapid and dose-dependent process (Anderson and Graves, 1994; Anderson, 1998). The initial effect usually occurs within 24 h from the addition of the inhibitor, though the time to reach maximal inhibition will depend on the elimination half-lives of the affected drug and of the inhibiting agent. When the inhibitor is withdrawn, restoration of baseline (pre-interaction) conditions is also dependent on the rates of the elimination of the affected drug and of the inhibitor. With non-competitive and uncompetitive inhibition, the time course of the interaction may be more complex, and a significant role may be played by the turnover (re-synthesis) rate of the enzyme.

Inhibitors of drug metabolism usually interfere with only a limited number of isoenzymes and, therefore, they may be used to discriminate between different isoenzymes (Guengerich, 1997b). Compounds acting as inhibitors of different CYPs are listed in Table 5.1. Some potent inhibitors of a given enzyme are substrates of the same enzyme, but this is generally not the case. For example, quinidine is a potent inhibitor of CYP2D6, but it is metabolized by CYP3A4. Inhibition of non-oxidative phase I and conjugating phase II enzymes has also been documented.

Among AEDs, those acting most commonly as enzyme inhibitors are valproic acid and felbamate (Perucca and Richens, 1995). Valproic acid is considered as a broad-spectrum inhibitor of various enzymes. In particular, studies in human liver microsomes demonstrated that, at clinically relevant concentrations, valproic acid competitively inhibits CYP2C9 activity, inhibits only weakly CYP2C19 and CYP3A4, and it has no appreciable effect on CYP2D6 and CYP2E1 (Wen *et al.*, 2001). This is consistent with clinical evidence that valproic acid may significantly increase the plasma concentrations of CYP2C9 substrates such as phenytoin and phenobarbital (Scheyer, 2002). Studies in human liver microsomes also indicated that valproic acid inhibits EH, which explains its ability to increase the plasma concentration of carbamazepine-10,11-epoxide in carbamazepine-treated patients (Kerr *et al.*, 1989). Valproic acid also has an important inhibitory effect on UGTs, as indicated by its ability to inhibit in vivo the glucuronide conjugation of lamotrigine, lorazepam and zidovudine, as well as the *N*-glucosidation of phenobarbital (Liston *et al.*, 2001). The specific UGT isoform involved in these metabolic reactions is known only for lamotrigine, whose glucuronidation is metabolized by UGT1A4.

Felbamate is a selective inhibitor of CYP2C19 (Glue *et al.*, 1997), which is consistent with the observation that felbamate reduces the clearance and increases the plasma concentration of phenytoin (Fuerst *et al.*, 1988). Moreover, felbamate has been reported to increase the plasma concentrations of phenobarbital (Gidal and Zupanc, 1994), clobazam, carbamazepine-10,11-epoxide (concomitantly with a reduction in plasma carbamazepine levels) and valproic acid (Patsalos *et al.*, 2002): with the possible exception of the increase in carbamazepine-10,11-epoxide, which may be related to induction of carbamazepine metabolism, these interactions are also ascribed to inhibition of the metabolism of the corresponding compounds, though the precise molecular mechanisms have not been elucidated. In the case of valproic acid, there is evidence that the increase in its plasma levels after addition of felbamate can be ascribed at least in part to inhibition of mitochondrial β-oxidation (Hooper *et al.*, 1996).

Other AEDs may at times act as enzyme inhibitors. Topiramate has been reported to be a modest inhibitor of the activity of CYP2C19 in vitro, though at concentrations higher than those usually found in therapeutic practice (Sachdeo *et al.*, 2002). Whether this mechanism is responsible for the moderate rise in plasma phenytoin concentration which is seen in a small subset of phenytoin-treated patients given topiramate is unclear. Other inhibitors of CYP2C19 are carbamazepine and oxcarbazepine: in particular, CYP2C19 inhibition explains the ability of oxcarbazepine, especially when used at high dosages, to increase by up to 40% the plasma concentrations of phenytoin (Patsalos *et al.*, 2002). Phenobarbital concentrations may also be increased by oxcarbazepine, though to a lesser extent compared with phenytoin. Interestingly, oxcarbazepine is an inducer of UGT and CYP3A4, as demonstrated by its ability to increase the metabolism of lamotrigine and oral contraceptives respectively (Perucca, 2001): this illustrates the important concept that a compound may act as an inducer or as an inhibitor depending on which isoenzyme is being considered. There are also situations where a drug may induce and inhibit the same isoenzyme simultaneously: for example, at low doses phenobarbital tends to induce the metabolism of phenytoin, probably through induction of CYP2C9 and/or CYP2C19, whereas at higher doses it may competitively inhibit phenytoin metabolism (Patsalos *et al.*, 2002). The extent of these differential interactions may vary across individuals, which may explain the unpredictable and bi-directional changes in plasma phenytoin concentration after addition or removal of phenobarbital therapy.

Most AEDs undergo extensive biotransformation, and their metabolism is, therefore, vulnerable to inhibition by a large number of competitive substrates and enzyme inhibitors.

In vitro systems for testing drug metabolism and metabolic drug interactions

The potential for metabolic drug interactions is an important aspect to be considered during the development of new drugs. In the past, most drug interaction studies were performed relatively late in phase II and III studies, and investigations were focused on compounds chosen for their likelihood of concurrent use. Since susceptibility to involvement in drug interactions is an undesirable property of a drug, information on this should ideally be obtained already, in the preclinical phase. In recent years, different in vitro techniques have been developed and have become widely used as screening tools to predict potential drug interactions before a drug reaches the clinical phases of development. The techniques used for in vitro assessments are described concisely in the sections below. For more comprehensive information, the reader is referred to specialized reviews (Ring and Wrighton, 2000).

Enzyme-based techniques

Initially, the simplest approach to the in vitro study of drug metabolism was through use of purified enzymes. One could determine whether a drug is a substrate of a specific isoenzyme, and the ability of the drug to inhibit the same isoenzyme can be evaluated by investigating its effect on the in vitro biotransformation of a probe substrate. However, the complexity of the purification techniques required to isolate these enzymes and the need for detergents, lipids and other enzymes (e.g. cytochrome b_5 and P450 reductase) in the incubation system may limit the possible extrapolation of results obtained with purified enzyme systems to the in vivo situation (Ring and Wrighton, 2000).

Recent advances in molecular biology have allowed isolation of cDNA encoding for drug-metabolizing enzymes. In these systems, the cDNA encoding for a specific enzyme is transfected into a cell host (e.g. *Escherichia coli*, yeast, insect cells) and the expressed enzymes can be isolated and utilized in metabolic studies (Ring and Wrighton, 2000). Although recombinant human enzymes are routinely used, they have the same limitations as purified enzymes when trying to extrapolate results to the in vivo situation.

Microsomes or other subcellular fractions prepared from human livers represent a ready source of enzymes responsible for drug metabolism and, therefore, a primary tool for in vitro interaction studies (Ring and Wrighton, 2000). Human liver samples, frozen and stored at approximately $-80°C$, retain their metabolic potential over a long period of time. These microsomal preparations contain the various human cytochromes in proportion to their quantitative representation in human liver in vivo. In these systems, the contribution of a given isoenzyme to the metabolism of a test drug can be assessed by using different approaches such as the investigation of changes in biotransformation rate after addition of a specific inhibitor of that isoenzyme. Likewise, the potential ability of the test drug to act as an enzyme inhibitor can be investigated by assessing its effect on isoenzyme-specific metabolic pathways of probe substrates added in the system. The data obtained with microsomes from human liver may have a greater relevance to the in vivo situation than those obtained through the use of isolated enzyme systems (Ring and Wrighton, 2000). This is mainly due the similarity of the lipid and enzyme environment to the in vivo situation. It should be noted that microsomal fractions may also be prepared from tissues other than the liver, in order to investigate extrahepatic drug metabolism.

Cell-based techniques

The two cell-based systems most commonly utilized to study drug metabolism include cultured hepatocytes and liver slices. The use of an intact cell system is, at least in theory, ideal because of its greater physiologic relevance to the intact organism, as it contains both phase I and II enzymes along with the appropriate cofactors found in vivo. A major advantage of this system, with special reference to primary cultures of human hepatocytes, is the possibility of studying the induction potential of a test compound, an effect which cannot be evaluated in in vitro enzyme systems (Lin and Lu, 1998; Ring and Wrighton, 2000).

Primary cultures of human hepatocytes as a tool to predict enzyme-inducing potential at the preclinical level are advantageous over the use of animal models in vivo because interspecies differences in substrate specificity and regulation of expression preclude extrapolation of animal data to humans. On the other hand, a drawback in the use of primary hepatocytes is the requirement for fresh human tissue.

Prediction of metabolic drug interactions based on in vitro data

Two complementary approaches have been developed to predict potential drug interactions in vivo based on in vitro data: (a) identification of the enzymes (CYP isoforms or other drug-metabolizing enzymes) responsible for the biotransformation of a test drug; (b) determination of the potential of the test drug to inhibit or induce the activities of the various drug-metabolizing enzymes. The first approach allows prediction of interactions affecting the metabolism of the test compound (i.e. interactions affecting the test drug as a substrate), the second allows prediction of any effect that the test compound may have on the metabolism of other drugs (i.e. interactions where the test drug may act as an inducer or an inhibitor).

The test drug as a substrate (target for interactions)

Prediction of interactions that may affect the test drug requires (a) knowledge of the enzyme systems responsible for its biotransformation, and (b) knowledge of the influence of other drugs on such enzyme systems.

Identification of the enzymes responsible for the metabolism of the test drug

Identification of the isoenzyme(s) responsible for the metabolism of a given drug is the major prerequisite for rational prediction of metabolic drug interactions. To this purpose, however, it is also important to determine the relative contribution of each isoenzyme, and related metabolic pathways, to the overall elimination of that drug in vivo. Apart from prediction of drug interactions, this information may be used to anticipate the possible occurrence of genetic polymorphisms (in the case of involvement of CYP2D6, CYP2C9 or CYP2C19), as well as the likelihood of substantial extrahepatic contributions to drug metabolism, as most frequently seen with CYP3A substrates that may be biotransformed in part in the gastrointestinal mucosa (Dresser *et al.*, 2000).

Information on the CYP isoforms responsible for the oxidative metabolism can be obtained by using a general in vitro strategy (Lin and Lu, 1998; Ring and Wrighton, 2000). This may involve assessment of: (a) catalytic activity in human liver microsomes; (b) correlation of this activity with markers for known CYP isoforms; (c) catalytic activity in cDNA-based vector systems; (d) catalytic activity in purified enzymes; (e) effects of selective inhibitors; and (f) immunoinhibition with monoclonal or polyclonal antibodies against various CYP isoforms. Each approach has its advantages and disadvantages, and a combination of approaches is usually required.

Usually, studies begin with a kinetic analysis of the in vitro formation of metabolites in human liver microsomes. These analyses allow determination of the oxidative metabolite(s) of the test drug, and of the range of enzymes that may be able to form a particular metabolite (Lin and Lu, 1998). The formation of each of the metabolites is determined over a wide range of substrate concentrations. The apparent kinetic parameters such as K_M (Michaelis–Menten constant, representing the concentration of the substrate that results in half-maximal velocity) and V_{max} (maximal velocity of the reaction) for the enzyme(s) responsible for the formation of a particular metabolite may then be calculated. In this system, a first indication of the isoenzyme(s) involved in the production of the metabolite may subsequently be obtained through studies correlating the formation rate of the metabolite to the activities of various enzyme isoforms in microsomes from different individuals. Isoform-selective catalytic activities for the major CYPs involved in drug metabolism are reported in Table 5.1. Identification of the isoenzyme(s) responsible for the formation of the metabolite may also be obtained by using cDNA expressed enzymes or purified enzymes. Another approach to determine the role of the various drug-metabolizing enzymes is through use of isoenzyme-specific inhibitors. The capacity of a relatively specific chemical inhibitor (Table 5.1) to inhibit the biotransformation of a given drug to its initial metabolite constitutes evidence supporting the participation of the corresponding isoenzyme. A similar approach to confirm the role of specific enzymes makes use of antibodies with relatively specific inhibitory activity against individual isoenzymes.

In order to estimate the contribution of a given CYP isoform to total drug clearance, the information obtained in vitro must be combined with the results from preliminary in vivo quantitative metabolic studies (sometimes carried out with radiolabeled drug) that measure the fraction of dose eliminated by each pathway (including renal excretion).

Predicting interactions affecting the metabolism of the test drug

Once the contribution of different isoenzymes to the metabolism of a given drug has been elucidated, prediction of interactions affecting the clearance of that drug can easily be made. This prediction is based on existing knowledge of the influence that other drugs have on the activity of the same isoenzymes. Moreover, if the influence of a potential interfering agent is not known, this can be easily tested in the in vitro systems described above.

The main isoenzymes responsible for the metabolism of most AEDs have been identified (Riva *et al.*, 1996; Anderson, 1998) and available data are summarized in Table 5.2. Carbamazepine may serve as an example of how this information can be applied to prediction of drug interactions (Levy, 1995). Identification of CYP3A4 as the primary catalytic enzyme for the main clearance pathway of carbamazepine allows the anticipation that any compound known to inhibit CYP3A4 activity at therapeutically meaningful concentrations has the potential to decrease carbamazepine clearance and to increase plasma carbamazepine concentration at steady state. The validity of this prediction is supported by a large bulk of experimental and clinical studies. For example, different compounds known to inhibit CYP3A4 activity such as the calcium-channel blockers diltiazem and verapamil, the macrolide antibiotics troleandomycin and erythromycin, the antidepressants viloxazine and nefazodone, and the antifungals ketoconazole and fluconazole, have been reported

Table 5.2 Elimination pathways for the major AEDs. Fraction of absorbed dose cleared by metabolic and renal elimination refers to average values described for patients on monotherapy. CYP isoforms responsible for metabolic clearance of each drug are shown in brackets (bold characters identify enzymes involved in metabolic pathways responsible for a major proportion of total drug clearance)

Drug	Fraction cleared by			Renal
	CYPs	UGTs	Other enzymes	
Carbamazepine	75% (**CYP3A4**, CYP2C8, CYP1A2)	15%	Negligible	<5%
Ethosuximide	70% (**CYP3A4**)	Nil	Negligible	20%
Felbamate	15% (CYP3A4, CYP2E1)	10%	25% (hydrolysis)	50%
Gabapentin	Nil	Nil	Nil	100%
Lamotrigine	Nil	>80%	Negligible	<10%
Levetiracetam	Nil	Nil	30% (hydrolysis)	70%
Oxcarbazepine[a]	<5%	70%	Nil	30%
Phenobarbital	30% (**CYP2C9**, CYP2C19, CYP2E1)	Negligible	25% (*N*-glucosidation)	25%
Phenytoin	90% (**CYP2C9, CYP2C19**)	Nil	Negligible	<5%
Tiagabine	>95% (**CYP3A4**)	Nil	Not identified	2%
Topiramate	<25%	Nil	Not known	75%
Valproic acid[b]	10% (CYP2C9, CYP2A6, CYP2B6)	40%	35% (β-oxidation)	<5%
Vigabatrin	Nil	Nil	Nil	100%
Zonisamide	50% (**CYP3A4**, CYP2C19, CYP3A5)	Negligible	20% (acetylation)	<30%

[a] Data refer to the active monohydroxycarbazepine derivative (MHD). Oxcarbazepine is transformed to MHD by ketoreduction catalyzed by cytosolic arylketone reductase.

[b] Fractions metabolized through various pathways are dose dependent.

to cause a clinically significant elevation in plasma carbamazepine concentration (Perucca, 1982; Patsalos *et al.*, 2002). Similarly, it is known that CYP3A4 activity is stimulated by enzyme-inducing AEDs such as phenobarbital and phenytoin: this allows prediction of the ability of these compounds to increase carbamazepine clearance and to reduce plasma carbamazepine concentration in patients with epilepsy (Spina *et al.*, 1996).

There can be many other examples of how knowledge of the isoenzymes responsible for the metabolism of an AED can be used to predict interactions affecting the plasma clearance of that drug in vivo. In the case of phenytoin, which is a substrate of CYP2C9 and CYP2C19, clinically documented examples of interactions consistent with inhibition of CYP2C9 are those caused by amiodarone, phenylbutazone, propoxyphene, miconazole and valproic acid, while interactions probably due to inhibition of CYP2C19 are caused by ticlopidine, fluoxetine, omeprazole and felbamate (Raguenau-Majlessi *et al.*, 2002).

When utilizing only in vitro findings to predict in vivo changes in the pharmacokinetics of the affected drug, it is important to remember that the extent of inhibition or induction of a given pathway as assessed on the basis of in vitro data does not necessarily imply that the total clearance of the affected substrate in vivo will be affected to the same extent. In fact, any change in clearance of the affected substrate will also be influenced by other factors, including the degree of inhibition or induction of the affected pathway in vivo (which may not necessarily correspond to the in vitro situation, due to intervention of confounding variables); the contribution of the affected pathway to the overall elimination of the substrate; the pharmacokinetic characteristics of the substrate and its route of administration; any influence that the interfering drug may have on alternative metabolic pathways of the substrate. A more detailed discussion of how these factors impact on the prediction process, including potential pitfalls, is provided in the section 'Crucial factors in predicting in vitro–in vivo correlations'.

The test drug as a cause of interactions affecting the metabolism of other drugs

The first step in predicting what effect a test compound may have on the metabolism of other drugs consists in the investigation of the influence of that compound on the activity of the various drug-metabolizing isoenzymes. This information is then interpreted by taking into account existing knowledge on the range of drugs which are substrates of the affected enzymes.

Assessment of the influence of the test drug on the activity of drug-metabolizing isoenzymes

In vitro approaches similar to those described in the section 'Identification of the enzymes responsible for the metabolism of the test drug' are applicable to the evaluation of drugs as potential inhibitors of specific enzyme isoforms. Using human liver microsomes or individual enzymes, a series of drugs and/or their metabolites can be screened relatively quickly to determine quantitatively their potency in inhibiting reactions considered to reflect specifically the activity of individual enzyme isoforms. One approach involves the use of a fixed concentration of the probe substrate incubated with variable concentrations of the potential inhibitor (Greenblatt *et al.*, 1998). Evaluation of the decrease in metabolite formation rate as a function of the inhibitor's concentration allows calculation of the 50% inhibitory concentration (IC_{50}), i.e. the inhibitor's concentration at which the reaction rate is reduced by 50%. IC_{50} values are independent of the specific biochemical mechanism of inhibition and, therefore, they are suitable for comparing the relative potency of a series of inhibitors. On the other hand, when inhibition is competitive, IC_{50} values depend on substrate concentration: therefore, they cannot be directly applied to in vitro–in vivo scaling models, except when inhibition is established as having a non-competitive mechanism. A second approach to the assessment of inhibitory interactions is based on calculation of the inhibition constant (K_i), which reflects inhibitory potency in a reciprocal fashion (Segel, 1975). Determination of K_i is more time and labour consuming, since it requires the study of multiple substrate concentrations and multiple inhibitor concentrations. K_i is model dependent, since it depends upon the specific mechanism of inhibition, which may not be established. However, K_i is independent of substrate concentration and can be used under some defined conditions for the quantitative in vitro–in vivo scaling of drug interactions. Although K_i is less than or equal to IC_{50} as a general rule, K_i will be equal to IC_{50} if inhibition is non-competitive, or if inhibition is competitive and the substrate concentration is far below the reaction K_M (Segel, 1975). Both K_i and IC_{50} provide similar estimates of relative inhibitory potency for a series of inhibitors of a specific reaction.

As discussed in the section 'Cell-based techniques', in vitro systems can also be used to estimate enzyme-inducing potential. These experiments are far more complex, time consuming and expensive, as they involve the use of primary cultures of hepatocytes (Li *et al.*, 1997). Evaluation of changes in the activity of specific isoenzymes can be obtained by applying the techniques described in the sections above.

Predicting effects of the test drug on the metabolism of other drugs

The effects of the major AEDs on various drug-metabolizing enzymes are summarized in Table 5.3. Once it has been established that an AED inhibits or induces the activity of a given isoenzyme, then one can predict that the metabolism of substrates of the same isoenzyme will be correspondingly affected. A list of substrates of individual CYP isoenzymes is reported in Table 5.1: for example, if a drug inhibits CYP1A2, then one can predict that the CYP1A2-mediated pathways of substrates such as amitryptyline, fluvoxamine, mirtazepine, clozapine, olanzapine,

Table 5.3 Effects of AEDs on the most common drug-metabolizing enzyme systems

Drug	Effect	Enzymes involved
Carbamazepine	Inducer	CYP1A2, CYP2B6, CYP2C, CYP3A4 Microsomal EH UGT
Ethosuximide	None (?)	
Felbamate	Inhibitor	CYP2C19 β-oxidation
	Inducer	CYP3A4
Gabapentin	None	
Lamotrigine	Negligible	UGT (weak autoinduction)
Levetiracetam	None	
Oxcarbazepine	Inhibitor	CYP2C19
	Inducer	CYP3A4 (weaker induction compared with carbamazepine) UGT (weaker induction compared with carbamazepine)
Phenobarbital/ primidone	Inducer	CYP1A2, CYP2B6, CYP2C, CYP3A Microsomal EH UGT
Phenytoin	Inducer	CYP1A2, CYP2B6, CYP2C, CYP3A4 Microsomal EH UGT
Tiagabine	None	
Topiramate	Inhibitor	CYP2C19 (weak inhibition)
	Inducer	CYP3A4 (weaker induction compared with carbamazepine)
Valproic acid	Inhibitor	CYP2C9 Microsomal EH UGT
Vigabatrin	None	
Zonisamide	None (?)	

haloperidol, theophylline, caffeine and phenacetin will be inhibited. The extent of inhibition will depend on the inhibiting potency and on the concentration (dosage) of the inhibitor, but the concentration of the substrate may also play a role. Similar considerations apply to predictions of drug interactions mediated by enzyme induction.

A good correlation between the ability to inhibit various CYPs in vitro and the in vivo inhibitory interaction profile has been established for a number of AEDs, including valproic acid (Scheyer, 2002) and felbamate (Glue *et al.*, 1997). As discussed in the section 'Predicting interactions affecting the metabolism of the test drug', it should be noted that the predicted extent of inhibition or induction of a given pathway does not necessarily imply that the total clearance of the affected substrate in vivo will be affected to the same extent. In vivo changes may be influenced by a number of variables such as the action of other metabolites, the accessibility of the inhibitor or inducer to the enzyme, the contribution of the affected pathway to the overall elimination of the affected drug, the pharmacokinetics characteristics of the affected drug and its route of administration, and any influence that the interfering drug may have on alternative metabolic pathways. These factors are discussed concisely in the section below.

Crucial factors in predicting in vitro–in vivo correlations

Information on the drug-metabolizing enzyme systems and their substrates, inhibitors and inducers may be of a great value for clinicians to anticipate and eventually avoid potential interactions. Co-administration of two substrates of the same enzyme, or co-administration of a substrate with an inhibitor or an inducer, entails the possibility of a drug interaction. As a consequence, plasma concentrations of the co-administered drugs may be increased or decreased, resulting in clinical toxicity or diminished therapeutic effect. Dosage adjustments may then be required to avoid adverse effects or therapeutic failure. However, not all theoretically possible drug interactions that are predicted from in vitro studies will occur in vivo, and some may not be clinically significant anyway. As suggested by Sproule *et al.* (1997), different aspects including drug-related, patient-related and epidemiological factors must be taken into account when evaluating the potential occurrence, extent and clinical significance of a metabolic drug interaction.

With respect to prediction of whether an interaction will occur in the clinical situation, it should be pointed out that, although it is relatively easy to assess a drug interaction in vitro, the correct interpretation and extrapolation of in vitro data to the in vivo situation may be complicated by various factors and require a good understanding of pharmacokinetic principles (Bertz and Granneman, 1997; Lin and Lu, 1998; Levy and Trager, 2000). One of the most important factors to be considered is whether in vitro drug interaction studies have utilized clinically relevant concentrations of inhibitor (or inducer) and substrate. While the use of supratherapeutic concentrations may obviously result in a drug interaction in vitro but not in vivo, it may not be easy to determine whether a given range of concentrations tested in vitro is therapeutically relevant. For example, reference to drug concentrations measured at steady state in patients receiving therapeutic dosages may not provide an adequate estimate of the concentration of the interacting (or affected) drug at the site of metabolism in vivo, due to the confounding effect of binding to proteins, transport systems and presence of other interfering endogenous and exogenous metabolites. A potentially important factor affecting in vitro drug interaction studies is represented by the protein concentration of microsomes. The K_i values of an inhibitor may be overestimated at high microsomal protein concentrations as a result of the depletion of the inhibitor by non-specific binding to microsomal proteins and/or microsomal metabolism. Moreover, the specificity of chemical inhibitor probes is of concern for the interpretation of in vitro studies. No inhibitory probe is completely specific for its corresponding isoform and all ultimately become non-specific at high concentrations. In view of these considerations, no prediction can be expected to be 100% accurate, and both false positive and false negatives need to be anticipated.

While the above limitations should be understood, it is nevertheless true that consideration of a number of factors is essential in maximizing the probability of making accurate predictions about the occurrence, and potential clinical importance, of specific drug interactions. These factors will be briefly discussed in the remaining part of this chapter.

The therapeutic index of the substrate

In general, interactions affecting medications with a narrow therapeutic index (e.g. phenytoin, anticoagulants, immunosuppressants or anticancer drugs) are more likely to be clinically relevant than interactions affecting drugs with a broad margin of safety (e.g. gabapentin, penicillin). In fact, given the same degree of inhibition or induction, any change in the plasma levels of the affected substrate is more likely to result in toxic or subtherapeutic values if the substrate has a narrow therapeutic index. Of course, the importance of the interaction will also vary depending on whether at baseline the concentration of the affected agent was near the threshold associated with toxicity or therapeutic failure.

Extent of metabolism of the substrate through the affected enzyme

For interactions involving inhibition of drug metabolism, a clinically important change in the plasma concentration of the affected drug can only be expected if the inhibited pathway contributes to a major extent to total drug clearance. For example, inhibition of a pathway which accounts for only 10% of total drug clearance will only increase the concentration of the affected drug by no more than 10%. It should be noted that the relative contribution of a given metabolic pathway to the overall elimination of a drug may vary across individuals, an observation which may explain why some interactions show considerable interindividual variability in their occurrence or extent (Gatti *et al.*, 2001). In some cases, the relative contribution of a given isoenzyme to total drug clearance is concentration dependent.

A good example for this is phenytoin, whose major metabolic pathway, *p*-hydroxylation, is mediated by CYP2C9 and, to a lesser extent, CYP2C19 (Bajpai *et al.*, 1996). At high concentration, the activity of CYP2C9 becomes saturated and the contribution of CYP2C19 to the metabolism of the drug will correspondingly increase. Therefore, a significant impact of CYP2C19 inhibitors on phenytoin disposition will only be expected to occur at higher concentrations, when the CYP2C19-mediated pathway becomes increasingly important for the elimination of the drug.

For interactions involving enzyme induction, the situation is totally different from that described for enzyme inhibition. In fact, there is theoretically no limit to the increase in the efficiency of a given metabolic pathway when the corresponding isoenzyme(s) have been induced. In other words, enzyme induction could transform an initially minor metabolic pathway into a major contributor to the overall elimination of the drug, with a consequent important increase in total drug clearance.

The principles summarized above are well illustrated by the metabolic interactions described for felbamate and topiramate. Since CYP3A4 plays only a minor role in the metabolism of felbamate, inhibitors of this isoform would be expected to have only minimal effects on the overall clearance of this drug and, in line with this prediction, felbamate pharmacokinetics have been found not to be significantly affected by the potent CYP3A4 inhibitor erythromycin (Glue *et al.*, 1997). On the other hand, the total plasma clearance of felbamate is significantly increased and its plasma concentrations are significantly decreased by concomitant treatment with the CYP3A4-inducers phenytoin, phenobarbital and carbamazepine. A similar situation is observed with topiramate, a drug which in healthy subjects is primarily excreted unchanged in urine. Because metabolism is of minor importance in the overall clearance of topiramate, no significant changes in its plasma concentration are expected when an enzyme inhibitor is added for patients receiving topiramate monotherapy. On the other hand, metabolic elimination becomes an important determinant of topiramate clearance in patients treated with enzyme-inducing AEDs, an observation which explains the ability of the latter to decrease plasma topiramate concentration by 40–50% (Perucca and Bialer, 1996). It should be noted that, theoretically, the plasma concentration of felbamate and topiramate could be significantly affected by an enzyme inhibitor only when the latter is added on as a third agent in a patient who is already taking an enzyme inducer. This is because it is only in enzyme-induced patients that the contribution of metabolism to the overall clearance of these drugs becomes clinically significant.

Role of metabolites

A factor to be considered is whether metabolites have any enzyme inducing or inhibiting effects independent of those of the parent drug. For example, if a metabolite has an inhibiting effect on a given isoenzyme that is not shared by the parent drug, in vitro experiments designed to test the enzyme-inhibiting potential of the parent drug may fail to identify a clinically important interaction.

As discussed above, many metabolites are biologically active and this needs to be considered when predicting the clinical consequence of a drug interaction. If the affected drug has a pharmacologically active (or toxic) metabolite, enzyme inhibition may paradoxically result in decreased pharmacological (or toxicological) effect, while the reverse will be true for enzyme induction. It is also important to consider what influence the interaction is expected to have on the subsequent biotransformation of the metabolites.

Pharmacokinetic characteristics of the drug and route of drug administration

An example of how pharmacokinetic characteristics can influence the consequences of metabolic drug interactions has already been provided in the section 'Extent of metabolism of the substrate through the affected enzyme' when discussing the implications of the concentration-dependent pharmacokinetics of phenytoin.

An even more important aspect to be considered is whether the affected drug shows a low or a high extraction ratio in the organ (usually the liver) responsible for its metabolism. In the case of highly extracted drugs, clearance is mainly determined by the blood flow through the eliminating organ, and changes in enzyme activity will have little or no effect on their pharmacokinetics after parenteral administration. However, if metabolism takes place mainly in the liver or in the gut, enzyme induction or inhibition can have a marked effect on the first-pass extraction of these agents and, hence, on their oral bioavailability. These considerations provide an explanation for the marked reduction in the bioavailability of high clearance drugs such as ethinylestradiol (Perucca, 1982), lidocaine (Perucca and Richens, 1979) and nisoldipine (Michelucci *et al.*, 1998) in patients taking the enzyme-inducers phenobarbital, carbamazepine or phenytoin.

The pharmacokinetics of drugs which show a low metabolic clearance are not influenced by changes in blood flow, and their plasma concentration is largely determined by drug-metabolizing enzyme activity irrespective of the route of intake. Therefore, enzyme induction and inhibition are expected to affect the steady-state plasma concentration of these drugs after both parenteral and oral administration. For a detailed discussion of these principles, the reader is referred to the seminal work of Wilkinson and Shand (1975).

Complex or biphasic interactions

Enzyme induction and inhibition are not mutually exclusive and may occur at the same time. The ability of a given compound to act as an inducer and as an inhibitor at the same time provides an explanation for the inconsistent and apparently contradictory nature of certain drug interactions. As discussed above, for example, phenobarbital may either decrease or increase the plasma concentration of phenytoin depending on whether induction or inhibition of phenytoin metabolism prevails in an individual patient (Perucca, 1982). Even more complex is the interaction between phenytoin and warfarin. When phenytoin is started in a patient stabilized on warfarin therapy, phenytoin may initially competitively inhibit the metabolism of warfarin because both phenytoin and S-warfarin are substrates for CYP2C9 and phenytoin has a K_M (and therefore a K_i) within its therapeutic range. After an initial increase, the plasma concentration of S-warfarin will then decline within 1–2 weeks because of CYP2C9 induction (Cropp and Bussey, 1997).

Even more complex situations may be observed when other mechanisms of interaction, e.g. altered gastrointestinal absorption, drug displacement from binding sites, or pharmacodynamic interactions, occur simultaneously with changes in enzyme activity. Other complex situations arise in patients receiving combinations of three or more drugs, and in this case direct and indirect interactions may become difficult to predict. At times, interactions may actually cancel out reciprocally: for example, the clearance of lamotrigine is markedly enhanced by co-administration of enzyme-inducing AEDs (phenobarbital, carbamazepine and phenytoin) and inhibited by valproate. However, patients receiving lamotrigine in a triple therapy regimen that includes valproate and an enzyme inducer show lamotrigine clearance values comparable with those observed in patients on lamotrigine monotherapy (Jawad *et al.*, 1989).

Other sources of variability

There is a large intersubject variability in the extent and clinical relevance of metabolic drug interactions. As discussed above, enzyme induction and inhibition are usually dose dependent, and differences in dosage (or plasma concentration) of the interfering drug are important in determining the occurrence or extent of a drug interaction. Additional sources of variability relate to interindividual differences in the contribution of specific metabolic pathways to overall drug clearance. Age has also been reported to affect response to drug interactions: for example, it has been suggested that the elderly may be less sensitive to enzyme induction (Twum-Barima *et al.*, 1984), even though in a recent study auto- and heteroinduction of carbamazepine metabolism was not found to differ between elderly patients and younger adults (Battino *et al.*, 2003). The role of confounding factors (e.g. the additional influence of enzyme inducers or inhibitors found in the diet or in voluctuary substances) also varies considerably across individuals.

In patients receiving drugs metabolized by a polymorphic enzyme, the effects of inhibitors or inducers may vary between phenotypes/genotypes. EMs are generally more susceptible to enzyme inhibition or induction than PMs. For inhibition, this has been most clearly documented for CYP2D6: interactions caused by potent inhibitors of this isoform, i.e. quinidine, are not observed in PMs, who show a genetically determined lack of functional CYP2D6 in their liver (Steiner *et al.*, 1987). Likewise, PMs for CYP2C19 and CYP2C9, which play a role in the metabolism of phenytoin, are not expected to be vulnerable to the inhibition of phenytoin metabolism caused by selective inhibitors of the corresponding enzymes. More complex effects can be expected when the genotype/phenotype influences susceptibility to drug interactions in an indirect way: for example, the enzyme-inducing effects of 40 mg/day omeprazole (a CYP2C19 substrate) on CYP1A2 activity only occurs in PMs for CYP2C19, because only these subjects achieve plasma omeprazole concentrations which are sufficiently high to cause enzyme induction (Rost *et al.*, 1992).

For any given extent of interaction, clinical consequences also vary widely across individuals. As discussed above, interactions are more likely to be clinically significant when the plasma concentration of the affected drug at baseline is closest to the threshold for toxicity or therapeutic failure. Pharmacodynamic factors affecting response to any drug concentration are also important. Elderly patients in general are more prone to adverse drug interactions, not only because they more frequently receive multiple drug therapy but also because they may show increased pharmacodynamic sensitivity to drugs.

Conclusions

Metabolic drug interactions may have important clinical consequences. In the case of AEDs, these interactions are particularly common, due to the fact that many of these agents are potent inducers (or in some case, inhibitors) of the drug-metabolizing enzymes, and they are usually administered chronically, often in combination therapy. In recent years, an improved understanding of the nature of the main isoenzymes responsible for drug metabolism, coupled with advances in methodology for the in vitro assessment of metabolic reactions and interactions, has resulted in major breakthroughs in our ability to predict the occurrence and the in vivo implications of drug interactions. While the methodology still requires some refinement to improve the predictive power, available knowledge is already applied successfully not only in drug discovery (through design and selection of new agents devoid of undesirable interaction potential) and in drug development (though rational identification of drug interactions to be assessed in the clinical setting), but also in making informed decisions when adding or withdrawing co-medications in routine clinical practice.

REFERENCES

Anderson GD. A mechanistic approach to antiepileptic drug interactions. *Ann Pharmacother* 1998; **32**: 554–563.

Anderson GD, Graves NM. Drug interactions with antiepileptic agents: prevention and management. *CNS Drugs* 1994; **2**: 268–279.

Bajpai M, Roskos LK, Shen DD, *et al.* Roles of cytochrome P4502C9 and cytochrome P4502C19 in stereoselective metabolism of phenytoin to its major metabolite. *Drug Metab Dispos* 1996; **24**: 1401–1403.

Battino D, Croci D, Rossini A, *et al.* Serum carbamazepine concentrations in elderly patients: a case-matched pharmacokinetic evaluation. *Epilepsia* 2003; **44**: 923–929.

Bertilsson L, Dahl ML, Dalen P, *et al.* Molecular genetics of CYP2D6: clinical relevance with focus on psychotropic drugs. *Br J Clin Pharmacol* 2002; **53**: 111–122.

Bertz RJ, Granneman GR. Use of in vitro and in vivo data to estimate the likelihood of metabolic pharmacokinetic interactions. *Clin Pharmacokinet* 1997; **32**: 210–258.

Bock KW, Gschaidmeier H, Heel H, *et al.* Functions and transcriptional regulation of PAV-inducible human UDP-glucuronosyltransferases. *Drug Metab Rev* 1999; **31**: 411–422.

Brandolese R, Scordo MG, Spina E, *et al.* Severe phenytoin intoxication in a subject homozygous for CYP2C9*3. *Clin Pharmacol Ther* 2001; **70**: 391–394.

Cropp JS, Bussey HI. A review of enzyme induction of warfarin metabolism with recommendations for patient management. *Pharmacotherapy* 1997; **17**: 917–928.

Dickins M, Chen C. Lamotrigine. Chemistry, biotransformation and pharmacokinetics. In *Antiepileptic Drugs*, 5th edn. R. H. Levy, R. H. Mattson, B. S. Meldrum, E. Perucca, eds. Philadelphia: Lippincott Williams & Wilkins, 2002: 370–379.

Doose DR, Wang SS, Padmanabhan, *et al.* Effect of topiramate or carbamazepine on the pharmacokinetics of an oral contraceptive containing norethindrone and ethinyl estradiol in healthy obese and non-obese female subjects. *Epilepsia* 2003; **44**: 540–549.

Dresser GK, Spence D, Bailey DG. Pharmacokinetic–pharmacodynamic consequences and clinical relevance of cytochrome P450 3A4 inhibition. *Clin Pharmacokinet* 2000; **38**: 41–57.

Evans DAP, Mahgoub A, Sloan TP, *et al.* A family and population study of the genetic polymorphism of debrisoquine oxidation in a white British Population. *J Med Genet* 1980; **17**: 102–105.

Fattore C, Cipolla G, Gatti G, *et al.* Induction of ethinylestradiol and levonorgestrel metabolism by oxcarbazepine in healthy women. *Epilepsia* 1999; **40**: 783–787.

Fuerst RH, Graves NM, Leppik IE, *et al.* Felbamate increases phenytoin but decrease carbamazepine concentrations. *Epilepsia* 1988; **29**: 488–491.

Fuhr U. Induction of drug metabolizing enzymes: pharmacokinetic and toxicological consequences in humans. *Clin Pharmacokinet* 2000; **38**: 493–504.

Gatti G, Furlanut M, Perucca E. Interindividual variability in the metabolism of antiepileptic drugs and its clinical implications. In *Interindividual Variability in Human Drug Metabolism*. G. M. Pacifici, O. Pelkonen, eds. London: Taylor and Francis Ltd, 2001: 157–180.

Gidal BE, Zupanc ML. Potential pharmacokinetic interaction between felbamate and phenobarbital. *Ann Pharmacother* 1994; **28**: 455–458.

Glue P, Banfield CR, Perhach JL, *et al.* Pharmacokinetic interactions with felbamate: in vitro–in vivo correlation. *Clin Pharmacokinet* 1997; **33**: 214–224.

Goldstein JA. Clinical relevance of genetic polymorphism in the human CYP2C subfamily. *Br J Clin Pharmacol* 2001; **52**: 349–355.

Gonzalez FJ, Ueno T, Umeno M, *et al.* Microsomal ethanol oxidizing system: transcriptional and posttranscriptional regulation of cytochrome P450, CYP2E1. *Alcohol Alcohol* 1991; **1**(Suppl.): 97–101.

Greenblatt DJ, Von Moltke LL, Harmatz JS, *et al.* Drug interactions with newer antidepressants: role of human cytochromes P450. *J Clin Psychiat* 1998; **59**(Suppl. 15): 19–27.

Guengerich FP. Comparisons of catalytic selectivity of cytochrome P450 subfamily enzymes from different species. *Chem Biol Interact* 1997a; **106**: 161–182.

Guengerich FP. Role of cytochrome P450 enzymes in drug–drug interactions. *Adv Pharmacol* 1997b; **43**: 7–35.

Hiller A, Nguyen N, Strassburg CP, *et al.* Retigabine *N*-glucuronidation and its potential role in enterohepatic circulation. *Drug Metab Dispos* 1999; **27**: 605–612.

Hooper WD, Franklin ME, Glue P, *et al.* Effect of felbamate on valproic acid disposition in healthy volunteers: inhibition of beta-oxidation. *Epilepsia* 1996; **37**: 91–97.

Jawad S, Richens A, Goodwin G, *et al.* Controlled trial of lamotrigine (Lamictal) for refractory partial seizures. *Epilepsia* 1989; **30**: 356–363.

Jin C, Miners JO, Lillywhite KJ, *et al.* Complementary deoxyribonucleic acid cloning and expression of a human liver uridine diphosphate-glucuronosyltransferase glucuronidating carboxylic acid-containing drugs. *J Pharmacol Exp Ther* 1993; **264**: 475–479.

Johansson I, Lundqvist E, Bertilsson L, *et al.* Inherited amplification of an active gene in the cytochrome P450 CYP2D locus as a cause of ultrarapid metabolism of debrisoquine. *Proc Natl Acad Sci* 1993; **90**: 11825–11829.

Kerr BM, Rettie AE, Eddy AC, *et al.* Inhibition of human liver microsomal epoxide hydrolase by valproate and valpromide: in vitro/in vivo correlation. *Clin Pharmacol Ther* 1989; **46**: 82–93.

Kerr BM, Thummel KE, Wurden CJ, *et al.* Human liver carbamazepine metabolism: role of CYP3A4 and CYP2C8 in the 10,11-epoxide formation. *Biochem Pharmacol* 1994; **47**: 1969–1979.

Kondo T, Otani K, Hirano T, *et al.* The effects of phenytoin and carbamazepine in serum concentrations of mono-unsaturated metabolites of valproic acid. *Br J Clin Pharmacol* 1990; **29**: 116–119.

Kroetz DL, Loiseau P, Guyot M, *et al.* In vivo and in vitro correlation of microsomal epoxide hydrolase inhibition by progabide. *Clin Pharmacol Ther* 1993; **54**: 485–497.

Lamba JK, Lin YS, Schuetz EG, *et al.* Genetic contribution to variable human CYP3A-mediated metabolism. *Adv Drug Deliv Rev* 2002; **54**(10): 1271–1294.

Levy RH. Cytochrome P450 isozymes and antiepileptic drug interactions. *Epilepsia* 1995; **36**(Suppl. 5): S8–S13.

Levy RH, Trager WF. From in vitro to in vivo: an academic perspective. In *Metabolic Drug Interactions*. R. H. Levy, K. E. Thummel, W. F. Trager, P. D. Hansten, M. Eichelbaum, eds. Philadelphia: Lippincott Williams & Wilkins, 2000: 21–27.

Li AP, Maurel P, Gomez-Lechon MJ, *et al.* Preclinical evaluation of drug–drug interaction potential: present status of the application of primary human hepatocytes in the evaluation of cytochrome P450 induction. *Chem Biol Interact* 1997; **107**: 5–16.

Lin JH, Lu AYH. Inhibition and induction of cytochrome P450 and the clinical implications. *Clin Pharmacokinet* 1998; **35**: 361–390.

Lindhout D. Pharmacogenetics and drug interactions: role in antiepileptic-drug-induced teratogenesis. *Neurology* 1992; **42**: 43–47.

Liston HL, Markowitz JS, Devane L. Drug glucuronidation in clinical psychopharmacology. *J Clin Psychopharmacol* 2001; **21**: 500–515.

Mackenzie PI, Owens IS, Burchell B, *et al.* The UDP glycosyltransferase gene superfamily: recommended nomenclature update based on evolutionary divergence. *Pharmacogenetics* 1997; **7**: 255–269.

May TW, Rambeck B, Jurgens U. Influence of oxcarbazepine and methsuximide on lamotrigine concentrations in epileptic patients with and without valproic acid co-medication: results of a retrospective study. *Ther Drug Monit* 1999; **21**: 175–181.

Meyer UA. The molecular basis of genetic polymorphism of drug metabolism. *J Pharm Pharmacol* 1994; **46**(Suppl. 1): 409–415.

Michelucci R, Cipolla R, Passatelli D, *et al.* Reduced plasma nisoldipine concentrations in phenytoin-treated patients with epilepsy. *Epilepsia* 1998; **37**: 1107–1110.

Miners JO, Birkett DJ. Cytochrome P4502C9: an enzyme of major importance in human drug metabolism. *Br J Clin Pharmacol* 1998; **45**: 525–538.

Miners JO, McKinnon RA. CYP1A. In *Metabolic Drug Interactions*. R. H. Levy, K. E. Thummel, W. F. Trager, P. D. Hansten, M. Eichelbaum, eds. Philadelphia: Lippincott Williams & Wilkins, 2000: 61–73.

Nakajima M, Yokoy T, Mizutani M, *et al.* Genetic polymorphism in the 5'-flanking region of human CYP1A2 gene: effect on the CYP1A2 inducibility in humans. *J Biochem* 1999; **125**: 803–808.

Nallani SC, Glauser TA, Hariparsad N, *et al.* Dose-dependent induction of cytochrome P450 (CYP) 3A4 and activation of pregnane X receptor by topiramate. *Epilepsia* 2003; **44**: 1521–1528.

Nelson DR, Koymans L, Kamataki T, *et al.* P450 superfamily: update on new sequences, gene mapping, accession numbers and nomenclature. *Pharmacogenetics* 1996; **6**: 1–42.

Omcienski CJ. Epoxide hydrolases. In *Metabolic Drug Interactions*. R. H. Levy, K. E. Thummel, W. F. Trager, P. D. Hansten, M. Eichelbaum, eds. Philadelphia: Lippincott Williams & Wilkins, 2000: 205–214.

Parker AC, Pritchard P, Preston T, *et al.* Induction of CYP1A2 activity by carbamazepine in children using the caffeine breath test. *Br J Clin Pharmacol* 1998; **45**: 176–178.

Patsalos PN, Froscher W, Pisani F, *et al.* The importance of drug interactions in epilepsy therapy. *Epilepsia* 2002; **43**: 365–385.

Perucca E. Clinical consequences of microsomal enzyme induction by antiepileptic drugs. *Pharmaco Ther* 1978; **2**: 285–314.

Perucca E. Pharmacokinetic interactions with antiepileptic drugs. *Clin Pharmacokinet* 1982; **7**: 57–84.

Perucca E. Clinical implications of hepatic microsomal enzyme induction by antiepileptic drugs. *Pharmacol Ther* 1987; **33**: 139–144.

Perucca E. The clinical pharmacology and therapeutic use of the new antiepileptic drugs. *Fund Clin Pharmacol* 2001; **15**: 405–417.

Perucca E, Bialer M. The clinical pharmacokinetics of the newer antiepileptic drugs. Focus on topiramate, zonisamide and tiagabine. *Clin Pharmacokinet* 1996; **31**: 29–46

Perucca E, Richens A. Reduction of oral availability of lignocaine by induction of first-pass metabolism in epileptic patients. *Br J Clin Pharmacol* 1979; **8**: 21–31.

Perucca E, Richens A. Biotransformation. In *Antiepileptic Drugs*, 4th edn. R. H. Levy, R. H. Mattson, B. Meldrum, eds. New York: Raven Press, 1995: 31–50.

Perucca E, Hedges A, Makki KA, *et al.* A comparative study of the enzyme inducing properties of anticonvulsant drugs in epileptic patients. *Br J Clin Pharmacol* 1984; **18**: 401–410.

Pisani F, Haj-Yehia A, Fazio A, *et al.* Pharmacokinetics of valnoctamide in epileptic patients and its interaction with carbamazepine: in vitro/in vivo correlation. *Epilepsia* 1993; **34**: 954–959.

Raguenau-Majlessi I, Bajpai M, Levy RH. Phenytoin and other hydantoins: interactions with other drugs. In *Antiepileptic Drugs*, 5th edn. R. H. Levy, R. H. Mattson, B. S. Meldrum, E. Perucca, eds. Philadelphia: Lippincott Williams & Wilkins, 2002: 581–590.

Raucy J, Carpenter SP. CYP2E1. In *Metabolic Drug Interactions*. R. H. Levy, K. E. Thummel, W. F. Trager, P. D. Hansten, M. Eichelbaum, eds. Philadelphia: Lippincott Williams & Wilkins, 2000: 95–113.

Rendic S, Di Carlo FJ. Human cytochrome P450 enzymes: a status report summarizing their reactions, substrates, inducers, and inhibitors. *Drug Metab Rev* 1997; **29**: 413–580.

Rettie AE, Koop DR, Haining RL. CYP2C. In *Metabolic Drug Interactions*. R. H. Levy, K. E. Thummel, W. F. Trager, P. D. Hansten, M. Eichelbaum, eds. Philadelphia: Lippincott Williams & Wilkins, 2000: 75–86.

Ring BJ, Wrighton SA. Industrial viewpoint: application of in vitro drug metabolism in various phases of drug development. In *Metabolic Drug Interactions*. R. H. Levy, K. E. Thummel, W. F. Trager, P. D. Hansten, M. Eichelbaum, eds. Philadelphia: Lippincott Williams & Wilkins, 2000: 29–39.

Riva R, Albani F, Contin M, *et al.* Pharmacokinetic interactions between antiepileptic drugs: clinical considerations. *Clin Pharmacokinet* 1996; **31**: 470–493.

Rosenfeld WE, Doose DR, Walker SA, *et al.* Effect of topiramate on the pharmacokinetics of an oral contraceptive containing norethindrone and ethinyl estradiol in patients with epilepsy. *Epilepsia* 1997; **38**: 317–323.

Rost KL, Brosicke H, Brockmoller J, *et al.* Increase of cytochrome P450IIA activity by omeprazole: evidence by the ^{13}C-(N-3-methyl)-caffeine breath test in poor and extensive metabolizers of S-mephenytoin. *Clin Pharmacol Ther* 1992; **52**: 170–180.

Saano V, Glue P, Benfield CR, *et al.* Effects of felbamate on the pharmacokinetics of a low-dose combination oral contraceptive. *Clin Pharmacol Ther* 1995; **58**: 523–531.

Sachdeo RC, Sachdeo SK, Levy RH, *et al.* Topiramate and phenytoin pharmacokinetics during repetitive monotherapy and combination therapy to epileptic patients. *Epilepsia* 2002; **43**: 691–696.

Sachse C, Brockmoller J, Bauer S, *et al.* Functional significance of a C $\rightarrow$ A polymorphism in intron 1 of the cytochrome P450 CYP1A2 gene tested with caffeine. *Br J Clin Pharmacol* 1999; **47**: 445–449.

Scheyer RD. Valproic acid: drug interactions. In *Antiepileptic Drugs*, 5th edn. R. H. Levy, R. H. Mattson, B. S. Meldrum, E. Perucca, eds. Philadelphia: Lippincott Williams & Wilkins, 2002: 801–807.

Schuetz EG, Beck WT, Schuetz JD. Modulators and substrates of P-glycoprotein and cytochrome P4503A coordinately up-regulate these proteins in human colon carcinoma cells. *Mol Pharmacol* 1996; **49**: 311–318.

Segel IH. *Enzyme Kinetics*. New York, NY: John Wiley & Sons, 1975.

Shimada T, Yamazaki H, Mimura M, *et al.* Interindividual variations in human liver cytochrome P450 enzymes involved in oxidation of drugs, carcinogens, and toxic chemicals: studies with human liver microsomes of 30 Japanese and 30 Caucasians. *J Pharmacol Exp Ther* 1994; **270**: 414–423.

Sogawa K, Fujii-Kuriyama Y. Ah receptor, a novel ligand activated transcription factor. *J Biochem* 1997; **122**: 1075–1079.

Spina E, Pisani F, Perucca E. Clinically significant pharmacokinetic drug interactions with carbamazepine: an update. *Clin Pharmacokinet* 1996; **3**: 198–214.

Sproule BA, Naranjo CA, Bremner KE, *et al.* Selective serotonin reuptake inhibitors and CNS drug interactions: a critical review of the evidence. *Clin Pharmacokinet* 1997; **33**: 454–471.

Steiner E, Dumont E, Spina E, *et al.* Inhibition of desipramine 2-hydroxylation by quinidine and quinine in rapid and slow hydroxylators. *Clin Pharmacol Ther* 1987; **44**: 431–435.

Sueyoshi T, Kawamoto T, Zelko I, *et al.* The repressed nuclear receptor CAR respond to phenobarbital in activating the human CYP2B6 gene. *J Biol Chem* 1999; **274**: 6043–6046.

Thummel KE, Kunze KL, Shen DD. Metabolically-based drug–drug interactions: principles and mechanisms. In *Metabolic Drug Interactions*. R. H. Levy, K. E. Thummel, W. F. Trager, P. D. Hansten, M. Eichelbaum, eds. Philadelphia: Lippincott Williams & Wilkins, 2000: 3–19.

Twum-Barima Y, Finnigan T, Habasch AI, *et al.* Impaired enzyme induction by rifampicin in the elderly. *Br J Clin Pharmacol* 1984; **17**: 595–596.

Wen X, Wang JS, Kivisto KT, *et al.* In vitro evaluation of valproic acid as an inhibitor of human cytochrome P450 isoforms: preferential inhibition of cytochrome P450 2C9 (CYP2C9). *Br J Clin Pharmacol* 2001; **52**: 547–553.

Wilkinson GR, Shand DG. A physiological approach to hepatic drug clearance. *Clin Pharmacol Ther* 1975; **18**: 377–390.

Wrighton SA, Thummel KE. CYP3A. In *Metabolic Drug Interactions*. R. H. Levy, K. E. Thummel, W. F. Trager, P. D. Hansten, M. Eichelbaum, eds. Philadelphia: Lippincott Williams & Wilkins, 2000: 115–133.

Zaccara G, Gangemi PF, Bendoni L, *et al.* Influence of single and repeated doses of oxcarbazepine on the pharmacokinetics profile of felodipine. *Ther Drug Monit* 1993; **15**: 39–42.

Zanger UM, Eichelbaum M. CYP2D6. In *Metabolic Drug Interactions*. R. H. Levy, K. E. Thummel, W. F. Trager, P. D. Hansten, M. Eichelbaum, eds. Philadelphia: Lippincott Williams & Wilkins, 2000: 87–94.

6

Influence of food and drugs on the bioavailability of antiepileptic drugs

Carlos A. Fontes Ribeiro

Department of Pharmacology, Faculty of Medicine, University of Coimbra, Coimbra, Portugal

Introduction

Whenever two or more agents are used in combination the potential for interactions can occur. These interactions can occur at the pharmacodynamic and/or pharmacokinetic level. Pharmacokinetic interactions are by far the most frequent and result in the modification of blood or tissue drug concentration as a consequence of alterations in absorption, distribution, metabolism, or elimination of a drug.

Drugs with a narrow therapeutic range or low therapeutic index are more likely to be associated with clinically important interactions. As far as antiepileptic drugs (AEDs) are concerned, they may interact with each other when used in combination therapy, and with other non-epilepsy-related drugs or with over-the-counter medications. Furthermore, food and many excipient components of pharmaceutical formulations may also interact with AEDs. This chapter deals with interactions which occur before (pharmaceutical interactions) and during (pharmacokinetic interactions) absorption.

General principles

Since many AEDs are sparingly soluble in aqueous solutions, they are sensitive to any effects that alter solubility, dissolution, or gastrointestinal motility. The delivery of drugs into the circulation may be altered by physicochemical interactions that occur prior to absorption. For example, drugs may interact in an intravenous solution to produce an insoluble precipitate or may be damaged by light (Figueiredo *et al.*, 1993). Moreover, in the gut, drugs may chelate with metal ions or adsorb to resins. Thus the absorption of a particular drug is profoundly influenced by a great number of factors, which can be classified as follows:

(a) chemical characteristics and formulation,
(b) food and fluid intake,

(c) disease states,
(d) interaction with other drugs.

Absorption, regardless of the site, is dependent upon drug solubility. Drugs administered in an aqueous solution are more rapidly absorbed than those administered in an oily solution, a suspension, or in a solid form because they mix more readily with the aqueous phase at the absorptive site. For those drugs administered as a solid form, the rate of dissolution may be the limiting factor in their absorption.

Large fluid intake results in faster emptying of the stomach due to the distension of the stomach wall (Deutsch *et al.*, 1991). Thus, a drug that is ingested with large volume of fluid will travel faster into the small intestine, ensuring a better and more complete absorption.

Whilst the effect of large fluid volume on the absorption of a drug is predictable, the effect of food is unpredictable. As a general rule, after the ingestion of solid food, the emptying time of the stomach is decreased and intestinal motility and splanchnic blood flow are increased. However, an increase in the extent of drug dissolution in the stomach, as a result of meal prolongation of gastric residence time, does not appear to contribute substantially to fed-state increases in drug plasma concentrations that are observed when a lipid meal is co-administered (Miles *et al.*, 1997). One hypothesis is that the solid meal may enhance the pancreatic secretion thus providing a greater fluid volume for drug dissolution in the small intestine (Miles *et al.*, 1997).

Several drugs can also interfere with the physiologic conditions and function of the gastrointestinal tract and therefore alter the absorption of other drugs. These interactions might be the consequence of altered pH, decreased or increased motility, toxic effects on mucosa and changes in splanchnic blood flow. Therefore, antacids could raise the pH of gastric juice; metoclopramide and other gastrokinetic drugs (cisapride and domperidone) accelerate stomach emptying; propantheline retards stomach emptying; laxative agents decrease the intestinal transit time; cytostatic agents and antibiotics can damage the intestinal mucosa or the normal bacterial flora. Although all of these changes may result in a modified rate and/or extent of absorption, it is not possible to predict whether or not the interaction will be of clinical significance.

Another mechanism of interaction is via the cytochrome P450 (CYP) isoenzymes that are present in the gut and which contribute to the first-pass metabolism of some drugs. For instance, the isoenzyme CYP3A4 is abundant in the gut and can be stimulated by carbamazepine, phenytoin, phenobarbital and primidone thus reducing the plasma concentrations of drugs that are metabolized by CYP3A4. In contrast, CYP3A4 can be inhibited by acetazolamide, macrolide antibiotics, isoniazid, metronidazole, certain antidepressants, verapamil, diltiazem, cimetidine, danazol and propoxyphene (Spina *et al.*, 1996), increasing plasma concentrations of drugs that are metabolized by CYP3A4.

Disease states also influence absorption of drugs: in diseases accompanied by decreased motility of the stomach the absorption of drugs is generally delayed or reduced, while in diseases with faster gastric emptying absorption is enhanced. Subjects with an ileojejunal bypass are likely to require increase oral dosages (e.g. phenytoin) to achieve an optimal plasma concentration (Kennedy and Wade, 1979). When blood flow is reduced, as can occur in cardiac failure or shock, or after drugs, the rate of absorption is generally diminished, although the extent is unpredictable. In contrast, increased blood flow may serve to augment absorption.

On the other hand, if optimizing drug therapy aims at achieving and maintaining therapeutic and safe drug concentrations, the sustained release formulations can be useful. The sustained release formulations are designed to be absorbed by an efficient gastrointestinal system that is not limited to certain sites along the gastrointestinal tract. Nevertheless, in the gastrointestinal tract some interactions can occur, namely with drugs which modify intestinal motility. Thus it is possible for all the drug dose, which is encapsulated in the sustained release formulation, to be released at once through some accidental chemical or physiological mechanism. In this setting, the patient could be in danger of a drug overdose (Bialer, 1992). If the drug has a long half-life the probability of interactions during absorption is lower, as was verified for topiramate.

Regarding the formulation and administration of AEDs by the rectal route, there are only a few studies. Generally, drug administration by the rectal route is not acceptable to patients, particularly since absorption can be interrupted by defaecation (de Boer *et al.*, 1982).

Intramuscular drug absorption can be slow, erratic and incomplete, and this has been particularly demonstrated for phenytoin (Tuttle, 1977). Factors which play a role in the bioavailability of these medications include the water solubility of the drug, dispersion of the injected solution and blood flow at the muscle site.

Finally, chronovariability in absorption–elimination parameters (such as peak concentration and peak time) has been observed for many AEDs. Sometimes these changes had been attributed to interactions with food or drugs. The fasting-induced increase in hepatic glucuronidation during the night and the relative inactivity of the gut during this period may explain variations in circulation plasma drug concentrations (Chaudhary *et al.*, 1993). Loiseau *et al.* (1982) found diurnal variations in steady-state plasma concentrations of valproic acid, when administered by the oral route. Similar findings were observed by Yoshiyama *et al.* (1989) who reported that C_{max} tended to be higher and T_{max} shorter in the morning than in the evening. Such circadian variations of pharmacokinetic parameters have also been shown for carbamazepine (Bruguerolle *et al.*, 1981) but not for phenytoin (Petker and Morton, 1993).

Interactions with the established AEDs

Phenytoin

Phenytoin is the most studied of the AEDs, principally because it has been in use the longest. Much of the knowledge about this drug may be applied to other AEDs. Phenytoin, a weak acid with a pKa of 8.3, is practically insoluble in water. The salt is readily soluble in water but in the acidic medium of the stomach it precipitates after dissolving (Levy, 1976). In relation to the parenteral formulation of phenytoin, despite the fact that this phenytoin salt is water soluble, it precipitates in a large-volume, glucose-containing fluid.

The factors influencing the absorption rate are the particle size, nature of the filler, and whether the free acid or the sodium salt of phenytoin is the active ingredient. Thus, the rate of absorption varies considerably among dosage forms. Numerous studies (Cacek, 1986) have shown that phenytoin products from different manufacturers vary in absorption rate and differ in the time to reach maximum concentration, even if the area under the curve (AUC) is adequate. Many generic preparations are more rapidly absorbed and may produce an intolerable fluctuation in the plasma phenytoin concentration. In fact, differences in absorption significant enough to be associated with clinical toxicity have occurred with changes in the excipient (Bochner *et al.*, 1972; Carter *et al.*, 1981) – for instance, when calcium sulfate dihydrate was replaced by lactose, since the calcium compound interferes with phenytoin absorption. Therefore, changes in dosage form or manufacturer should be avoided once a patient's dosage requirements have been established, as a relatively small decrease or increase in bioavailability can greatly alter the steady-state plasma concentration during chronic administration.

Phenytoin suspensions of the acid have limited clinical utility for two reasons. First, unless well dispersed, precipitation of the drug in the bottle gives rise to doses lower-than-expected initially and higher-than-expected as the container is emptied. Second, the usual methods for measurements of liquids, especially with teaspoons, are inexact. When the phenytoin suspension is put into a unit-dose package, it is important to state on the label whether or not rinsing of the container is needed to ensure proper delivery of the intended dose.

The time to reach the maximum phenytoin plasma concentration after a single oral dose increases with the dose – the greater the dose, the longer the time to reach the peak (Tozer and Winter, 1990). The greatly increased peak time with dose is probably a consequence of two mechanisms. One is the relatively low solubility, slow dissolution and continued absorption of the drug; the other is the capacity-limited metabolism that is associated with phenytoin.

Burstein *et al.* (2000) reported that the absorption of phenytoin from polyethylene glycol rectal suppositories in healthy subjects is highly variable and unpredictable. Thus, this formulation is not recommended.

Food effect on phenytoin absorption

Food has been found to have variable but modest, usually enhancing, effects on phenytoin absorption (Cacek, 1986). The mechanisms include increased phenytoin dissolution in the stomach, saturation of the first-pass mechanisms, and increased splanchnic blood flow (Melander *et al.*, 1979). High-fat meals appear to increase phenytoin bioavailability (Sekikawa *et al.*, 1980), probably due to a combination of stimulation of bile flow and accelerated dissolution of phenytoin particles or by the delay of the gastric emptying time caused by the fat intake (Hamaguchi *et al.*, 1993). A protein-rich diet had the same effect on phenytoin acid but not on the sodium salt (Kennedy and Wade, 1982). Food may also enhance the delivery of phenytoin from prodrug formulations (e.g. 3-pentanonoyloxymethyl-5,5-diphenylhydantoin and 3-octanoyloxymethyl-5,5-diphenylhydantoin; Stella *et al.*, 1999).

Grapefruit juice, which inhibits the intestinal CYP3A4, does not affect the oral bioavailability of phenytoin (Kumar *et al.*, 1999). A possible explanation for this may relate to the fact that only a small amount (dose) of grapefruit juice was ingested by the subjects investigated in the study and also because phenytoin is not a substrate of CYP3A4.

The absorption of phenytoin is significantly impaired when given concurrently to epileptic patients receiving continuous nasogastric feeds (nutritional formulae). Substantial reduction in steady-state phenytoin plasma concentration have been reported in neurosurgery patients and in normal subjects (Bauer, 1982; Prichard *et al.*, 1987). The most likely mechanism is a reduced bioavailability due to rapid gastro-intestinal transit. In addition, it has been demonstrated that the presence of caseinate salts and calcium chloride may decrease phenytoin absorption (Smith *et al.*, 1988). Binding of phenytoin to the nasogastric tube apparatus has been largely excluded, since the tube is flushed after dosing (Cacek *et al.*, 1986). Decreased plasma phenytoin concentration associated with enteral feeding formulations may increase the risk of seizures (Au Yeung and Ensom, 2000).

Phenytoin and gastrointestinal diseases

The bioavailability of phenytoin may be reduced by gastrointestinal diseases, particularly those associated with increased intestinal motility. Thus, in cases of severe diarrhea, malabsorption syndromes, or gastric resection, decreased bioavailability should be considered (Tozer and Winter, 1990).

Drugs which may affect the gastrointestinal absorption of phenytoin

Activated charcoal

The absorption of phenytoin was almost completely prevented when given just before the oral ingestion of activated charcoal (Nation *et al.*, 1990). When a single dose of activated charcoal was administered 1 h after a dose of phenytoin, there was still an estimated 80% reduction in absorption (Welling, 1984).

Antacids and inhibitors of gastric hydrochloric acid secretion

Studies regarding the effect of antacids on the disposition of phenytoin have produced conflicting results. Overall, it appears that the influence of antacids is variable, both between antacid preparations and between subjects (Kutt, 1984). Moreover, both the timing of antacid dosing and the volume of antacid used may also contribute to this variability (D'Arcy and McElnay, 1987). The magnesium-containing antacids primarily increase gastric pH that enhances the solubility of weak acids and reduces the absorption rate from the stomach as it increases the ionization of the drug (Kutt, 1989). Aluminium-containing antacids, in addition, prolong gastric emptying time which under these circumstances further slows the rate of absorption (Marano *et al.*, 1985). Chelation or adsorption of phenytoin into the calcium-containing preparations has been suspected (Kutt, 1989; Nation *et al.*, 1990). On the whole, antacids containing aluminium hydroxide, magnesium hydroxide, and calcium carbonate decreased the bioavailability of phenytoin. It is generally recommended that, if antacids are to be used in patients receiving phenytoin, the administration of the two agents should be separated by a few hours.

Omeprazole does not affect the single-dose kinetics of phenytoin in healthy volunteers (Bachmann *et al.*, 1994). However, Prichard *et al.* (1987) have reported that the extent and rate of oral absorption of phenytoin is increased during omeprazole therapy. The mechanism of this is unknown but may relate to changes in gastric pH. Multiple doses (for 7 days) of pantoprazole were without effect on the rate or the extent of single-dose phenytoin absorption (Middle *et al.*, 1995). The hydrogen receptor antagonist cimetidine may increase the bioavailability of orally administered phenytoin (Hetzel *et al.*, 1981) through inhibition of CYP isoenzymes, although additional factors relating to absorption may also be involved.

Sucralfate

Concurrent administration of sucralfate significantly reduced the AUC of phenytoin (Hall *et al.*, 1986). Further studies are required to assess the effect of long-term sucralfate administration on phenytoin plasma concentrations.

Theophylline

It was suggested by Hendeles *et al.* (1979) that theophylline decreased the absorption of phenytoin when the two agents were administered at the same time.

Antineoplastic therapy

Some antineoplastics (e.g. cisplatinum, vinblastine, and bleomycin) impair the gastrointestinal absorption of phenytoin (Sylvester *et al.*, 1984).

Other drugs
Erythromycin, clarithromycin, and roxithromycin may increase the bioavailability of phenytoin (al-Humayyd, 1997). This effect may be due to an increased gastrointestinal motility induced by these macrolide antibiotics and subsequent augmented phenytoin absorption.

Co-administration of ciprofloxacin and phenytoin revealed a significant decrease in steady-state maximum and minimum concentrations and in the area under the plasma time concentration curve (Islam *et al.*, 1999). This finding warrants close monitoring of levels when these two agents are given simultaneously.

An approximately 30% reduction in dietary fat absorption induced by orlistat administered at doses of 120 mg three times daily did not significantly alter the pharmacokinetics of a single 300 mg oral dose of phenytoin in healthy volunteers (Melia *et al.*, 1996).

Interactions during phenytoin parenteral administration

Although phenytoin sodium could be given both intravenously and intramuscularly, both of these routes of administration have limitations.

The major disadvantage of the intravenous route is the requirement for slow administration of the propylene glycol/alcohol diluent which is adjusted to pH 12 with sodium hydroxide (Tozer and Winter, 1990). This vehicle is required to maintain phenytoin in solution at a concentration of 50 mg of the sodium salt per milliliter. Due to the inconvenience of administering the drug slowly, there is often a desire to give phenytoin with other intravenous fluids. If phenytoin admixtures are to be used, only normal saline or lactated Ringer's solution should be used, since admixtures with other solutions could result in phenytoin precipitation (Tozer and Winter, 1990).

The intramuscular route of administration should be avoided because phenytoin precipitates at the site of injection. Consequently, absorption from the injection site tends to be rather erratic and slow, often continuing for 5 days or more (Tozer and Winter, 1990).

Phenytoin actions affecting the pharmacokinetics and/or pharmacodynamics of other drugs

It seems that phenytoin does not alter the absorption of other drugs. However, epileptic patients receiving phenytoin have been reported to exhibit a significantly smaller diuretic response to furosemide (Williamson, 1986). Furthermore, the time to peak diuretic response was considerably delayed in these patients. This was attributed to delayed oral absorption of furosemide, perhaps the result of a phenytoin-induced decrease in the spontaneous activity of gastrointestinal smooth muscle (Williamson, 1986). However, other factors may be involved, such as the reduction of the sensitivity of the renal tubule to the diuretic action of furosemide

(Ahmad, 1974). In contrast with the observations with furosemide, Keller *et al.* (1981) have reported that pre-treatment with phenytoin did not alter the disposition of orally administered hydrochlorothiazide. There is some evidence that phenytoin treatment may decrease the gastrointestinal absorption of thyroxin and folic acid (Nation *et al.*, 1990). Phenytoin can act as folate antagonist and precipitate folic acid deficiency (Matsui and Rozovski, 1982). Finally, Rowland and Gupta (1987) suggested that the treatment with phenytoin leads to decreased gastrointestinal absorption of cyclosporine.

Carbamazepine

The gastrointestinal absorption of carbamazepine formulations is slow, erratic and unpredictable (Morselli, 1989). The mechanisms that are associated with these characteristics may be:

(a) low water solubility ($<$200 mg/ml) and other physicochemical properties of the molecule (a neutral drug which cannot be converted to a soluble salt), leading to a very slow dissolution rate in gastrointestinal fluid,
(b) anticholinergic properties of the drug which may become more evident during prolonged treatment and which modify its gastrointestinal transit time (Morselli, 1989).

It has been suggested that the rate and extent of its absorption may be dose-dependent.

Carbamazepine usually peaks 3–8 h after oral dosing, but the addition of propylene glycol, polysorbate, or ethanol can accelerate the absorptive process and reduce the time to peak to 1.5–4 h and increase its bioavailability (Leppik and Wolff, 1993). There is evidence that the dissolution rate of tablets can be affected by moisture (Wang *et al.*, 1993). Furthermore, absorption of the suspension is more rapid than that of tablets, resulting in peak concentrations at 1–3 h (Morselli, 1989). Therefore, liquid oral carbamazepine dosage formulations are typically associated with a doubling in their oral bioavailability compared with tablet formulations (Brewster *et al.*, 1997). However, the relative bioavailability of carbamazepine suspension with enteral or nasogastric feeding administration is slightly diminished and generally slower than during fasting (Bass *et al.*, 1989). Changes in gastric pH induced by ranitidine in healthy adults did not affect the bioavailability of carbamazepine (Dalton *et al.*, 1985).

Carbamazepine induces the CYP3A4 catalyzed sulfoxidation of omeprazole, apparently without major clinical implication, and it has no or less effect on hydroxylation via the CYP2C19 (Bertilsson *et al.*, 1997). CYP3A4 isoenzyme exists in the gut and liver. Carbamazepine half-life and 24 h post dose concentration increased significantly during erythromycin administration (Miles and Tennison,

1989). These effects are not only due to changed absorption but also to inhibition of metabolic pathways (Miles and Tennison, 1989).

Aminophylline reduced the bioavailability of carbamazepine which may be of clinical significance (Kulkarni *et al.*, 1995); 400 mg pentoxifylline administered at 22:00 h reduced the rate but not the extent of carbamazepine absorption (Poondru *et al.*, 2001). Interestingly, these effects were not observed when pentoxifylline was administered at 10:00 h.

Valproic acid

Valproic acid is a branched-chain fatty acid which is rapidly and completely absorbed once it is released from its pharmaceutical formulation. In spite of differences in populations and pharmaceutical formulations, the absolute bioavailability of valproate is consistently found to be close to unity. This observation indicates that valproate is not subject to a first-pass effect which is consistent with its low metabolic clearance.

Meals can have a profound effect on the time to peak concentration for the enteric-coated tablets; however, the long peak times represent delayed, rather than prolonged, absorption. Ramadan, with its changes in eating and rest/activity rhythms, significantly influences the pharmacokinetics of valproic acid. A significant decrease in the bioavailability of valproic acid was found at the end of the 3rd week of Ramadan, compared to the control period (Aadil *et al.*, 2000).

Carbapenem antibiotics induce a decrease in plasma concentration of valproic acid in epileptic patients (Torii *et al.*, 2002). By using Caco-2 cell monolayers, the influence of carbapenems was tested on the transepithelial transport of valproic acid (Torii *et al.*, 2002); it was found that carbapenems may inhibit the absorption of valproic acid at the basolateral membrane of intestinal epithelial cells. The same authors had verified that imipenem inhibits the intestinal absorption of valproic acid but not through an inhibition of a carrier-mediated transport of valproic acid (Torii *et al.*, 2001).

Repeat charcoal administered several hours after sodium valproate ingestion appears not to impair the absorption of valproic acid or indeed its pharmacokinetics (al-Shareef *et al.*, 1997). Aminophylline also seems not to alter the pharmacokinetic parameters of valproic acid (Kulkarni *et al.*, 1995).

Phenobarbital

Phenobarbital has a pKa of 7.2 and is more water soluble than phenytoin or carbamazepine. Early work on the rate and extent of absorption of phenobarbital indicated the potential for dissolution-rate-limited absorption after oral administration (Rust and Dodson, 1989). More recent studies have found that phenobarbital (acid and tablets) is absorbed rapidly and completely. The absolute bioavailability of phenobarbital has been found to be close to unity.

The bioavailability of phenobarbital appears to be greater in protein malnourished subjects (Syed *et al.*, 1986). Activated charcoal reduces phenobarbital absorption, a characteristic that is exploited clinically in the early treatment of phenobarbital overdose (Neuvonen and Elonen, 1980; Welling, 1984). However, colestipol hydrochloride, a hypocholesterolemic bile acid-binding anion-exchange polymer, does not change phenobarbital absorption (Phillips *et al.*, 1976).

Is has been suggested that the absorption of griseofulvin may be reduced by phenobarbital (Riegelman *et al.*, 1970), perhaps as a result of diminished dissolution. Phenobarbital may cause a modest reduction of cimetidine absorption (Somogyi and Gugler, 1982), mainly due to induction of its gastrointestinal metabolism (Somogyi *et al.*, 1981). Patients receiving phenobarbital have been reported to exhibit a significantly smaller diuretic response to furosemide and this may be the consequence of reduced absorption (Williamson, 1986).

Ethosuximide

Ethosuximide is relatively water soluble and is rapidly absorbed from tablets. The time required to reach peak plasma concentration is less than 3 h (Chang, 1989). Due to its very low clearance, no first-pass effect is expected. Ethosuximide has not been associated with any interactions at the gastrointestinal site of absorption.

Interactions with other AEDs

Over the past few years, eight new AEDs (felbamate, gabapentin, lamotrigine, oxcarbazepine, topiramate, zonisamide, vigabatrin, and levetiracetam) have reached the market and are licensed for clinical use. Due to the risks associated with the use of an unproved new drug as monotherapy, current guidelines for AED trials require that the test drug be evaluated as add-on therapy. Thus, drug interactions are important considerations. Very dramatic pharmacokinetic interactions were observed with some new AEDs that were evaluated during the 1980s. For example, nafimidone is a potent inhibitor of both carbamazepine and phenytoin (Leppik *et al.*, 1993); the inhibition is of such magnitude that clinical toxicity is observed, and this limited the development of the drug. Another example is that of MK-801 (Leppik *et al.*, 1993). These examples underscore the need for evaluating pharmacokinetic interactions in the early stage of new AED development. However, in general, AED interactions with food are not studied during preclinical studies (phases I–III) and therefore information in this regard is sparse.

Vigabatrin

Vigabatrin is a synthetic gamma aminobutyric acid (GABA) derivative which was designed to increase brain GABA concentrations by inhibiting GABA transaminase, the enzyme responsible for the breakdown of GABA. Vigabatrin is a racemic mixture but only the $S(+)$ enantiomer is pharmacologically active. However, the R enantiomer does not interfere with the disposition of the S enantiomer, nor does it undergo chemical inversion in vivo (Haegle and Schechter, 1986; Richens, 1989; Rey *et al.*, 1992).

The bioavailability of vigabatrin is considered to be at least 60–80% (Haegle and Schechter, 1986). The AUC for fasted and fed volunteers is not significantly different, indicating that food does not affect the extent of absorption (Frisk-Holmberg *et al.*, 1989). Overall the interaction potential of vigabatrin is minimal.

Tiagabine

This AED, a nipecotic acid derivative, increases brain GABA concentrations through inhibition of GABA re-uptake (Natsch *et al.*, 1997). After oral ingestion tiagabine is rapidly absorbed with peak plasma concentrations occurring within 1 h. Its bioavailability is 90% (Jansen *et al.*, 1995). Whilst the rate of tiagabine ingestion is slowed by food co-ingestion (T_{max} increases from 0.9 to 2.6 h), the extent of absorption remains the same (Mengel *et al.*, 1991). To date there are no data on the effects of drugs on the absorption of tiagabine.

Felbamate

Felbamate is a lipophilic dicarbamate which is only very slightly soluble in water. After oral ingestion felbamate is rapidly absorbed with a bioavailability of over 90% (Shumaker *et al.*, 1990). Food co-ingestion has no significant effect on either the rate or extent of absorption of felbamate (Graves *et al.*, 1989; Leppik *et al.*, 1993). To date there are no data on the effects of drugs on the absorption of felbamate.

Gabapentin

Gabapentin is a GABA-related amino acid with properties of an amino acid, but unlike GABA it readily penetrates the blood–brain barrier. Gabapentin is a substrate of intestinal large neutral amino acid carriers (Gidal *et al.*, 1998b). A consequence of this type of transport is the dose-dependent oral absorption of gabapentin, with saturation at high doses (McLean, 1994). Thus, the bioavailability of gabapentin which is reported to be only 35% at a steady dosage of 1500 mg t.i.d., may be improved by ingesting the drug more frequently (e.g. from t.i.d. to q.i.d.; Gidal *et al.*, 1998a).

High-protein meals do not seem to interfere with the absorption of gabapentin in spite of the fact that amino acids could interfere with the carrier system (Benetello *et al.*, 1997). In contrast, a trend was noted for a modest increase in both C_{max} and AUC values when gabapentin was ingested with a fat-free chocolate pudding

(Gidal *et al.*, 1998b), which led these authors to state that dietary macronutrient composition (i.e. protein) may favourably influence gabapentin absorption. However, this conclusion is not in accordance with the transport of gabapentin though an amino acid carrier. Overall, it can be concluded that the bioavailability of gabapentin is not significantly affected by food.

An interaction between gabapentin and antacids containing aluminium and magnesium hydroxide has been reported (Turnheim, 2004). The gastrointestinal absorption of gabapentin appears to be reduced and typically gabapentin plasma concentrations are approximately 15% lower; this interaction is not considered to be of clinical significance. To date there are no other data on the effects of drugs on the absorption of gabapentin.

Lamotrigine

Lamotrigine is a phenyltriazine derivative which was initially developed as an antifolate compound. Following oral ingestion, lamotrigine is rapidly well absorbed with peak plasma concentrations occurring at 1–3 h post ingestion (Cohen *et al.*, 1987; Yuen, 1991; Leppik *et al.*, 1993). The absolute bioavailability of lamotrigine after a 75-mg oral dose is 98 ± 5% (Yuen, 1991). Whereas food co-ingestion slightly delays the occurrence of the peak plasma lamotrigine concentration, it does not affect the extent of absorption (Goa *et al.*, 1993). To date there are no data on the effects of drugs on the absorption of lamotrigine.

Topiramate

Topiramate is a sulfamate-substituted monosaccharide which is structurally distinct from other AEDs. It is rapidly absorbed, with peak plasma concentrations occurring within 2 h to 4 h after oral ingestion. The bioavailability of topiramate is estimated to be 81–95% (Easterling *et al.*, 1988). Co-administration with food moderately slows absorption (11–13% decreased mean maximum absorption) whereas the extent of absorption is unaffected (Doose *et al.*, 1996). Thus topiramate can be ingested without due regard to meal times. To date there are no data on the effects of drugs on the absorption of topiramate.

Oxcarbazepine

Oxcarbazepine, a keto compound chemically related to carbamazepine, has a similar therapeutic profile to that of carbamazepine but is associated with an improved tolerability profile (Jensen and Dam, 1990). Following oral ingestion, oxcarbazepine is rapidly absorbed with peak plasma concentrations of its pharmacologically active metabolite (a monohydroxylated derivative), occurring 4–6 h later. Its bioavailability is 89% (Feldmann *et al.*, 1978). After a fat- and protein-rich breakfast there was a moderate increase in the monohydroxylated derivative AUC (16%) and C_{max} (23%)

values but with no changes in $T_{\max}$ and terminal half-life values (Degen *et al.*, 1994). These changes should be of little therapeutic consequence. To date there are no data on the effects of drugs on the absorption of oxcarbazepine.

Zonisamide

Zonisamide is a benzisoxazole compound which is structurally different to other AEDs. Absorption is rapid after oral ingestion with peak plasma concentrations occurring after 2.4–3.6 h. The bioavailability of zonisamide is estimated to be 65%. The bioavailability of zonisamide is unaffected by food co-ingestion although there is a delay in peak plasma concentration values to 4–6 h. To date there are no data on the effects of drugs on the absorption of zonisamide.

Levetiracetam

Levetiracetam is the *S* enantiomer of the ethyl analog of piracetam and as such is structurally unrelated to other AEDs. The absorption of levetiracetam after oral ingestion is rapid with peak plasma concentrations occurring approximately 1 h later. Its bioavailability is considered to be essentially 100% (Patsalos, 2002). Although food co-ingestion slows the rate of absorption of levetiracetam, the extent is unaffected (Patsalos, 2003). To date there are no data on the effects of drugs on the absorption of levetiracetam.

REFERENCES

Aadil N, Fassi-Fihri A, Houti I, *et al.* Influence of Ramadan on the pharmacokinetics of a single oral dose of valproic acid administered at two different times. *Method Find Exp Clin Pharmacol* 2000; **22**: 109–114.

Ahmad S. Renal insensitivity to frusemide caused by chronic anticonvulsant therapy. *Br Med J* 1974; **3**: 657–659.

al-Humayyd MS. Pharmacokinetic interactions between erythromycin, clarithromycin, roxithromycin and phenytoin in the rat. *Chemotherapy* 1997; **43**: 77–85.

al-Shareef A, Buss DC, Shetty HG, *et al.* The effect of repeated-dose activated charcoal on the pharmacokinetics of sodium valproate in healthy volunteers. *Br J Clin Pharmacol* 1997; **43**: 109–111.

Au Yeung SC, Ensom MH. Phenytoin and enteral feedings: does evidence support an interaction? *Ann Pharmacother* 2000; **34**: 896–905.

Bachmann KA, Sullivan TJ, Jauregui L, *et al.* Drug interactions of H_2-receptor antagonists. *Scand J Gastroenterol* 1994; **206**(Suppl.): 14–19.

Bass J, Miles MV, Tennison MB, *et al.* Effects of enteral tube feeding on the absorption and pharmacokinetic profile of carbamazepine suspension. *Epilepsia* 1989; **30**: 364–369.

Bauer LA. Interference of oral phenytoin absorption by continuous nasogastric feedings. *Neurology* 1982; **32**: 570–572.

Benetello P, Furlanut M, Fortunato M, *et al.* Oral gabapentin disposition in patients with epilepsy after a high-protein meal. *Epilepsia* 1997; **38**: 1140–1142.

Bertilsson L, Tybring G, Widen J, *et al.* Carbamazepine treatment induces the CYP3A4 catalysed sulphoxidation of omeprazole, but has no or less effect on hydroxylation via CYP2C19. *Br J Clin Pharmacol* 1997; **44**: 186–189.

Bialer M. Pharmacokinetic evaluation of sustained release formulations of antiepileptic drugs. Clinical implications. *Clin Pharmacokinet* 1992; **22**: 11–21.

Bochner F, Hooper WD, Tyrer J, *et al.* Factors involved in an outbreak of phenytoin intoxication. *J Neurol Sci* 1972; **16**: 481–487.

Brewster ME, Anderson WR, Meinsma D, *et al.* Intravenous and oral pharmacokinetic evaluation of a 2-hydroxypropyl-beta-cyclodextrin-based formulation of carbamazepine in the dog: comparison with commercially available tablets and suspensions. *J Pharm Sci* 1997; **86**: 335–339.

Bruguerolle B, Valli M, Bouyard L, *et al.* Circadian effect on carbamazepine kinetics in rat. *Eur J Drug Metab Pharmacokinet* 1981; **6**: 189–193.

Burstein AH, Fisher KM, McPherson ML, *et al.* Absorption of phenytoin from rectal suppositories formulated with a polyethylene glycol base. *Pharmacotherapy* 2000; **20**: 562–567.

Cacek AJ. Review of alterations in oral phenytoin bioavailability associated with formulations, antacids and food. *Ther Drug Monit* 1986; **8**: 166–171.

Cacek AT, DeVito JM, Koonce JR. In vitro evaluation of nasogastric administration methods for phenytoin. *American J Hosp Pharm* 1986; **43**: 689–692.

Carter BL, Garnett WR, Pellock JM, *et al.* Effect of antacid on phenytoin bioavailability. *Ther Drug Monit* 1981; **3**: 333–340.

Chaudhary A, Lane RA, Woo D, *et al.* Multiple-dose lorazepam kinetics: shuttling of lorazepam glucuronide between the circulation and the gut during day- and night-time dosing intervals in response to feeding. *J Pharmacol Exp Ther* 1993; **267**: 1034–1038.

Chang T. Ethosuximide: absorption, distribution, and excretion. In *Antiepileptic Drugs*. R. H. Levy, R. H. Mattson, B. Meldrum, J. K. Penry, F. E. Dreifuss, eds. New York: Raven Press, 1989: 671–678.

Cohen AF, Land GS, Bramer DD, *et al.* Lamotrigine, a new anticonvulsant: Pharmacokinetics in normal humans. *Clin Pharmacol Ther* 1987; **42**: 535–541.

Dalton MJ, Powell JR, Messenheimer JA Jr. Ranitidine does not alter single-dose carbamazepine pharmacokinetics in healthy adults. *Drug Intell Clin Pharm* 1985; **19**: 941–944.

D'Arcy PF, McElnay JC. Drug–antacid interactions of clinical importance. *Drug Intel Clin Pharm* 1987; **21**: 607–617.

de Boer AG, Moolenaar F, de Leede LG, *et al.* Rectal drug administration: clinical pharmacokinetic considerations. *Clin Pharmacokinet* 1982; **7**: 285–311.

Degen PH, Flesch G, Cardot JM, *et al.* The influence of food on the disposition of the antiepileptic oxcarbazepine and its major metabolites in healthy volunteers. *Biopharm Drug Dispos* 1994; **15**: 519–526.

Deutsch T, Ludwig E, Gráber H, *et al.* Basic clinical pharmacokinetics. In *Human Pharmacology*. H. Kuemmerle, T. Shibuya, J.-P. Tillement, eds. Amsterdam: Elsevier Science Publishers, 1991: 307–535.

Doose DR, Walker SA, Gisclon LG, *et al.* Single-dose pharmacokinetics and effect of food on the bioavailability of topiramate, a novel antiepileptic drug. *J Clin Pharmacol* 1996; **36**: 884–891.

Easterling DE, Zakszewski T, Moyer MD, *et al.* Plasma pharmacokinetics of topiramate, a new anticonvulsant in humans. *Epilepsia* 1988; **29**: 662.

Feldmann KF, Brechbuhler S, Faigle JW, *et al.* Pharmacokinetics and metabolism of GP 47680, a compound related to carbamazepine, in animals and man. In *Advances in Epileptology.* H. Meinardi, A. J. Rowan, eds. Amsterdam: Swets and Zeitlinger, 1978: 290–294.

Figueiredo A, Fontes Ribeiro CA, Gonçalo M, *et al.* Experimental studies on the mechanisms of tiaprofenic acid photosensitization. *J Photochem Photobiol B: Biol* 1993; **18**: 161–168.

Frisk-Holmberg M, Kerth P, Meyer P. Effect of food on the absorption of vigabatrin. *Br J Clin Pharmacol* 1989; **27**: 23S–25S.

Gidal BE, DeCerce J, Bockbrader HN, *et al.* Gabapentin bioavailability: effect of dose and frequency of administration in adult patients with epilepsy. *Epilepsy Res* 1998a; **31**: 91–99.

Gidal BE, Maly MM, Kowalski JW, *et al.* Gabapentin absorption: effect of mixing with foods of varying macronutrient composition. *Ann Pharmacother* 1998b; **32**: 405–409.

Goa KL, Ross SR, Chrisp P. Lamotrigine—A review of its pharmocological properties and clinical efficacy in epilepsy. *Drugs* 1993; **46**: 152–176.

Graves NM, Ludden TM, Holmes GB, *et al.* Pharmacokinetics of felbamate, a novel antiepileptic drug: Application of mixed-effect modelling to clinical trials. *Pharmacotherapy* 1989; **9**: 372–376.

Haegle KD, Schechter PJ. Kinetics of the enantiomers of vigabatrin after an oral dose of the racemate or the active S-enantiomer. *Clin Pharmacol Therap* 1986; **40**: 581–585.

Hall TG, Cuddy PG, Glass CJ, *et al.* Effect of sucralfate on phenytoin bioavailability. *Drug Intell Clin Pharm* 1986; **20**: 607–611.

Hamaguchi T, Shinkuma D, Irie T, *et al.* Effect of a high-fat meal on the bioavailability of phenytoin in a commercial powder with a large particle size. *Int J Clin Pharmacol Ther Toxicol* 1993; **31**: 326–330.

Hendeles L, Wyatt R, Weinberger M, *et al.* Decreased oral phenytoin absorption following concurrent theophylline administration. *J Allergy Clin Immunol* 1979; **63**: 156.

Hetzel DJ, Bochner F, Hallpike JF, *et al.* Cimetidine interaction with phenytoin. *Br Med J* 1981; **282**: 1512.

Islam AF, Garg SK, Bhargava VK. Effect of ciprofloxacin on steady state pharmacokinetics of phenytoin in rabbits. *Ind J Exp Biol* 1999; **37**: 86–88.

Jansen JA, Oliver S, Dirach J, *et al.* Absolute bioavailability of tiagabine. *Epilepsia* 1995; **36**(Suppl. 3): S159.

Jensen PK, Dam M. Oxcarbamazepine. In *Comprehensive Epileptology.* M. Dam, L. Gram, eds. New York: Raven Press, 1990: 621–629.

Keller E, Sulzer U, Brennes M. Disposition of hydrochlorothiazide during phenytoin treatment. *Klin Wochenschr* 1981; **59**: 1223–1224.

Kennedy MC, Wade DN. Phenytoin absorption in patients with ileojejunal bypass. *Br J Clin Pharmacol* 1979; **7**: 515–518.

Kennedy MC, Wade DN. The effect of food on the absorption of phenytoin. *Aust NZ J Med* 1982; **12**: 258–261.

Kulkarni C, Vaz J, David J, *et al.* Aminophylline alters pharmacokinetics of carbamazepine but not that of sodium valproate – a single dose pharmacokinetic study in human volunteers. *Ind J Physiol Pharmacol* 1995; **39**: 122–126.

Kumar N, Garg SK, Prabhakar S. Lack of pharmacokinetic interaction between grapefruit juice and phenytoin in healthy male volunteers and epileptic patients. *Method Find Exp Clin Pharmacol* 1999; **21**: 629–632.

Kutt H. Interactions between anticonvulsants and other commonly prescribed drugs. *Epilepsia* 1984; **25**(Suppl. 2): S118–S131.

Kutt H. Phenytoin – Interactions with Other Drugs. In *Antiepileptic Drugs*. R. H. Levy, R. H. Mattson, B. Meldrum, J. K. Penry, F. E. Dreifuss, eds. New York: Raven Press, 1989: 215–232.

Leppik IE, Wolff DL. Antiepileptic medication interactions. *Neurol Clin* 1993; **11**: 905–921.

Leppik IE, Graves N, Devinsky O. New antiepileptic medications. *Neurol Clin* 1993; **11**: 923–949.

Levy G. Clinical implications of interindividual differences in plasma protein binding of drugs and endogenous substances. In *The Effect of Disease States on Drug Pharmacokinetics*. L. Z. Benet, ed. Washington: American Pharmaceutical Association, 1976: 137–151.

Loiseau P, Cenraud B, Levy RH, *et al.* Diurnal variations in steady-state plasma concentrations of valproic acid in epileptic patients. *Clin Pharmacokinet* 1982; **7**(6): 544–552.

Marano AR, Caride VJ, Prokop EK. Effect of sucralfate and an aluminum hydroxide gel on gastric emptying of solids and liquids. *Clin Pharmacol Ther* 1985; **37**: 629–632.

Matsui MS, Rozovski SJ. Drug–nutrient interaction. *Clin Ther* 1982; **4**: 423–440.

McLean MJ. Clinical pharmacokinetics of gabapentin. *Neurology* 1994; **44**(Suppl. 5): S17–S22.

Melander A, Brante G, Johansson O, *et al.* Influence of food on the absorption of phenytoin in man. *Eur J Clin Pharmacol* 1979; **15**: 269–274.

Melia AT, Mulligan TE, Zhi J. The effect of orlistat on the pharmacokinetics of phenytoin in healthy volunteers. *J Clin Pharmacol* 1996; **36**: 654–658.

Mengel HB, Gustavson LE, Soerensen HJ, *et al.* Effect of food on the bioavailability of tiagabine HCl. *Epilepsia* 1991; **32**(Suppl. 3): 6.

Middle MV, Muller FO, Scall R, *et al.* No influence of pantoprazole on the pharmacokinetics of phenytoin. *Int J Clin Pharmacol Ther* 1995; **33**: 304–307.

Miles MV, Tennison MB. Erythromycin effects on multiple-dose carbamazepine kinetics. *Ther Drug Monit* 1989; **11**: 47–52.

Miles C, Dickson P, Rana K, *et al.* CCK antagonist pre-treatment inhibits meal-enhanced drug absorption in dogs. *Regul Pept* 1997; **68**: 9–14.

Morselli PL. Carbamazepine absorption, distribution and excretion. In *Antiepileptic Drugs*. R. H. Levy, R. H. Mattson, B. Meldrum, J. K. Penry, F. E. Dreifuss, eds. New York: Raven Press, 1989: 473–490.

Nation RL, Evans AM, Milne RE. Pharmacokinetic drug interactions with phenytoin (Part I). *Clin Pharmacokinet* 1990; **18**: 37–60.

Natsch S, Hekster YA, Keyser A, *et al.* Newer anticonvulsant drugs: role of pharmacology, drug interactions and adverse reactions in drug choice. *Drug Saf* 1997; **17**: 228–240.

Neuvonen PJ, Elonen E. Effect of activated charcoal on absorption and elimination of phenobarbitone, carbamazepine and phenylbutazone in man. *Eur J Clin Pharmacol* 1980; **17**: 51–57.

Patsalos PN. Pharmacokinetic profile of levetiracetam: toward ideal characteristics. *Pharmacol Ther* 2002; **85**: 77–85.

Patsalos PN. The pharmacokinetic characteristics of levetiracetam. *Method Find Exp Clin Pharmacol* 2003; **25**: 123–129.

Petker MA, Morton DJ. Comparison of the effectiveness of two oral phenytoin products and chronopharmacokinetics of phenytoin. *J Clin Pharm Ther* 1993; **18**: 213–217.

Phillips WA, Ratchford JM, Schultz JR. Effects of colestipol hydrochloride on drug absorption in the rat. *J Pharm Sci* 1976; **65**: 1285–1291.

Poondru S, Devaraj R, Boinpally, RR, *et al.* Time-dependent influence of pentoxifylline on the pharmacokinetics of orally administered carbamazepine in human subjects. *Pharmacol Res* 2001; **43**: 301–305.

Prichard PJ, Walt RP, Kitchingman GK, *et al.* Oral phenytoin pharmacokinetics during omeprazole therapy. *Br J Clin Pharmacol* 1987; **24**: 543–545.

Rey E, Pons G, Olive G. Vigabatrin: clinical pharmacokinetics. *Clin Pharmacokinet* 1992; **23**: 267–278.

Richens A. Vigabatrin. In *Antiepileptic Drugs*. R. H. Levy, R. H. Mattson, B. Meldrum, J. K. Penry, F. E. Dreifuss, eds. New York: Raven Press, 1989: 937–946.

Riegelman S, Rowland M, Epstein WL. Griseofulvin–phenobarbital interactions in man. *J Amer Med Assoc* 1970; **213**: 426–341.

Rowland M, Gupta SK. Cyclosporin–phenytoin interaction: re-evaluation using metabolite data. *Br J Clin Pharmacol* 1987; **24**: 329–334.

Rust RS, Dodson WE. Phenobarbital: absorption, distribution, and excretion. In *Antiepileptic Drugs*. R. H. Levy, R. H. Mattson, B. Meldrum, J. K. Penry, F. E. Dreifuss, eds. New York: Raven Press, 1989: 293–304.

Sekikawa H, Nakano M, Takada M. Influence of dietary components on the bioavailability of phenytoin. *Chem Pharm Bull* 1980; **22**: 2443–2449.

Shumaker RC, Fantel C, Kelton E, *et al.* Evaluation of the elimination of [^{14}C] felbamate in healthy men. *Epilepsia* 1990; **31**: 642.

Smith OB, Longe RL, Altman RE, *et al.* Recovery of phenytoin from solutions of caseinate salts and calcium chloride. *Am J Hosp Pharm* 1988; **45**: 365–368.

Somogyi A, Thielscher S, Gugler R. Influence of phenobarbital treatment on cimetidine kinetics. *Eur J Clin Pharmacol* 1981; **19**: 343–347.

Somogyi A, Gugler R. Drug interaction with cimetidine. *Clin Pharmacokinet* 1982; **7**: 23–41.

Spina E, Pisani F, Perucca E. Clinically significant pharmacokinetic drug interactions with carbamazepine. An update. *Clin Pharmacokinet* 1996; **31**: 198–214.

Stella VJ, Martodihardjo S, Rao VM. Aqueous solubility and dissolution rate does not adequately predict in vivo performance: a probe utilizing some *N*-acyloxymethyl phenytoin prodrugs. *J Pharm Sci* 1999; **88**: 775–779.

Syed GB, Sharma DB, Raina RK. Pharmacokinetics of phenobarbitone in protein energy malnutrition. *Dev Pharmacol Ther* 1986; **9**: 317–322.

Sylvester RK, Lewis FB, Caldwell KC, *et al.* Impaired phenytoin bioavailability secondary to cisplatinum, vinblastine, and bleomycin. *Ther Drug Monit* 1984; **6**: 302–305.

Torii M, Takiguchi Y, Saito F. Inhibition by carbapenem antibiotic imipenem of intestinal absorption of valproic acid in rats. *J Pharm Pharmacol* 2001; **53**: 823–829.

Torii M, Takiguchi Y, Izumi M. Carbapenem antibiotics inhibit valproic acid transport in Caco-2 cell monolayers. *Int J Pharm* 2002; **233**: 253–256.

Tozer TN, Winter ME. Phenytoin. In *Applied Pharmacokinetics – Principles of Therapeutic Drug Monitoring*. W. E. Evans, J. J. Schentag, W. J. Jusko, eds. San Francisco: Applied Therapeutics, 1990: 275–314.

Turnheim K. Drug interactions with antiepileptic agents. *Wien Klin Wochenshr* 2004; **116**: 112–118.

Tuttle CB. Intramuscular injections and bioavailability. *Am J Hosp Pharm* 1977; **34**(9): 965–968.

Wang JT, Shiu GK, Ong-Chen T, *et al.* Effects of humidity and temperature on in vitro dissolution of carbamazepine tablets. *J Pharm Sci* 1993; **82**: 1002–1005.

Welling PG. Interactions affecting drug absorption. *Clin Pharmacokinet* 1984; **9**: 404–434.

Williamson HE. Interaction of furosemide and phenytoin in the rat. *Proc Soc Exp Biol Med* 1986; **182**: 322–324.

Yoshiyama Y, Nakano S, Ogawa N. Chronopharmacokinetic study of valproic acid in man: comparison of oral and rectal administration. *J Clin Pharmacol* 1989; **29**: 1048–1052.

Yuen WC. Lamotrigine. In *New Antiepileptic Drugs* (Epilepsy Research Suppl. 3). F. Pisani, E. Perucca, G. Avanzini, eds. Amsterdam: Elsevier, 1991: 115–123.

7

Interactions between antiepileptic drugs

Bernhard Rambeck and Theodor W. May

Biochemisches Labor der Gesellschaft für Epilepsieforschung, Maraweg 13, Bielefeld, Germany

Summary

Old and new antiepileptic drugs (AEDs) are associated with a wide range of pharmacokinetic drug–drug interactions. The classic AEDs exert important inducing and inhibiting effects on old and new AEDs.

Phenobarbital (PB) concentrations are significantly increased by valproic acid (VPA) and to a variable degree also by phenytoin (PHT). PHT levels may be decreased or increased by PB, depending on the PB concentration. The protein binding of PHT is decreased by VPA. Enzyme-inducing AEDs decrease primidone concentrations, but increase the levels of its metabolite PB. Carbamazepine (CBZ) concentrations are decreased by PB and PHT, whereas its metabolite CBZ-10,11-epoxide (CBZ-E) may be increased by VPA. Concentrations of VPA are considerably decreased by enzyme-inducing AEDs such as PB, PHT or CBZ. Sulthiame, a rarely used AED, increases PHT levels. Methsuximide (MSM), another rarely used AED, inhibits the metabolism of PB and PHT, but induces the metabolism of lamotrigine (LTG) and oxcarbazepine (OXC).

New AEDs exert relatively few inhibiting or inducing effects on the classic AEDs and hardly any on the new AEDs. However, felbamate (FBM) increases concentrations of PHT, PB, VPA and of CBZ-E, but reduces concentrations of CBZ. OXC (and some other new AEDs) may also increase PHT, whereas vigabatrin reduces the serum levels of PHT by approximately 20%. OXC has less pronounced enzyme-inducing effects than CBZ; however, topiramate (TPM) and LTG may be lowered by OXC.

On the other hand, enzyme-inducing AEDs reduce serum concentrations of FBM, LTG, tiagabine (TGB), TPM, zonisamide (ZWS) and to a minor extent of 10-hydroxy-carbazepine, the clinically relevant metabolite of OXC. VPA markedly increases LTG and FBM. In comparison to other AEDs the potential for clinically relevant interactions associated with gabapentin and levetiracetam is low.

Introduction

Antiepileptic therapy has been associated with a wide range of drug–drug interactions. Classical pharmacokinetic interactions are enzyme induction, enzyme inhibition and displacement from protein binding. From the pharmacological point of view monotherapy with AEDs is often considered as the treatment regime of choice for epileptic patients in order to avoid undesirable consequences of drug interactions such as side effects by increased AED concentrations or inefficacy of the therapy due to decreased serum levels. But for clinical reasons, in practice, many patients have to be treated with AED combinations. Furthermore, newly introduced AEDs are licensed usually as comedication.

Correspondingly, the knowledge of pharmacokinetic interactions is most important. Countless papers have been published about interactions of AEDs. However, many of these interactions are hardly clinically relevant in so far as they concern only weak influences or they have no practical consequences. This overview will deal especially with the clinically important interactions of AEDs. Of course, the extent and the significance of an interaction can vary individually, as it often depends not only on the relative dosages of the interacting drugs, but also on previous drug exposure and on pharmacogenetic factors.

Benzodiazepines are not regarded in this review. The effects of these drugs are minimal as they usually occur only in relatively low concentrations in the serum compared to AED concentrations. Possibly enzyme-inducing drugs may reduce their serum concentrations, but there are hardly any investigations on this topic.

Interactions between classic AEDs (phenobarbital, phenytoin, primidone, carbamazepine, valproic acid, ethosuximide, methsuximide) and other AEDs

Phenobarbital

Phenobarbital (PB) is about one-third metabolized to a p-hydroxylated derivative. It is partially (50–60%) bound to serum proteins.

Effect of phenobarbital on other drugs

PB is the prototype among inducers of the hepatic mixed-function oxidase system. Numerous studies have been performed showing that PB decreases concentrations of other concomitantly given AEDs. Particularly impressive is the effect of PB on CBZ and VPA. A typical investigation, which documents the influence of PB on CBZ metabolism, is a detailed study with data of 609 epileptic patients (Rambeck *et al.*, 1987). PB decreases CBZ levels by about 34% when compared to levels of patients on CBZ alone. The inducing effect was thereby comparable with that of PHT and primidone (PRM).

PB shows not only inducing effects, but also inhibiting effects on some enzyme systems. In some cases, such as for the influence of PB on PHT, results are controversial as two apparently contradictory mechanisms, competitive metabolic inhibition and enzyme induction may play a role (Inoue and Chambers, 1985). There are studies which show that PB tends to lower PHT levels when the two drugs are used simultaneously (Abarbanel *et al.*, 1978) and others which demonstrate a significant increase of PHT in the presence of PB, but returning to prevalues some weeks later (Müller *et al.*, 1977). Another study with stable isotope tracer techniques concluded that PB does not alter PHT steady-state concentration or kinetics (Browne *et al.*, 1988a). A statistical investigation of a large collective with 1992 epileptic patients indicated that low levels of PB induce PHT metabolism and thereby decrease PHT concentrations, but higher PB levels inhibit PHT metabolism in a competitive manner and thereby increase PHT concentrations (May *et al.*, 1982).

PB increases the clearance of VPA. For example, in a representative study with 259 epileptic patients, VPA levels were about 24% lower when VPA was given concomitantly with PB than when it was given alone (May and Rambeck, 1985). The inducing effect in this case was smaller than that of CBZ and PHT, where reductions of 34% and 50% respectively were found.

PB shows its inducing effect also in the presence of some new AEDs. PB reduces LTG levels considerably. A typical study with data of 302 epileptic patients documented that LTG levels are decreased by PB by 48% (May *et al.*, 1996a). The inducing effect was somewhat stronger than that of CBZ (43%) but smaller than that of PHT (68%). TGB levels are reduced by PB (see section on TGB), and TPM metabolism is increased (see section on TPM); furthermore, PB induces the metabolism of ZNS (see section on ZNS). There is also a study (Tartara *et al.*, 1993) which indicates that the biotransformation of OXC and its metabolite 10-hydroxy-carbazepine (or monohydroxy-derivative, MHD) may be accelerated by concomitant treatment with PB, but the magnitude of this effect is unlikely to be of great clinical significance. PB does not seem to influence FBM levels (Kelley *et al.*, 1997) or gabapentin (GBP) levels (Hooper *et al.*, 1991).

Effect of other drugs on phenobarbital

The metabolism of PB itself is inhibited by some other AEDs when given in combination. VPA increases PB concentrations and often thereby causes side effects such as sedation and drowsiness. In a study with 186 epileptic patients, PB levels were about 40% higher when VPA was given additionally. This effect was independent whether PB was directly given or occurred as a metabolite of PRM (Rambeck *et al.*, 1979). Wilder *et al.* (1978) documented a comparable influence for 25 epileptic adults. Various studies showed a reduced hydroxylation of PB (Bruni *et al.*, 1980) and a prolongation of the half-life of PB by VPA by about 50% (Patel *et al.*, 1980; Kapetanovic *et al.*, 1981).

As PHT and PB are metabolized by the same phenyl hydroxylating enzyme system, PHT may inhibit PB metabolism in a competitive manner. PB concentrations are then increased (Windorfer and Sauer, 1977). Correspondingly, Duncan *et al.* (1991) found a decrease in PB concentrations when the concomitant PHT medication was stopped. A study with 121 patients (Eadie *et al.*, 1976) failed to find any significant elevations of plasma levels attributable to PHT. But there is also a study (Encinas *et al.*, 1992) which concludes that PHT may interact with PB as an inducer or an inhibitor of metabolism depending on the length of treatment with the combination of the two drugs.

An important interaction is the competitive inhibition of PB metabolism by methsuximide or its clinically relevant metabolite *N*-desmethyl-MSM, whereby PB concentrations are increased by about 40% (Rambeck, 1979).

FBM increases PB levels by a reduction of its p-hydroxylation (Reidenberg *et al.*, 1995a; Glue *et al.*, 1997). Furthermore, OCBZ may increase PB but to a minor extent (Barcs *et al.*, 2000). The other new AEDs do not show clinically relevant influences on PB; these facts are discussed in the respective sections.

Phenytoin

PHT is nearly completely metabolized to p-hydroxy-PHT and glucuronidated derivatives. It is bound to serum proteins to about 92%. Due to its saturable non-linear Michaelis–Menten kinetics, even moderate influences of other drugs on its metabolism may lead to considerable increases of PHT serum concentration.

Effect of phenytoin on other drugs

PHT has enzyme-inducing properties and decreases drug concentrations of concomitant AEDs.

CBZ metabolism is increased by PHT to a considerable extent. The above-mentioned study with 609 epileptic patients indicated a reduction of CBZ levels by 40% (Rambeck *et al.*, 1987). As already mentioned the interaction between PHT and PB is controversial as different effects may play a role. Some studies found an increase of PB concentrations by about 30% (Windorfer and Sauer, 1977; Duncan *et al.*, 1991), others found no influence of PHT on PB levels (Eadie *et al.*, 1976). PHT induces the metabolism of PRM to its important metabolite PB. The ratio between PRM and its metabolite PB which is usually about 1:1 in monotherapy is then changed to about 1:4 (Fincham *et al.*, 1973).

Addition of PHT to a VPA therapy leads to a considerable decrease in VPA levels. An analysis of data from 259 epileptic patients on polytherapy with AEDs indicated that PHT was a strong inducer (reduction 50%) of VPA levels (May and Rambeck, 1985).

LTG levels are also reduced by PHT. This was shown in the already mentioned study with 302 epileptic patients on LTG where LTG levels were reduced by 68%

when patients were on PHT comedication (May *et al.*, 1996a). PHT exerts its inducing effect also on some other new AEDs such as TGB (see section on TGB), TPM (see section on TPM) and ZNS (see section on ZNS).

The influence of PHT on FBM is not quite clear. In a study by Kelley *et al.* (1997) PHT increased the clearance of FBM by about 40%, whereas Troupin *et al.* (1997) found no appreciable changes in FBM clearance for comedication with PHT.

Effect of other drugs on phenytoin

The metabolism of PHT itself may be increased or decreased by comedicated drugs; in some cases even by the same substance, depending on the serum concentration of the interacting drug. These effects have been discussed exemplarily for the influence of PB on PHT in the section 'Effect of PB on other drugs'.

An investigation by Browne *et al.* (1988b) of six otherwise healthy men found that CBZ increases PHT serum concentrations. Concomitant therapy with MSM often leads to a remarkable increase in PHT concentrations (mean 78%) and thereby disturbing side effects may occur (Rambeck, 1979). Sulthiame also inhibits PHT metabolism and increases PHT levels (Hansen *et al.*, 1968). Although today sulthiame is only rarely used, this interaction is noteworthy as it may induce severe side effects. Furthermore, this was one of the first important drug interactions observed in the treatment of epilepsy.

The interaction of PHT with VPA is somewhat complex as it primarily concerns protein binding. VPA displaces PHT from serum proteins and increases the free fraction of this drug from normally 8% in the absence of VPA to 20%, depending on the VPA concentration (May *et al.*, 1991). But, as the total concentration of PHT decreases, the actually important free concentration of PHT often remains unchanged. Lai and Huang (1993) concluded that there are at least two mechanisms involved in this interaction. Whereas VPA displacing PHT from plasma protein decreased the total drug concentration of PHT, the enzyme inhibition by VPA increased both the total and unbound concentration of PHT. A detailed analysis of data from 237 patients on PHT with and without VPA comedication indicated a significant decrease in total PHT concentration by VPA (Rambeck *et al.*, 1979). The interaction between PHT and VPA may even be time dependent as the plasma concentration of VPA fluctuates during the day, resulting in variable displacement of PHT from its protein binding (Riva *et al.*, 1985; May and Rambeck, 1990).

The new AEDs show no or only small effects on PHT metabolism. LTG does not influence the disposition of PHT (Grasela *et al.*, 1999) and no significant effect by ZNS on the serum concentration or protein binding of PHT was found (Tasaki *et al.*, 1995). As expected, the addition of levetiracetam (LEV) did not bring about clinically relevant changes in PHT pharmacokinetic parameters (Browne *et al.*, 2000).

Total PHT plasma concentrations increased with coadministered FBM (Fuerst *et al.*, 1988), accordingly the PHT dosage should be reduced by about 20% (Sachdeo *et al.*, 1999). OXC also seems to inhibit the metabolism of PHT (Barcs *et al.*, 2000). Some studies showed that vigabatrin (VGB) decreases serum PHT concentrations, but the mechanism is unknown (Gatti *et al.*, 1993).

Primidone

PRM is metabolized to PB and phenyl-ethyl-malonamide (PEMA). The ratio of PRM to PB and PEMA depends not only on auto-induction but also on induction by other AED.

Effect of primidone on other drugs

As PRM is metabolized to a great extent to PB, it shows the same influences on other drugs as PB itself. This means that it decreases levels of VPA, CBZ, LTG and many other drugs.

Effect of other drugs on primidone

When discussing influences of other AEDs on PRM metabolism two effects have to be considered. Primarily, the degradation of PRM to PB is induced by drugs such as PHT or CBZ and furthermore other comedicated AEDs may increase the resulting metabolite PB (Porro *et al.*, 1982).

In the first days of a PRM monotherapy, only PRM is found in the serum. Then the auto-induction of its own metabolism leads to increasing PB concentrations. After some weeks, in steady-state conditions, PB/PRM ratios of about 1:1 are reached. In the presence of other inducing AEDs such as PHT or CBZ the PB/PRM ratio is further increased to 5:1. This has been documented in various studies (Fincham *et al.*, 1973; Schmidt, 1975).

But, it must also be considered that the same drugs that increase PB levels also increase levels of PB occurring as a metabolite of PRM. This has been shown for PHT (Lambie and Johnson, 1981), MSM (Rambeck, 1979) and VPA (Rambeck *et al.*, 1979). A further increase of the PB/PRM ratio to 10:1 may be the consequence. In such cases, it is questionable how far or whether the anticonvulsant effect of a PRM therapy is still exerted by PRM itself or more or less by PB.

Carbamazepine

CBZ is largely metabolized to CBZ-E and then to CBZ-10, 11-diol. CBZ-E seems to contribute to the side effects of a CBZ therapy whilst the diol is physiologically inactive. CBZ and CBZ-E are bound by about 40% to serum proteins.

Effect of carbamazepine on other drugs

CBZ has enzyme-inducing properties and correspondingly decreases concentrations of other concomitantly given AEDs.

The influence of CBZ on PHT is not quite clear. Lai *et al.* (1992) showed in a study with volunteers that CBZ may decrease PHT levels possibly by decreased bioavailability of PHT when CBZ was co-administered. As mentioned above CBZ may induce the metabolism of PRM.

VPA is considerably reduced by CBZ. In a study with 259 patients on VPA, CBZ reduced VPA levels by about 34%. Its inducing effect was larger than that of PB but smaller than that of PHT (May and Rambeck, 1985). Comparable results were found in a study of Reunanen *et al.* (1980) with epileptic patients and in a study of Bowdle *et al.* (1979) with healthy volunteers.

CBZ reduces LTG levels (Bartoli *et al.*, 1997; Battino *et al.*, 1997). In a study of 302 patients on LTG, patients on CBZ comedication had LTG levels that were about 50% lower than that of patients on LTG monotherapy. The inducing effect was comparable with that of PB but less than that of PHT (May *et al.*, 1996a). Furthermore, CBZ reduces FBM levels (Kelley *et al.*, 1997; Troupin *et al.*, 1997), TGB levels (Brodie, 1995; So *et al.*, 1995; Snel *et al.*, 1997), TPM levels (Sachdeo *et al.*, 1996) and ZNS concentrations (Ojemann *et al.*, 1986). GBP concentrations are not influenced (Radulovic *et al.*, 1994).

Effect of other drugs on carbamazepine

Besides the impressive inducing effect of CBZ it has to be borne in mind that CBZ itself is subject to enzyme induction. Various studies have documented that simultaneously given AEDs reduce CBZ concentrations.

An investigation by Michele *et al.* (1985) with 58 patients showed that PB reduces CBZ levels to a considerable extent. Christiansen and Dam (1973) showed in 123 epileptic patients that PB and PHT reduce CBZ concentrations. In a study with 609 epileptic patients on CBZ therapy (Rambeck *et al.*, 1987), the mean serum concentration of CBZ was reduced when given in combination with PHT by 42%, with PB by 34% and with VPA by 17%.

Besides the inducing effect on CBZ metabolism some drugs inhibit the degradation of CBZ-E. In the above-mentioned study (Rambeck *et al.*, 1987) the mean concentration of CBZ-E was increased by VPA (+45%), PRM (+19%) and a combination of the latter (+67%) compared to CBZ monotherapy. These effects are reflected by the ratios between CBZ and its CBZ-E. In CBZ monotherapy a ratio of about 7:1 is found in adults (Rambeck *et al.*, 1987). In the presence of inducing AEDs the ratio is lowered to 3:1, and in the presence of inducing AEDs in combination with VPA it is 2:1. VPA appears to inhibit the conversion of CBZ-E to the trans-diol derivative and furthermore the glucuronidation of this CBZ-10,11-diol

(Bernus *et al.*, 1997). In the special case of adding CBZ to a basic VPA therapy, the inhibiting effect of VPA on the metabolism of CBZ-E is particularly impressive, especially in children. CBZ-E concentrations of up to 13 µg/ml have been observed, accompanied by side effects such as vomiting and tiredness, although the CBZ levels were in the usually accepted effective range (Rambeck *et al.*, 1990). After a few days the CBZ-E concentration decreases, but CBZ/CBZ-E ratios of 3:1 remain.

FBM appears to induce CBZ metabolism and decrease CBZ levels (Liu and Delgado, 1997), whereby CBZ-E levels are increased (Wagner *et al.*, 1993). In a study by Jedrzejczak *et al.* (2000), VGB increased CBZ concentrations. There was no significant change in the serum concentrations of CBZ when LTG was added to a CBZ therapy (Eriksson and Boreus, 1997; Gidal *et al.*, 1997b; Besag *et al.*, 1998). Data regarding the influence of LTG on CBZ-E are conflicting. TPM (Sachdeo *et al.*, 1996) and GBP (Radulovic *et al.*, 1994) also do not influence CBZ levels.

Valproate

VPA is metabolized to a series of saturated and unsaturated carbonic acids and glucuronidated derivatives. It is largely bound to serum proteins.

Effect of valproate on other drugs

As already discussed, VPA shows an inhibiting effect on the CBZ metabolite CBZ-E. When VPA is given in combination with CBZ, CBZ-E is increased (Sälke-Treumann *et al.*, 1988; Rambeck *et al.*, 1990; Bernus *et al.*, 1997).

VPA increases PB levels by about 40% (Rambeck *et al.*, 1979). Regarding PHT, there seem to be two mechanisms involved in the interaction of VPA with PHT. Whereas VPA displacing PHT from the plasma protein decreased the total drug concentration of PHT, the enzyme inhibition by VPA increased both the total and unbound concentration of PHT (Lai and Huang, 1993).

VPA increases levels of LTG in an impressive manner (Yuen *et al.*, 1992; Anderson *et al.*, 1996; May *et al.*, 1996a; Battino *et al.*, 1997; Kanner and Frey, 2000). In our study with 302 epileptic patients the LTG levels of patients on a combination of LTG with VPA were increased by a factor of 3.6 in comparison to patients on LTG monotherapy (May *et al.*, 1996a). This could benefit the patient with epilepsy not only by attaining higher plasma LTG concentrations with 'standard' dosages of LTG, but also possibly by achieving better seizure control through providing a less variable peak-to-trough fluctuation in LTG concentrations as a result of extending the half-life of LTG (Morris *et al.*, 2000).

VPA decreased the clearance of FBM by about 21% (Kelley *et al.*, 1997). Although VPA seems to decrease the protein binding of TGB, the relevance of this effect is unclear. VPA does not influence the metabolism of other new AEDs.

Effect of other drugs on valproate

Inducing AEDs such as PB (May and Rambeck, 1985), PHT (May and Rambeck, 1985) or CBZ (May and Rambeck, 1985; Yukawa *et al.*, 1997) decrease VPA levels considerably. In accordance with our own observations (Mataringa *et al.*, 2002) Besag *et al.* (2001) reported that MSM also significantly decreases VPA levels. Besides the inducing effects of other AEDs on VPA, it has to be considered that the kinetics of VPA is non-linear, resulting in a lower than proportional increase of the serum concentration when increasing the dose. These two facts are the reason why in polytherapy even with high dosages of up to 6 g VPA per day, morning concentrations higher than 100 µg/ml are rarely exceeded.

Ethosuximide (ESM) seems to reduce VPA levels by an unknown mechanism (Sälke-Kellermann *et al.*, 1997).

VPA levels rose by 12.7% when FBM was added (Wagner *et al.*, 1994; Hooper *et al.*, 1996; Siegel *et al.*, 1999). In a study with human volunteers, the addition of LTG was associated with a small but significant decrease in steady-state VPA plasma concentration (Anderson *et al.*, 1996). Mataringa *et al.* (2002) observed also a slight decreasing effect of LTG on VPA (-7%) in a retrospective study. However, in clinical studies such an effect was not documented (Jawad *et al.*, 1987; Eriksson *et al.*, 1996). The effect of TPM on VPA kinetics seems to be negligible (Rosenfeld *et al.*, 1997). GBP (Radulovic *et al.*, 1994) or VGB (Armijo *et al.*, 1992) do not influence the kinetics of VPA.

Ethosuximide

ESM is a simple aliphatic compound which is metabolized to hydroxylated compounds. It is not bound to proteins. Besides a weak decreasing effect on VPA, ESM does not influence other drugs.

The metabolism of ESM itself may be induced to some degree by PB and PHT, but this is hardly of clinical relevance (Sälke-Kellermann *et al.*, 1997).

Methsuximide

MSM is rapidly metabolized to the therapeutically active derivative *N*-desmethyl-MSM and then to hydroxylated and glucuronidated derivatives.

Effect of methsuximide on other drugs

MSM inhibits the metabolism of PHT and PB. In a study with 94 epileptic patients MSM increased concentrations of PB by 38%, of PB as metabolite of PRM by 40% and of PHT by 78%, in many cases with ensuing side effects (Rambeck, 1979).

But MSM also has enzyme-inducing effects and lowers LTG (May *et al.*, 1999; Besag *et al.*, 2000), VPA (Besag *et al.*, 2001) and TPM levels (May *et al.*, 2002).

Effect of other drugs on methsuximide

PB and PHT can increase concentrations of *N*-desmethyl-MSM, the metabolite of MSM, in a competitive manner as these substances are metabolized by the same hydroxylating liver enzymes (Rambeck, 1979).

Interactions between new AEDs and other AEDs

In the last decade, a series of new AEDs have become available for the treatment of epileptic patients. One of the basic reasons to develop new AEDs was the aim of finding agents which are not or only to a small degree interactive with other drugs; but this aim has only partially been reached.

Felbamate

FBM is partly bound to plasma proteins (24–35%) and eliminated by renal excretion, hydroxylation and conjugation.

Effect of felbamate on other drugs

Early studies (Wilensky *et al.*, 1985; Fuerst *et al.*, 1988) with only a few patients showed that adding FBM resulted in an increase in PHT concentrations and a small decrease in CBZ concentrations. These effects were also found in a clinical trial with FBM by Graves *et al.* (1989) where 32 patients received concomitant PHT and CBZ treatment. All patients required a PHT dose reduction of 10–30% during FBM treatment to maintain stable PHT concentrations. CBZ serum concentrations decreased (mean 1.3 μg/ml) in nearly all patients. Theodore *et al.* (1991) also found a significant reduction (24%) of CBZ concentrations in a clinical study with FBM. Albani *et al.* (1991) reported on a controlled trial where FBM was added to a stable CBZ monotherapy of 22 patients. CBZ total concentrations were lower during FBM treatment (mean reduction 25%). Wagner *et al.* (1993) evaluated the effect of FBM on CBZ and its major metabolites during a trial in 26 patients. Mean CBZ concentrations decreased from 7.5 μg/ml during placebo treatment to 6.1 μg/ml during FBM treatment. Mean CBZ-E concentrations increased from 1.8 to 2.4 μg/ml. The effects of FBM on the kinetics of PB and its hydroxylated metabolite were assessed in a study with 24 healthy volunteers by Reidenberg *et al.* (1995a). FBM increased the area under the curve (AUC) of PB by 22% and the maximum concentration (C_{max}) by 24%.

Wagner *et al.* (1994) showed that VPA doses may require reduction when FBM is added to a regimen of VPA. Co-administration of FBM increased the mean AUC, C_{max} and average steady-state concentrations (from 67 to 103 μg/ml) of VPA in 10 epileptic patients who received FBM in addition to a stable VPA dosage. This effect has also been documented by Hooper *et al.* (1996) in a study of 18 healthy volunteers.

FBM has only a small increasing effect (Colucci *et al.*, 1996) or no effect on LTG (Gidal *et al.*, 1997a). Reidenberg *et al.* (1995b) found no clinically relevant interactions between FBM and VGB in a study of 18 healthy volunteers. The influence of FBM on the multiple dose kinetics of monohydroxy and dihydroxy metabolites of OCBZ was assessed in healthy volunteers (Hulsman *et al.*, 1995). FBM had no effect on MHD kinetics.

Effect of other drugs on felbamate

PHT and CBZ induce the metabolism of FBM resulting in lower than expected steady-state concentrations. Wagner *et al.* (1991) performed a controlled discontinuation study of PHT and CBZ in five patients with FBM. As PHT dosages were reduced, FBM clearance decreased by 21% and as the CBZ dosages were reduced, FBM clearance decreased by an additional 16.5%.

In a study by Kelley *et al.* (1997), PB had no influence on FBM, and VPA reduced the clearance of FBM by about 21%.

Reidenberg *et al.* (1995b) did not find any clinically relevant influence of VGB on FBM. Furthermore, LTG has no influence on FBM (Troupin *et al.*, 1997). However, a study indicated that the half-life of FBM is increased by GBP via an unknown mechanism (Hussein *et al.*, 1996).

Gabapentin

GBP shows dose-dependent absorption kinetics. It is not bound to plasma proteins and it is eliminated unchanged in the urine.

Effect of gabapentin on other drugs

The US Gabapentin Study Group (1994) found no influence of GBP on CBZ, PHT and VPA concentrations in a study with GBP as add-on therapy.

When administered over a period of 3 days, GBP had no statistically significant effect on PB concentrations in 12 healthy volunteers (Hooper *et al.*, 1991). Clinical studies have also documented a lack of interaction between GBP and PB (Crawford *et al.*, 1987; Goa and Sorkin, 1993). Radulovic *et al.* (1994) investigated the effect of GBP co-administration for more than 3 days on steady-state CBZ concentrations (12 epileptic patients) and for more than 5 days on VPA concentrations (14 epileptic patients). Mean CBZ and CBZ-E and mean VPA concentrations before, during and after GBP administration were not significantly different.

Crawford *et al.* (1987) performed a dose-ranging study with 300, 600 and 900 mg/day GBP as add-on therapy. No significant drug interactions were seen, although there was a trend towards elevation of serum PHT concentration in patients taking 900 mg/day of GBP.

There is also a case report about a considerable PHT increase after the addition of low doses of GBP (300 and 600 mg/day) to PHT with CBZ and clobazam as comedication (Tyndel, 1994). The authors conclude that the unusual step of adding GBP to three AEDs may have allowed this unusual interaction. But, it seems rather problematic to draw such a conclusion from a single clinical observation with few serum level determinations since, for example, irregular drug intake prior to addition of GBP may also result in an increase of serum concentrations.

As mentioned above, GBP might elevate FBM levels.

Effect of other drugs on gabapentin

The above-mentioned investigation by Hooper *et al.* (1991) found no statistically significant influences of PB on GBP kinetics. There are no special studies about PHT, but according to our own experience PHT does not significantly influence GBP concentrations. In the study by Radulovic *et al.* (1994), GBP pharmacokinetic parameters during CBZ or VPA co-administration were similar to data reported in healthy subjects. The authors conclude that no pharmacokinetic interaction exists between CBZ or VPA and GBP.

Lamotrigine

LTG is about 55% bound to to plasma proteins and is extensively metabolized by glucuronidation.

Effect of lamotrigine on other drugs

Concentrations of concomitant VPA, PHT or CBZ were unaltered by 1 week of LTG administration in 22 patients examined by Jawad *et al.* (1987). Loiseau *et al.* (1990) reported on a controlled add-on trial of LTG in 23 patients. Concentrations of PHT, CBZ and PB remained unchanged. Sander *et al.* (1990) also performed a controlled add-on trial of LTG in 21 epileptic patients. Serum concentrations of CBZ, PHT, VPA and PB were unaffected by LTG treatment. Jawad *et al.* (1989) assessed the antiepileptic effects of LTG in a crossover trial in 24 adult patients. No statistically significant changes in concentrations of PHT, CBZ, PRM or PB were found between the two treatment periods. Schapel *et al.* (1993) performed a controlled trial of LTG as add-on therapy in 41 patients. Concomitant AEDs (CBZ, PHT and VPA) concentrations were virtually unchanged. Moreover, no clinically important changes in plasma concentrations of CBZ, VPA, ESM and PB were observed in epileptic children during LTG therapy (Eriksson *et al.*, 1996).

In contrast, an interaction between LTG and CBZ metabolism resulting in an increase of CBZ-E of 45% was reported by Warner *et al.* (1992). These observations are at variance with those of Wolf (1992). He added LTG to a subtoxic, just tolerated dose of CBZ in nine patients. Cerebellar toxicity developed in eight of them. In the total group, a small (about 10%) but significant increase of CBZ-E was found, whereas no consistent change could be detected in CBZ. The increase in the CBZ-E, however, was too small and too inconsistent to explain the toxicity in all cases. These results indicate that the interaction of CBZ and LTG may be primarily pharmacodynamic rather than pharmacokinetic. Pisani *et al.* (1994) found no effect of LTG on CBZ-E. They compared the pharmacokinetics of a single dose of 100 mg CBZ-E in 10 patients on chronic LTG monotherapy and in 10 drug-free healthy control subjects. CBZ-E kinetic parameters were similar in subjects on LTG and in controls.

Effect of other drugs on lamotrigine

Binnie *et al.* (1986) reported on short-term effects of a single dose of LTG in 16 persons with epilepsy. Comedication with CBZ and/or PHT reduced the elimination half-life to a mean of 15 h and comedication with VPA prolonged the half-life to a mean of 59 h. In a study by Jawad *et al.* (1987), patients receiving LTG together with enzyme-inducing AEDs showed as LTG plasma elimination half-life of 14 ± 7 h (mean $\pm$ SD). Those receiving LTG plus an inducing AED plus VPA exhibited a mean LTG half-life of 30 ± 10 h.

Yuen *et al.* (1992) studied six healthy volunteers who received LTG as a single dose alone or together with VPA. Concomitant administration of VPA reduced LTG total clearance by approximately 21% and increased the elimination half-life and AUC. Renal elimination of LTG was not impaired.

May *et al.* (1996a) studied the influence of comedication on LTG concentrations in 588 blood samples of 302 epileptic patients. The LTG serum concentration in relation to LTG dose per body weight (level-to-dose ratio, LDR, μg/ml per mg/kg) was calculated and compared for different drug combinations. The results showed that comedication had a highly significant influence on the LTG serum concentrations. The mean LDR for LTG was as follows: 0.32 (LTG + PHT) < 0.52 (LTG + PB) $\cong$ 0.57 (LTG + CBZ) < 0.98 (LTG monotherapy) $\cong$ 0.99 (LTG + VPA + PHT) < 1.67 (LTG + VPA + CBZ) $\cong$ 1.80 (LTG + VPA + PB) < 3.57 (LTG + VPA). The considerable influence of various AED and their combinations on LTG concentrations is shown in Figure 7.1. It is interesting that a comparable study by Battino *et al.* (1997) with 482 LTG determinations form 106 epileptic patients found nearly the same values. The LDR of LTG for patients on VPA was 3.2, for patients on enzyme-inducing drugs 0.6 and on VPA in combination with enzyme-inducing drugs 1.9. These data furthermore were confirmed in a prospective study with epileptic children (Bartoli *et al.*, 1997).

As already mentioned, several studies (May *et al.*, 1999; Besag *et al.*, 2000) found that MSM lowers LTG levels by about 50–70%.

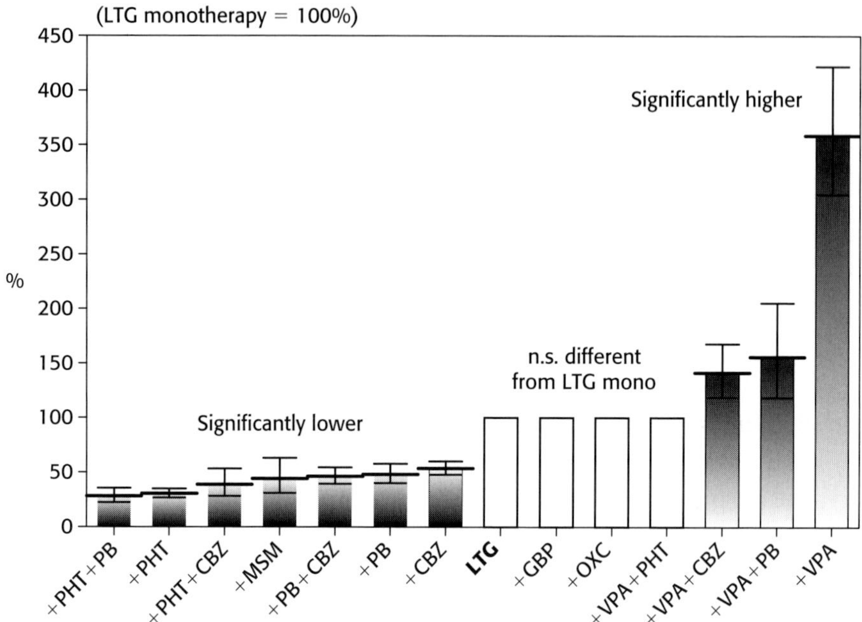

Figure 7.1   Influence of PHT, PB, CBZ, MSM, GBP, OCBZ, VPA and of their combinations on serum concentrations of LTG. LTG monotherapy is taken as 100% (n.s.: not significantly; bars ±95% confidence intervals); data of 302 patients (May *et al.*, 1996a)

The decreasing effect of OXC on LTG levels (29%) is less than that of CBZ but statistically significant (May *et al.*, 1999). FBM and TPM (Berry *et al.*, 1998; Doose *et al.*, 2003) have no important influence on LTG.

Oxcarbazepine

OXC is the 10-keto analogue of CBZ. OXC is a prodrug for MHD, and is rapidly converted to this substance. MHD is approximately 40% bound to serum proteins and is excreted mainly by direct conjugation to glucuronic acid.

Effect of oxcarbazepine on other drugs

McKee *et al.* (1994) investigated the interaction between OXC and other AEDs in three groups of 12 epileptic patients taking CBZ, VPA or PHT as monotherapy. No differences in the median AUC at steady-state of CBZ and its metabolite CBZ-E, as well as VPA and PHT, were observed during additional treatment with OXC at steady-state compared with the AUC calculated for the placebo phase, suggesting an absence of metabolic interference with these AEDs. In contrast, Barcs *et al.* (2000) found in an OXC dose-ranging trial a slight decrease in CBZ levels of 13%, an increase in PB levels of 15% and an increase of PHT levels of 40% in patients with high MHD concentrations, compared to placebo. The in vitro study by Lakehal *et al.* (2002) indicated that MHD inhibited CYP2C19-mediated PHT metabolism at therapeutic concentrations. Thus, administration of OXC with CYP2C19 substrates with narrow therapeutic ranges should be done cautiously.

Battino *et al.* (1992) investigated changes of unbound and total VPA concentrations after replacement of CBZ with OXC in four epileptic patients. In confirmation of the above results, total and free VPA concentrations rose when the medication was switched from CBZ to OXC. Houtkooper *et al.* (1987) also observed a statistically significant increase of concomitant VPA and PHT concentrations in a crossover trial with 48 patients when CBZ was replaced by OXC. The increase in the serum concentrations during OXC therapy can be explained by a decrease in the prior enzyme induction caused by CBZ (Houtkooper *et al.*, 1987).

The inducing properties of OXC on the metabolism of LTG and TPM are less pronounced than that of CBZ but the inducing effect is statistically significant (May *et al.*, 1999, 2002). A mean decrease in LTG levels of about 30% compared to LTG monotherapy was found. A comparable effect was also found on TPM metabolism, patients on OXC comedication had about 30% lower TPM levels than patients on TPM monotherapy (May *et al.*, 2002).

Effect of other drugs on oxcarbazepine

Kumps and Wurth (1990) analyzed the concentrations of MHD and of the inactive metabolite CBZ-diol in 15 epileptic patients, six of them receiving PB and/or PHT as comedication. The results indicate that MHD concentrations are unaffected by the comedication, but oxidation of MHD to its inactive metabolite may be induced. However, this seems to be of little clinical significance. In the above-mentioned study of McKee *et al.* (1994), patients taking CBZ or PHT had lower MHD concentrations compared with control patients without CBZ or PHT, the difference being small and statistically significant only for the CBZ-treated group. VPA had no effect at all in this study. In contrast, the OXC dose-ranging study of Barcs *et al.* (2000) found that patients receiving concomitant treatment with PHT and PB had statistically lower MHD levels than patients not receiving these AEDs.

The absence of an effect of VPA was confirmed by Tartara *et al.* (1993). The kinetics of OXC and MHD after a single oral OXC dose were comparable in healthy control subjects and in epileptic patients treated with VPA. However, in patients on PB the AUC values of both OXC and MHD were lower and the MHD half-life marginally shorter than in controls. But the magnitude of this effect was judged to be only of minor clinical significance. In combination with VPA the free fraction of MHD (64%) was slightly, but significantly, higher than in monotherapy (52%) with OXC (May *et al.*, 1996b).

The study of Hulsman *et al.* (1995) documented the absence of an influence of FBM on MHD and its metabolite. Further observations indicate that LTG and GBP have no influence on MHD (Sallas, 1999; Viola *et al.*, 2000).

Vigabatrin

VGB does not bind to plasma proteins, does not appear to undergo metabolic transformation and is excreted extensively in urine in its unchanged form.

Effect of vigabatrin on other drugs

In an early double-blind study (Grant and Heel, 1991) of VGB in epileptic patients, serum concentrations of PHT were about 20% lower during VGB treatment than during placebo, but concentrations of other concomitant AEDs did not change. In a study with 89 epileptic patients, Browne *et al.* (1989) also found a statistically significant decrease of 20% in PHT concentrations when VGB was added. Furthermore, minor decreases in PB (7%) and PRM (11%) were observed. Dalla Bernardina *et al.* (1995) performed a study in 46 epileptic children. Serum concentrations of associated AEDs (CBZ, PB and VPA) showed no significant changes, except for PHT which decreased from 19.3 ± 8.0 to $11.9 \pm 5.2\,\mu g/ml$ on VGB treatment. The effect of VGB on PHT has been further studied by Rimmer and Richens (1989). When VBG was added to the PHT therapy of eight epileptic patients, mean plasma PHT concentrations fell significantly by 23% during the 5th week. No change was found in plasma protein binding of PHT, the urinary ratio of PHT to its metabolite p-hydroxy-PHT, and the antipyrine clearance before and at the end of the treatment period. It is not clear why the fall in PHT levels may show a delay of a few weeks. This slight, but unequivocal, effect was confirmed in 21 epileptic patients by Gatti *et al.* (1993). By switching from oral to intravenous PHT for 5 days before and after combined treatment with VGB and by measuring p-hydroxy-PHT, it could be demonstrated that the oral availability of PHT is unaffected by VGB. So the mechanism of the VGB-induced decrease in serum PHT is still unclear. A dose–response study of VGB in 20 children aged 2 months to 18 years also showed a modest decrease in PHT plasma levels (Herranz *et al.*, 1991), but no changes in CBZ and VPA levels.

Armijo *et al.* (1992) investigated the effects of adding VGB to the antiepileptic regimens of 16 children. In the eight patients receiving VPA, no significant changes of VPA concentrations were observed.

Furthermore, several controlled trials have shown that VGB has no significant effect on serum concentrations of CBZ and VPA (Gram *et al.*, 1985), CBZ, PB, PHT and VPA (Loiseau *et al.*, 1986) or CBZ and PB (Cocito *et al.*, 1989).

On the other hand, Jedrzejczak *et al.* (2000) found in a study with 66 epileptic patients a small increasing influence (of about 10%) of VGB on CBZ. Some patients responded with adverse, toxic symptoms. Also Sanchez-Alcaraz *et al.* (2002) reported higher CBZ concentrations during comedication with VGB compared to CBZ mono-therapy in 15 patients.

As already mentioned, the study of Reidenberg *et al.* (1995b) found no clinically relevant influence of VGB on FBM in healthy volunteers.

Effect of other drugs on vigabatrin

In the study of Armijo *et al.* (1992) no differences were found in VGB concentrations between patients with and without VPA. In a retrospective study (Armijo *et al.*, 1997), patients with and without enzyme-inducing AEDs (PHT, PB and CBZ) had comparable VGB levels. One study (Sanchez-Alcaraz *et al.*, 1996) reported on a small decreasing influence of CBZ.

An investigation by Reidenberg *et al.* (1995b) concluded that FBM does not influence the inactive $R(-)$-VGB enantiomer, but produced a 13% increase in AUC and an 8% increase in urinary excretion of the active $S(+)$ enantiomer.

Topiramate

TPM is only 15% plasma protein bound and it is mainly excreted unchanged in the urine (80%), but significant metabolism occurs when TPM is administered in conjunction with enzyme-inducing AEDs.

Effect of topiramate on other drugs

TPM has no significant or only little effect on the serum concentrations of CBZ or its metabolite CBZ-E (Sachdeo *et al.*, 1996) or on PB, PRM and LTG, except for an occasional moderate increase in plasma PHT levels (Walker and Patsalos, 1995), and a small mean decrease of VPA levels, but this is hardly clinically relevant (Rosenfeld *et al.*, 1997).

LTG does not influence TPM levels to a clinically relevant extent (Berry *et al.*, 1998; Doose *et al.*, 2003).

Effect of other drugs on topiramate

The elimination half-life of TPM of approximately 20–30 h may be shortened considerably in the presence of concomitant treatment with enzyme inducers such as PB, PHT or CBZ and lead to a decrease in TPM levels (Sachdeo *et al.*, 1996; Glauser *et al.*, 1999; Rosenfeld *et al.*, 1999; May *et al.*, 2002). Furthermore, MSM and to a lesser degree OXC reduces TPM levels (May *et al.*, 2002). VPA (Rosenfeld *et al.*, 1999), LTG and GBP (Contin *et al.*, 2002; May *et al.*, 2002; Doose *et al.*, 2003) have no significant influence on TPM.

Tiagabine

TGB is 96% protein bound. It is metabolized in the liver and only small portions are excreted unchanged.

Effect of tiagabine on other drugs

TGB does not influence serum concentrations of other AEDs, as was shown in studies for CBZ and PHT (Gustavson *et al.*, 1998a), VPA (Gustavson *et al.*, 1998b) and for CBZ, PHT, VPA, VGB (Richens *et al.*, 1995). This lack of interactions is understandable because of its low concentration, in the nanogram range.

Effect of other drugs on tiagabine

Enzyme inducers such as CBZ, PB and PHT reduce the elimination half-life of TGB considerably (So *et al.*, 1995; Snel *et al.*, 1997).

Levetiracetam

LEV is a new AED with a nearly ideal pharmacokinetic profile. It shows a high bioavailability, linear and time-invariant kinetics, minimal protein binding and a low metabolism to an inactive metabolite.

In some clinical trials, the addition of LEV increased PHT levels to variable degrees in a few patients (Sharief *et al.*, 1996; Patsalos, 2000), but this effect could not be confirmed by trials with deuterium-labeled PHT (Browne *et al.*, 2000). Besides this unexplained effect no clinically relevant interactions are known. Perucca *et al.* (2000) found no interactions between other AED and LEV. However, more recent studies indicate that enzyme-inducing AEDs (May *et al.*, 2003; Perucca *et al.*, 2003) and OCBZ (May *et al.*, 2003) slightly decrease LEV concentrations.

Zonisamide

ZNS is rapidly and completely absorbed. It is approximately 50% bound to proteins and has a relatively long half-life of about 63–69 h. It is partly metabolized with non-linear kinetics.

Effect of zonisamide on other drugs

Conflicting results have been found regarding the influence of ZNS on comedicated AEDs. Sackellares *et al.* (1985) showed a consistent rise in concentrations of the comedication, particularly of CBZ, when ZNS was administered to 10 adult patients in a pilot study. In contrast, in a study by Minami *et al.* (1994) the average LDR of CBZ was lower in patients with ZNS than in patients without ZNS. Other studies could not demonstrate a relevant influence of ZNS on concentrations or protein binding of concomitant AEDs such as CBZ, PHT, PB, PRM or VPA (Schmidt *et al.*, 1993) and PHT or VPA (Tasaki *et al.*, 1995).

Table 7.1 Pharmacokinetic interactions of AEDs

Effect of/on …	CBZ	PB	PHT	PRM	ESM	MSM	VPA	VGB	GBP	LEV	TGB	TPM	LTG	OXC[e]	FBM	ZNS
CBZ		=	↓/↑	↓ PB ↑	↓		↓↓	=(↓)	=	=/↓	↓↓	↓↓	↓↓	↓	↓↓	↓↓
PB	↓↓[a]		↓/↑[b]		↓	↑	↓↓	=	=	=/↓	↓↓	↓	↓↓	=/↓	=/↓	↓↓
PHT	↓↓[a]	=/↑		↓ PB ↑	↓	↑	↓↓	=	=	=/↓	↓↓	↓↓	↓↓	=/↓	↓↓	↓↓
PRM	↓↓ CBZ-E ↑						↓↓			=/↓	↓↓	↓	↓↓		↓	
ESM		=		=			↓							=		
MSM		↑↑	↑↑	↓ PB ↑			↓↓			↓		↓↓	↓↓			
VPA	↓ CBZ-E ↑↑	↑↑	↓[c]	(↓) PB ↑	=			=	=	=	=[d]	=	↑↑	=[f]	=/↑	=[g]
VGB	=/↑	=(↓)	↓/↓↓	=(↓)			=								=	
GBP	=	=	=(↑)				=			=		=	=	=	(↑)	
LEV	=	=	=(↑)	=			=		=			=				
TGB	=	=	=				=	=								
TPM	=	=	↑/↑↑	=			=(↓)			=			=			
LTG	=(CBZ-E ↑)	=	=	=			=/↓		=		=			=		
OXC	=/↓	=/↑	↑/↑↑	=(↑)			=			=/↓		↓	↓			
FBM	↓ CE ↓↓	↑↑	↑↑				↑↑	=/↑						=(↑)	=	
ZNS	↑/↓ CE ↑	=	=(↑)				=									

=: no relevant or statistically significant interaction. ↑ and ↓: increase and decrease, respectively, of serum concentrations mostly without clinical relevance. ↑↑ and ↓↓: clinically relevant increase and decrease, respectively, of serum concentrations. Different symbols (e.g. =/↑): indication of inconsistent or contradictory observations. Arrows in parentheses: indication of interactions based on case reports or on a small number of patients. Empty cells: no data available.

[a] CBZ decreases, ratio CBZ-E/CBZ increases.

[b] Dependent on concentration of PB.

[c] VPA decreases PHT total concentration; however, as VPA simultaneously increases the free fraction of PHT, these effects cancel each other to a great extent.

[d] VPA probably increases the free fraction of TGB.

[e] Data regarding the clinically relevant 10-hydroxy-carbazepine (MHD).

[f] VPA slightly increases the free fraction of 10-hydroxy-carbazepine (MHD).

[g] VPA slightly increases the free fraction of ZNS.

For clarity, bromide, sulthiame and benzodiazepines are not listed. Clinically relevant interactions of bromide with other AEDs are unlikely and were not reported. Sulthiame can increase concentrations of PHT markedly; other clinically relevant interactions with sulthiame are unknown. For benzodiazepines, relatively few interactions with other AEDs are reported.

Effect of other drugs on zonisomide

The study of Shinoda *et al.* (1996) indicated that enzyme-inducing AEDs (PB, PHT and CBZ) reduce the ZNS LDR. Ojemann *et al.* (1996) investigated the influence of CBZ and PHT on kinetics of a single dose of ZNS in epileptic patients. Plasma half-life of ZNS was significantly higher in patients on CBZ (36.4 h) than in those on PHT therapy (27.1 h), but both values were shorter than half-life values (50–68 h) usually found after administration of single oral doses on ZNS in healthy volunteers.

VPA has no clinically relevant influence on ZNS levels (Shinoda *et al.*, 1996).

Therapeutic implications

The experience of several decades with the classic AEDs has shown that interactions may have severe clinical consequences. However, in the case of the pharmaco-kinetic interactions of the new AEDs their clinical importance is less clear. This is because the relevance of serum concentrations and of therapeutic drug monitoring for avoidance of side effects or for reduction of seizures has not yet been definitively established for most of the new AEDs. For FBM, LTG, OXC, TPM and GBP, a relation between serum concentrations and antiepileptic effect probably exists, but further studies are necessary to clarify this important topic. This seems also to be true for the correlation between serum concentrations and side effects of FBM, LTG and OXC. In contrast, in the case of VGB the antiepileptic effect and side effects seem to be unrelated to the serum concentration of the drug.

Reports on AED interactions usually focus on the increase or decrease of serum concentrations. But, it should be borne in mind that interactions moreover influence the whole pharmacokinetic properties of an AED. For example, changes of the half-life time also affect daily fluctuations of serum levels and furthermore the time to reach steady-state concentrations or the speed of elimination after withdrawal of a drug.

The pharmacokinetic interactions (summarized in Table 7.1) of the old and new AEDs have been investigated by many studies. Most interactions correspond to the pharmacokinetic properties of the compounds, but it should be borne in mind that rare interactions may also play an important role in the individual.

REFERENCES

Abarbanel J, Herishanu Y, Rosenberg P, *et al.* In vivo interaction of anticonvulsant drugs. The mathematical correlation of plasma levels of anticonvulsant drugs in epileptic patients. *J Neurol* 1978; **218**: 137–144.

Albani F, Theodore WH, Washington P, *et al.* Effect of felbamate on plasma levels of carbamazepine and its metabolites. *Epilepsia* 1991; **32**: 130–132.

Anderson GD, Yau MK, Gidal BE, *et al.* Bidirectional interaction of valproate and lamotrigine in healthy subjects. *Clin Pharmacol Ther* 1996; **60**: 145–156.

Armijo JA, Arteaga R, Valdizan EM, *et al.* Coadministration of vigabatrin and valproate in children with refractory epilepsy. *Clin Neuropharmacol* 1992; **15**: 459–469.

Armijo JA, Cuadrado A, Bravo J, *et al.* Vigabatrin serum concentration to dosage ratio: influence of age and associated antiepileptic drugs. *Ther Drug Monit* 1997; **19**: 491–498.

Barcs G, Walker EB, Elger CE, *et al.* Oxcarbazepine placebo-controlled, dose-ranging trial in refractory partial epilepsy. *Epilepsia* 2000; **41**: 1597–1607.

Bartoli A, Guerrini R, Belmonte A, *et al.* The influence of dosage, age, and comedication on steady state plasma lamotrigine concentrations in epileptic children: a prospective study with preliminary assessment of correlations with clinical response. *Ther Drug Monit* 1997; **19**: 252–260.

Battino D, Croci D, Granata T, *et al.* Changes in unbound and total valproic acid concentrations after replacement of carbamazepine with oxcarbazepine. *Ther Drug Monit* 1992; **14**: 376–379.

Battino D, Croci D, Granata T, *et al.* Lamotrigine plasma concentrations in children and adults: influence of age and associated therapy. *Ther Drug Monit* 1997; **19**: 620–627.

Bernus I, Dickinson RG, Hooper WD, *et al.* The mechanism of the carbamazepine–valproate interaction in humans. *Br J Clin Pharmacol* 1997; **44**: 21–27.

Berry DJ, Besag C, Pool F, *et al.* Does topiramate change lamotrigine serum concentrations when added to treatment? An audit of a dose-escalation study. *Epilepsia* 1998; **39**(Suppl. 6): 56–57.

Besag FM, Berry DJ, Pool F, *et al.* Carbamazepine toxicity with lamotrigine: pharmacokinetic or pharmacodynamic interaction? *Epilepsia* 1998; **39**: 183–187.

Besag FM, Berry DJ, Pool F. Methsuximide lowers lamotrigine blood levels: a pharmacokinetic antiepileptic drug interaction. *Epilepsia* 2000; **41**: 624–627.

Besag FMC, Berry DJ, Vasey M. Methsuximide reduces valproic acid serum levels. *Ther Drug Monit* 2001; **23**: 694–697.

Binnie CD, van Emde Boas W, Kasteleijn-Nolste-Trenite DG, *et al.* Acute effects of lamotrigine (BW430C) in persons with epilepsy. *Epilepsia* 1986; **27**: 248–254.

Bowdle TA, Levy RH, Cutler RE. Effects of carbamazepine on valproic acid kinetics in normal subjects. *Clin Pharmacol Ther* 1979; **26**: 629–634.

Brodie MJ. Tiagabine pharmocology in profile. *Epilepsia* 1995; **36**(Suppl. 6): S7 S9.

Browne TR, Szabo GK, Evans J, *et al.* Phenobarbital does not alter phenytoin steady-state serum concentration or pharmacokinetics. *Neurology* 1988a; **38**: 639–642.

Browne TR, Szabo GK, Evans J, *et al.* Carbamazepine increases phenytoin serum concentration and reduces phenytoin clearance. *Neurology* 1988b; **38**: 1146–1150.

Browne TR, Mattson RH, Penry JK, *et al.* A multicentre study of vigabatrin for drug-resistant epilepsy. *Br J Clin Pharmacol* 1989; **27**(Suppl. 1): S95–S100.

Browne TR, Szabo GK, Leppik IE, *et al.* Absence of pharmacokinetic drug interaction of levetiracetam with phenytoin in patients with epilepsy determined by new technique. *J Clin Pharmacol* 2000; **40**: 590–595.

Bruni J, Wilder BJ, Perchalski RJ, *et al.* Valproic acid and plasma levels of phenobarbital. *Neurology* 1980; **30**: 94–97.

Christiansen J, Dam M. Influence of phenobarbital and diphenylhydantoin on plasma carbamazepine levels in patients with epilepsy. *Acta Neurol Scand* 1973; **49**: 543–546.

Cocito L, Maffini M, Perfumo P, *et al*. Vigabatrin in complex partial seizures: a long-term study. *Epilepsy Res* 1989; **3**: 160–166.

Colucci R, Glue P, Holt B, *et al*. Effect of felbamate on the pharmacokinetics of lamotrigine. *J Clin Pharmacol* 1996; **36**: 634–638.

Contin M, Riva R, Albani F, *et al*. Topiramate therapeutic monitoring in patients with epilepsy: effect of concomitant antiepileptic drugs. *Ther Drug Monit* 2002; **24**(3): 332–337.

Crawford P, Ghadiali E, Lane R, *et al*. Gabapentin as an antiepileptic drug in man. *J Neurol Neurosurg Psychiat* 1987; **50**: 682–686.

Dalla Bernardina B, Fontana E, Vigevano F, *et al*. Efficacy and tolerability of vigabatrin in children with refractory partial seizures: a single-blind dose-increasing study. *Epilepsia* 1995; **36**: 687–691.

Doose DR, Brodie MJ, Wilson EA, *et al*. Topiramate and lamotrigine pharmacokinetics during repetitive monotherapy and combination therapy in epilepsy patients. *Epilepsia* 2003; **44**: 917–922.

Duncan JS, Patsalos PN, Shorvon SD. Effects of discontinuation of phenytoin, carbamazepine, and valproate on concomitant antiepileptic medication. *Epilepsia* 1991; **32**: 101–115.

Eadie MJ, Lander CM, Hooper WD, *et al*. The effects of phenobarbitone dose on plasma phenobarbitone levels in epileptic patients. *Proc Aust Assoc Neurol* 1976; **13**: 89–96.

Encinas MP, Santos Buelga D, Alonso Gonzalez AC, *et al*. Influence of length of treatment on the interaction between phenobarbital and phenytoin. *J Clin Pharm Ther* 1992; **17**: 49–50.

Eriksson AS, Hoppu K, Nergardh A, *et al*. Pharmacokinetic interactions between lamotrigine and other antiepileptic drugs in children with intractable epilepsy. *Epilepsia* 1996; **37**: 769–773.

Eriksson AS, Boreus LO. No increase in carbamazepine-10,11-epoxide during addition of lamotrigine treatment in children. *Ther Drug Monit* 1997; **19**: 499–501.

Fincham RW, Schottelius DD, Sahs AL. The influence of diphenylhydantoin on primidone metabolism. *Trans Am Neurol Assoc* 1973; **98**: 197–199.

Fuerst RH, Graves NM, Leppik IE, *et al*. Felbamate increases phenytoin but decreases carbamazepine concentrations. *Epilepsia* 1988; **29**: 488–491.

Gatti G, Bartoli A, Marchiselli R, *et al*. Vigabatrin-induced decrease in serum phenytoin concentration does not involve a change in phenytoin bioavailability. *Br J Clin Pharmacol* 1993; **36**: 603–606.

Gidal BE, Kanner A, Maly M, *et al*. Lamotrigine pharmacokinetics in patients receiving felbamate. *Epilepsy Res* 1997a; **27**: 1–5.

Gidal BE, Rutecki P, Shaw R, *et al*. Effect of lamotrigine on carbamazepine epoxide/carbamazepine serum concentration ratios in adult patients with epilepsy. *Epilepsy Res* 1997b; **28**: 207–211.

Glauser TA, Miles MV, Tang P, *et al*. Topiramate pharmacokinetics in infants. *Epilepsia* 1999; **40**: 788–791.

Glue P, Banfield CR, Perhach JL, *et al.* Pharmacokinetic interactions with felbamate. In vitro-in vivo correlation. *Clin Pharmacokinet* 1997; **33**: 214–224.

Goa KL, Sorkin EM. Gabapentin – a review of its pharmacological properties and clinical potential in epilepsy. *Drugs* 1993; **46**: 409–427.

Gram L, Klosterskov P, Dam M. γ-Vinyl GABA: a double-blind placebo-controlled trial in partial epilepsy. *Ann Neurol* 1985; **17**: 262–266.

Grant SM, Heel RC. Vigabatrin – a review of its pharmacodynamic and pharmacokinetic properties, and therapeutic potential in epilepsy and disorders of motor control. *Drugs* 1991; **41**: 889–926.

Grasela TH, Fiedler-Kelly J, Cox E, *et al.* Population pharmacokinetics of lamotrigine adjunctive therapy in adults with epilepsy. *J Clin Pharmacol* 1999; **39**: 373–384.

Graves NM, Holmes GB, Fuerst RH, *et al.* Effect of felbamate on phenytoin and carbamazepine serum concentrations. *Epilepsia* 1989; **30**: 225–229.

Gustavson LE, Boellner SW, Granneman GR, *et al.* A single-dose study to define tiagabine pharmacokinetics in pediatric patients with complex partial seizures. *Neurology* 1997; **48**: 1032–1037.

Gustavson LE, Cato A, Boellner SW, *et al.* Lack of pharmacokinetic drug interactions between tiagabine and carbamazepine or phenytoin. *Am J Ther* 1998a; **5**: 9–16.

Gustavson LE, Sommerville KW, Boellner SW, *et al.* Lack of a clinically significant pharmacokinetic drug interaction between tiagabine and valproate. *Am J Ther* 1998b; **5**: 73–79.

Hansen JM, Kristensen M, Skovsted L. Sulthiame (ospolot) as inhibitor of diphenylhydatoin metabolism. *Epilepsia* 1968; **9**: 17–22.

Herranz JL, Arteaga R, Farr IN, *et al.* Dose–response study of vigabatrin in children with refractory epilepsy. *J Child Neurol Suppl* 1991; **2**: S45–S51.

Hooper WD, Kavanagh MC, Herkes GK, *et al.* Lack of a pharmacokinetic interaction between phenobarbitone and gabapentin. *Br J Clin Pharmacol* 1991; **31**: 171–174.

Hooper WD, Franklin ME, Glue P, *et al.* Effect of felbamate on valproic acid disposition in healthy volunteers: inhibition of beta-oxidation. *Epilepsia* 1996; **37**: 91–97.

Houtkooper MA, Lammertsma A, Meyer JW, *et al.* Oxcarbazepine (GP 47.680): a possible alternative to carbamazepine? *Epilepsia* 1987; **28**: 693–698.

Hulsman JA, Rentmeester TW, Banfield CR, *et al.* Effects of felbamate on the pharmacokinetics of the monohydroxy and dihydroxy metabolites of oxcarbazepine. *Clin Pharmacol Ther* 1995; **58**: 383–389.

Hussein G, Troupin AS, Montouris G. Gabapentin interaction with felbamate. *Neurology* 1996; **47**: 1106.

Inoue F, Chambers DN. The effect of phenobarbital on the pharmacokinetics of phenytoin – a case report. *Can J Hos Pharm* 1985; **38**: 147–148.

Jawad S, Yuen WC, Peck AW, *et al.* Lamotrigine: single-dose pharmacokinetics and initial 1 week experience in refractory epilepsy. *Epilepsy Res* 1987; **1**: 194–201.

Jawad S, Richens A, Goodwin G, *et al.* Controlled trial of lamotrigine (lamictal) for refractory partial seizures. *Epilepsia* 1989; **30**: 356–363.

Jedrzejczak J, Dlawichowska E, Owczarek K, *et al.* Effect of vigabatrin addition on carbamazepine blood serum levels in patients with epilepsy. *Epilepsy Res* 2000; **39**: 115–120.

Kanner AM, Frey M. Adding valproate to lamotrigine: a study of their pharmacokinetic interaction. *Neurology* 2000; **55**: 588–591.

Kapetanovic IM, Kupferberg HJ, Porter RJ, *et al*. Mechanism of valproate–phenobarbital interaction in epileptic patients. *Clin Pharmacol Ther* 1981; **29**: 480–486.

Kelley MT, Walson PD, Cox S, *et al*. Population pharmacokinetics of felbamate in children. *Ther Drug Monit* 1997; **19**: 29–36.

Kumps A, Wurth C. Oxcarbazepine disposition: preliminary observations in patients. *Biopharm Drug Dispos* 1990; **11**: 365–370.

Lai ML, Lin TS, Huang JD. Effect of single- and multiple-dose carbamazepine on the pharmacokinetics of diphenylhydantoin. *Eur J Clin Pharmacol* 1992; **43**: 201–203.

Lai ML, Huang JD. Dual effect of valproic acid on the pharmacokinetics of phenytoin. *Biopharm Drug Dispos* 1993; **14**: 365–370.

Lakehal F, Wurden CJ, Kalhorn TF, *et al*. Carbamazepine and oxcarbazepine decrease phenytoin metabolism through inhibition of CYP2C19. *Epilepsy Res* 2002; **52**: 79–83.

Lambie DG, Johnson RH. The effects of phenytoin on phenobarbitone and primidone metabolism. *J Neurol Neurosurg Psychiat* 1981; **44**: 148–151.

Liu H, Delgado MR. Effect of valproate and felbamate on carbamazepine and its metabolite in epileptic children. *J Epilepsy* 1997; **10**: 37–41.

Loiseau P, Hardenberg JP, Pestre M, *et al*. Double-blind, placebo-controlled study of vigabatrin (gamma-vinyl GABA) in drug-resistant epilepsy. *Epilepsia* 1986; **27**: 115–120.

Loiseau P, Yuen AW, Duche B, *et al*. A randomised double-blind placebo-controlled crossover add-on trial of lamotrigine in patients with treatment-resistant partial seizures. *Epilepsy Res* 1990; **7**: 136–145.

Mataringa MI, May TW, Rambeck B. Does lamotrigine influence valproate concentrations? *Ther Drug Monit* 2002; **24**: 631–636.

May T, Stenzel E, Rambeck B. Phenytoin serum concentration in epileptic patients: influence of therapeutic and physiological factors. *Nervenarzt* 1982; **53**: 291–296.

May T, Rambeck B. Serum concentrations of valproic acid: influence of dose and comedication. *Ther Drug Monit* 1985; **7**: 387–390.

May T, Rambeck B. Fluctuations of unbound and total phenytoin concentrations during the day in epileptic patients on valproic acid comedication. *Ther Drug Monit* 1990; **12**: 124–128.

May TW, Rambeck B, Nothbaum N. Nomogram for the prediction of unbound phenytoin concentrations in patients on a combined treatment of phenytoin and valproic acid. *Eur Neurol* 1991; **31**: 57–60.

May TW, Rambeck B, Jürgens U. Serum concentrations of lamotrigine in epileptic patients: the influence of dose and comedication. *Ther Drug Monit* 1996a; **18**: 523–531.

May TW, Rambeck B, Sälke-Kellermann A. Fluctuations of 10-hydroxy-carbazepine during the day in epileptic patients. *Acta Neurol Scand* 1996b; **93**(6): 393–397.

May TW, Rambeck B, Jürgens U. Influence of oxcarbazepine and methsuximide on lamotrigine concentrations in epileptic patients with and without valproic acid comedication: results of a retrospective study. *Ther Drug Monit* 1999; **21**: 175–181.

May TW, Rambeck B, Jürgens U. Serum concentrations of topiramate in patients with epilepsy: influence of dose, age, and comedication. *Ther Drug Monit* 2002; **24**: 366–374.

May TW, Rambeck B, Jürgens U. Serum concentrations of levetiracetam in patients with epilepsy: influence of dose and comedication. *Ther Drug Monit* 2003; **25**: 690–699.

McKee PJ, Blacklaw J, Forrest G, *et al.* A double-blind, placebo-controlled interaction study between oxcarbazepine and carbamazepine, sodium valproate and phenytoin in epileptic patients. *Br J Clin Pharmacol* 1994; **37**: 27–32.

De Michele G, Brescia Morra V, Pisanti N, *et al.* Carbamazepine serum levels in epileptics. Influence of age, sex, body weight and interaction with phenobarbital. *Acta Neurol (Napoli)* 1985; **7**: 228–234.

Minami T, Ieiri I, Ohtsubo K, *et al.* Influence of additional therapy with zonisamide (excegran) on protein binding and metabolism of carbamazepine. *Epilepsia* 1994; **35**: 1023–1025.

Morris RG, Black AB, Lam E, *et al.* Clinical study of lamotrigine and valproic acid in patients with epilepsy: using a drug interaction to advantage? *Ther Drug Monit* 2000; **22**: 656–660.

Müller FO, Aucamp AK, Hundt HK, *et al.* Evaluation of serum levels during prolonged combination therapy with phenytoin and phenobarbitone. *S Afr Med J* 1977; **52**: 356–358.

Ojemann LM, Shastri RA, Wilensky AJ, *et al.* Comparative pharmacokinetics of zonisamide (CI-912) in epileptic patients on carbamazepine or phenytoin monotherapy. *Ther Drug Monit* 1986; **8**: 293–296.

Patel IH, Levy RH, Cutler RE. Phenobarbital–valproic acid interaction. *Clin Pharmacol Ther* 1980; **27**: 515–521.

Patsalos PN. Pharmacokinetic profile of levetiracetam: toward ideal characteristics. *Pharmacol Ther* 2000; **85**: 77–85.

Perucca E, Gidal BE, Ledent E, *et al.* Levetiracetam does not interact with other antiepileptic drugs. *Epilepsia* 2000; **41**(Suppl. 7): 254–255.

Perucca E, Gidal BE, Baltes E. Effects of antiepileptic comedication on levetiracetam pharmacokinetics: a pooled analysis of data from randomized adjunctive therapy trials. *Epilepsy Res* 2003; **53**: 47–56.

Pisani F, Xiao B, Fazio A, *et al.* Single dose pharmacokinetics of carbamazepine-10,11-epoxide in patients on lamotrigine monotherapy. *Epilepsy Res* 1994; **19**: 245–248.

Porro MG, Kupferberg HJ, Porter RJ, *et al.* Phenytoin: an inhibitor and inducer of primidone metabolism in an epileptic patient. *Br J Clin Pharmacol* 1982; **14**: 294–297.

Radulovic LL, Wilder BJ, Leppik IE, *et al.* Lack of interaction of gabapentin with carbamazepine or valproate. *Epilepsia* 1994; **35**: 155–161.

Rambeck B. Pharmacological interactions of mesuximide with phenobarbital and phenytoin in hospitalized epileptic patients. *Epilepsia* 1979; **20**: 147–156.

Rambeck B, Boenigk HE, May T. Pharmacological influence of valproate on phenobarbitone and phenytoin serum concentrations in epileptic patients. *Nervenarzt* 1979; **50**: 743–746.

Rambeck B, May T, Juergens U. Serum concentrations of carbamazepine and its epoxide and diol metabolites in epileptic patients: the influence of dose and comedication. *Ther Drug Monit* 1987; **9**: 298–303.

Rambeck B, Sälke-Treumann A, May T, *et al.* Valproic acid-induced carbamazepine-10,11-epoxide toxicity in children and adolescents. *Eur Neurol* 1990; **30**: 79–83.

Reidenberg P, Glue P, Banfield CR, *et al.* Effects of felbamate on the pharmacokinetics of phenobarbital. *Clin Pharmacol Ther* 1995a; **58**: 279–287.

Reidenberg P, Glue P, Banfield C, Colucci R, *et al*. Pharmacokinetic interaction studies between felbamate and vigabatrin. *Br J Clin Pharmacol* 1995b; **40**: 157–160.

Reunanen MI, Luoma P, Myllyla VV, Hokkanen E. Low serum valproic acid concentrations in epileptic patients on combination therapy. *Curr Ther Res Clin Exp* 1980; **28**: 456–462.

Richens A, Chadwick DW, Duncan JS, *et al*. Adjunctive treatment of partial seizures with tiagabine: A placebo-controlled trial. *Epilepsy Res* 1995; **21**: 37–42.

Rimmer EM, Richens A. Interaction between vigabatrin and phenytoin. *Br J Clin Pharmacol* 1989; **27**(Suppl. 1): 27S–33S.

Riva R, Albani F, Contin M, *et al*. Time-dependent interaction between phenytoin and valproic acid. *Neurology* 1985; **35**: 510–515.

Rosenfeld WE, Liao S, Kramer LD, *et al*. Comparison of the steady-state pharmacokinetics of topiramate and valproate in patients with epilepsy during monotherapy and concomitant therapy. *Epilepsia* 1997; **38**: 324–333.

Rosenfeld WE, Doose DR, Walker SA, *et al*. A study of topiramate pharmacokinetics and tolerability in children with epilepsy. *Pediatr Neurol* 1999; **20**: 339–344.

Sachdeo RC, Sachdeo SK, Walker SA, *et al*. Steady-state pharmacokinetics of topiramate and carbamazepine in patients with epilepsy during monotherapy and concomitant therapy. *Epilepsia* 1996; **37**: 774–780.

Sachdeo R, Wagner ML, Sachdeo S, *et al*. Coadministration of phenytoin and felbamate: evidence of additional phenytoin dose-reduction requirements based on pharmacokinetics and tolerability with increasing doses of felbamate. *Epilepsia* 1999; **40**: 1122–1128.

Sackellares JC, Donofrio PD, Wagner JG, *et al*. Pilot study of zonisamide (1,2-benzisoxazole-3-methanesulfonamide) in patients with refractory partial seizures. *Epilepsia* 1985; **26**: 206–211.

Sälke-Kellermann RA, May TW, Boenigk HE. Influence of ethosuximide on valproic acid serum concentrations. *Epilepsy Res* 1997; **26**: 345–349.

Sälke-Treumann A, Rambeck B, May TW, *et al*. Nebenwirkungen durch carbamazepin-epoxid bei kindern. *Epilepsie-Blätter* 1988; (**1**): 39–41.

Sallas W. Population pharmacokinetics analysis of oxcarbazepine (trileptal) in children with epilepsy. *Epilepsia* 1999; **40**(Suppl. 7): 102.

Sanchez-Alcaraz A, Quintana B, Rodriguez I, *et al*. Plasma concentrations of vigabatrin in epileptic patients. *J Clin Pharm Ther* 1996; **21**: 393–398.

Sanchez-Alcaraz A, Quintana MB, Lopez E, *et al*. Effect of vigabatrin on the pharmacokinetics of carbamazepine. *J Clin Pharm Ther* 2002; **27**: 427–430.

Sander JW, Patsalos PN, Oxley JR, *et al*. A randomised double-blind placebo-controlled add-on trial of lamotrigine in patients with severe epilepsy. *Epilepsy Res* 1990; **6**: 221–226.

Schapel GJ, Beran RG, Vajda FJ, *et al*. Double-blind, placebo controlled, crossover study of lamotrigine in treatment resistant partial seizures. *J Neurol Neurosurg Psychiat* 1993; **56**: 448–453.

Schmidt D. The effect of phenytoin and ethosuximide on primidone metabolism in patients with epilepsy. *J Neurol* 1975; **209**: 115–123.

Schmidt D, Jacob R, Loiseau P, *et al*. Zonisamide for add-on treatment of refractory partial epilepsy: a European double-blind trial. *Epilepsy Res* 1993; **15**: 67–73.

Sharief MK, Singh P, Sander JWAS, *et al.* Efficacy and tolerability study of ucb L059 in patients with refractory epilepsy. *J Epilepsy* 1996; **9**: 106–112.

Shinoda M, Akita M, Hasegawa M, *et al.* The necessity of adjusting the dosage of zonisamide when coadministered with other anti-epileptic drugs. *Biol Pharm Bull* 1996; **19**: 1090–1092.

Siegel H, Kelley K, Stertz B, *et al.* The efficacy of felbamate as add-on therapy to valproic acid in the Lennox–Gastaut syndrome. *Epilepsy Res* 1999; **34**: 91–97.

Snel S, Jansen JA, Mengel HB, *et al.* The pharmacokinetics of tiagabine in healthy elderly volunteers and elderly patients with epilepsy. *J Clin Pharmacol* 1997; **37**: 1015–1020.

So EL, Wolff D, Graves NM, *et al.* Pharmacokinetics of tiagabine as add-on therapy in patients taking enzyme-inducing antiepilepsy drugs. *Epilepsy Res* 1995; **22**: 221–226.

Tartara A, Galimberti CA, Manni R, *et al.* The pharmacokinetics of oxcarbazepine and its active metabolite 10-hydroxy-carbazepine in healthy subjects and in epileptic patients treated with phenobarbitone or valproic acid. *Br J Clin Pharmacol* 1993; **36**: 366–368.

Tasaki K, Minami T, Ieiri I, *et al.* Drug interactions of zonisamide with phenytoin and sodium valproate: serum concentrations and protein binding. *Brain Dev* 1995; **17**: 182–185.

The US Gabapentin Study Group. The long-term safety and efficacy of gabapentin (neurontin) as add-on therapy in drug-resistant partial epilepsy. *Epilepsy Res* 1994; **18**: 67–73.

Theodore WH, Raubertas RF, Porter RJ, *et al.* Felbamate: a clinical trial for complex partial seizures. *Epilepsia* 1991; **32**: 392–397.

Troupin A, Montouris G, Hussein G. Felbamate: therapeutic range and other kinetic information. *J Epilepsy* 1997; **10**: 26–31.

Tyndel F. Interaction of gabapentin with other antiepileptics. *Lancet* 1994; **343**: 1363–1364.

Viola MS, Bercellini MA, Saidon P, *et al.* Pharmacokinetic variability of oxcarbazepine in epileptic patients. *Medicina Buenos Aires* 2000; **60**(6): 914–918.

Wagner ML, Graves NM, Marienau K, *et al.* Discontinuation of phenytoin and carbamazepine in patients receiving felbamate. *Epilepsia* 1991; **32**: 398–406.

Wagner ML, Remmel RP, Graves NM, *et al.* Effect of felbamate on carbamazepine and its major metabolites. *Clin Pharmacol Ther* 1993; **53**: 536–543.

Wagner ML, Graves NM, Leppik IE, *et al.* The effect of felbamate on valproic acid disposition. *Clin Pharmacol Ther* 1994; **56**: 494–502.

Walker MC, Patsalos PN. Clinical pharmacokinetics of new antiepileptic drugs. *Pharmacol Therapeutics* 1995; **67**: 351–384.

Warner T, Patsalos PN, Prevett M, *et al.* Lamotrigine-induced carbamazepine toxicity: an interaction with carbamazepine-10,11-epoxide. *Epilepsy Res* 1992; **11**: 147–150.

Wilder BJ, Willmore LJ, Bruni J, *et al.* Valproic acid: interaction with other anticonvulsant drugs. *Neurology* 1978; **28**(9 Pt 1): 892–896.

Wilensky AJ, Friel PN, Ojemann LM, *et al.* Pharmacokinetics of W-554 (ADD 03055) in epileptic patients. *Epilepsia* 1985; **26**: 602–606.

Windorfer Jr A, Sauer W. Drug interactions during anticonvulsant therapy in childhood: diphenylhydantoin, primidone, phenobarbitone, clonazepam, nitrazepam, carbamazepine and dipropylacetate. *Neuropädiatrie* 1977; **8**: 29–41.

Wolf P. Lamotrigine: preliminary clinical observations on pharmacokinetics and interactions with traditional antiepileptic drugs. *J Epilepsy* 1992; **5**: 73–79.

Yuen AW, Land G, Weatherley BC, *et al.* Sodium valproate acutely inhibits lamotrigine metabolism. *Br J Clin Pharmacol* 1992; **33**: 511–513.

Yukawa E, Honda T, Ohdo S, *et al.* Detection of carbamazepine-induced changes in valproic acid relative clearance in man by simple pharmacokinetic screening. *J Pharm Pharmacol* 1997; **49**: 751–756.

8

Interaction between antiepileptic and non-antiepileptic drugs

Jerzy Majkowski[1] and Philip N. Patsalos[2]

[1] Center for Epilepsy Diagnosis and Treatment Foundation of Epileptology, Warsaw, Poland
[2] Pharmocology and Therapeutics Unit, Department of Clinical and Experimental Epilepsy, Institute of Neurology, London; The National Society for Epilepsy, Chalfont St Peter, UK

Introduction

Clinically important drug interactions occur essentially at two levels – at the pharmacokinetic level and at the pharmacodynamic level (Patsalos *et al.*, 2002; Patsalos and Perucca, 2003a). By far the most important interactions are pharmacokinetic in nature and this is partly due to the fact that they are particularly prevalent in relation to antiepileptic drug (AED) use and also because they are more readily detected and quantitated. Whilst pharmacodynamic interactions are also of clinical significance they are less well documented and indeed difficult to quantitate. Pharmacokinetic interactions are associated with a change in blood concentration as a consequence of alterations in absorption, protein binding, distribution, metabolism or elimination of a drug.

Since AEDs are frequently used for years, decades or even throughout a patient's life, it is inevitable that drugs for the treatment of concurrent diseases will be co-prescribed. In this setting the potential for interactions is high and there are many such interactions that have been described (Patsalos and Perucca, 2003b). By far the most important and clinically significant interactions occur either as the consequence of hepatic enzyme inhibition or hepatic enzyme induction of cytochrome P450 (CYP) isoenzymes. Enzyme induction results in reduction in blood concentrations and possibly a loss of an adequate therapeutic response whilst enzyme inhibition results in an elevation in blood concentrations and possibly toxicity.

The characterization of the isoenzymes involved in the metabolism of individual drugs during the past decade has greatly enhanced our ability to predict whether or not a metabolic interaction will occur and this is covered in more detail in Chapter 5. In clinical practice it is best to avoid prescribing drugs that have a high propensity to interact. However, it is sometimes necessary to co-prescribe such drugs. In this setting, it is advisable to undertake therapeutic monitoring and to measure plasma drug concentrations, particularly after an interacting drug is introduced or withdrawn but also when a dosage change has occurred. Occasionally, it may be necessary to measure the free (pharmacologically active) concentration in plasma so as to aid a dose change and dose optimization. This would apply to drug interactions that involve the displacement of a drug that is highly protein bound (>90%) from its plasma protein-binding site combined with an inhibition of its metabolism (e.g. phenytoin (PHT) and phenylbutazone).

In this chapter, clinically significant interactions between AEDs and non-AEDs are described. Interactions between AEDs and oral contraceptives, and between AEDs and psychoactive drugs are not described here as they are discussed in detail in Chapters 16 and 19, respectively. The interactions are presented in alphabetical order and are divided into those affected by a particular AED and those that affect the AED. However, in some instances we discuss interactions within a drug class. With regard to the new AEDs, because of the scarcity of available information, all interactions are highlighted regardless of whether or not a significant interaction was identified. In contrast, non-interaction drug combinations with the established AEDs are not reported.

It should be remembered that for interactions that are associated with an increase in clearance, a reduction in plasma concentrations and a reduction in area under the concentration versus time curve (AUC) values would probably require that a dose increase be undertaken so as to maintain an adequate therapeutic response. Conversely, interactions that are associated with a decrease in clearance, an increase in plasma concentrations and an increase in AUC values would probably require that a dose reduction be undertaken so as to prevent drug toxicity. In both settings it is appropriate that patients are closely monitored and that plasma concentrations are measured.

Carbamazepine

Carbamazepine is extensively metabolized to carbamazepine-10,11-epoxide and then to carbamazepine-10,11-diol by CYPP450 enzymes. The formation of the epoxide is mediated primarily via CYP3A4, with some contribution by CYP2C8, whilst the metabolism of the epoxide is via the enzyme epoxide hydrolase. Plasma protein binding is 70%.

Interactions affecting carbamazepine

Antibiotics

As the macrolide antibiotics are metabolized by CYP3A4 they have the propensity to interact with carbamazepine. The interactions can be classified into three groups according to their risk of interaction with AEDs (Periti *et al.*, 1992). The first group comprises clarithromycin, erythromycin and troleandomycin and these drugs have a high propensity to inhibit the metabolism of carbamazepine (Babany *et al.*, 1988). Typically, plasma carbamazepine concentrations increase by up to four-fold (Mesdjian *et al.*, 1980; Majkowski, 1995).

The second group compromises flurithromycin, josamycin, midecamycin, miocamycin and roxithromycin. These antibiotics are less potent CYP3A4 inhibitors and are usually associated with only a modest increase in plasma carbamazepine concentrations (Albin *et al.*, 1982; Vincon *et al.*, 1987; Barzaghi *et al.*, 1988; Couet *et al.*, 1990; Levy, 1995). For example, the addition of clarithromycin (500 mg/day) to carbamazepine, can result in an increase in plasma carbamazepine concentration of 30–50%, and a concurrent decrease of carbamazepine-epoxide concentrations (Albani *et al.*, 1993; O'Connor and Fris, 1994; Yasui *et al.*, 1997). In one study roxithromycin was not associated with any interaction (Saint-Salvi *et al.*, 1987).

Azitromycin, dirithromycin, rokitamycin and spiramycin comprise the third group of macrolide antibiotics and these do not have any effect on CYP3A4 and therefore do not interact with carbamazepine (Periti *et al.*, 1992; Principi and Esposito, 1999).

Antiviral agents

The antiviral agents delavirdine, indinavir and ritonavir are potent CYP3A4 inhibitors. Thus, their co-administration with carbamazepine can result in carbamazepine toxicity. Indeed, there are reports of ritonavir causing a two- to three-fold increase in plasma carbamazepine concentration (Burman and Orr, 2000; Garcia *et al.*, 2000; Kato *et al.*, 2000; von Moltke *et al.*, 2000; Mateu-de Antonio *et al.*, 2001). Carbamazepine toxicity was similarly observed in a patient taking ritonavir and efavirenzin in combination (Burman and Orr, 2000).

Cimetidine

During combination therapy with cimetidine, carbamazepine intoxication has been reported. However, the interaction does not occur consistently and is probably of little clinical significance since the effect on carbamazepine is small (17% increase in plasma concentrations) and possibly transient (Dalton *et al.*, 1986; Spina *et al.*, 1996).

Cisplatin

It has been reported that a young woman with epilepsy had seizures during antineoplastic therapy and that the seizures were the consequence of a reduced plasma carbamazepine concentration (Neef and de Voogd-van der Straaten, 1988). The mechanism of this interaction may be induction of metabolism or an increased volume of distribution.

Danazol

Co-administration of danazol with carbamazepine results in a clinically significant increase (50–100%) in plasma carbamazepine concentrations. Moreover, danazol inhibits carbamazepine-epoxide elimination via an action on epoxide hydrolase and this too can contribute to the associated carbamazepine toxicity (Krämer *et al.*, 1986; Zielinski *et al.*, 1987; Hayden and Buchanan, 1991; Spina *et al.*, 1996).

Diltiazem

Plasma carbamazepine concentration can increase by up to 50% during combination therapy with diltiazem (Brodie and MacPhee, 1986; Eimer and Carter, 1987; Bahls *et al.*, 1991; Maoz *et al.*, 1992). Diltiazem is metabolized to two metabolites (*N*-desmethyl-diltiazem and *N,N*-didesmethyl-diltiazem) and both are potent inhibitors of CYP3A4-mediated testosterone-6-β-hydroxylation (11 and 200 times, respectively), compared to that of diltiazem. This would suggest that the major contribution to this interaction is the consequence of the two metabolites.

Fluconazole

Many imidazole antifungals are potent inhibitors of CYP isoenzymes and these drugs commonly interact with carbamazepine. Fluconazole is a strong inhibitor of carbamazepine metabolism and a mean 120% increase in plasma carbamazepine concentration has been reported (Nair and Morris, 1999). During combination therapy carbamazepine intoxication can occur.

Isoniazid

Isoniazid can inhibit the metabolism of carbamazepine, via an action on CYP3A4, resulting in elevated plasma concentrations and associated toxicity (Valsalan and Cooper, 1982). The clearance of carbamazepine can be decreased by up to 45% (Block, 1982; Wright *et al.*, 1982; Spina *et al.*, 1996).

Ketoconazole

Like fluconazole, ketoconazole is also a strong inhibitor of carbamazepine metabolism. The administration of ketoconazole to patients taking carbamazepine has been found to result in a significant (mean 29%) increase in plasma carbamazepine concentrations and possibly in carbamazepine intoxication (Spina *et al.*, 1997).

Metronidazole

The metabolism of carbamazepine can be inhibited by metronidazole. This results in an increase in plasma carbamazepine concentration and possible adverse events (Patterson, 1994).

Nicotinamide

Nicotinamide has been reported to increase plasma carbamazepine concentrations (Bourgeois *et al.*, 1982).

Propoxyphene

Propoxyphene appears to reduce the activity of CYP3A4 and consequently inhibits the metabolism of carbamazepine (Abernethy *et al.*, 1985). Thus during combination therapy, plasma carbamazepine concentrations can increase by 45–77% (Dam and Christensen, 1977; Hansen *et al.*, 1980). In addition, plasma carbamazepine-epoxide concentrations are significantly reduced (Bergendal *et al.*, 1997).

Quinine

In healthy volunteers, single doses of the antimalarial agent quinine have been reported to increase plasma carbamazepine concentrations (Amabeoku *et al.*, 1993).

Ticlopidine

Ticlopidine increased plasma carbamazepine concentrations which resulted in symptoms of neurological intoxication in a patient with epilepsy undergoing coronary stenting (Brown and Cooper, 1997).

Verapamil

Verapamil is extensively metabolized in the liver to several metabolites by numerous CYP isoenzymes: CYPCA4, CYP2C8 and CYP1A2 (Kroemer *et al.*, 1993; Spina *et al.*, 1996; Tracy *et al.*, 1999). Verapamil inhibits CYP3A4 and it has been reported that plasma carbamazepine concentrations can increase by a mean of 46% resulting in neurotoxicity (MacPhee *et al.*, 1986). Interestingly, an increase in free carbamazepine concentrations can also occur (mean rise of 33% in five of six patients) (MacPhee *et al.*, 1986).

Interactions affected by carbamazepine

Carbamazepine is a potent hepatic enzyme inducer and, as well as inducing its own metabolism via an action on CYP3A4, it also induces the metabolism of many other drugs that are CYP3A4 substrates. There is also evidence to suggest that it induces CYP2C9, CYP2C19 and CYP1A2.

Antihypertensive drugs

Carbamazepine enhances the metabolic clearance of the β-adrenoceptor blocking agents propranolol, metropronol and alprenolol, and the dihydropyridine calcium antagonists nimodipine, nifedipine, felodipine and nisoldipine as well as verapamil (Tartara *et al.*, 1991; Flockart and Tanus-Santos, 2002). In relation to nimodipine, nifedipine, felodipine and nisoldipine, the magnitude of the interaction is so substantial (e.g. with nimodipine, plasma concentrations can decline seven-fold) that the usefulness of these agents in patients co-medicated with carbamazepine, and indeed other enzyme inducing AEDs, is questionable (Tartara *et al.*, 1991).

Cyclosporin

Cyclosporin is metabolized by CYP3A4 and consequently during combination therapy with carbamazepine the metabolism of cyclosporin A is enhanced (Alvarez *et al.*, 1991). Typically, plasma cyclosporin concentrations can be expected to decline by 65% (Cooney *et al.*, 1995).

Dicoumarol

Carbamazepine reduces the anticoagulant effect of dicoumarol by enhancing its metabolism, possibly via an action on CYP2C9 (Freedman and Olatidoye, 1994). Overall, whenever there is a change in carbamazepine therapy (and indeed that of any other enzyme inducing AED; see sections later) it is advisable to monitor internationalized normalized ratio (INR) because all anticoagulants are associated with a narrow therapeutic ratio (Cropp and Bussey, 1997).

Doxycycline

The half-life of the antibiotic doxycycline is reduced two-fold when co-administered with carbamazepine (Penttila *et al.*, 1974).

Fentanyl

The anaesthetic fentanyl is primarily metabolized by CYP3A4 and its metabolism is enhanced by carbamazepine. Consequently, induction of anaesthesia requires substantially higher doses of fentanyl in patients taking carbamazepine (Tempelhoff *et al.*, 1990; Feierman and Lasker, 1996).

Indinavir

In one case report, the addition of carbamazepine (200 mg/day) to indinavir treatment (800 mg t.i.d.) resulted in a reduction in plasma indinavir concentration by up to 16 times (Bonay *et al.*, 1993). This interaction has recently been reported in another case report (Hugen *et al.*, 2000).

Itraconazole

Co-administration of carbamazepine with itraconazole results in a clinically significant reduction in plasma itraconazole concentrations (Bonay *et al.*, 1993).

Methotrexate

The clearance of methotrexate is significantly enhanced by carbamazepine, resulting in a clinically significant reduction in the therapeutic efficacy of methotrexate (Relling *et al.*, 2000).

Phenprocoumon

Carbamazepine induces the metabolism of phenprocoumon and consequently reduces its anticoagulant effect (Schlienger *et al.*, 2000). Overall, whenever there is a change in carbamazepine therapy (and indeed that of any other enzyme inducing AED; see sections later) it is advisable to monitor INR because all anticoagulants are associated with a narrow therapeutic ratio (Cropp and Bussey, 1997).

Rocuronium

Carbamazepine, through its induction of CYP3A4, CYP2C19 and CYP1A2, enhances the metabolism of rocuronium, and some other neuromuscular blocking agents, and therefore reduces their efficacy (Soriano *et al.*, 2000).

Steroids

Carbamazepine enhances the metabolic clearance of a variety of steroids including prednisolone, methylprednisolone and dexamethasone (Spina *et al.*, 1996).

Teniposide

Carbamazepine enhances the clearance of teniposide and consequently reduces the efficacy of teniposide (Relling *et al.*, 2000).

Vincristine

During co-medication with carbamazepine, vincristine clearance was increased by 63% when compared to a control group (Villikka *et al.*, 1999). As vincristine is metabolized in part by CYP3A4, induction of this isoenzyme by carbamazepine is the most likely explanation of this interaction.

Warfarin

The metabolism of warfarin is significantly enhanced by carbamazepine and this is associated with an increase in prothrombin time and a reduced anticoagulant effect (Schlienger *et al.*, 2000). The interaction is mediated via an action on CYP2C9, although some induction of CYP3A4 may also occur (Rettie *et al.*, 1992; Kunze *et al.*, 1996). Overall, whenever there is a change in carbamazepine therapy (and indeed that of any other enzyme inducing AED; see sections later) it is advisable to monitor INR because all anticoagulants are associated with a narrow therapeutic ratio (Cropp and Bussey, 1997).

Ethosuximide

Ethosuximide is eliminated primarily by metabolism with 30–60% of an administered dose recovered in urine. Metabolism is primarily mediated by CYP3A and to
a lesser extent by CYP2E and CYP2B/C. Approximately 20% of an administered
dose is excreted unchanged in urine. Ethosuximide is not bound to plasma
proteins.

Interactions affecting ethosuximide

Isoniazid

Isoniazid may increase plasma ethosuximide concentrations resulting in clinical
signs of intoxication (Van Wieringen and Vrijlandt, 1983).

Rifampicin

In adult healthy volunteers, rifampicin has been observed to decrease plasma ethosuximide concentrations by induction of its metabolism (Bachmann and Jauregui,
1993).

Interactions affected by ethosuximide

There are no clinical data to suggest ethosuximide induces or inhibits the metabolism of other non-AEDs.

Felbamate

Approximately 50% of an administered dose is metabolized to form two hydroxylated metabolites. Felbamate is a substrate of CYP3A4 and CYP2E1. Approximately
40–50% of an absorbed dose is excreted unchanged in urine. Plasma protein binding
is 23%.

As a new AED, knowledge of the interaction profile of felbamate with non-AEDs
is rather limited. Only interactions with specific drugs have been investigated.

Interactions affecting felbamate

Erythromycin, a potent CYP3A4 inhibitor is without effect on the metabolism of
felbamate and indeed plasma felbamate concentrations are not significantly
affected during combination therapy (Glue *et al.*, 1997).

Interactions affected by felbamate

To date there are no clinical data to suggest that felbamate induces or inhibits
the metabolism of other non-AEDs. However, interactions may conceivably occur
with drugs that are substrates for the same isoenzymes as occur with felbamate.

Gabapentin

Gabapentin is not metabolized and is exclusively eliminated as unchanged gabapentin in urine. It is not protein bound. Consequently, gabapentin should have little propensity to interact with other drugs and indeed this is the case.

As a new AED, knowledge of the interaction profile of gabapentin with non-AEDs is rather limited. Only interactions with specific drugs have been investigated.

Interactions affecting gabapentin

Antacids

Antacids containing aluminium and magnesium hydroxide reduce the absorption of gabapentin by approximately 15% (Busch *et al.*, 1992). This interaction is of little clinical significance.

Cimetidine

Cimetidine appears to decrease plasma gabapentin concentrations by approximately 15%. The mechanism appears to be renal in nature and is considered not to be of clinical significance.

Interactions affected by gabapentin

To date there are no clinical data to suggest that gabapentin affects the metabolism of other non-AEDs.

Lamotrigine

Lamotrigine undergoes extensive metabolism via glucuronidation and the primary metabolite is *N*-2 glucuronide (71% of dose). Glucuronidation is a major conjugation reaction that is catalyzed by a number of different isoforms of uridine 5′ diphosphate (UDP)-glucuronosyl transferase (UGT). The *N*-2 glucuronidation of lamotrigine is catalyzed by UGT1A4. Plasma protein binding is 50%.

As a new AED, knowledge of the interaction profile of lamotrigine with non-AEDs is rather limited. Only interactions with specific drugs have been investigated.

Interactions affecting lamotrigine

Acetaminophen (paracetamol)

Since acetaminophen is excreted by glucuronidation, as is indeed lamotrigine, it was anticipated that an interaction between the two drugs would occur. In a healthy volunteer study acetaminophen enhanced the clearance of lamotrigine (15%) and decreased AUC (20%) and half-life values (15%) (Depot *et al.*, 1990).

Bupropion

In healthy volunteers, bupropion was observed not to interact with lamotrigine (Odishaw and Chen, 2000).

Cimetidine

In healthy volunteers, cimetidine was observed not to interact with lamotrigine (Ebert *et al.*, 2000).

Rifampicin

Rifampicin is a potent inducer of CYPP450 and of the UGT enzyme system. In adult healthy volunteers, rifampicin enhanced the clearance of lamotrigine and the amount of lamotrigine excreted as a glucuronide was increased by 36% when compared to placebo (Ebert *et al.*, 2000). The corresponding half-life and AUC values for lamotrigine were significantly reduced (60% and 56%, respectively) compared to placebo.

Interactions affected by lamotrigine

To date there are no clinical data to suggest that lamotrigine affects the metabolism of other non-AEDs.

Levetiracetam

Levetiracetam undergoes minimal metabolism with approximately 30% being metabolized non-hepatically in blood to an inactive metabolite. Furthermore, the elimination of levetiracetam is predominantly renal with approximately 70% of a levetiracetam dose excreted unchanged in urine. It is not protein bound, consequently levetiracetam should have little propensity to interact with other drugs and indeed this is the case.

As a new AED, knowledge of the interaction profile of levetiracetam with non-AEDs is rather limited. Only interactions with specific drugs have been investigated.

Interactions affecting levetiracetam

Digoxin

No clinically relevant effect of digoxin on the pharmacokinetics of levetiracetam was observed in a study of 11 healthy adult volunteers (Levy *et al.*, 2000).

Probenecid

The pharmacokinetics of levetiracetam were unaffected by co-administration of probenecid (Patsalos, 2000). However, the plasma concentration of the primary pharmacologically inactive metabolite of levetiracetam (ucb LO 57) was increased 2.5-fold. The clinical significance of the latter effect is unknown.

Warfarin

The co-administration of warfarin with levetiracetam did not result in any significant change in the pharmacokinetics of levetiracetam (Ragueneau-Majlessi *et al.*, 2001).

Interactions affected by levetiracetam

Digoxin

Plasma digoxin concentrations are not significantly affected by levetiracetam (Levy *et al.*, 2000).

Warfarin

Levetiracetam does not alter the anticoagulant effect or the pharmacokinetics of warfarin (Ragueneau-Majlessi *et al.*, 2001).

Oxcarbazepine

Although oxcarbazepine is clinically related to carbamazepine, its pharmaco-kinetic and interaction profiles are substantially different. Oxcarbazepine undergoes rapid and extensive metabolism to its pharmacologically active metabolite, 10-hydroxycarbazepine, which is subsequently eliminated by glucuronidation or undergoes hydroxylation to form a dihydrodiol metabolite. Only the latter reaction depends on CYP isoenzymes (Patsalos and Duncan, 1993; Baruzzi *et al.*, 1994; Tecoma, 1999). Oxcarbazepine can induce CYP3A4 and CYP3A5 activities and inhibit CYP2C19. Plasma protein binding is 40%.

As a new AED, knowledge of the interaction profile of oxcarbazepine with non-AEDs is rather limited. Only interactions with specific drugs have been investigated.

Interactions affecting oxcarbazepine

Cimetidine

Co-administration of cimetidine and oxcarbazepine in healthy volunteers was not associated with any significant change in the pharmacokinetics of oxcarbazepine (Keränen *et al.*, 1992b).

Dextropropoxyphene

In a study of eight patients taking oxcarbazepine, dextropropoxyphene administration was without effect on steady-state plasma 10-hydroxycarbazepine concentrations (Mogensen *et al.*, 1992).

Erythromycin

Co-administration of erythromycin and oxcarbazepine to eight healthy volunteers over a 1-week period did not result in any major change in oxcarbazepine or 10-hydroxycarbazepine pharmacokinetic parameters (Keränen *et al.*, 1992a).

Verapamil

The potential interaction between verapamil and oxcarbazepine was investigated in 10 healthy volunteers (Krämer *et al.*, 1991). A 20% decrease in 10-hydroxycarbazepine AUC values was observed and the investigators concluded that this interaction may be of clinical relevance in some patients.

Interactions affected by oxcarbazepine

Felodipine

The potential interaction of oxcarbazepine and felodipine, a calcium antagonist, was studied in eight healthy volunteers (Zaccara *et al.*, 1993). It was observed that the bioavailability of felodipine was reduced by 28% but the clinical relevance of this observation is as yet not clear.

Warfarin

The influence of oxcarbazepine on the anticoagulant effect of warfarin was studied in 10 adult healthy volunteers (Krämer *et al.*, 1992). Oxcarbazepine was without any significant effect as measured by prothrombin time.

Phenobarbital

Phenobarbital is extensively metabolized to two major metabolites, *p*-hydroxyphenobarbital, and 9-D-glucopyranosylphenobarbital. CYP2C9 plays a major role in the metabolism of phenobarbital with minor metabolism by CYP2C19 and CYP2E1. Phenobarbital is a potent enzyme inducer. Plasma protein binding is 50%.

Interactions affecting phenobarbital

Activated charcoal

Co-administration of activated charcoal with phenobarbital results in reduction of phenobarbital absorption (Neuvonen and Elonen, 1980). This interaction is used clinically to treat those patients that have overdosed with phenobarbital. After phenobarbital intravenous administration, repeated administration of charcoal over 2–4 days results in an increased phenobarbital clearance (60–270%) whilst half-life values are decreased 2.5–8-fold (Berg *et al.*, 1982, 1987; Frenia *et al.*, 1996).

This effect is considered to be the consequence, in part, of impaired phenobarbital enterohepatic recirculation (Wakabayashi *et al.*, 1994).

Chloramphenicol

Co-administration of chloramphenicol and phenobarbital results in a significant decrease (40%) in phenobarbital clearance (Koup *et al.*, 1978).

Ethanol

During chronic use, alcohol enhances the metabolism of phenobarbital (Sands *et al.*, 1993). In contrast, the acute effect of alcohol is to inhibit the metabolism of phenobarbital (Forney and Hughes, 1964).

Interactions affected by phenobarbital

Cefotaxime

High dose phenobarbital administration to children along with β-lactam antibiotics results in toxic exanthematous skin reactions in about 50% of cases (Harder *et al.*, 1990). This potentiating of antibiotic-related allergic features is particularly prevalent in children receiving phenobarbital and cefotaxime in combination. This interaction may be pharmacodynamic in nature.

Cimetidine

Phenobarbital enhances the metabolism and clearance (15%) of cimetidine (Somogyi *et al.*, 1981).

Cyclosporin

Phenobarbital can significantly enhance the metabolism of cyclosporin in a dose-dependent manner (Carstensen *et al.*, 1986; Nishioka *et al.*, 1990). Withdrawal of phenobarbital from a paediatric renal transplant patient resulted in a 70% reduction in cyclosporin clearance (Burckart *et al.*, 1984).

Dexamethasone

The administration of dexamethasone intravenously to asthmatic patients receiving phenobarbital was associated with significantly shorter dexamethasone half-life values (45%) and increased clearance (87%), when compared to values before phenobarbital administration (Brooks *et al.*, 1972).

Felodipine

The clearance of felodipine can be significantly enhanced (~9-fold) by phenobarbital co-administration (Capewell *et al.*, 1988).

Fentanyl

Phenobarbital enhances the metabolism of fentanyl and decreases its plasma concentration (Tempelhoff *et al.*, 1990).

Folic acid

As phenobarbital is a potent hepatic enzyme inducer, it enhances the metabolism of folic acid and, typically, folate concentrations can be reduced by 24% during long-term treatment (Reynolds, 1974). Consequently, folic acid supplementation is mandatory if one is to avoid adverse foetal outcome (e.g. neural tube defects) that is associated with low plasma folate concentrations (Kishi *et al.*, 1997).

Ifosfamide

A reversible toxic encephalopathy was reported in a girl with epilepsy who was taking phenobarbital. The symptoms presented after a single dose of ifosfamide/mesna and the authors concluded that it was the consequence of an interaction with phenobarbital (Ghosn *et al.*, 1988).

Itraconazole

Phenobarbital decreases plasma itraconazole concentrations (Bonay *et al.*, 1993).

Metronidazole

Phenobarbital enhances the metabolism of metronidazole resulting in significant decreases in metronidazole half-life (23%) and AUC (30%) values (Eradiri *et al.*, 1988). This drug interaction is associated with clinical failure of metronidazole treatment in women with vaginal trichomoniasis and gardiasis (Mead *et al.*, 1982; Gupte, 1983).

Methylprednisolone

The co-administration of methylprednisolone with phenobarbital results in pharmacokinetic changes to methylprednisolone, which are similar in magnitude to that described for dexamethasone (Stjernholm and Katz, 1975; Wassner *et al.*, 1976).

Nifedipine

The clearance of nifedipine can be significantly (270%) enhanced by phenobarbital co-administration (Schellens *et al.*, 1989).

Nimodipine

The clearance of nimodipine can be significantly enhanced (nine-fold) by phenobarbital co-administration (Tartara *et al.*, 1991). Thus clinically relevant reduced nimodipine efficacy can be observed.

Prednisolone

Phenobarbital enhances the metabolism of prednisolone resulting in significantly shorter (32%) prednisolone half-life values and increased (44%) clearance values. Co-administration of prednisolone with phenobarbital in patients with rheumatoid arthritis has resulted in shorter (25%) half-life values and marked worsening of clinical symptoms (Brooks, S., *et al.*, 1972; Brooks, P., *et al.*, 1976).

Teniposide

Phenobarbital co-administered with teniposide results in a two- to three-fold increase in clearance of teniposide (Baker *et al.*, 1992). The resultant reduced efficacy of teniposide (Relling *et al.*, 1994) is the consequence of induction of CYP3A4 and possibly CYP3A5 (Relling *et al.*, 2000).

Theophylline

Phenobarbital enhances (34%) the clearance of theophylline in older children and adults (Landay *et al.*, 1978; Saccar *et al.*, 1985; Yazdani *et al.*, 1987). However, in premature neonates this interaction does not occur (Kandrotas *et al.*, 1990).

Tirilazad

Phenobarbital significantly decreases plasma concentrations of tirilazad by 50–69% (Fleishaker *et al.*, 1996).

Tolbutamide

Phenobarbital increases the free fraction of tolbutamide by displacing it from plasma protein-binding sites (Fernandez *et al.*, 1985). The clinical significance of this interaction is not established.

Verapamil

The clearance of orally ingested verapamil can be enhanced five fold during combination therapy with phenobarbital. When verapamil was administered intravenously, the clearance of verapamil was enhanced two-fold (Rutledge *et al.*, 1988).

Warfarin

Co-administration of warfarin and phenobarbital results in a significant increase (~50%) in warfarin clearance and a decrease in its half-life (~40%) (Orme and Breckenridge, 1976). These changes are accompanied by a 25% reduction in prothrombin time which may persist for 3–4 weeks after phenobarbital discontinuation (Udall, 1975; Cropp and Bussey, 1997). This prolonged effect requires that patients are closely monitored.

Phenytoin

PHT is eliminated almost entirely by metabolic transformation. Metabolism is via the isoenzymes CYP2C9 and CYP2C19. PHT is an enzyme inducer (CYP2A, CYP2C and CYP3A) and has a high propensity to interact with other drugs. Plasma protein binding is 92%.

Interactions affecting phenytoin

Activated charcoal

Co-administration of activated charcoal with PHT results in reduction of PHT absorption (Welling, 1984). This interaction is used clinically to treat those patients that have overdosed with PHT.

Acyclovir

Co-administration of PHT and acyclovir may result in a reduction in PHT plasma concentrations (Permeggiani *et al.*, 1995).

Amiodarone

Amiodarone is potent inhibitor of CYP2C9. In healthy subjects, amiodarone has been observed to increase the half-life of PHT several fold (Nolan *et al.*, 1989), whilst in patients, plasma PHT concentrations have been increased two- to three-fold (McGovern *et al.*, 1984), resulting in possible PHT intoxication.

Antacids

The gastrointestinal absorption of PHT may be reduced by co-ingestion with antacids such as aluminium or magnesium hydroxides and calcium bicarbonate. This interaction is avoided if the ingestion of PHT and the antacid is separated by a few hours. Sucralfate, a complex of aluminium hydroxide and sulphated sucrose, which has minimal antacid properties but acts by protecting the mucosa from acid–pepsin attack, can similarly impede the absorption of PHT.

Antineoplastic agents

It has been reported that antineoplastic agents such as adriamycin, bleomycin, cis-platin or vinblastine can decrease plasma PHT concentrations (Bollini *et al.*, 1983; Sylvester *et al.*, 1984; Neef and de Voogd-van der Straaten, 1988). It has been reported that a young woman with epilepsy had seizures during antineoplastic therapy and that the seizures were the consequence of a reduced (37%) plasma PHT concentration (Neef and de Voogd-van der Straaten, 1988). The mechanism of this interaction may be induction of metabolism or an increased volume of distribution. In contrast, tamoxifen has been associated with increased plasma PHT concentrations and signs of PHT toxicity (Rabinowicz *et al.*, 1995).

Bishydroxycoumarin

Plasma bishydroxycoumarin concentrations can increase in some patients co-administered with PHT (Skovsted *et al.*, 1974).

Calcium channel blockers

Whilst verapamil and nifedipine have little or no effect on plasma PHT concentrations, diltiazem may cause an elevation and cause PHT intoxication in some patients (Bahls *et al.*, 1991).

Chloramphenicol

Whilst chloramphenicol may cause only modest elevations of plasma PHT concentrations in some patients, it may produce marked elevations in others (Koup, 1978; Nation *et al.*, 1990).

Cimetidine

Cimetidine inhibits the metabolism of PHT thereby increasing plasma PHT concentrations and this may result in clinical intoxication (Salem *et al.*, 1983; Phillips and Hansky, 1984; Levine *et al.*, 1985).

Disulfiram

Disulfiram inhibits the metabolism of PHT and increases its plasma concentration. This can result in signs of PHT intoxication in the majority of patients (Olesen, 1967; Levy, 1995). In healthy volunteers, disulfiram was shown to reduce PHT clearance by 30% (Svendsen *et al.*, 1976).

Ethanol

Chronic use of alcohol decreases plasma PHT concentrations, probably as a consequence of enzyme induction (Sandor *et al.*, 1981), whereas occasional moderate or heavy alcohol consumption can result in an increase in PHT plasma concentration and this can result in PHT toxicity (Kutt, 1984).

Fluconazole

Fluconazole inhibits both CYP2C9 and CYP2C19 activities and consequently would be expected to inhibit the metabolism of PHT. Indeed there are several case reports, both of healthy volunteers and patients, that describe significant increases in plasma PHT concentrations and toxicity during combination therapy with fluconazole (Howit and Oziemski, 1989; Mitchell and Holland, 1989; Blum *et al.*, 1990; Lazar and Wilner, 1990; Cadle *et al.*, 1994; Levy, 1995).

Isoniazid

PHT metabolism is inhibited by isoniazid. In patients taking isoniazid and PHT, significant PHT accumulation with consequent intoxication has been reported in 10–15% of patients (de Wolff *et al.*, 1983; Witmer and Ritschel, 1984). This interaction would be particularly prevalent in patients that exhibit slow acetylation. In the Groote Schuur Hospital, South Africa, where 74% of patients with epilepsy are taking PHT, it has been observed that ~12% of patients have plasma PHT concentrations in the toxic range because they are taking antituberculous medication of which the primary drug is isoniazid (Walubo and Aboo, 1995).

Miconazole

As miconazole is an inhibitor of CYP2C9, it inhibits the metabolism of PHT resulting in elevated plasma PHT concentrations and symptoms of PHT toxicity (Rolan *et al.*, 1983; Levy, 1995).

Omeprazole

In healthy subjects, the co-administration of omeprazole with PHT has been shown to result in a significant increase in PHT plasma concentrations (Gugler and Jensen, 1985; Prichard *et al.*, 1987).

Phenylbutazone

When PHT and phenylbutazone are co-administered, the half-life of PHT is significantly increased and this may be accompanied by clinical intoxication (Levy, 1995). The mechanism of this interaction involves the displacement of PHT from plasma albumin binding sites and a concurrent inhibition of PHT metabolism (Skovsted *et al.*, 1974). Thus, the interaction can present as an increase in the free pharmacologically active concentration of PHT in the absence of a change in the total PHT concentration. Dosage adjustment may be needed and should be based on the measurement of free PHT concentrations.

Propoxyphene

Propoxyphene inhibits the metabolism of PHT via an action on CYP2C9 (Levy, 1995). The consequent increase in plasma PHT concentrations can result in intoxication (Dam *et al.*, 1980; Kutt, 1984).

Rifampin

Rifampin may significantly increase the clearance of PHT by as much as two-fold and consequently decrease plasma PHT concentrations (Kay *et al.*, 1985). It should be noted that rifampin minimizes the inhibitory effect of isoniazid on PHT, even in patients that are slow acetylators.

Salicylates

Although salicylates can displace PHT from its plasma protein-binding site so that the unbound fraction of PHT is increased from 10% to 16%, the concurrent increase in PHT clearance makes this interaction of little clinical significance for the majority of patients (Fraser *et al.*, 1980).

Sulfonamides

Numerous bacteriostatic sulpfonamides (sufadiazine, sulfamethiazole, sulfamethoxazole and sulfaphenazole) are inhibitors of PHT metabolism and can decrease its clearance and prolong its half-life (Molhom Hansen *et al.*, 1979). Sulfaphenazole is particularly potent in this regard.

Ticlopidine

Ticlopidine is a potent CYP2C19 inhibitor. Consequently, when co-administered with PHT the clearance of PHT is decreased and PHT intoxication can occur (Privitera and Welty, 1996; Klaassen, 1998; Denahue *et al.*, 1999).

Tolbutamide

Tolbutamide displaces PHT from its plasma protein-binding sites and this can result in lower plasma PHT concentrations (Wesseling and Molsthurkow, 1975). However, as free PHT concentrations are unaffected, this interaction is not of clinical significance.

Interactions affected by phenytoin

Acetaminophen (paracetamol)

PHT enhances the metabolism of acetaminophen and reduces its plasma concentration (Nation *et al.*, 1990).

Chloramphenicol

During combination therapy with PHT and chloramphenicol, plasma chloramphenicol concentrations have been observed to decline significantly (Krasinski *et al.*, 1982).

Cyclophosphamide

It has been reported that PHT increases the clearance of both the *R*- and *S*-isomers of cyclophosphamide by 100% and 150%, respectively (Williams, M., *et al.*, 1999).

Cyclosporin

PHT significantly enhances the metabolism of cyclosporin and reduces its maximal plasma concentration as well as AUC and half-life values, resulting in a reduction of the clinical efficacy of cyclosporin (Freeman *et al.*, 1984).

Dexamethasone

The metabolism of dexamethasone is substantially enhanced by PHT, probably via enzyme induction. In one study the elimination half-life of dexamethasone was reduced from 3.5 to 1.8 h (Chalk *et al.*, 1984). In another patient study, plasma dexamethasone concentrations were reduced by 50% (Wong *et al.*, 1985).

Dicoumarol

PHT can decrease blood dicoumarol concentrations, probably via induction of metabolism (Hansen, J., *et al.*, 1971). Overall, whenever there is a change in PHT therapy (and indeed that of any other enzyme-inducing AED) it is advisable to monitor INR because all anticoagulants are associated with a narrow therapeutic ratio (Cropp and Bussey, 1997).

Digitoxin

In some patients, PHT is associated with a modest reduction in plasma digitoxin concentrations (Solomon *et al.*, 1971).

Digoxin

In healthy volunteers, PHT increased digoxin clearance by 27% and this was associated with a significant decrease in its half-life (Rameis, 1985).

Disopyramide

Although PHT enhances the metabolism of disopyramide and therefore reduces plasma disopyramide concentrations, the fact that plasma concentration of its pharmacologically active metabolite is also increased, may not necessarily result in a loss of effectiveness (Aitio *et al.*, 1981).

Doxycycline

PHT enhances the metabolism of doxycycline and decreases its plasma concentration (Neuvonen *et al.*, 1975).

Fluconazole

Plasma fluconazole concentrations are substantially reduced during co-medication with PHT probably via induction of fluconazole metabolism (Tucker *et al.*, 1992).

Folic acid

As PHT is a potent hepatic enzyme inducer, it enhances the metabolism of folic acid (Lewis *et al.*, 1995). Consequently, folic acid supplementation is mandatory if one is to avoid adverse fetal outcomes (e.g. neural tube defects) that are associated with low plasma folate concentrations (Kishi *et al.*, 1997).

Furosemide

The diuretic effect of furosemide is reduced when PHT is co-administered. The interaction is primarily due to a reduction in furosemide absorption from the alimentary tract but a pharmacodynamic interaction in the kidneys may also occur (Ahmad, 1974).

Itraconazole

In healthy volunteers, PHT has been observed to decrease itraconazole AUC values by 93% and half-life values by 83% (Tucker *et al.*, 1992; Ducharme *et al.*, 1995).

Ketoconazole

Plasma ketoconazole concentrations are substantially reduced during co-medication with PHT probably via induction of ketoconazole metabolism (Tucker *et al.*, 1992).

Methadone

Plasma methadone concentrations were decreased by ∼50% during co-medication with PHT (Tong *et al.*, 1981). In this setting patients may experience symptoms of methadone withdrawal.

Meperidine (pethidine)

During combination therapy with PHT and meperidine, the half-life of meperidine was reduced by ∼30% and the AUC of its primary metabolite was increased (Pond and Kretschzmar, 1981).

Methotrexate

PHT increases the clearance of methotrexate. This interaction has been reported to compromise the efficacy of methotrexate in the treatment of lymphoblastic leukemia in children (Relling *et al.*, 2000).

Mexiletine

In healthy volunteers, PHT increased the metabolism of mexiletine and reduced the AUC of mexiletine by 55% (Begg *et al.*, 1982).

Misonidazole

PHT enhances the metabolism of misonidazole and reduces its half-life. Therefore, lower plasma misonidazole concentrations are achieved which may serve to reduce the toxicity of misonidazole whilst not reducing its effectiveness as a therapeutic adjunct in radiation therapy (Williams, K., *et al.*, 1983).

Nisoldipine

In patients with epilepsy, PHT has been observed to significantly enhance the metabolism of nisoldipine with a mean reduction in nisoldipine AUC values of ~90% (Nation *et al.*, 1990; Michelucci *et al.*, 1996).

Praziquantel

PHT induces the metabolism of praziquantel, a drug used to treat neurocysticercosis. The interaction results in a two- to three-fold reduction in plasma praziquantel concentrations (Bittencourt *et al.*, 1992).

Prednisolone

PHT enhances the clearance of prednisolone and consequently reduces the effectiveness of this corticosteroid (Nation *et al.*, 1990).

Quinidine

PHT decreases the half-life of quinidine by 50% (Nation *et al.*, 1990).

Rocuronium

In patients taking PHT chronically, muscle relaxation after rocuronium administration was only achieved at higher doses of rocuronium and also it was necessary to administer rocuronium more frequently (Soriano *et al.*, 2000). This effect is considered to be the consequence of enzyme induction.

Teniposide

PHT induces the metabolism and enhances the clearance of teniposide and this interaction is of clinical significance (Baker *et al.*, 1992; Relling *et al.*, 2000).

Theophylline

In healthy volunteers, PHT administration (300–400 mg/day) was associated with an enhanced clearance and a 40% reduction in theophylline half-life values after intravenously administered theophylline (Jonkman and Upton, 1984; Sklar and Wagner, 1985).

Tirilazad

In healthy volunteers PHT enhanced the clearance of tirilazad by ~92% (Fleishaker *et al.*, 1998). The mechanism of this interaction is probably enzyme induction.

Vecuronium

In patients taking PHT chronically, muscle relaxation after vecuronium administration was only achieved at higher doses of vecuronium and it was necessary to administer vecuronium more frequently (Platt and Thackery, 1993). This effect is considered to be the consequence of enzyme induction.

Warfarin

The effect of PHT on warfarin is variable. Overall, the observed interaction involves a reduction in warfarin blood concentrations, via hepatic induction of warfarin metabolism. However, an increase in anticoagulant effect has been reported in some patients (Nappi, 1979). Overall, whenever there is a change in PHT therapy (and indeed that of any other enzyme-inducing AED) it is advisable to monitor INR because all anticoagulants are associated with a narrow therapeutic ratio (Cropp and Bussey, 1997).

Primidone

Primidone is metabolized to two pharmacologically active metabolites, namely phenylethylmalonamide and phenobarbital. Phenobarbital, the primary metabolite, subsequently undergoes oxidation to form *p*-hydroxyphenobarbital. Primidone, via its metabolite phenobarbital, is an enzyme inducer. Plasma protein binding of primidone is 15%. The interactions of primidone are primarily those involving phenobarbital.

Interactions affecting primidone

Acetazolamide

Acetazolamide may impair the absorption of primidone (Syverson *et al.*, 1977). Similar effects can be expected with other drugs that alter gastric pH (antacids) or motility.

Isoniazid

Isoniazid decreases the conversion of primidone to phenobarbital resulting in increased plasma primidone concentrations. The interaction is considered to be a consequence of CYP inhibition (Sutton and Kupferberg, 1975).

Nicotinamide

Nicotinamide decrease the conversion of primidone to phenobarbital resulting in increased plasma primidone concentrations. The interaction is considered to be a consequence of CYP inhibition (Bourgeois *et al.*, 1982).

Interactions affected by primidone

Folic acid

The absorption of folic acid appears to be hindered by primidone (Reynolds *et al.*, 1972).

Tiagabine

Tiagabine is extensively metabolized by CYP3A and is also extensively protein bound (98%).

As a new AED, knowledge of the interaction profile of tiagabine with non-AEDs is rather limited. Only interactions with specific drugs have been investigated.

Interactions affecting tiagabine

Cimetidine

A multiple-dose crossover study of the effect of cimetidine on the pharmaco-kinetics of tiagabine showed a small ($\sim$5%) increase in tiagabine plasma concentrations (Mengel *et al.*, 1995). This is not considered to be of clinical significance.

Erythromycin

The effect of erythromycin on the pharmacokinetics of tiagabine in 13 healthy volunteers was investigated and it was observed that erythromycin was without effect (Thompson *et al.*, 1997).

Other drugs

The effects of numerous other drugs on the pharmacokinetics of tiagabine have been investigated. Triazolam (Richens *et al.*, 1998), ethanol (Kastberg *et al.*, 1998), theophylline (Mengel *et al.*, 1995), digoxin (Snel *et al.*, 1998) or warfarin (Mengel *et al.*, 1995) showed no effect.

In vitro studies have shown that tiagabine is displaced from its protein-binding sites by the analgesics naproxen and salicylate (Brodie, 1995; Gustavson and Mengel 1995; Patsalos *et al.*, 2002). The clinical significance of these interactions is not known.

Interactions affected by tiagabine

Digoxin

Tiagabine was without effect on the pharmacokinetics of digoxin in a series of 13 healthy volunteers (Snel *et al.*, 1998).

Ethanol

Tiagabine was without effect on the pharmacokinetics of ethanol in a series of 20 healthy volunteers (Mengel *et al.*, 1995; Kastberg *et al.*, 1998).

Theophylline

Tiagabine was without effect on the pharmacokinetics of theophylline in healthy volunteers (Mengel *et al.*, 1995).

Triazolam

Tiagabine was without effect on the pharmacokinetics of triazolam in healthy volunteers (Mengel *et al.*, 1995).

Warfarin

The pharmacokinetics of warfarin are unaffected by warfarin (Mengel *et al.*, 1995).

Tiagabine does not appear to displace other highly protein-bound drugs, such as amitriptyline, tolbutamide and warfarin, from their plasma protein-binding sites (Brodie, 1995).

Topiramate

In the absence of hepatic enzyme inducers, only 40% of topiramate is metabolized, whilst in the presence of inducers this value is doubled. Although the specific CYP isoenzymes responsible for the metabolism of topiramate have not been identified, it is evident that isoenzymes induced by carbamazepine (CYP3A4) and PHT (CYP2C9 and CYP2C19) play a major role. Elimination occurs both via hepatic metabolism and renal excretion. Plasma protein binding is 10%.

As a new AED, knowledge of the interaction profile of topiramate with non-AEDs is rather limited. Only interactions with specific drugs have been investigated.

Interactions affecting topiramate

There have been no clinical studies to investigate the effect of non-AEDs on the pharmacokinetics of topiramate.

Interactions affected by topiramate

Digoxin

In a study of 12 healthy volunteers the pharmacokinetics of a single oral dose of digoxin were compared during monotherapy and in combination with topiramate (Liao and Palmer, 1993). Digoxin plasma concentrations were reduced by 16% and clearance was increased by 13% during topiramate administration when compared with administration of digoxin alone.

Valproic acid

The metabolism of valproic acid is both extensive and complex in that it involves multiple metabolic pathways, including β- and ω-oxidation, CYP2A6, CYP2C9, CYP2C19 and CYP2B6 isoenzymes and glucuronidation by UGT. To date, in excess of 25 metabolites of valproic acid have been identified. Valproic acid is 92% protein bound.

Interactions affecting valproic acid

Cholestyramine

There is a report suggesting that cholestyramine may decrease valproic acid plasma concentrations during combination therapy (Malloy *et al.*, 1996).

Cimetidine

Cimetidine inhibits the metabolism of valproic acid and increases its plasma concentrations (Webster *et al.*, 1984).

Cisplatin

It has been reported that a young woman with epilepsy presented with seizures during antineoplastic therapy and that the seizures were the consequence of a reduced valproic acid plasma concentration (Neef and de Voogd-van der Straaten, 1988). The mechanism of this interaction may be induction of metabolism or an increased volume of distribution.

Doxorubicin

Doxorubicin (adryamicin) can decrease plasma valproic acid concentrations (Neef and de Voogd-van der Straaten, 1988).

Ibuprofen

In vitro data show that ibuprofen can significantly displace valproic acid from its plasma protein-binding sites and increase the free concentration of valproic acid

(Dasgupta and Volk, 1996). The clinical significance of this interaction is not known.

Isoniazid

Isoniazid may increase valproic acid plasma concentrations resulting in clinically significant intoxication (Jonville *et al.*, 1991).

Ketoconazole

In vitro data show that ketoconazole can significantly displace valproic acid from its plasma protein-binding sites and increase the free concentration of valproic acid (Dasgupta and Luke, 1997). The clinical significance of this interaction is not known.

Mefenamic acid

In vitro data show that mefenamic acid can significantly displace valproic acid from its plasma protein-binding sites and increase the free concentration of valproic acid (Dasgupta and Volk, 1996). The clinical significance of this interaction is not known.

Methotrexate

Methotrexate significantly decreases (75%) plasma valproic acid concentrations (Schroder and Ostergaard, 1999).

Naproxen

In vitro data show that naproxen can significantly displace valproic acid from its plasma protein-binding sites and increase the free concentration of valproic acid (Dasgupta and Volk, 1996). The clinical significance of this interaction is not known.

Rifampicin

Rifampicin enhances the metabolism of valproic acid and its clearance can increase by 40%.

Salicylic acid

Salicylic acid displaces valproic acid from its protein-binding sites on albumin and consequently higher unbound concentrations occur (Fleitman *et al.*, 1980; Abbott *et al.*, 1986). In addition, salicylic acid inhibits the metabolism of valproic acid (Schobben *et al.*, 1978; Goulden *et al.*, 1987). The combination of these two effects can result in elevated valproic acid plasma concentrations and consequent toxicity.

Tolbutamide

Tolbutamide can displace valproic acid from its plasma protein-binding sites and increase the free concentration of valproic acid (Fernandez *et al.*, 1985). The clinical significance of this interaction is not known.

Tolmetin

In vitro data show that tolmetin can significantly displace valproic acid from its plasma protein-binding sites and increase the free concentration of valproic acid (Dasgupta and Volk, 1996). The clinical significance of this interaction is not known.

Interactions affected by valproic acid

Warfarin

Valproic acid can displace warfarin from its plasma protein-binding sites but this is not considered to be of clinical significance (Panjehshahin *et al.*, 1991).

Zidovudine

The clearance of zidovudine is significantly reduced by valproic acid resulting in elevated plasma (Lertora *et al.*, 1993) and cerebrospinal fluid concentrations (Akula *et al.*, 1997). The probable mechanism of this effect is by inhibition of zidovudine glucuronidation (Lertora *et al.*, 1993).

Vigabatrin

Vigabatrin is not metabolized and is exclusively eliminated as unchanged vigabatrin in urine. It is not protein bound. Consequently vigabatrin should have little propensity to interact with other drugs and indeed this is the case.

As a new AED, knowledge of the interaction profile of vigabatrin with non-AEDs is rather limited. Only interactions with specific drugs have been investigated.

Interactions affecting vigabatrin

To date there have been no reports of non-AEDs affecting the pharmacokinetics of vigabatrin.

Interactions affected by vigabatrin

To date there have been no reports of vigabatrin affecting the pharmacokinetics of non-AEDs.

Zonisamide

Zonisamide undergoes extensive metabolism, via CYP3A4, and approximately 30% of zonisamide is excreted in urine as unchanged zonisamide. Plasma protein binding is 50%.

As a new AED, knowledge of the interaction profile of zonisamide with non-AEDs is rather limited. Only interactions with specific drugs have been investigated.

Interactions affecting zonisamide

Sulfonamides

In vitro studies show that sulpfonamides can readily displace zonisamide from its binding to erythrocytes (Matsumoto *et al.*, 1989) but not from albumin (Matsumoto *et al.*, 1983). The clinical significance of this interaction is not known.

Other drugs

In vitro studies have shown that the metabolism of zonisamide is inhibited in descending order of potency by ketoconazole, cyclosporin, dihydroergotamine, itraconazole, miconazole, triazolam and fluconazole (Sugihara *et al.*, 1996). The clinical significance of these interactions is not known.

Interactions affected by zonisamide

To date there are no reports of zonisamide affecting the pharmacokinetics of non-AEDs.

REFERENCES

Abbott FS, Kassam J, Orr JM, *et al*. The effect of aspirin on valproic acid metabolism. *Clin Pharmacol Ther* 1986; **40**: 94–100.

Abernethy DR, Greenblatt DJ, Morse DS, *et al*. Interaction of propoxyphene with diazepam, alprazolam and lorazepam. *Br J Clin Pharmacol* 1985; **19**: 51–57.

Ahmad S. Renal insensitivity to furosemide caused by chronic anticonvulsant therapy. *Br Med J* 1974; **3**: 657–659.

Aitio ML, Mansbury L, Tala E, *et al*. The effect of enzyme induction on the metabolism of disopyramide in man. *Br J Clin Pharmacol* 1981; **11**: 279–286.

Akula SK, Rege AB, Dreisbach AW, *et al*. Valproic acid increases cerebrospinal fluid zidovudine levels in a patient with AIDS. *Am Med Sci* 1997; **313**: 244–246.

Albani F, Riva R, Baruzzi A. Clarithromycin–carbamazepine interaction: a case report. *Epilepsia* 1993; **34**: 161–162.

Albin H, Vincan G, Pehourcq F, *et al*. Influence of josamycin treatment on carbamazepine kinetics (in French). *Therapie* 1982; **37**: 151–156.

Alvarez JS, Del Castillo JAS, Ortiz MJA. Effect of carbamazepine on cyclosporin blood level. *Nephron* 1991; **58**: 235–236.

Amabeoku GJ, Chikuni O, Akino C, *et al.* Pharmacokinetic interaction of single doses of quinine and carbamazepine, phenobarbitone and phenytoin in healthy volunteers. *East Afr Med J* 1993; **70**: 90–93.

Babany G, Larrey D, Pessayre D. Macrolide antibiotics as inducers and inhibitors of cytochrome P450 in experimental animals and man. *Prog Drug Metab* 1988; **11**: 61–98.

Bachmann KA, Jauregui L. Use of simple clearance estimates of cytochrome P450 substrates to characterize human hepatic CYP status in vivo. *Xenobiotica* 1993; **3**: 307–315.

Bahls FH, Ozuma J, Ritchie DE. Interactions between calcium channel blockers and anticonvulsants carbamazepine and phenytoin. *Neurology* 1991; **41**: 470–472.

Baker DK, Relling MV, Pui CH, *et al.* Increased teniposide clearance with concomitant anticonvulsant therapy. *J Clin Oncol* 1992; **10**: 311–315.

Baruzzi A, Albani F, Riva R. Oxcarbazepine: pharmacokinetic interactions and their clinical relevance. *Epilepsia* 1994; **35**(Suppl. 3): S14–S19.

Barzaghi N, Gatti G, Crema F, *et al.* Effect of flurithromycin, a new macrolide antibiotic, on carbamazepine disposition in normal subjects. *Int J Clin Pharmacol Res* 1988; **8**: 101–105.

Begg EJ, Chinwah PM, Webb C, *et al.* Enhanced metabolism of mexiletine after phenytoin administration. *Br J Clin Pharmacol* 1982; **14**: 219–223.

Berg MJ, Berlinder WG, Goldberg MJ, *et al.* Acceleration of the body clearance of phenobarbital by oral activated charcoal. *New Engl J Med* 1982; **307**: 642–644.

Berg MJ, Rose JQ, Wurster DE, *et al.* Effect of charcoal and corbitol–charcoal suspension on the elimination of intravenous phenobarbital. *Ther Drug Monit* 1987; **9**: 41–47.

Bergendal L, Friberg A, Schaffrath AM, *et al.* The clinical relevance of the interaction between carbamazepine and dextropropoxyphene in elderly patients in Gothenburg, Sweden. *Eur J Clin Pharmacol* 1997; **53**: 203–206.

Bittencourt PRM, Gracia CM, Martins R, *et al.* Phenytoin and carbamazepine decrease oral bioavailability of praziquantel. *Neurology* 1992; **42**: 492–496.

Block SH. Carbamazepine-isoniazid interaction. *Paediatrics* 1982; **69**: 494–495.

Blum RA, Wilton JH, Hilligross DM, *et al.* Effect of fluconazole on disposition of phenytoin. *Clin Pharmacol Ther* 1990; **47**: 182.

Bollini P, Riva R, Albani F, *et al.* Decreased phenytoin level during antineoplastic therapy: a case report. *Epilepsia* 1983; **24**: 75–78.

Bonay M, Jonville-Bera AP, Diot P, *et al.* Possible interaction between phenobarbital, carbamazepine and itraconazole. *Drug Saf* 1993; **9**: 309–311.

Bourgeois BF, Dodson WE, Ferrendelli JA. Interactions between primidone, carbamazepine and nicotinamide. *Neurology* 1982; **32**: 1122–1126.

Brodie MJ. Tiagabine pharmacology in profile. *Epilepsia* 1995; **36**(Suppl. 6): S7–S9.

Brodie MJ, MacPhee GJ. Carbamazepine neurotoxicity precipitated by diltiazem. *Br Med J* 1986; **292**: 1170–1171.

Brooks S, Werk E, Ackerman S, *et al.* Adverse effects of phenobarbital on corticosteroid metabolism in patients with bronchial asthma. *New Engl J Med* 1972; **286**: 1125–1128.

Brooks P, Buchanan W, Grove M, *et al*. Effects of enzyme induction on metabolism of prednisolone: clinical and laboratory study. *Ann Rheum Dis* 1976; **35**: 339–343.

Brown RI, Cooper TG. Ticlopidine–carbamazepine interaction in a coronary stent patient. *Can J Cardiol* 1997; **13**: 853–854.

Burckart G, Venkataramanan R, Starzl T, *et al*. Cyclosporin clearance in children following organ transplantation. *J Clin Pharmacol* 1984; **24**: 412.

Burman W, Orr L. Carbamazepine toxicity after starting combination antiretroviral therapy including ritonavir and efavirenz. *AIDS* 2000; **14**: 2793–2794.

Busch JA, Radulovic LI, Bockbrader HN, *et al*. Effect of Maalox TC on single-dose pharmacokinetics of gabapentin capsules in healthy subjects. *Pharm Res* 1992; **9**(Suppl. 10): S315.

Cadle RM, Zenon III GJ, Rodriguez-Barradas MC, *et al*. Fluconazole-induced symptomatic phenytoin toxicity. *Ann Pharmacother* 1994; **28**: 191–195.

Capewell S, Freestone S, Critchley J, *et al*. Reduced felodipine bioavailability in patients taking anticonvulsants. *Lancet* 1988; 480–482.

Carstensen H, Jacobsen N, Dieperink H. Interaction between cyclosporin A and phenobarbitone. *Br J Clin Pharmacol* 1986; **21**: 550–551.

Chalk JB, Ridgeway K, Brophy T, *et al*. Phenytoin impairs the bioavailability of dexamethasone in neurological and neurosurgical patients. *J Neurol Neurosurg Psychiatr* 1984; **47**: 1087–1090.

Coniglia AA, Garnett WR, Pellock JH, *et al*. Effect of acute and chronic terfenadine on free and total serum concentration in epileptic patients. *Epilepsia* 1989; **30**: 611–616.

Cooney GF, Mochon M, Kaiser B, *et al*. Effects of carbamazepine on cyclosporine metabolism in pediatric renal transplant recipients. *Pharmacotherapy* 1995; **15**: 353–356.

Couet W, Istin B, Ingrand I, *et al*. Effect of ponsinomycin on single-dose kinetics and metabolism of carbamazepine. *Ther Drug Monit* 1990; **12**: 144–149.

Cropp JS, Bussey HJ. A review of enzyme induction of warfarin metabolism with recommendations for patient management. *Pharmacotherapy* 1997; **17**: 917–928.

Dalton MJ, Powell JR, Messenheimer Jr JA, *et al*. Cimetidine and carbamazepine: a complex drug interaction. *Epilepsia* 1986; **27**: 553–558.

Dam M, Christensen J. Interaction of propoxyphene with carbamazepine. *Lancet* 1977; **2**: 509.

Dam M, Christensen JM, Brandt J, *et al*. Antiepileptic drugs: interaction with dextropropoxyphene. In *Antiepileptic Therapy: Advances in Drug monitoring*. S. I. Johannessen, P. L. Morselli, C. E. Pippenger, *et al.*, eds. New York: Raven Press, 1980: 299–304.

Dasgupta A, Luke M. Valproic acid–ketoconazole interaction in normal, hypoalbuminemic, and uremic sera: lack of interaction in uremic serum caused by the presence of inhibitor. *Ther Drug Monit* 1997; **19**: 281–285.

Dasgupta A, Volk A. Displacement of valproic acid and carbamazepine from protein binding in normal and uremic sera by tolmetin, ibuprofen, and naproxen: presence of inhibitor in uremic serum that blocks valproic acid–naproxen interactions. *Ther Drug Monit* 1996; **18**: 284–287.

Denahue S, Flockart DA, Albernethy DR. Ticlopidine inhibits phenytoin clearance. *Clin Pharmacol Ther* 1999; **66**: 563–568.

Depot M, Powell JR, Messenheimer Jr JA, *et al*. Kinetic effects of multiple oral doses of acetaminophen on a single oral dose of lamotrigine. *Clin Pharmacol Ther* 1990; **48**: 346–355.

de Wolff F, Vermeij P, Ferrari MD, *et al.* Impairment of phenytoin parahydroxylation as a cause of severe intoxication. *Ther Drug Monit* 1983; **5**: 213–215.

Ducharme MP, Slaughter RL, Warbasse LH. Itraconazole and hydroxyitraconazole serum concentrations are reduced more than tenfold by phenytoin. *Clin Pharmacol Ther* 1995; **58**: 617–624.

Ebert U, Thong NQ, Oertel R, *et al.* Effects of rifampicin and cimetidine on pharmacokinetics and pharmacodynamics of lamotrigine in healthy subjects. *Eur J Clin Pharmacol* 2000; **56**: 299–304.

Eimer M, Carter BL. Elevated serum carbamazepine concentrations following diltiazem initiation. *Drug Intel Clin Pharm* 1987; **21**: 340–342.

Eradiri O, Jamali F, Thomson A. Interaction of metronidazole with phenobarbital, cimetidine, prednisone, and sulfasalazine in Crohn's disease. *Biopharm Drug Dispos* 1988; **9**: 219–227.

Feierman DE, Lasker JM. Metabolism of fentanyl, a synthetic opioid analgesic, by human liver microsomes: role of CYP3A4. *Drug Metab Dispos* 1996; **24**: 932–939.

Fernandez MC, Erill S, Lucena MI, *et al.* Serum protein binding of tolbutamide in patients treated with antiepileptic drugs. *Clin Pharmacokin* 1985; **10**: 451–455.

Fleishaker JC, Pearson LK, Peters GR. Gender does not affect the degree of induction of tirilazad clearance by phenobarbital. *Eur J Clin Pharmacol* 1996; **50**: 139–145.

Fleishaker JC, Pearson LK, Peters GR. Induction of tirilazad clearance by phenytoin. Biopharm *Drug Dispos* 1998; **19**: 91–96.

Fleitman JS, Bruni J, Perrin JH, *et al.* Albumin-binding interactions of sodium valproate. *J Clin Pharmacol* 1980; **20**: 514–517.

Flockart DA, Tanus-Santos JE. Implications of cytochrome P450 interactions when prescribing medication for hypotension. *Arch Intern Med* 2002; **162**: 405–412.

Forney RB, Hughes FW. Meprobamate, ethanol or meprobamate–ethanol combinations on performance of human subjects under delayed autofeedback (DAF). *J Psychol* 1964; **57**: 431–436.

Fraser DG, Ludden TM, Evens RP, *et al.* Displacement of phenytoin from plasma binding sites by salicylate. *Clin Pharmacol Ther* 1980; **27**: 165–169.

Freedman MD, Olatidoye AG. Clinically significant drug interactions with anticoagulants. *Drug Saf* 1994; **10**: 381–394.

Freeman DJ, Laupacis A, Keown A, *et al.* Evaluation of cyclosporin and phenytoin interaction with observations on cyclosporin metabolites. *Br J Clin Pharmacol* 1984; **18**: 887–893.

Frenia ML, Schauben JL, Wears RL, *et al.* Multiple-dose activated charcoal compared to urinary alkalinization for the enhancement of phenobarbital elimination. *J Toxicol Clin Toxicol* 1996; **34**: 169–175.

Garcia BA, Latorre IA, Porta EJ, *et al.* Protease inhibitor-induced carbamazepine toxicity. *Clin Neuropharmacol* 2000; **23**(4): 216–218.

Ghosn M, Carde P, Leclerq B, *et al.* Ifosfamide/mesna related encephalopathy: a case report with a possible role of phenobarbital in enhancing neurotoxicity. *Bull Cancer* 1988; **75**: 391–392.

Glue P, Banfield CR, Perhach JL, *et al.* Pharmacokinetic interactions with felbamate: in vitro–in vivo correlation. *Clin Pharmacokinet* 1997; **33**: 214–223.

Goulden KI, Dooley IM, Camfield PR, *et al.* Clinical valproate toxicity induced by acetylsalicylic acid. *Neurology* 1987; **37**: 1392–1394.

Gugler R, Jensen JC. Omeprazole inhibits oxidative drug metabolism. *Gastroenterology* 1985; **89**: 1235–1241.

Gupte S. Phenobarbital and metabolism of metronidazole. *New Engl J Med* 1983; **308**: 529.

Gustavson LE, Mengel HB. Pharmacokinetics of tiagabine; a γ-aminobutyric acid-uptake inhibitor, in healthy subjects after single and multiple doses. *Epilepsia* 1995; **36**: 605–611.

Hansen BS, Dam M, Brandt J, *et al*. Influence of dextropropoxyphene on steady state serum levels and protein binding of three anti-epileptic drugs in man. *Acta Neurol Scand* 1980; **61**: 357–367.

Hansen JJM, Siersbaek-Nielsen K, Kristensen M, *et al*. Effect of diphenylhydantoin on the metabolism of dicoumarol in man. *Acta Med Scand* 1971; **189**: 15–19.

Harder S, Schneider W, Bae ZU, *et al*. Undesirable drug reactions in simultaneous administration of high-dosage phenobarbital and beta-lactam antibiotics. *Klinische Padiatrie* 1990; **202**: 404–407.

Hayden M, Buchanan N. Danazol–carbamazepine interaction (Letter). *Med J Aust* 1991; **155**: 851.

Howitt KM, Oziemski MA. Phenytoin toxicity induced by fluconazole. *Med J Aust* 1989; **151**: 603–604.

Hugen PW, Burger DM, Brinkman K, *et al*. Carbamazepine–indinavir interaction causes antiretroviral therapy failure. *Ann Pharmacother* 2000; **34**(4): 465–470.

Jonkman JHG, Upton RA. Pharmacokinetic drug interactions with theophylline. *Clin Pharmacokinet* 1984; **9**: 309–334.

Jonville AP, Gauchez AS, Autret E, *et al*. Interaction between isoniazid and valproate: a case of valproate overdosage. *Eur J Clin Pharmacol* 1991; **40**: 197–198.

Kandrotas R, Cranfield T, Gal P, *et al*. Effect of phenobarbital administration on theophylline clearance in premature neonates. *Ther Drug Monit* 1990; **12**: 139–143.

Kastberg H, Jansen JA, Cole G, *et al*. Tiagabine: absence of kinetic or dynamic interactions with ethanol. *Drug Metabol Drug Interact* 1998; **14**: 259–273.

Kato Y, Fujii T, Mizoguchi N, *et al*. Potential interaction between ritonavir and carbamazepine. *Pharmacotherapy* 2000; **20**: 851–854.

Kay L, Kampmann JP, Svendsen TL, *et al*. Influence of rifampin and isoniazid on the kinetics of phenytoin. *Br J Clin Pharmacol* 1985; **20**: 323–326.

Keränen T, Jolkkonen J, Jensen PK, *et al*. Absence of interaction between oxcarbazepine and erythromycin. *Acta Neurol Scand* 1992a; **86**: 20–23.

Keränen T, Jolkkonen J, Klosterskov Jensen P, *et al*. Oxcarbazepine does not interact with cimetidine in healthy volunteers. *Acta Neurol Scand* 1992b; **85**: 239–242.

Kishi T, Fujita N, Eguchi T, *et al*. Mechanism for reduction of serum folate by antiepileptic drugs during prolonged therapy. *J Neurol Sci* 1997; **145**: 109–112.

Klaassen SL. Ticlopidine-induced phenytoin toxicity. *Ann Pharmacother* 1998; **32**: 1295–1298.

Koup JR. Interaction of chloramphenicol with phenytoin and phenobarbital: a case report. *Clin Pharmacol Ther* 1978; **24**: 571–575.

Koup JR, Gibaldi M, McNamara P, *et al*. Interaction of chloramphenicol with phenytoin and phenobarbital. *Clin Pharmacol Ther* 1978; **24**: 571–575.

Krämer G, Theisohn M, von Unruh GE, *et al*. Carbamazepine–danazol drug interaction: its mechanism examined by a stable isotope technique. *Ther Drug Monit* 1986; **8**: 387–392.

Krämer G, Tettenborn B, Flesch G. Oxcarbazepine–verapamil drug interaction in healthy volunteers. *Epilepsia* 1991; **32**(Suppl. 1): S70–S71.

Krämer G, Tettenborn B, Klosterskov Jensen P, *et al*. Oxcarbazepine does not affect the anticoagulant activity of warfarin. *Epilepsia* 1992; **33**: 1145–1148.

Krasinski K, Kusmiesz M, Nelson JD. Pharmacologic interactions among chloramphenicol, phenytoin and phenobarbital. *Pediat Infect Dis* 1982; **1**: 232–235.

Kroemer HK, Gautier JC, Beaune P, *et al.* Identification of P450 enzymes involved in metabolism of verapamil in humans. *Naunyn Schmiedebergs Arch Pharmacol* 1993; **348**: 332–337.

Kunze KL, Wienkers LC, Thummel KE, *et al.* Warfarin-fluconazole: I. Inhibition of the human cytochrome P450-dependent metabolism of warfarin by fluconazole: in vitro studies. *Drug Metab Dispos* 1996; **24**: 414–421.

Kutt H. Interactions between anticonvulsants and other commonly prescribed drugs. *Epilepsia* 1984; **25**(Suppl. 2): S118–S131.

Landay R, Gonzalez M, Taylor J. Effect of phenobarbital on theophylline disposition. *J Aller Clin Immunol* 1978; **62**: 27–29.

Lazar JD, Wilner KD. Drug interactions with fluconazole. *Rev Infect Dis* 1990; **12**: S327–S333.

Lertora JJ, Greenspan DL, Rege AB, *et al.* Valproic acid inhibits glucuronidation of zidovudine (AZT) in HIV-infected patients. *Clin Pharmacol Ther* 1993; **53**: 197.

Levine M, Jones MW, Sheppard I. Differential effect of cimetidine on serum concentrations of carbamazepine and phenytoin. *Neurology* 1985; **35**: 562–565.

Levy RH. Cytochrome P450 isozymes and antiepileptic drug interactions. *Epilepsia* 1995; **36**(Suppl. 5): S8–S13.

Levy RH, Ragueneau-Majlessi I, Baltes E. Repeated administration of the novel antiepileptic agent levetiracetam does not alter digoxin pharmacokinetics and pharmacodynamics in healthy volunteers. *Epilepsia* 2001; **46**: 93–99.

Lewis DP, Van Dyke DC, Willhite LA, *et al.* Phenytoin–folic acid interactions. *Ann Pharmacother* 1995; **29**: 726–735.

Liao S, Palmer M. Digoxin and topiramate drug interaction study in male volunteers. *Pharm Res* 1993; **10**(Suppl. 1): S405.

MacPhee GJ, McInnes GT, Thompson GG, *et al.* Verapamil potentiates carbamazepine neurotoxicity: a clinically important inhibitory interaction. *Lancet* 1986; **1**: 700–703.

Majkowski J. Carbamazepine and erythromycin interaction resulting in myoclonic seizures in epileptic patients. Case report. *Epileptologia* 1995; **3**: 57–62.

Malloy MJ, Ravis WR, Pennell AT, *et al.* Effect of cholestyramine resin on single dose valproate pharmacokinetics. *Int J Clin Pharmacol Ther* 1996; **34**: 208–211.

Maoz E, Grossman E, Thaler M, *et al.* Carbamazepine neurotoxic reaction after administration of diltiazem. *Arch Intern Med* 1992; **152**: 2503–2504.

Mateu-de Antonio J, Grau S, Gimeno-Bayon JL, *et al.* Ritonavir induced carbamazepine toxicity. *Ann Pharmacother* 2001; **35**: 125–126.

Matsumoto K, Miyazaki H, Fujii T, *et al.* Absorption, distribution and excretion of 3-(sulfamoyl[^{14}C]methyl)-1,2-benzisoxazole (AD-810) in rats, dogs and monkeys and of AD-810 in men. *Arzneimittelforschung* 1983; **33**: 961–968.

Matsumoto K, Miyazaki H, Fujii T, *et al.* Binding of sulfonamides to erythrocyte proteins and possible drug–drug interaction. *Chem Pharm Bull (Tokyo)* 1989; **37**: 2807–2810.

Mattson RH, Gallagher BB, Reynolds EH, *et al.* Folate therapy in epilepsy: a controlled study. *Arch Neurol* 1973; **29**: 78–81.

McGovern B, Geer VR, Laraia PJ, *et al*. Possible interaction between amiodarone and phenytoin. *Ann Intern Med* 1984; **101**: 650–651.

Mead P, Gibson M, Schentag J, *et al*. Possible alteration of metronidazole metabolism by phenobarbital. *New Engl J Med* 1982; **306**.

Mengel H, Jansen JA, Sommerville KW, *et al*. Tiagabine evaluation of the risk of interaction with theophylline, warfarin, digoxin, cimetidine, oral contraceptives, traizolam, or ethanol. *Epilepsia* 1995; **36**(Suppl. 3): S160.

Mesdjian E, Dravet C, Cenraud B, *et al*. Carbamazepine intoxication due to triacetyloleandomycin administration in epileptic patients. *Epilepsia* 1980; **21**: 489–496.

Michelucci R, Cipolla G, Passarelli D, *et al*. Reduced plasma nisoldipine concentrations in phenytoin-treated patients with epilepsy. *Epilepsia* 1996; **37**: 1107–1110.

Mitchell AS, Holland JT. Fluconazole and phenytoin: a predictable interaction. *Br Med J* 1989; **298**: 1315.

Mogensen PH, Jorgensen L, Boas J, *et al*. Effects of dextropropoxyphene on the steady-state kinetics of oxcarbazepine and its metabolites. *Acta Neurol Scand* 1992; **85**: 14–17.

Molholm Hansen J, Kampmann JP, Siersbaek-Nielsen K, *et al*. The effect of different sulfonamides on phenytoin metabolism in man. *Acta Med Scand* 1979; **624**(Suppl. 1): S106–S110.

Nair DR, Morris HH. Potential fluconazole-induced carbamazepine toxicity. *Ann Pharmacother* 1999; **33**: 790–792.

Nappi J. Warfarin and phenytoin interaction. *Ann Intern Med* 1979; **90**: 852.

Nation RL, Evans AM, Milne RW. Pharmacokinetic interactions with phenytoin. *Clin Pharmacokinet* 1990; **18**: 37–60.

Neef C, de Voogd-van der Straaten I. An interaction between cytostatic and anticonvulsant drugs. *Clin Pharmacol Therapeut* 1988; **43**: 372–375.

Neuvonen PJ, Elonen E. Effect of activated charcoal on absorption and elimination of phenobarbitone, carbamazepine and phenylbutazone in man. *Eur J Clin Pharrnacol* 1980; **17**: 51–57.

Neuvonen PJ, Penttila O, Lehtovaara R, *et al*. Effects of antiepileptic drugs on the elimination of various tetracycline derivatives. *Eur J Clin Pharmacol* 1975; **9**: 147–154.

Nishioka T, Ikegami M, Imanishi M, *et al*. Interaction between phenobarbital and ciclosporin following renal transplantation: a case report. *Hinyokikia Kiyo Acta Urol Jap* 1990; **36**: 447–450.

Nolan PE, Marcus FI, Hoyer GL, *et al*. Pharmacokinetic interaction between intravenous phenytoin and amiodarone in healthy volunteers. *Clin Pharmacol Ther* 1989; **46**: 43–50.

O'Connor NK, Fris J. Clarithromycin–carbamazepine interaction in a clinical setting. *Am Board Family Pract* 1994; **7**: 489–492.

Odishaw J, Chen C. Effects of steady-state bupropion on the pharmacokinetics of lamotrigine in healthy subjects. *Pharmacotherapy* 2000; **20**: 1448–1453.

Olesen OV. The influence of disulfiram and calcium carbamide on the serum diphenylhydantoin. *Arch Neurol* 1967; **16**: 642–644.

Orme M, Breckenridge A. Enantiomers of warfarin and phenobarbital. *New Engl J Med* 1976; **295**: 1482.

Panjehshahin MR, Bowmer CJ, Yates MS. Effect of valproic acid, its unsaturated metabolites and some structurally related fatty acids on the binding of warfarin and dansylsarcosine to human albumin. *Biochem Pharmacol* 1991; **41**: 1227–1233.

Patsalos PN. Pharmacokinetic profile of levetiracetam: toward ideal characteristics *Pharmacol Ther* 2000; **85**: 77–85.

Patsalos PN, Duncan JS. Antiepileptic drugs: a review of clinically significant drug interactions. *Drug Saf* 1993; **9**: 156–184.

Patsalos PN, Elyas AA, Ratnaraj N, *et al.* Concentration-dependent displacement of tiagabine by valproic acid. *Epilepsia* 2002; **43**(Suppl. 8): S143.

Patsalos PN, Froscher W, Pisani F, *et al.* The importance of drug interactions in epilepsy therapy. *Epilepsia* 2002; **43**: 365–385.

Patsalos PN, Perucca E. Clinically important interactions in epilepsy: general features and interactions between antiepilepticdrugs. *Lancet Neurol* 2003a; **2**: 347–356.

Patsalos PN, Perucca E. Clinically important interactions in epilepsy: interactions between antiepileptic drugs and other drugs. *Lancet Neurol* 2003b; **2**: 473–481.

Patterson BD. Possible interaction between metronidazole and carbamazepine. *Ann Pharmacother* 1994; **28**: 1303–1304.

Penttila O, Neuvonen PJ, Aho K, *et al.* Interaction between doxycycline and some antiepileptic drugs. *Br Med J* 1974; **2**: 470–472.

Periti P, Mazzei T, Mini E, *et al.* Pharmacokinetic drug interactions of macrolides. *Clin Pharmacokinet* 1992; **23**: 106–131.

Permeggiani A, Riva R, Posar A, *et al.* Possible interaction between acyclovir and antiepileptic treatment. *Ther Drug Monit* 1995; **17**: 312–315.

Pessayre D, Larrey D, Funck-Brentano C, *et al.* Drug interactions and hepatitis produced by some macrolide antibiotics. *J Antimicrob Chemother* 1985; **16**(Suppl. A): S181–S194.

Phillips P, Hansky J. Phenytoin toxicity secondary to cimetidine administration. *Med J Aust* 1984; **141**: 602.

Platt PR, Thackery NM. Phenytoin-induced resistance to vecuronium. *Anesth Intens Care* 1993; **21**: 185–191.

Pond SM, Kretschzmar KM. Effect of phenytoin on meperidine clearance and normeperidine formation. *Clin Pharmacol Ther* 1981; **30**: 680–686.

Posner J, Webster H, Yuen AWC. Investigation of the ability of lamotrigine, a novel antiepileptic drug, to induce mixed function oxygenase enzymes. *Br J Clin Pharmacol* 1991; **32**: 658.

Prichard PJ, Walt RP, Kitchingman GK, *et al.* Oral phenytoin pharmacokinetics during omeprazole therapy. *Br J Clin Pharmacol* 1987; **24**: 543–545.

Principi N, Espasito S. Comparative tolerability of erythromycin and newer macrolide antibacterials in paediatric patients. *Drug Saf* 1999; **20**: 25–41.

Privitera M, Welty TE. Acute phenytoin toxicity followed by seizure breakthrough from a ticlopidine–phenytoin interaction. *Arch Neurol* 1996; **53**: 1191–1192.

Rabinowicz AL, Hinton DR, Dyck P, *et al.* High-dose tamoxifen in treatment of brain tumours: interaction with antiepileptic drugs. *Epilepsia* 1995; **36**: 513–515.

Ragueneau-Majlessi I, Levy RH, Meyerhoff C. Lack of effect of repeated administration of levetiracetam on the pharmacodynamics and pharmacokinetic profile of warfarin. *Epilepsy Res* 2001; **47**: 55–63.

Rameis H. On the interaction between phenytoin and digoxin. *Eur J Clin Pharmacol* 1985; **29**: 49–53.

Relling MV, Nemec J, Schuetz EG, *et al.* O-demethylation of epipodophyllotoxins is catalyzed by human cytochrome P450 3A4. *Mol Pharmacol* 1994; **45**: 352–358.

Relling MV, Pui CH, Sandlund JT, *et al.* Adverse effect of anticonvulsants on efficacy of chemotherapy for acute lymphoblastic leukaemia. *Lancet* 2000; **356**: 285–290.

Rettie AE, Korzekwa KR, Kunze KL, *et al.* Hydroxylation of warfarin by human cDNA-expressed cytochrome P-450; a role for P-4502C9 in the etiology of (S)-warfarin–drug interactions. *Chem Res Toxicol* 1992; **5**: 54–59.

Reynolds EH. Chronic antiepileptic toxicity: a review. *Epilepsia* 1974; **16**: 319–352.

Reynolds EH, Mattson RH, Gallagher BB. Relationship between serum and cerebrospinal fluid anticonvulsant drug and folic acid concentrations in epileptic patients. *Neurology* 1972; **22**: 841–844.

Richens A, Marshall RW, Dirach J. Absence of interaction between tiagabine, a new antiepileptic drug, and the benzodiazepine triazolam. *Drug Metabol Drug Interact* 1998; **14**: 159–177.

Roe TF, Podosin RL, Blaskovics ME. Drug interaction: diazoxide and diphenylhydantoin. *J Pediatr* 1975; **87**: 480–484.

Rolan PE, Somogy AA, Drew MR, *et al.* Phenytoin intoxication during treatment with parenteral miconazole. *Br Med J* 1983; **287**: 1760.

Rutledge DR, Pieper JA, Mirvis DM. Effects of chronic phenobarbital on verapamil disposition in humans. *J Pharmacol Exp Ther* 1988; **246**: 7–13.

Saccar C, Danish M, Ragni M, *et al.* The effect of phenobarbital on theophylline disposition in children with asthma. *J Allergy Clin Immunol* 1985; **75**: 716–719.

Saint-Salvi B, Tremblay D, Surjus A, *et al.* A study of the interaction of roxithromycin with theophylline and carbamazepine. *J Antimicrob Chemother* 1987; **20**(Suppl. B): S121–S129.

Salem RB, Breland BD, Mishra SK, *et al.* Effect of cimetidine on phenytoin serum level. *Epilepsia* 1983; **24**: 284–288.

Sandor P, Sellers EM, Dumbell M, *et al.* Effect of long and short term alcohol on phenytoin kinetics in chronic alcoholics. *Clin Pharmacol Ther* 1981; **30**: 390–397.

Sands BF, Knapp CM, Ciraulo DA. Medical consequences of alcohol–drug interactions. *Alcohol Health Res World* 1993; **17**(4): 316–320.

Schellens JH, van der Wart JH, Brugman M, *et al.* Influence of enzyme induction and inhibition on the oxidation of nifedipine, sparteine, mephenytoin and antipyrine in humans as assessed by a "cocktail" study design. *J Pharmacol Exp Ther* 1989; **249**: 638–645.

Schlienger R, Kurmann ML, Drewe J, *et al.* Inhibition of phenprocoumon anticoagulation by carbamazepine. *Eur Neuropsychopharmacol* 2000; **10**: 219–221.

Schroder H, Ostergaard JR. Interference of high-dose methotrexate in the metabolism of valproate? *Pediatr Hematol* 1994; **11**: 445–449.

Schobben F, Vree TB, van der Kleijn D. Pharmacokinetics, metabolism and distribution of 2-N-propyl pentanoate (sodium valproate) and the influence of salicylate comedication. In *Advances in Epileptology*. H. Meinardi, A. J. Rowan, eds. Amsterdam: Swets & Zeitlinger, 1978: 271–277.

Sklar SJ, Wagner JC. Enhanced theophylline clearance secondary to phenytoin therapy. *Drug Intell Clin Pharm* 1985; **19**: 34–36.

Skovsted L, Hansen JM, Kristensen M, *et al.* Inhibition of drug metabolism in man. In *Drug Interactions*. P. L. Morselli, S. Garattini, S. N. Cohen, eds. New York: Raven Press, 1974: 81–90.

Snel S, Jansen JA, Pedersen PC, *et al.* Tiagabine, a novel antiepileptic agent: lack of pharmacokinetic interaction with digoxin. *Eur J Clin Pharmacol* 1998; **54**: 355–357.

Solomon HM, Reich S, Spirt N, *et al.* Interaction between digitoxin and other drugs in vitro and in vivo. *Ann NY Acad Sci* 1971; **79**: 362–369.

Somogyi A, Thielscher S, Gugler R. Influence of phenobarbital on cimetidine kinetics. *Eur J Clin Pharmacol* 1981; **19**: 343–347.

Soriano SG, Kaus SJ, Sullivan LJ, *et al.* Onset and duration of action of rocuronium in children receiving chronic anticonvulsant therapy. *Pediatr Anaesth* 2000; **10**: 133–136.

Spina E, Pisani F, Perucca E. Clinically significant pharmacokinetic drug interactions with carbamazepine: an update. *Clin Pharmacokinet* 1996; **31**: 198–214.

Spina E, Arena D, Scordo MG, *et al.* Elevation of plasma carbamazepine concentrations by ketoconazole in patients with epilepsy. *Ther Drug Monit* 1997; **19**: 535–538.

Stjernholm M, Katz F. Effects of diphenylhydantoin, phenobarbital, and diazepam on the metabolism of methylprednisolone and its sodium succinate. *J Clin Endocrinol Metab* 1975; **41**: 887–893.

Sugihara K, Kitamura S, Tatsumi K. Involvement of mammalian liver cytosols and aldehyde oxidase in reductive metabolism of zonisamide. *Drug Metab Dispos* 1996; **24**: 199–202.

Sutton G, Kupferberg HJ. Isoniazid as an inhibitor of primidone metabolism. *Neurology* 1975; **25**: 1179–1181.

Svendsen TL, Kristensen M, Hansen JM, *et al.* The influence of disulfiram on the half-life and metabolic clearance rate of diphenylhydantoin and tolbutamide in man. *Eur J Clin Pharmacol* 1976; **9**: 439–441.

Sylvester RK, Lewis FB, Caldwell KC, *et al.* Impaired phenytoin bioavailability secondary to cisplatinum, vinblastin and bleomycine. *Ther Drug Monit* 1984; **6**: 302–305.

Syverson GB, Morgan JP, Weintraub M, *et al.* Acetazolamide-induced interference with primidone absorption. *Arch Neurol* 1977; **34**: 80–84.

Tartara A, Galimberti CA, Manni R, *et al.* Differential effects of valproic acid and enzyme-inducing anticonvulsants on nimodipine pharmacokinetics in epileptic patients. *Br J Clin Pharmacol* 1991; **32**: 335–340.

Tecoma ES. Oxcarbazepine. *Epilepsia* 1999; **40**(Suppl. 5): S37–S46.

Tempelhoff R, Modica PA, Spitznagel EL. Anticonvulsant therapy increases fentanyl requirements during anaesthesia for craniotomy. *Can J Anaesth* 1990; **37**: 327–332.

Thompson MS, Groes L, Schwietert HR, *et al.* An open label sequence listed two period crossover pharmacokinetic trials evaluating the possible interaction between tiagabine and erythromycin during multiple administration to healthy volunteers. *Epilepsia* 1997; **38**(Suppl. 3): S64.

Tong TG, Pond SM, Kreek MJ, *et al.* Phenytoin induced methadone withdrawal. *Ann Intern Med* 1981; **94**: 349–351.

Tracy TS, Korzekwa KR, Gonzalez FJ, *et al.* Cytochrome P450 isoforms involved in metabolism of the enantiomers of verapamil and norverapamil. *Br J Clin Pharmacol* 1999; **47**: 545–552.

Tucker RM, Denning DW, Hanson LH, *et al.* Interaction of azoles with rifampin, phenytoin, and carbamazepine: in vitro and clinical observation. *Clin Infect Dis* 1992; **14**: 165–174.

Udall J. Clinical implications of warfarin interactions with five sedatives. *Am J Cardiol* 1975; **35**: 67–71.

Valsalan VC, Cooper GL. Carbamazepine intoxication caused by interaction with isoniazid. *Br Med J* 1982; **285**: 261–262.

Van Wieringen A, Vrijlandt CM. Ethosuximide intoxication caused by interaction with isoniazid. *Neurology* 1983; **33**: 1227–1228.

Villikka K, Kivisto KT, Maenpaa H, *et al.* Cytochrome P450-inducing antiepileptics increase the clearance of vincristine in patients with brain tumors. *Clin Pharmacol Ther* 1999; **66**: 589–593.

Vincon G, Albin H, Demotes-Mainard F, *et al.* Effects of josamycin on carbamazepine kinetics. *Eur J Clin Pharmacol* 1987; **32**: 321–323.

von Moltke LL, Durol AL, Duan SX, *et al.* Potent mechanism based inhibition of human CYP3A in vitro by amprenavir and ritonavir: comparison with ketoconazole. *Eur J Clin Pharmacol* 2000; **56**: 259–261.

Wakabayashi Y, Maruyama S, Hachimura K, *et al.* Activated charcoal interrupts enterohepatic circulation of phenobarbital. *J Toxicol Clin Toxicol* 1994; **32**: 419–424.

Walubo A, Aboo A. Phenytoin toxicity, due to concomitant antituberculosis therapy. *South Afr Med J* 1995; **85**: 1175–1176.

Wassner S, Pennisi A, Malekzadeh M, *et al.* The adverse effect of anticonvulsant therapy on renal allograft survival: a preliminary report. *J Pediatr* 1976; **88**: 134–137.

Webster LK, Michaly GW, Jones DB. Effect of cimetidine and ranitidine on carbamazepine and sodium valproate pharmacokinetics. *Eur J Clin Pharmacol* 1984; **27**: 341–343.

Welling PG. Interactions affecting drug absorption. *Clin Pharmacokinet* 1984; **9**: 404–434.

Wesseling H, Molsthurkow I. Interaction of diphenylhydantoin (DPH) and tolbutamide in man. *Eur J Clin Pharmacol* 1975; **8**: 75–78.

Williams K, Begg E, Wade D, *et al.* Effects of phenytoin, phenobarbital and ascorbic acid on misonidazole elimination. *Clin Pharmacol Ther* 1983; **33**: 314–321.

Williams ML, Wainer IW, Embree L, *et al.* Enantioselective induction of cyclophosphamide metabolism by phenytoin. *Chirality* 1999; **11**: 569–574.

Witmer DR, Ritschel WA. Phenytoin and isoniazid interaction: a kinetic approach to management. *Drug Intell Clin Pharm* 1984; **18**: 483–486.

Wong DD, Longenecer RG, Liepman M, *et al.* Phenytoin–dexamethasone: a possible drug–drug interaction. *J Am Med Assos* 1985; **254**: 2062–2063.

Wright JM, Stokes EF, Sweeney VP. Isoniazid-induced carbamazepine toxicity and vice versa: a double drug interaction. *New Engl J Med* 1982; **307**: 1325–1327.

Yasui N, Otani K, Kaneko S. Carbamazepine toxicity induced by clarithromycin coadministration in psychiatric patients. *Intern Clin Psychopharmacol* 1997; **12**: 225–229.

Yazdani M, Kissling GE, Tran TH. Phenobarbital increases the theophylline requirement of premature infants being treated of apnea. *Am J Dis Child* 1987; **141**: 97–99.

Zaccara G, Gangemi PF, Bendoni L, *et al.* Influence of single and repeated doses of oxcarbazepine on the pharmacokinetic profile of felodipine. *Ther Drug Monit* 1993; **15**: 39–42.

Zielinski JJ, Lichten EM, Haidukewych D. Clinically significant danazol–carbamazepine interaction. *Ther Drug Monit* 1987; **9**: 24–27.

Part III

Pharmacodynamic interactions

9

Pharmacodynamic principles and mechanisms of drug interactions

Blaise F. D. Bourgeois

Harvard Medical School, Division of Epilepsy and Clinical Neurophysiology, Children's Hospital, Boston, MA, USA

Distinction between pharmacodynamic and pharmacokinetic drug interactions

The term pharmacokinetics refers to mostly quantitative assessments of what happens to a drug in the body following its administration by any route. The processes that are assessed include absorption into the blood, serum protein binding, distribution into various tissues or compartments, biotransformation, and elimination from the body. The drug can be eliminated unchanged through the kidneys or in the form of a conjugate or metabolite following conjugation or enzymatic biotransformation in the liver. Metabolites can be eliminated through the kidneys or through the bile. Pharmacokinetics rely on measurements of drug concentrations in various body fluids or tissues (in practice mostly in the blood, urine, or saliva) and assessments of changes in these concentrations over time. The clinical relevance of pharmacokinetics is based on the fact that optimal treatment with a drug requires achieving and maintaining certain levels in the target organs, and corresponding levels in the blood.

The term pharmacodynamics refers to qualitative and quantitative assessments of all possible effects of a drug in various organs of the body. These effects may include:

1 one or more desirable therapeutic effects (e.g. seizure reduction, prevention of migraine headaches or a positive psychotropic effect);
2 one or more undesirable/harmful adverse effects (e.g. sedation or an allergic reaction);
3 side effects that may be either desirable or undesirable (e.g. weight loss);
4 side effects that are neither desirable nor undesirable (e.g. elevation of gamma-glutamyl transpeptidase (gamma-GT), lowering of bilirubin levels).

Some desirable and undesirable pharmacodynamic drug effects can be assessed quantitatively (e.g. seizure reduction, excessive weight gain, and hyponatremia), some can be assessed semi-quantitatively (e.g. decreased seizure severity, sedation or gum hypertrophy), and some can virtually not be assessed quantitatively (mostly idiosyncratic reactions). Obviously, pharmacodynamics are more complex and more difficult to assess than pharmacokinetics. Also, since many pharmacodynamic effects of drugs are related to concentrations, pharmacodynamic observations may be influenced by pharmacokinetics. However, pharmacodynamics have no influence on pharmacokinetics, with the exception of hepatic enzyme induction and inhibition.

Based on the above concepts, there is a fundamental difference between pharmacokinetic and pharmacodynamic interactions. Pharmacokinetic interactions consist of alterations in the concentration of a drug that are caused by the presence of another drug in the body. This may include competition for absorption, displacement from protein-binding sites, enzymatic induction, enzymatic inhibition, or competition for renal excretion. Pharmacokinetic interactions are relatively easy to assess quantitatively. They are mostly undesirable but, when they are known, they can be anticipated and corrected. Any pair of drugs may or may not have pharmacokinetic interactions.

Pharmacodynamic interactions consist of the quantitative or qualitative alterations of any effect of a drug on any organ when these alterations are caused by the presence of another drug in the body. Pharmacodynamic interactions are much more difficult to assess quantitatively. They can be desirable (enhancement of a therapeutic effect or reduction of an adverse effect) or undesirable (enhancement of an adverse effect or reduction of a therapeutic effect). However, even when they are known and predicted, pharmacodynamic interactions cannot be influenced, corrected, or avoided. By altering drug concentrations, pharmacokinetic interactions may cause apparent pharmacodynamic interactions in the absence of a true pharmacodynamic interaction. However, pharmacodynamic interactions will never cause an apparent pharmacokinetic interaction.

Types of pharmacodynamic interaction

In order for two drugs to have a pharmacodynamic interaction, they have to share at least one common pharmacodynamic property or, more specifically, they have to share an identifiable clinical effect. Just as pharmacokinetic interactions may result in a drug concentration that is greater or smaller than expected, a pharmacodynamic interaction may result in a measurable response that is greater or smaller than expected. In general, it is assumed that each drug alone could elicit that response to some extent. However, it is conceivable that a specific effect of a drug could be enhanced or inhibited by another drug that does not have that particular effect by itself, even in the absence of a pharmacokinetic interaction. Nevertheless, for most pairs of drugs that do not share a common effect, the

Table 9.1 Basic pharmacodynamic interactions

Additive	$C = A + B$
Supra-additive	$C > A + B$
Infra-additive	$C < A + B$
Indifferent	$C = A$ and/or B

A, effect of drug A alone; B, effect of drug B alone;
C, combined effect of drugs A and B administered together;
A + B, expected sum of individual effects of drugs A and B.

pharmacodynamic interaction will be absent or indifferent. For instance, in the absence of a pharmacokinetic interaction, an antiepileptic drug (AED) is unlikely at any dose to alter the antimicrobial effect of an antibiotic, and an antibiotic is unlikely to alter the seizure protection provided by an AED. Of course, if that antibiotic is known to lower the seizure threshold by itself, it could diminish the seizure protection provided by the AED and this would represent a pharmacodynamic interaction.

The various types of pharmacodynamic interaction are listed in Table 9.1. If the combined effect C of drug A and B administered together corresponds to the expected sum of the effects of drug A alone and drug B alone, the interaction is said to be additive. If the combined effect is greater than the expected sum, the interaction is said to be supra-additive. A supra-additive effect is also called potentiation and the terms can be considered to be synonymous. The term synergism is used by some synonymously with a supra-additive effect, but it has been argued that synergism means literally that drugs just work together. Therefore, the term synergism should be used preferably for any type of pharmacodynamic interaction that is not indifferent. When the combined effect of two drugs is greater than that of each drug alone at the same concentration, but less than the expected sum of the two actions, the pharmacodynamic interaction is said to be infra-additive. As there is no other reason why a drug should be less effective in combination than when it is given alone, this type of pharmacodynamic interaction is also called antagonistic. This implies that at least one of the two drugs somehow decreases the effectiveness of the other. Antagonism may exist between two drugs with a common pharmacological effect and, of course, between two drugs with an opposite pharmacological effect (for instance elevation and lowering of the seizure threshold).

These definitions raise one obvious question: what is the expected sum of the effects of two drugs that are administered together and how is it determined? The difficulty of quantifying individual and combined drug actions is the main reason why pharmacodynamic interactions are much more difficult to assess than the pharmacokinetic interactions. For most AEDs the relationship between dose and level is linear, such as the relationship between single dose and peak level, or

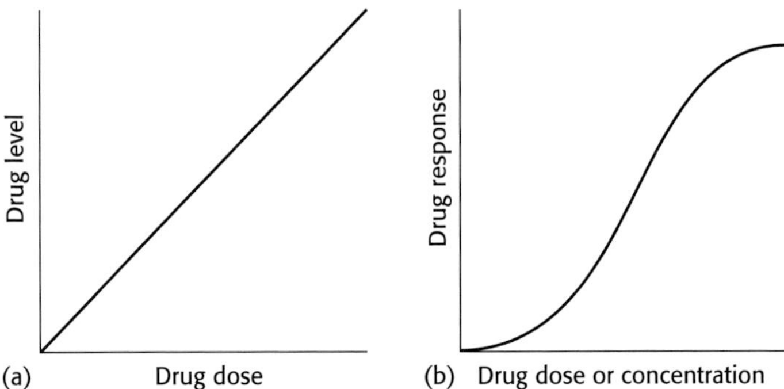

Figure 9.1   Relationship between (a) drug dose and drug level and (b) drug dose or drug concentration and the magnitude of response to the drug

between maintenance dose and steady-state level (the main exception to this rule is phenytoin). If the administered dose is doubled, this will result in a level that is twice as high. In contrast, the magnitude of the response to a drug as a function of its dose or of its concentration usually follows a sigmoid curve (see Figure 9.1). Therefore, at twice the dose or level of drug A, the magnitude of the response is not twice as high. It may be less or it may be greater. Similarly, the magnitude of the response to combined doses of two drugs that produce the same effect individually will not be twice the magnitude of the individual effect. These issues will be addressed in detail in the next chapter devoted to the methods for assessing pharmacodynamic interactions.

Clinical significance of pharmacodynamic interactions

Whenever a patient takes two or more medications simultaneously, there is the potential for some type of pharmacodynamic interaction. If, in the absence of a pharmacokinetic interaction, any clinical response to one of the drugs is enhanced or reduced by another drug, a pharmacodynamic interaction can be assumed. For the desirable primary effect of either drug, and for the desirable and undesirable secondary effect of either drug, the interaction can be additive, supra-additive or infra-additive. The clinical spectrum of possible pharmacodynamic interactions is summarized in Table 9.2:

1 The common primary therapeutic effect of two drugs can be enhanced when they are administered together. An obvious example would be further seizure reduction when a second AED is added to the first.
2 A common adverse effect of two drugs can be enhanced when they are administered together. An example would be increased sedation when a second potentially sedative AED is added to the first.

Table 9.2 Clinical spectrum of pharmacodynamic interactions

1 Enhancement of common (primary) therapeutic effect
2 Enhancement of common adverse effect
3 Reduction of or less than additive common therapeutic effect
4 Reduction of or less than additive common adverse effect
5 Enhancement of a therapeutic effect that is not shared by the drugs
6 Enhancement of an adverse effect that is not shared by the drugs
7 Reduction of a therapeutic effect that is not shared by the drugs
8 Reduction of an adverse effect that is not shared by the drugs

3 The common primary therapeutic effect can be reduced, or less than additive, when two drugs are administered together. An example would be a lack of further seizure reduction, or even an increase in seizure frequency, when two AEDs are administered together, compared with each one administered alone.

4 A common adverse effect of two drugs can be reduced, or less than additive, when they are administered together. For example, there may be no increase in sedation when a second potentially sedative AED is added to the first.

5 The therapeutic effect of a drug could be enhanced by a drug that does not by itself possess this property. For instance, the seizure protection by an AED could be enhanced by adding another drug for which no antiepileptic efficacy has been demonstrated.

6 Inversely, an adverse effect of a drug could be enhanced by the addition of a second drug that does not by itself cause this adverse effect. For instance, the incidence of liver failure could be higher when a drug is combined with other drugs that do not cause liver failure.

7 The therapeutic effect of a drug can be reduced after the addition of a second drug that does not share this therapeutic effect or that has an opposite effect. For example, the seizure frequency can increase when an AED is combined with a drug that potentially can lower the seizure threshold, such as certain psychoactive drugs.

8 Finally, an adverse effect of a drug can be reduced by the addition of a drug that does not share this side effect, or that has an opposite effect. For example, the sedative effect of an AED could be reduced after the addition of a psychostimulant.

Whenever two or more drugs are taken simultaneously by a patient, more than one pharmacodynamic interaction may occur, and any combination of the interactions listed in Table 9.3 is possible. Whether or not a drug combination is therapeutically more desirable than the individual drugs taken alone will ultimately not depend on a single pharmacodynamic interaction between the drugs, but on the ultimate clinical result of all the pharmacodynamic interactions that exist between the drugs.

Table 9.3 Desirable and undesirable pharmacodynamic interactions

Potential advantages of drug combinations
Better effectiveness (higher-therapeutic index)
Milder or absent (subthreshold) side effects
Broader spectrum of seizure control

Potential disadvantages of drug combinations
Potentiation of side effects (lower-therapeutic index) or more, different
   side effects
Idiosyncratic toxicity
Seizure exacerbation

Desirable and undesirable pharmacodynamic interactions

Desirable interactions

Potential clinical advantages and disadvantages of drug combinations over single drug therapy are listed in Table 9.3. Although enhancement of the primary therapeutic efficacy seems to be the obvious pharmacodynamic interaction that will render a particular drug combination desirable, other considerations will have to be included in order to take into account clinical realities. For instance, in the treatment of epilepsy, further seizure reduction could be achieved by increasing the dose of an AED in monotherapy. However, even if the efficacy of the drug continues to increase as its dose is increased, there will come a point when the patient will no longer tolerate a further dosage increase because of dose-related adverse effects. The maximal tolerated dose is an easily defined clinical therapeutic endpoint. The clinical value of a drug will be determined not only by its efficacy, but also by its tolerability. This relationship between efficacy and tolerability can be expressed as the therapeutic index (for instance the ratio between toxic dose and therapeutic dose). It can also be expressed as clinical effectiveness, which reflects both efficacy and tolerability (Deckers *et al.*, 2000). If a drug is more efficacious at a high dose but not tolerated, it will not be more effective at a higher dose. These considerations that apply to increases in the dosage of a single drug also apply to the addition of a second drug. In order for a combination of two drugs to be more desirable than either drug taken alone, the combination has to be more effective than either drug alone. In other words, either the combination provides better seizure protection at the maximal tolerated dose, or it is better tolerated at the same level of seizure protection than either drug alone. In both cases, the combination can be said to be more effective or to have a better therapeutic index. Whether or not this is the case for a certain combination of two drugs will depend on the ultimate result of all possible pharmacodynamic interactions that occur between the two drugs. Specifically, this may be the case if the common therapeutic effect (for instance seizure protection) is supra-additive and the dose-related adverse effects are additive or infra-additive, or if the therapeutic effect is additive and the dose-related adverse effects are infra-additive. If, however, the therapeutic effect and the adverse effects are both supra-additive, or both additive, the combination is unlikely to be clinically more effective than either drug taken alone.

A drug combination could be superior to either drug used alone by causing milder side effects or no side effects, even if the actual seizure protection is not better. The reason is that all AEDs share an antiepileptic effect, whereas they do not share all of their adverse effects. In addition, many side effects are dose related and may occur only once a certain dosage threshold is attained. When two AEDs are combined, a certain degree of seizure protection could be achieved at a dose of both drugs that is below their individual threshold for this specific side effect. That same degree of seizure protection with either drug alone might require a dose that is above their threshold dose. This represents a concept that is opposite to the widespread concept of high-dose monotherapy, namely low-dose polytherapy. For example, a patient may become seizure free on valproate, but only at a dose that causes thrombocytopenia and tremor. In the same patient, topiramate alone may then fully control the seizures, but only at a dose that causes undesired weight loss or word finding difficulties. It is conceivable that this patient's seizures might be controlled on valproate and topiramate in combination at lower doses that cause none of these side effects. This concept of low-dose polytherapy is supported by the literature analysis of Deckers *et al.* (1997). These authors concluded that it is the total drug load of a patient that determines the number of adverse effects, and not just the number of AEDs that the patient is taking (see section 'Undesirable interactions').

An obvious potential advantage of combining AEDs is a broadening of the spectrum of activity. This applies only to patients who have more than one seizure type and in whom no single drug is fully effective against all seizure types and also well tolerated. For example, in patients with juvenile myoclonic epilepsy, the generalized tonic–clonic seizures might come under full control with either valproate, lamotrigine or topiramate, but the myoclonic seizures may persist. Inversely, clonazepam has been shown to be more effective against the myoclonic seizures than against the generalized tonic–clonic seizures in patients with juvenile myoclonic epilepsy (Obeid and Panayiotopoulos, 1989). In some patients, only a combination of clonazepam with one of the above three drugs may provide full control of the generalized tonic–clonic and the myoclonic seizures.

Undesirable interactions

There can be little doubt that one of the main disadvantages of antiepileptic combination therapy is an increase in the intensity or the number of side effects. In general, decreasing the number of AEDs will be associated with a decrease in side effects. This decrease in side effects involves a reduction in their severity, in their number, or both. Several studies have suggested that a reduction in the number of AEDs reduces the overall occurrence of side effects, in particular the sedative effects and the dose-related neurological side effects in general (Fischbacher, 1982; Bennett *et al.*, 1983; Schmidt, 1983; Theodore and Porter, 1983; Albright and Bruni, 1985; Pellock and Hunt, 1996). Interestingly, there was little or no increase in seizure frequency among the patients enrolled in these studies, and a reduction in seizures was actually not uncommon. When patients undergoing a temporal lobe resection were randomized to ongoing polytherapy or reduction to carbamazepine monotherapy, the seizure recurrence rate was the same for both groups, but side effects were more common in the polytherapy group (30%) than in the monotherapy group (10%). Also, controlled monotherapy trials with some of the newer AEDs have shown lower incidence of side effects than for the same drug in add-on trials.

Deckers *et al.* (1997) studied the relationship between AED polytherapy and adverse effects by analyzing published data from a literature review. They introduced a concept that they called total AED load. This concept is based on the ratio PDD/DDD, or prescribed daily dose (PDD) divided by the usual or defined daily dose (DDD). The total antiepileptic load in a patient is then calculated as the sum of the PDD/DDD ratios for all AEDs taken by the patient. For instance, if a patient takes 1.5 times the usual dose of two different AEDs, that patient's total drug load is three, whereas a patient taking the usual dose of one drug has a total drug load of one. This type of analysis takes into account not only the number of drugs taken by a patient, but also the total relative dosage of these drugs. In 15 selected articles, the authors found a relationship between total drug load and number of adverse effects, but they found no relationship between just the number of AEDs prescribed and these adverse effects. This finding was later confirmed in a randomized study (Deckers *et al.*, 2001). In this study, 130 adult patients with untreated generalized tonic–clonic and/or partial seizures were randomized to equal drug loads of monotherapy with carbamazepine, 400 mg/day, or combination therapy with carbamazepine 200 mg/day and valproate 300 mg/day. The study was designed to detect differences in neurotoxicity, and no such difference was found between the two groups. There was also no difference in efficacy, but this was not the primary outcome variable.

In addition to the dose-related central nervous system side effects of AEDs, there is no doubt that eliminating drugs from the regimen will eliminate the various individual and specific side effects of those drugs that are discontinued, such as excessive weight gain or tremor from valproate, behavioural problems from levetiracetam, or cognitive impairment from topiramate.

Exacerbation of side effects by combination therapy is not limited to central nervous system toxicity of AEDs. For instance, ammonia levels following a first dose of valproate were significantly higher than baseline in patients treated with phenobarbital, phenytoin, or both, whereas ammonia levels did not differ from baseline in patients receiving no other medication (Zaccara *et al.*, 1985). Also, the rates of fatality from valproate hepatotoxicity have been found to be substantially higher in polytherapy than in monotherapy for all age groups (Bryant and Dreifuss, 1996). In patients less than 3 years old, the rate was 1 in 618 on polytherapy, whereas there was no death in this age group among 4533 patients on monotherapy. For all ages, the rate of death was 6–7 times higher on polytherapy than on monotherapy.

At times, combining two AEDs may increase the likelihood of an idiosyncratic toxic reaction. For instance, treatment with valproate can be associated with an acute encephalopathy characterized by a change in mental status that can evolve to stupor or coma, as well as by seizure exacerbation (Sackellares *et al.*, 1979; Marescaux *et al.*, 1982). It has been shown that this encephalopathic reaction to valproate is more likely to occur in the presence of another AED, and it is invariably reversible after valproate is discontinued. This reaction can also subside after another AED is removed from the drug regimen, although that drug itself may never have been associated with such an encephalopathic reaction (Sackellares *et al.*, 1979; Marescaux *et al.*, 1982).

Antiepileptic combination therapy can at times cause seizure exacerbation. As mentioned above, a reduction in the number of AEDs has been at times found to be associated with a decrease rather than an increase in seizure frequency. Besides a spontaneous fluctuation, there are possible explanations for this observation:

(a) *Seizure aggravation by AEDs, paradoxical intoxication.* There is a growing body of literature supporting the notion that certain drugs can cause or aggravate certain seizures in certain types of epilepsy. This is particularly common in generalized epilepsies. For instance, carbamazepine can cause or aggravate absence seizures (Snead and Hosey *et al.*, 1985; Liporace *et al.*, 1994), myoclonic seizures (Shield and Saslow, 1983), seizures in patients with Lennox–Gastaut syndrome or with benign rolandic epilepsy (Corda *et al.*, 2001). It can also aggravate or cause de novo generalized spike-wave discharges in the electroencephalogram (EEG) (Talwar *et al.*, 1994). In patients with juvenile myoclonic epilepsy, myoclonic seizures have been shown to be potentially exacerbated by carbamazepine and phenytoin (Genton *et al.*, 2000), and by lamotrigine (Biraben *et al.*, 2000). In the Lennox–Gastaut syndrome, certain seizures can be aggravated by carbamazepine, phenytoin, gabapentin, vigabatrin, benzodiazepines and lamotrigine (Guerrini *et al.*, 1999). In patients with severe myoclonic epilepsy of infancy (Dravet syndrome), seizure aggravation was reported with carbamazepine, lamotrigine and vigabatrin (Guerrini *et al.*, 1998). The higher the number of AEDs taken by a patient, the more likely it is that one of them may actually be exacerbating certain seizures and that its elimination might lead to improved seizure control.

(b) *Pharmacodynamic antagonism.* Whenever a patient takes two or more AEDs, there is a pharmacodynamic interaction. In relation to seizure protection, this interaction can be purely additive, it can be supra-additive (this represents potentiation), or it can be infra-additive (this represents antagonism). In case of antagonism, one drug actually prevents or decreases the efficacy of the other drug. There is experimental and clinical evidence suggesting that antagonism may exist between AEDs. In an animal model, the combined seizure protection provided by carbamazepine and lamotrigine was found to be infra-additive (Czuczwar, S. J., personal communication, 2002). In a study of the efficacy of vigabatrin in children with infantile spasms (Elterman *et al.*, 2001), the efficacy of vigabatrin was reduced in patients taking valproate and in those taking carbamazepine, and it was even lower in those taking valproate and carbamazepine (Shields, W. D., personal communication, 2002). Based on such evidence, it is conceivable that removing an AED involved in an antagonistic antiepileptic pharmacodynamic interaction will result in improved seizure control.

Clinical relevance of pharmacodynamic interactions: monotherapy versus combination therapy

There has been a shift in practice regarding the treatment of epilepsy with drug combinations or with one drug alone. After decades during which patients were treated with multiple drugs, monotherapy has been considered to be the gold standard for over 20 years (Deckers *et al.*, 2001). More recently, the concept of rational polytherapy has been proposed and debated. The clinical significance of pharmacodynamic interactions and their advantages and disadvantages have been discussed in detail earlier in this chapter. There are three potential advantages of combination drug therapy:

1 better seizure control with similar or fewer side effects,
2 same seizure control with fewer side effects,
3 reduction of two or more different seizure types that respond only to different drugs.

Clinical studies of pharmacodynamic interactions between AEDs are discussed in Chapter 13. There is a paucity of clinical studies documenting the superiority of specific AED combinations. Whether or not to use combination therapy and the selection of a combination will often have to be based on an educated guess or on careful clinical observations in each individual patient (Meinardi, 1995). Considerations may include the mechanism of action of the drugs, the clinical spectrum of activity, and potential pharmacokinetic interactions. It has been suggested that drugs to be combined should have different mechanisms of action which would be complementary (Perucca, 1995; Macdonald, 1996). Although elegant, this hypothesis has never been proven experimentally or clinically. A literature review of data in animals and in humans was used to determine whether appropriate AED combinations can be selected on the basis of their mechanism of action (Deckers *et al.*, 2000). There was some evidence that efficacy could be enhanced by combining a sodium channel blocker with a drug enhancing GABAergic inhibition, or by combining two gamma amino butyric acid (GABA) mimetic drugs, or by combining an alpha-amino-3-hydroxy-5-methyl-4-isoxazolepropionic acid (AMPA) antagonist with an *N*-methyl-D-aspartate (NMDA) antagonist. At the present time, the basis for choosing a drug combination based on the mechanisms of actions is purely hypothetical and no specific combination can be recommended. When a patient has two or more different seizure types that cannot be controlled by one drug alone, two drugs can be selected according to their spectrum of efficacy. Although the absence of pharmacokinetic interactions between two drugs will certainly make it easier and safer to use them together, the interactions are known and predictable, and therefore largely correctable. Therefore, pharmacokinetic interactions should not be a reason to avoid a potentially beneficial drug combination. Finally, as discussed earlier, there are arguments in favor of the concept of low-dose polytherapy as opposed to the common practice of high-dose monotherapy. The rationale for this concept is that AEDs share an antiepileptic effect, but do not necessarily share their side effects.

In conclusion, rational polytherapy can rarely be predicted. In any given patient, a rational AED combination will have been identified if the patient does better in terms of seizure control versus side effects while taking drugs A and B together (at any doses) than the patient had done on drug A alone and on drug B alone at their respective optimal doses. There may be instances in which it would be appropriate to maintain a drug combination beyond the above definition. For instance, a patient may respond partially to a first drug and may experience further improvement after addition of a second drug, or the patient becomes seizure free after addition of the second drug, despite lack of response to the first drug. It is understandable in such a case that the patient and the physician may be reluctant to make any change.

REFERENCES

Albright P, Bruni J. Reduction of polytherapy in epileptic patients. *Arch Neurol* 1985; **42**: 797–799.

Bennett HS, Dunlop T, Ziring P. Reduction of polypharmacy for epilepsy in an institution for the retarded. *Dev Med Child Neurol* 1983; **25**: 735–737.

Biraben A, Allain H, Scarabin JM, *et al*. Exacerbation of juvenile myoclonic epilepsy with lamotrigine. *Neurology* 2000; **55**: 1758.

Bryant III AE, Dreifuss FE. Valproic acid hepatic fatalities. III. U.S. experience since 1986. *Neurology* 1996; **46**: 465–469.

Corda D, Gelisse P, Genton P, *et al.* Incidence of drug-induced aggravation in benign epilepsy with centrotemporal spikes. *Epilepsia* 2001; **42**: 754–759.

Deckers CL, Hekster YA, Keyser A, *et al.* Reappraisal of polytherapy in epilepsy: a critical review of drug load and adverse effects. *Epilepsia* 1997; **38**(5): 570–575.

Deckers CL, Czuczwar SJ, Hekster YA, *et al.* Selection of antiepileptic drug polytherapy based on mechanisms of action: the evidence reviewed. *Epilepsia* 2000; **41**: 1364–1374.

Deckers CL, Hekster YA, Keyser A, *et al.* Monotherapy versus polytherapy for epilepsy: a multicenter double-blind randomized study. *Epilepsia* 2001; **42**: 1387–1394.

Elterman RD, Shields WD, Mansfield KA, *et al.* Randomized trial of vigabatrin in patients with infantile spasms. *Neurology* 2001; **57**: 1416–1421.

Fischbacher E. Effect of reduction of anticonvulsants on wellbeing. *Br Med J* 1982; **285**: 423–424.

Genton P, Gelisse P, Thomas P, *et al.* Do carbamazepine and phenytoin aggravate juvenile myoclonic epilepsy? *Neurology* 2000; **55**: 1106–1109.

Guerrini R, Belmonte A, Genton P. Antiepileptic drug-induced worsening of seizures in children. *Epilepsia* 1998; **39**: S2–S10.

Guerrini R, Belmonte A, Parmeggiani L, *et al.* Myoclonic status epilepticus following high-dosage lamotrigine therapy. *Brain Dev* 1999; **21**: 420–424.

Liporace JD, Sperling MR, Dichter MA. Absence seizures and carbamazepine in adults. *Epilepsia* 1994; **35**: 1026–1028.

Macdonald R. Is there a mechanistic basis for rational polypharmacy? *Epilepsy Res* 1996; **11**: 79–93.

Marescaux C, Warter JM, Micheletti G, *et al.* Stuporous episodes during treatment with sodium valproate: report of seven cases. *Epilepsia* 1982; **23**: 297–305.

Meinardi H. Use of combined antiepileptic drug therapy. In *Antiepileptic Drugs*, 4th edn. R. H. Levy, R. H. Mattson, B. S. Meldrum, eds. New York: Raven Press, 1995: 91–97.

Obeid T, Panayiotopoulos CP. Clonazepam in juvenile myoclonic epilepsy. *Epilepsia* 1989; **30**: 603–606.

Pellock JM, Hunt PA. A decade of modern epilepsy therapy in institutionalized mentally retarded patients. *Epilepsy Res* 1996; **25**(3): 263–268.

Perucca E. Pharmacological principles as a basis for polytherapy. *Acta Neurol Scand* 1995; **162**(Suppl.): 31–34.

Sackellares JC, Lee SI, Dreifuss FE. Stupor following administration of valproic acid to patients receiving other antiepileptic drugs. *Epilepsia* 1979; **20**: 697–703.

Schmidt D. Reduction of two-drug therapy in intractable epilepsy. *Epilepsia* 1983; **24**: 368–376.

Shield WD, Saslow E. Myoclonic, atonic, and absence seizures following institution of carbamazepine therapy in children. *Neurology* 1983; **33**: 1487–1489.

Snead OC, Hosey LC. Exacerbation of seizures in children by carbamazepine. *New Engl J Med* 1985; **313**: 916–921.

Talwar D, Arora MS, Sher PK. EEG changes and seizure exacerbation in young children treated with carbamazepine. *Epilepsia* 1994; **35**: 1154–1159.

Theodore WH, Porter RJ. Removal of sedative-hypnotic antiepileptic drugs from the regimen of patients with intractable epilepsy. *Ann Neurol* 1983; **13**: 320–324.

Zaccara G, Paganini M, Campostrini R, *et al.* Effect of associated antiepileptic treatment on valproate-induced hyperammonemia. *Ther Drug Monit* 1985; **7**: 185–190.

10

Methods for assessing pharmacodynamic interactions

Blaise F. D. Bourgeois

Harvard Medical School, Division of Epilepsy and Clinical Neurophysiology, Children's Hospital, Boston, MA, USA

Experimental methods

Basic principles

Overall, it is much easier to assess and quantify pharmacokinetic interactions than pharmacodynamic ones. In the case of pharmacokinetic interactions, one drug will alter the pharmacokinetics of another drug. Changes in pharmacokinetic parameters can be assessed quantitatively by single dose pharmacokinetic studies, by changes in steady-state levels, or by changes in protein binding, etc. Measuring levels and calculating pharmacokinetic parameters is relatively straightforward. Assessing a pharmacodynamic interaction between two drugs requires a valid quantitative measurement of a specific drug effect for the two drugs individually, as well as a quantitative measurement of the effect of the two drugs administered together. Finally, it is necessary to determine the nature of the pharmacodynamic interaction that has occurred between the two drugs. Also, before the two drugs are administered together, one has to determine for each of the two drugs the appropriate dose to be administered for an assessment of the pharmacodynamic interaction to be possible. Once the response to the two drugs given together has been measured, the interaction has to be analyzed and categorized according to its type. As discussed and defined in Chapter 9 (see Table 9.1), there are four possible types of pharmacodynamic interactions: additive, supra-additive (potentiation), infra-additive (antagonism), and indifferent. Methods have been developed that make it possible to determine the type of interaction in experimental animal models. None of these methods can be applied directly to clinical studies.

It is important to realize that determining the type of pharmacodynamic interaction is only the first step. Whether the pharmacodynamic interaction (for instance seizure protection by two drugs) is additive or supra-additive may be of no interest whatsoever unless the therapeutic relevance of this interaction can be assessed.

For instance, does the fact that the combined seizure protection achieved by two drugs in combination is supra-additive compared to their individual effects have therapeutic relevance? Not necessarily. One could envision that the same seizure protection that is provided by the two drugs together could possibly be achieved by administering sufficiently high doses of either one of the two drugs alone. However, the limiting factor to progressive increases of the dose of the drugs (alone or in combination) will be the dose-related toxicity. Consequently, the therapeutic relevance of a pharmacodynamic interaction between two drugs providing seizure protection will depend not only on the nature of their antiepileptic interaction, but also on the type of their pharmacodynamic interaction in relation to their dose-related neurotoxicity. If the neurotoxic interaction is also supra-additive, it may be that the seizure protection afforded by the two drugs together at their subtoxic doses is no better than the seizure protection afforded by either drug alone at its subtoxic dose. In other words, what is really relevant about the pharmacodynamic interactions between two drugs is how and to what extent the therapeutic index of the combination differs from the individual therapeutic indices of the two drugs. As early as 1955, while discussing the concepts delineated by Loewe, Weaver *et al.* (1955) addressed this issue quite appropriately:

Loewe (1953) has examined the characteristics of the dose–effect relationship of combined drugs acting in an additive manner and has given attention to the meaning of the common terms which are used to describe deviations from simple additive effects. He indicates that the terms synergism and antagonism, and analogous terms for supra-additive and infra-additive effects of combined drugs are usually imaginary terms and are meaningful only when they are clearly defined … He further states that it is more important to study the ratio between the intensities of various effects of the same combination, i.e., to know whether these ratios (margins of safety or therapeutic indices) assume a larger or smaller value for the combinations than for the components.

Isobolographic analysis

The concept of the isobolographic analysis has been developed about half a century ago (Loewe, 1953; Hewlett, 1969). The isobolographic analysis is currently widely used to determine the various types of pharmacodynamic interaction in experimental animal models, in particular for antiepileptic drugs (see also Chapter 11). It is a relatively simple and accurate method, which can be represented as a diagram in which concentrations or doses of drugs a and b used in a given experiment are plotted. The principle and the name of the method are best understood by analyzing additive interactions (Figure 10.1-I). The effective concentrations or doses of drugs a and b administered alone are plotted as A and B, respectively. This could be, for instance, the minimal effective dose or plasma concentration (MED,

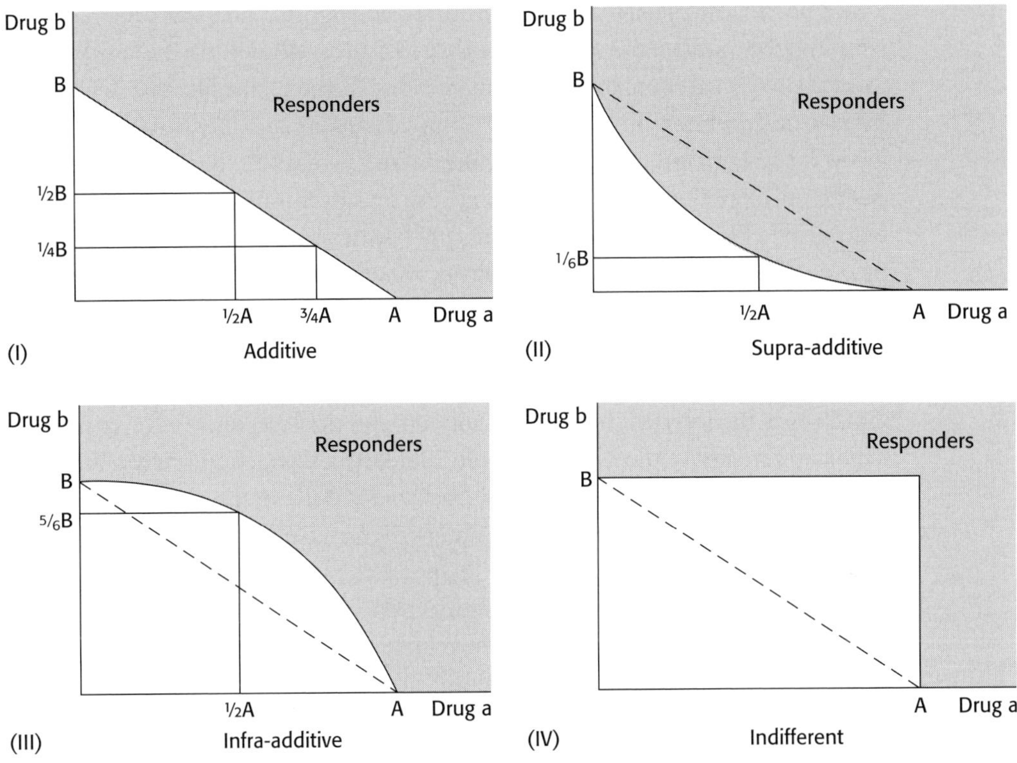

Figure 10.1   Isobolographic analysis of different types of pharmacodynamic interactions. The abscissa and the ordinate represent the dose or concentration of drugs a and b. A and B represent the effective doses or concentrations of drugs a and b. See text for additional explanations

MEC), or the median effective dose or concentration (ED_{50}, EC_{50}) against maximal electroshock (MES). If the interaction between drugs a and b is purely additive, ½ of A combined with ½ of B will achieve the same effect as A or B alone. Similarly, ¾ of A and ¼ of B will also achieve the same effect as A or B alone. In both cases, the plot of the doses or concentrations of drugs a and b will fall on the straight line connecting A and B. Whenever plots of effective doses or concentrations of drugs a and b administered together fall on this straight line, the pharmacodynamic interaction is additive. This additive interaction implies that ½ of A can replace ½ of B, and ¼ of A can replace ¼ of B. Therefore, the 'drug bolus' consisting of ½A plus ½B, or ¾A plus ¼B, is equivalent in efficacy to A or B alone. Hence the term isobologram. The straight line between A and B represents the isobole for additive interaction. Any dose or concentration pair of a and b that plots above this line will be effective (responders) and any pair that plots below this line will be ineffective (non-responders).

If a pharmacodynamic interaction is supra-additive, the bolus of drugs a and b administered together that will be necessary to achieve efficacy may be smaller than would be expected from an additive interaction. Therefore, the line that defines the interface between responders and non-responders is a curve that bends downward below the straight isobole for additive interaction (Figure 10.1-II). For instance, ½ of A with only ⅙ of B may be effective. Any dose or concentration pair of a and b that plots above this downward curving line will be effective (responders) and any pair that plots below this downward curving line will be ineffective (non-responders).

Inversely, if a pharmacodynamic interaction is infra-additive, the bolus of drugs a and b administered together that will be necessary to achieve efficacy may be greater than would be expected from an additive interaction. Therefore, the line that defines the interface between responders and non-responders is a curve that bends upward above the straight isobole for additive interaction (Figure 10.1-III). For instance, ½ of A and ⅚ of B may be required to achieve the response provided by A or B alone. Any dose or concentration pair of a and b that plots above this upward curving line will be effective (responders) and any pair that plots below this upward curving line will be ineffective (non-responders).

Finally, an interaction can be indifferent. In this case, the drugs do not act together at all and no amount of drug b will replace any amount of drug a. Therefore, the drug combination will be effective only if the amount of drug a is $\geq$A, or the amount of drug b is $\geq$B (Figure 10.1-IV). If the administered amounts of drugs a and b are smaller than A and B, respectively, there will be no response.

The isobolographic analysis can be applied in at least two different ways (Figure 10.2). One application consists of plotting doses or concentrations for individual animals receiving different doses and different ratios of drugs a and b (Figure 10.2-I). On this diagram, responders and non-responders must be identified as such. In Figure 10.2-I, one can see that there are several responders whose plots fall below the isobole for additive interaction. This is evidence that this particular interaction is supra-additive. An example of such an application is provided by a study on the anticonvulsant interaction between phenytoin and phenobarbital (Masuda *et al.*, 1981).

The isobolographic analysis can also be applied by using a single plot for values obtained from a group of animals. For instance, once the median effective dose (ED_{50}) has been determined for drugs a and b, the ED_{50} can be determined for the combination of the two drugs. In order to do so, the two drugs must be administered together at increasing doses until the ED_{50} in the combination is determined. For this purpose, it is crucial to maintain constant ratios of doses or concentrations of drugs a to b at any level. It is probably best to choose a ratio of dose a:b that is equal to ED_{50}a:ED_{50}b. Such an example is provided in Figure 10.2-II. If the ED_{50} of the two

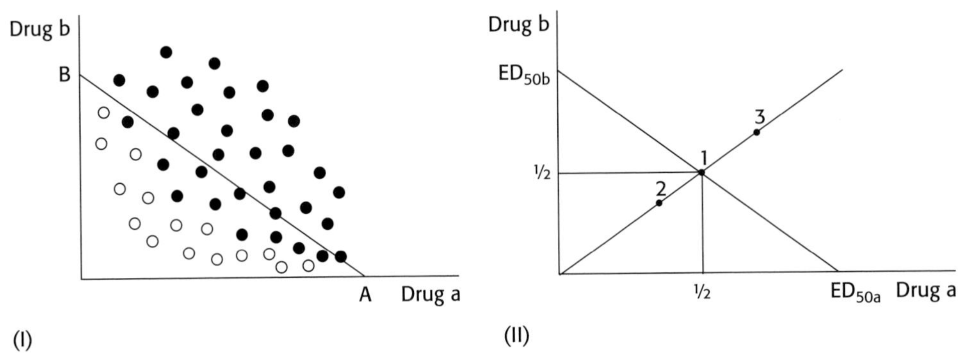

Figure 10.2   Two types of application of the isobolographic analysis. (I) Scatter plot of the results from individual animals, supra-additive interaction (closed symbols represent responders, open symbols represent non-responders). (II) Determination of median effective dose (ED_{50}) of the combination of drugs a and b, using a dosage ratio A:B. Point 1: ED_{50} in case of additive interaction. Points 2 and 3: ED_{50} in case of supra-additive (2) and infra-additive (3) interaction. Symbols A, B, a and b as in Figure 10.1. See text for additional explanations

drugs in combination is equal to 1/2 of each drug's respective ED_{50}, the interaction is additive and the point will fall on the straight isobole line for additive interaction (point 1). If the interaction is supra-additive, smaller doses will be sufficient to achieve the same effect, and the ED_{50} of the two drugs in combination will plot below the straight isobole (point 2). Inversely, if the interaction is infra-additive, larger doses will be necessary and the combined ED_{50} values will plot above the straight isobole (point 3). Again, the dose ratio of drug a to b in combination does not have to be equal to the ratio of the respective ED_{50} or equivalent values, but the ratio must be constant throughout the dosage range used to determine the ED_{50} or equivalent value of the two drugs in combination.

As discussed earlier, the practical relevance of pharmacodynamic interactions may be limited to their effect on the therapeutic index. The therapeutic index of individual drugs and of drug combinations can be expressed as a ratio of a certain toxic dose or concentration divided by the effective dose or concentration, for instance TD_{50}/ED_{50}. The isobolographic analysis in its traditional form does not allow comparison of the therapeutic index of a drug combination with the therapeutic indices of individual drugs. In order for that, it is necessary that first, the dose or concentration ratio of the two drugs be similar when efficacy and toxicity are measured and, secondly, that the sum of the two drug doses or concentrations be used. For this purpose, a modified version of the isobolographic analysis was

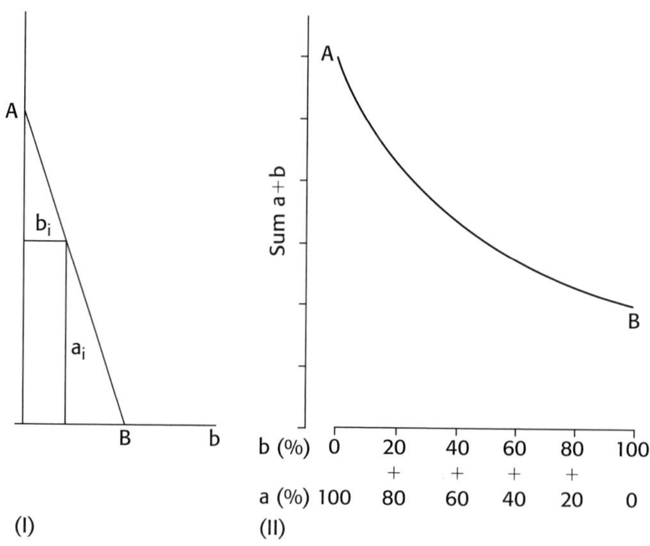

Figure 10.3   Modified form of the isobolographic analysis taking into account the sum of the amounts of drugs a and b (ordinate), and the relative concentrations of the drugs a and b (abscissa). A and B are equivalent effective amounts of the drugs. The curve drawn between points A and B corresponds to an additive interaction according to Eq. (10.1). Reproduced, with permission, from Bourgeois, 1986

developed (Bourgeois, 1986) (Figure 10.3). This modified version takes into account the dose or concentration ratio (abscissa) and the sum of the doses or concentrations of the two drugs (ordinate). The sum of the doses or concentrations in case of additive interaction would then be:

$$a_i + b_i = A\,\frac{1 + r_i}{1 + r_i R} \tag{10.1}$$

where a_i and b_i are the median effective or toxic concentrations of drugs a and b, respectively, in a given combination i, A and B are the corresponding effective or toxic concentrations of drugs a or b given alone, r_i is the ratio b_i/a_i (concentration ratio), and R is A/B (potency ratio). When A ≠ B, the line formed by all values for additive interaction at various concentration ratios is no longer straight. An example of such an application is provided in Figure 10.4 for the combination of carbamazepine and phenobarbital (Bourgeois and Wad, 1988). As can be seen, the interactions are additive for seizure protection (lower points) as well as for neurotoxicity (upper points). In this study, the therapeutic index of phenobarbital was 1.6, the therapeutic index of carbamazepine was 4.4, and the therapeutic index of the combination was 2.8 (higher than for phenobarbital but lower than for carbamazepine).

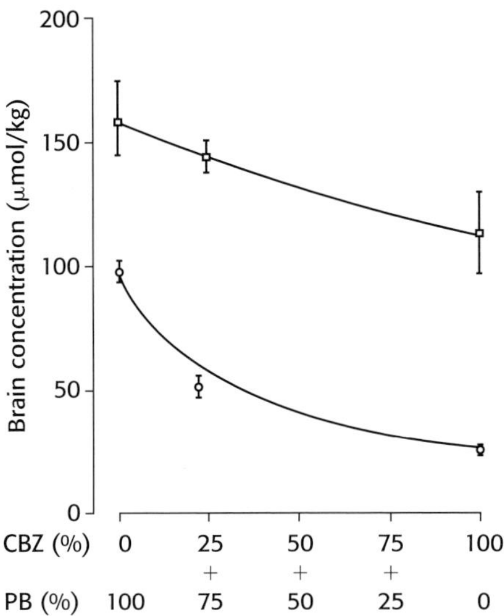

Figure 10.4 Median effective brain concentrations against maximal electroshock (circles) and
median toxic brain concentrations (squares) for phenobarbital (PB) alone (left) and
for carbamazepine (CBZ) alone (right), as well as for the sum of the two drugs in
combination. Solid lines represent expected values for purely additive interaction
according to Eq. (10.1), and vertical bars represent 95% confidence limits. Both the
anticonvulsant and the neurotoxic interactions are purely additive. Reproduced, with
permission, from Bourgeois and Wad, 1988

A different example is provided in Figure 10.5 (Bourgeois, 1988). In this case,
the anticonvulsant interaction between valproate and ethosuximide (lower points)
was purely additive, whereas the neurotoxic interaction (upper points) was infra-
additive. In this study, the therapeutic index of valproate alone was 1.8, the therapeutic index of ethosuximide alone was 2.4, and the therapeutic index of the combination
was 3.1, superior to both individual values.

A similar diagram expressing the effective dose or concentration (ordinate) as a
function of the drug concentration ratio (abscissa) was later proposed by Levasseur
et al. (1998). Their mathematical analysis also includes a quantification of the
intensity of the pharmacodynamic interaction.

Other methods

Besides the isobolographic analysis, various other methods have been used to
assess pharmacodynamic interactions. One of them is the fractional effective concentration index (Elison *et al.*, 1954; Kerry *et al.*, 1975). The first step for this
method is to determine the fractional effective concentration (FEC) for drugs a

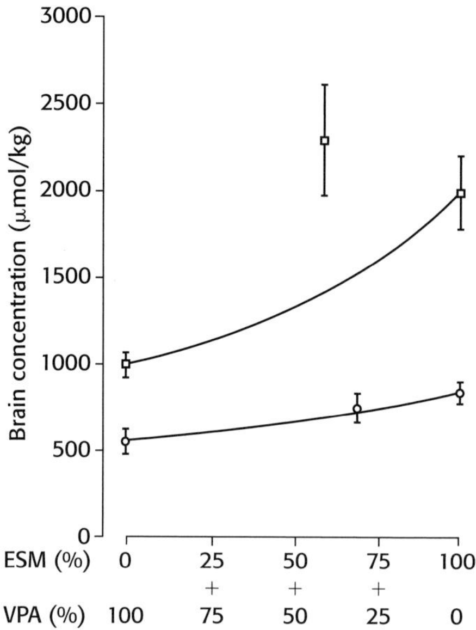

Figure 10.5   Median effective brain concentrations against pentylenetetrazole (circles) and median toxic brain concentrations (squares) for valproate (VPA) alone (left) and ethosuximide (ESM) alone (right), as well as for the sum of the two drugs in combination. Solid lines represent expected values for purely additive interaction according to Eq. (10.1), and vertical bars represent 95% confidence limits. The anticonvulsant interaction is purely additive, whereas the neurotoxic is clearly infra-additive. Reproduced, with permission, from Bourgeois, 1988

and b. The FEC is the ratio between the effective amount of a drug used in combination with a second drug and the effective amount of the drug used alone. For instance, it could be the ratio between the median effective concentration (EC_{50}) of the drug in the presence of the other drug, divided by the corresponding EC_{50} of the drug alone ($FEC_a = EC_{50a}$ in combination with drug b/EC_{50a} alone). The sum of the FEC value for drugs a and b represents the FEC index. It has been suggested that an FEC index of 0.7–1.3 can be considered to represent an additive interaction (Kerry *et al.*, 1975). FEC index values below 0.7 are indicative of a supra-additive interaction, and FEC index values above 1.3 are indicative of infra-additive interactions. An example of additive interactions by FEC index is provided in Table 10.1. This FEC index analysis is based on the same study as Figure 10.4, and addresses the seizure protection and the neurotoxicity of carbamazepine and phenobarbital, alone and in combination (Bourgeois and Wad, 1988). The isobolographic analysis had revealed a purely additive interaction for both seizure protection and neurotoxicity (Figure 10.4). Analysis of the interaction using the

Table 10.1 Fractional effective concentration (FEC) and FEC indices of phenobarbital (PB) and carbamazepine (CBZ)

	FEC^a		FEC index[b]
	PB	CBZ	
MES	$\dfrac{39.5}{97.1} = 0.41$	$\dfrac{11.3}{25.2} = 0.45$	0.86
Rotorod	$\dfrac{107.5}{157.9} = 0.68$	$\dfrac{35.5}{111.3} = 0.32$	1.00

[a] FEC: EC_{50} or TC_{50} in combination/EC_{50} or TC_{50} alone.

[b] FEC index: sum of FEC values for PB and CBZ. A value of 1.0 ± 0.3 indicates an additive interaction, lower values being indicative of synergism and higher values indicating antagonism.

Table 10.2 FEC and FEC indices of valproate (VPA) and ethosuximide (ESM)

	FEC^a		FEC index[b]
	VPA	ESM	
PTZ	$\dfrac{225.0}{549} = 0.41$	$\dfrac{507.8}{826.3} = 0.61$	1.02
Rotorod	$\dfrac{921.7}{986.9} = 0.93$	$\dfrac{1348.6}{2001.0} = 0.67$	1.60

[a] FEC: EC_{50} or TC_{50} in combination/EC_{50} or TC_{50} alone.

[b] FEC index: sum of FEC values for VPA and ESM. A value of 1.0 ± 0.3 indicates an additive interaction, lower values being indicative of synergism and higher values indicating antagonism.

FEC index also indicates additive interaction for efficacy and neurotoxicity, both FEC indices being >0.7 and <1.3 (Table 10.1). Another example is provided in Table 10.2. The data are from the same study as Figure 10.5, and are based on seizure protection and neurotoxicity of valproate and ethosuximide, alone and in combination (Bourgeois, 1988). The isobolographic analysis had revealed an additive anticonvulsant interaction and an infra-additive neurotoxic interaction (Figure 10.5). The FEC indices confirm these findings. The FEC index of 1.60 for neurotoxicity is considered to be in the infra-additive range.

Another method of analysis of pharmacodynamic interactions consists of administering an inactive dose of one drug and determining the effect of this inactive dose on the potency of the other drug. Examples and definitions of ineffective doses may include the dose that is effective for 1% or less of the animals, i.e. ED_1 or $ED_{0.1}$ (Bourgeois *et al.*, 1983), or a dose that is ineffective in a group of animals (for instance 25–50 animals) (Gordon *et al.*, 1993; Borowicz *et al.*, 1999). The ED_1 or the $ED_{0.1}$ can be determined by extrapolation of the probit analysis used to determine the ED_{50} of a compound.

When drug a is administered at a sub-effective dose together with drug b, the potency of drug b can be modified, such as a significant decrease of its ED_{50} compared to the administration of b alone. This has been shown to be the case for the effect of nicotinamide on the anticonvulsant activity of phenobarbital (Bourgeois *et al.*, 1983). It has also been shown that inactive doses of phenytoin, valproate, carbamazepine, and phenobarbital can significantly lower the ED_{50} of felbamate (Gordon *et al.*, 1993), or that a sub-protective dose of melatonin can enhance the effect of carbamazepine and phenobarbital on the electroconvulsive threshold in mice (Borowicz *et al.*, 1999). Such an effect has been considered to represent evidence of potentiation. Whether or not this is valid will be addressed in the section on 'Methodological pitfalls'.

Methodological pitfalls

Considering how complex and elaborate the assessment of pharmacodynamic interactions can be, it is not surprising that there may be several methodological pitfalls. One potential pitfall has already been alluded to earlier in this chapter, mainly attributing a certain relevance to a given pharmacodynamic interaction where there may be none. A good example would be the finding of a supra-additive anticonvulsant interaction between two drugs being interpreted as an argument for the combined use of these two drugs. In fact, the finding may be totally irrelevant, unless it can be shown that the combination has a superior therapeutic index.

Another potential methodological pitfall is the use of drug doses to quantify a pharmacodynamic interaction between two drugs when there is also a pharmacokinetic interaction between the drugs. What is interpreted as a pharmacodynamic interaction may actually only be a pharmacokinetic interaction. The interaction between phenytoin and phenobarbital is a good example. It has been concluded from several studies, based on the analysis of doses, that the anticonvulsive pharmacodynamic interaction between phenytoin and phenobarbital is supra-additive (Chen and Ensor, 1954; Weaver *et al.*, 1955; Wallin *et al.*, 1970; Consroe *et al.*, 1977). However, there is a pharmacokinetic interaction between the two drugs. It was shown independently in rats (Leppik and Sherwin, 1977) and in mice (Bourgeois, 1986) that brain concentrations of phenytoin following a single dose are higher in relation to the dose when phenytoin is administered with phenobarbital than when it is administered alone. If doses only are analyzed, this may lead to the conclusion that the interaction between the two drugs is supra-additive, because of the higher brain concentration of phenytoin when the combination is tested. In rats and in mice (Leppik and Sherwin, 1977; Bourgeois, 1986), assessment of the anticonvulsive pharmacodynamic interaction based on brain concentrations was shown to be consistent with a purely additive interaction.

Using an ineffective or sub-protective dose of one drug and measuring its effect on the potency of another drug has been presented earlier as one possible method for the assessment for pharmacodynamic interactions. In particular, it has been concluded that, if an inactive dose of a drug significantly reduces the ED_{50} of another drug, this represents a supra-additive interaction. The reasoning is that adding 0 to any number should not increase that number. In the case of pharmacodynamic interactions between drugs this conclusion is open to criticism and may actually be wrong. The main reason is that the relationship between dose and response (or concentration and response) is not a straight line, but a sigmoid curve (see Chapter 9, Figure 9.1). Also, based on the isobolographic analysis, ¼ of the ED_{50} of drug a can be replaced by ¼ of the ED_{50} of drug b, etc. Yet, it may be that ¼ of the ED_{50} of either drug is in itself ineffective. Therefore, a dose that is ineffective in itself is not necessarily ineffective when added to another drug, or when added to another dose of the same drug for that matter, even if the interaction is purely additive. Let us assume that the anticonvulsant ED_{50} of a drug is 50 mg/kg and that a dose of 10 mg/kg of that drug is found to be ineffective. However, if one adds the ineffective dose of 10 mg/kg to the ED_{50} of 50 mg/kg of the drug, the resulting dose of 60 mg/kg will protect >50% of the animals. Inversely, one could argue that, since 10 mg/kg is ineffective, 40 mg/kg should be just as effective as 50 mg/kg, which is obviously not true. Although the method of assessing the change in potency of one drug by an ineffective dose of another drug may not help to distinguish between a supra-additive and an additive interaction, this approach is still valid for the study of drug combinations. The reason is that this method does allow an assessment of the effect of one drug on the therapeutic index of another drug.

Clinical methods

Basic principles

The difficulties encountered in the assessment of pharmacodynamic interactions in experimental animals are compounded when interactions are to be studied clinically in patients, especially for antiepileptic drugs. The isobolographic analysis can be applied clinically under certain circumstances, but it is difficult to apply to patients with epilepsy. The interaction between anesthetics has been studied in patients using the isobolographic analysis. For instance, the propofol–thiopental hypnotic interaction was analyzed in patients undergoing eye surgery (Vinik *et al.*, 1999). The abolition of the ability to open the eyes on command was used as an endpoint. The ED_{50} was determined by probit analysis for thiopental alone, for propofol alone, and for three different dosage ratios of the two drugs. All ED_{50} values were on the straight isobole, indicating a purely additive interaction. In this study, the FEC index analysis was also used, resulting in values equal to or close to 1.0.

Populations of patients with seizures are not homogeneous and cannot be compared with groups of healthy animals in whom standardized seizures are elicited, e.g. with MES or pentylenetetrazole. Therefore, values for median effective doses or for median toxic doses, or equivalent values, cannot be determined in patients with seizures, and isobolograms are therefore difficult or impossible to create. A more reproducible and quantifiable endpoint would actually be the maximal tolerated dose (MTD) or sub-toxic dose. In the end, determining the type of pharmacodynamic interaction between two antiepileptic drugs (mainly whether it is supra-additive or not) in patients may be a moot point. As stated earlier, what is of interest is not so much the type of interaction, but the practical relevance of the interaction. Translated into clinical terms, the practical relevance is whether a certain combination of two antiepileptic drugs, compared to each drug alone, can provide better seizure protection with the same level of toxicity or the same degree of seizure protection with fewer side effects. Therefore, clinical studies should be designed to address this issue rather than whether the anticonvulsant interaction between two antiepileptic drugs is supra-additive or not.

Trial designs

The discussion on designs of clinical trials to study pharmacodynamic interactions between antiepileptic drugs will be based on the assumption that the studies are to be clinically relevant. They should be aimed at demonstrating that, compared with the individual drug effects, a given combination offers better seizure protection at the same level of toxicity or the same seizure protection with less toxicity. Possible study designs will be divided into four groups: optimal, probably valid, questionably valid, and invalid.

Optimal design

Among a cohort of patients with uncontrolled seizures, a group is to be identified whose seizures are not fully controlled at the MTD of drug a in monotherapy. The MTD is a dose that causes no persistent side effects and is just below a dose that does cause persistent side effects. This group of patients should be switched to monotherapy with drug b. The dose of drug b should be increased until seizures subside, or to the MTD. Those patients who do not benefit significantly from drug b, even at the MTD, should have drug a re-introduced while maintained on drug b. The dose of drug b may be maintained at the MTD or, if necessary, it may be lowered somewhat in order to allow an increase in the dose of drug a. To what extent the combination of drugs a and b is superior will be determined by the percentage of patients receiving this combination that will have a >50% reduction in their seizure frequency. As can be seen, the essential component of an optimal study design is that all patients receive an appropriate monotherapy trial with both drugs before being treated with a combination.

Probably valid design

1 The initial step here would also be to identify patients whose seizures have failed to come under control at the MTD of drug a. At that point, drug b is added to drug a, if necessary to the MTD. In those patients who experience a >50% reduction in seizure frequency after the addition of drug b, an attempt is made to gradually taper and discontinue drug a. To what extent the combination of drugs a and b is superior will be determined by the percentage of patients whose seizure control deteriorates as drug a is tapered or discontinued and whose seizure control improves after drug a is re-introduced.

2 Patients are identified whose seizures are not controlled on monotherapy at the MTD. Some may be on drug a, some on drug b, and some on drug c. In these patients, drug d is added as a second drug and the dose of drug d is increased as necessary and as tolerated. It is conceivable that, after the addition of drug d, a substantial number of patients on drug b, for example, may experience a >50% seizure reduction whereas few or none of the patients taking drug a or c benefit. This would represent fairly good evidence that drugs b and d may have a favorable pharmacodynamic interaction profile and that they represent a desirable drug combination. An effect of drug d alone is unlikely with the present design, if a good response after the addition of drug d is not observed in patients taking drug a or c, assuming that the patient groups do not differ significantly in terms of their seizure types.

Questionably valid design

1 Clinical studies have been carried out for the use of designs outlined above as optimal or probably valid; the only difference being that patients were not on monotherapy and then on a combination of only two drugs, but took additional baseline antiepileptic drugs. Even though these baseline antiepileptic drugs remain constant, they introduce different variables and more potential for pharmacodynamic interactions.

2 Pharmacodynamic interactions between antiepileptic drugs can also be assessed by using a design based on the concept of the isobolographic analysis. As in the optimal design described above, patients are identified who have failed to

respond to the MTD of drugs a or b in monotherapy. Trough serum levels of drugs a and of drug b are determined at the MTD. The patients then receive drugs a and b in combination at doses that are adjusted to achieve 1/2 of the trough serum levels that were reached at the MTDs. Theoretically, if the antiepileptic pharmacodynamic interaction between the two drugs is supra-additive, the patients as a group should experience a reduction in their seizure frequency. However, this method does not necessarily address the issue of the clinical superiority of the combination, i.e. whether the combination has a better efficacy to toxicity ratio than either drug alone.

Invalid design

At times, conclusions regarding the value of drug combinations have been drawn from studies that were not designed to properly address this question. For instance, if patients improve with the addition of drug b after failure of drug a, this cannot be interpreted as evidence that this improvement is due to a combination of the two drugs. The improvement could just as well been entirely due to the effect of drug b only, in which case it might be maintained after discontinuation of drug a. Also, the combination cannot be assessed unless the doses of the two drugs in monotherapy have been increased to the MTD. Since the combination may be at the MTD, it is possible that improved seizure control could also have been achieved at the MTD of the two drugs in monotherapy. Finally, as in experimental studies, possible pharmacokinetic interactions between drugs have to be taken into account and they must be corrected or compensated.

REFERENCES

Borowicz KK, Rafal K, Gasior M, *et al.* Influence of melatonin upon the protective action of conventional anti-epileptic drugs against maximal electroshock in mice. *Eur Neuropsychopharmacol* 1999; **9**: 185–190.

Bourgeois BFD. Antiepileptic drug combinations and experimental background: the case of phenobarbital and phenytoin. *Naunyn-Schmiedeberg's Arch Pharmacol* 1986; **333**: 406–411.

Bourgeois BFD. Combination of valproate and ethosuximide: antiepileptic and neurotoxic interaction. *J Pharmacol Exp Ther* 1988; **237**: 1128–1132.

Bourgeois BFD, Wad N. Combined administration of carbamazepine and phenobarbital: effect on anticonvulsant activity and neurotoxicity. *Epilepsia* 1988; **29**: 482–487.

Bourgeois BFD, Dodson WE, Ferrendelli JA. Potentiation of the antiepileptic activity of phenobarbital by nicotinamide. *Epilepsia* 1983; **23**: 238–244.

Chen G, Ensor CR. A study of the anticonvulsant properties of phenobarbital and dilantin. *Arch Int Pharmacodyn* 1954; **100**: 234–248.

Consroe P, Wolkin A. Cannabidiol – antiepileptic drug comparisons and interactions in experimentally induced seizures in rats. *J Pharmacol Exp Ther* 1977; **201**: 26–32.

Elison G, Singer S, Hitchings GH. Antagonists of nucleic acid derivatives. VIII. Synergism in combinations of biochemically related antimetabolites. *J Biol Chem* 1954; **208**: 477–488.

Gordon R, Gels M, Wichmann J, *et al.* Interaction of felbamate with several other antiepileptic drugs against seizures induced by maximal electroshock in mice. *Epilepsia* 1993; **34**: 367–371.

Hewlett PS. Measurement of the potencies of drug mixtures. *Biometrics* 1969; **25**: 477–487.

Kerry DW, Hamilton-Miller JMT, Brumfitt W. Trimethoprim and rifampicin: in vitro activities separately and in combination. *J Antimicrob Agents Chemother* 1975; **1**: 1417–1427.

Leppik IE, Sherwin AL. Anticonvulsant activity of phenobarbital and phenytoin in combination. *J Pharmacol Exp Ther* 1977; **200**: 570–575.

Levasseur LM, Delon A, Greco WR, *et al.* Development of a new quantitative approach for the isobolographic assessment of the convulsant interaction between pefloxacin and theophylline in rats. *Pharmaceut Res* 1998; **15**: 1069–1076.

Loewe S. The problem of synergism and antagonism of combined drugs. *Arzneimittelforsch* 1953; **3**: 285–290.

Masuda Y, Utsui Y, Shiraishi Y, *et al.* Evidence for a synergistic interaction between phenytoin and phenobarbital in experimental animals. *J Pharmacol Exp Ther* 1981; **217**: 805–811.

Vinik R, Bradley E, Kissin I. Isobolographic analysis of propofol–thiopental hypnotic interaction in surgical patients. *Anesth Analg* 1999; **88**: 667–670.

Wallin RF, Blackburn WH, Napoli. Pharmacological interactions of albutoin with other anticonvulsant drugs. *Pharmacol Exp Ther* 1970; **174**: 276–282.

Weaver LC, Swinyard EA, Woodbury LA, *et al.* Studies on anticonvulsant drug combinations: phenobarbital and diphenylhydantoin. *J Pharmacol Exp Ther* 1955; **113**: 359–370.

11

Experimental studies of pharmacodynamic interactions

Stanislaw J. Czuczwar

Department of Pathophysiology, Medical University and
Isotope Laboratory, Institute of Agricultural Medicine, Jaczewskiego, Lublin, Poland

Introduction

In most patients, the therapy of newly diagnosed epilepsy is initiated with a single antiepileptic drug. Approximately 60–70% of patients may experience a reasonable seizure control with monotherapy (Sander *et al.*, 1993; Czuczwar and Patsalos, 2001). However, monotherapy is not sufficient for the remainder of epileptic patients. Therefore, experimental background information may be helpful for an epileptologist to know what drug combinations can be considered preferentially for combination therapy or for controlled clinical trials. Animal studies evaluate the combinations of conventional antiepileptic drugs or combinations of a conventional antiepileptic drug with a novel (or potential) antiepileptic drug. The protective effect of a drug combination may be quantified with the isobolographic method on the basis of equieffective doses of individual drugs administered alone or in combination (Tallarida, 1992; Tallarida *et al.*, 1989). An alternative method evaluates the effect of one antiepileptic drug given in sub-protective doses upon the ED_{50} value (the effective dose of a drug necessary to protect 50% of the animals) of another drug against experimental seizures. The ED_{50} value of the second drug in combination with sub-protective doses of the first antiepileptic drug is compared to the control ED_{50} value, estimated for the second drug alone, according to the method of Litchfield and Wilcoxon (1949).

Interactions between conventional antiepileptic drugs

As already mentioned, the experimental background may provide clues regarding which drug combinations may actually have a significant therapeutic potential. There have been many experimental studies dealing with combinations of conventional antiepileptic drugs. For instance, Bourgeois (1986; 1988a, b), Bourgeois and Wad (1984), and Chez *et al.* (1994) studied the interactions between conventional antiepileptic drugs in two rapid and simple screening convulsive tests – the maximal electroshock and the pentylenetetrazol test. Practically, all existing conventional and novel antiepileptic drugs are effective in at least one of these tests, except for levetiracetam. According to Löscher and Schmidt (1988), maximal electroshock-induced seizures in rodents provide a good experimental model for generalized tonic–clonic convulsions while the pentylenetetrazol test may be regarded as a model for myoclonic seizures in humans.

On the basis of brain concentrations of phenytoin and phenobarbital, Bourgeois (1986), using the isobolographic analysis, concluded that the interaction between these antiepileptic drugs was purely additive against maximal electroshock in mice, while their neurotoxicity was infra-additive. However, because of the very poor therapeutic index of phenobarbital in this model, the therapeutic index of phenytoin alone was still better than the therapeutic index of the combination. For seizure protection, a purely additive interaction between phenytoin and phenobarbital, based on their brain concentration in rats, was also found by Leppik and Sherwin (1977). There are other reports pointing to a synergy between these two antiepileptic drugs in rodents. However, they were based on the analysis of doses (Chen and Ensor, 1954; Weaver *et al.*, 1955). On the other hand, an apparent synergy was found between phenobarbital and phenytoin in mice and rabbits with the use of maximal electroshock, and these results were verified with both plasma and brain concentrations of the antiepileptic drugs. However, the neurotoxicity of this combination was not evaluated (Masuda *et al.*, 1981).

Anticonvulsant efficacy and neurotoxicity of another combination of conventional antiepileptic drugs, carbamazepine and phenobarbital, was evaluated in mice against maximal electroshock by Bourgeois and Wad (1988). Brain concentrations of these drugs were taken into consideration. No supra-additive interaction was found. An additive effect was evident for both the anticonvulsant and the neurotoxic activity. In another model of experimental epilepsy – penicillin-induced epileptic foci in cats – no potentiation could be demonstrated between carbamazepine and phenobarbital (Monaco *et al.*, 1985). Also, only additive effects were reported when valproate was combined with phenobarbital or carbamazepine in maximal electroshock test in mice. Considering the neurotoxic effects of these combinations, additive and infra-additive interactions were evident, respectively (Bourgeois, 1988a). With the use of the same experimental approach, Chez *et al.* (1994) provided evidence for a supra-additive anticonvulsant interaction between valproate and diphenylhydantoin (while neurotoxicity was simply additive) that may be interpreted in terms of a potential benefit for antiepileptic treatment. Also, another combination of conventional antiepileptic drugs, valproate and ethosuximide, was found potentially beneficial in the pentylenetetrazol test in mice (Bourgeois, 1988b). Although isobolographic analysis of effective brain concentrations of both drugs was indicative of an additive anticonvulsant interaction, a less

Table 11.1 Antiepileptic drugs – mechanisms of action

Antiepileptic drug	Blockade of Na$^+$ channels	Blockade of T-type Ca^{2+} channels	Blockade of other Ca^{2+} channels	Enhancement of GABA-mediated events
Benzodiazepines	↑			↑↑
Carbamazepine	↑↑			
Ethosuximide		↑↑		
Felbamate	↑			
Gabapentin			↑↑	
Lamotrigine	↑↑			
Phenobarbital	↑			↑
Phenytoin	↑↑			
Tiagabine				↑↑
Topiramate	↑			↑
Valproate	↑			↑
Vigabatrin				↑↑

Data are from (see for review) Löscher (1998), Urbańska *et al.* (1998), Deckers *et al.* (2000), and Czuczwar and Patsalos (2001). Only the mechanisms were considered which are evident within therapeutic drug concentrations.

For the influence of antiepileptic drugs on glutamate-mediated events see Table 11.3.

GABA, γ-amino butyric acid. ↑, effective; ↑↑, very effective.

than additive neurotoxic interaction was found. These interactions resulted in a better therapeutic index for the combined treatment than for either drug alone.

A question that has been debated is whether there might be a general rule on how to combine antiepileptic drugs based on their mechanisms of action. According to Deckers *et al.* (2000), combining a sodium channel blocker (mechanisms of action of antiepileptic drugs are listed in Table 11.1) with a GABAergic drug seems more efficacious than two sodium channel blockers. Experimental data provided by Czuczwar *et al.* (1981) seem to support such a hypothesis. These authors observed a potent enhancement of diazepam's anti-pentylenetetrazol effect in mice by diphenylhydantoin, which is completely inactive in this seizure model. Although the plasma concentrations of these antiepileptic drugs were not measured, a pharmacokinetic mechanism does not seem probable since this very potent interaction was not observed against bicuculline- or isoniazid-induced seizures in mice (Czuczwar *et al.*, 1981). This may also point to different mechanisms of action of conventional antiepileptic drugs, which may result in a potentiation in some models of experimental epilepsy. On the other hand, some other models may require the involvement of different mechanisms.

Interactions between conventional and newer antiepileptic drugs

Shank *et al.* (1994) studied the protection offered by a newer antiepileptic drug, topiramate, alone and combined with standard antiepileptic drugs, phenytoin, phenobarbital, and carbamazepine against maximal electroshock-induced seizures in mice. Topiramate was combined with a conventional antiepileptic drug at fixed ratios (0.75/0.25, 0.50/0.50, and 0.25/0.75) of their respective ED_{50} values. To plot a dose–response curve, multiple doses of each combination were used. The results provided evidence that the combination of topiramate with phenytoin was additive in terms of anticonvulsant activity. However, a synergy was observed when topiramate was combined with either carbamazepine or phenobarbital. The second experimental approach (effect of sub-protective doses) was used to study the interactions between felbamate and carbamazepine, phenytoin, phenobarbital, or valproate against maximal electroshock in mice (Gordon *et al.*, 1993). It was evident that all conventional antiepileptic drugs in non-effective doses in this seizure test reduced the ED_{50} value of felbamate (42.9 mg/kg) – carbamazepine (4 mg/kg) by 70%, phenytoin (6 mg/kg) by 60%, phenobarbital (4 mg/kg) by 45%, and valproate (150 mg/kg) by 69%. It is noteworthy that the protective index of felbamate, defined as its TD_{50}/ED_{50}, was significantly elevated after combinations with each standard antiepileptic drug (TD_{50} is the dose of a drug necessary to cause neurotoxicity in 50% of the animals). Similarly to the former studies, a pharmacokinetic mechanism was unlikely to account for the observed interaction. Conversely, doses of felbamate sub-protective against electroconvulsions failed to affect the ED_{50} values of carbamazepine, phenytoin, phenobarbital and valproate against maximal electroshock in mice (Borowicz *et al.*, 2000c). This may emphasize the importance of dose ratios in the final quantitative analysis of an interaction between antiepileptic drugs. In fact, such a dose dependence was observed by Shank *et al.* (1994) with topiramate and conventional antiepileptic drugs. Swiader *et al.* (2000) combined topiramate (in sub-protective doses of 2.5 and 5 mg/kg in relation to the electroconvulsive threshold in mice) with conventional antiepileptic drugs. The convulsive test was maximal electro-shock. A possible pharmacokinetic interaction was identified on the basis of measurements of the free-plasma concentrations of the antiepileptic drugs. Topiramate's ED_{50} against maximal electroshock was 62.1 mg/kg. The most remarkable interaction was observed when topiramate (5 mg/kg) was co-administered with carbamazepine (its ED_{50} value was reduced by 41%). In the case of phenobarbital and phenytoin, the ED_{50} reductions were 30% and 28%, respectively. Much weaker effect was observed for the combination of topiramate (5 mg/kg) with valproate (its ED_{50} value was decreased by only 18%). However, topiramate (5 mg/kg) elevated the free-plasma concentration of carbamazepine by 47%. Thus, a pharmacokinetic factor is apparently responsible for the observed potentiation of the protective effect of carbamazepine. The free-plasma concentrations of the remaining antiepileptic drugs were not affected by topiramate. Although the interaction of topiramate with valproate was not remarkable (but still statistically significant) in terms of the anticonvulsant activity, the combined treatment did not disturb motor coordination or long-term memory of mice evaluated in the chimney test and passive avoidance task, respectively. In contrast, valproate alone at its ED_{50} value of 248 mg/kg against maximal electroshock impaired both motor performance and long-term memory (Swiader *et al.*, 2000). In the pentylenetetrazol test in mice, pronounced anticonvulsant activity was noted when topiramate was administered together with clobazam or phenobarbital, limited and/or variable effects being observed for its combinations with valproate, primidone, and ethosuximide (Sills *et al.*, 1999). Another newer anti-epileptic drug, gabapentin, at a sub-protective dose of 25 mg/kg, reduced the ED_{50} values of major conventional antiepileptic drugs: carbamazepine (by 28%), phenytoin (by 52%), phenobarbital (by 58%), and valproate (by 28%) against maximal electroshock in mice. In no case were the free-plasma concentrations of the conventional antiepileptic drugs affected by gabapentin. Therefore, a pharmacokinetic interaction is not probable (Czuczwar *et al.*, 1999). Isobolographic analysis revealed distinctly supra-additive interactions for the combinations of gabapentin with carbamazepine, valproate, phenytoin, or phenobarbital, since experimentally evaluated ED_{50} values were much lower than the additive ED_{50} values theoretically calculated from the line of additivity for the respective combinations. A pharmacokinetic interaction was at least partially involved in the interactions between gabapentin and phenobarbital. The adverse effects of the respective drug mixtures were only additive which suggests that the combinations are potentially promising for clinical studies (Borowicz *et al.*, 2002b). Gabapentin was also evaluated in this respect in a model of reflex epilepsy, sound-induced seizures in DBA/2 mice (De Sarro *et al.*, 1998). At a non-protective dose of 2.5 mg/kg, gabapentin enhanced the protective activity of carbamazepine, diazepam, phenytoin, phenobarbital, and valproate. The most remarkable potentiation of the anticonvulsant effect occurred for diazepam, phenobarbital, and valproate. In addition, the therapeutic indices of the combined treatments were better than for the respective antiepileptic drugs alone. A possible pharmacokinetic mechanism may be excluded because gabapentin did not significantly affect the plasma concentration of the antiepileptic drugs. Some combinations between newer and conventional antiepileptic drugs are listed in Table 11.2.

Interactions between newer antiepileptic drugs

Only limited experimental data are available on this issue. De Sarro *et al.* (1998) studied gabapentin and its combinations with felbamate or lamotrigine. However,

Table 11.2 Interactions between conventional and novel antiepileptic drugs in the maximal electroshock-induced convulsions in mice

Conventional antiepileptic drug	Novel antiepileptics		
	Felbamate	Gabapentin	Topiramate
Carbamazepine	0	↑↑[b]	↑↑[a,b]
Phenobarbital	0	↑↑[b]	↑↑[b]
Phenytoin	0	↑↑[b]	↑↑[b]
Valproate	0	↑↑[b]	↑↑

Novel antiepileptic drugs were given at non-protective doses, evaluated in the threshold electroconvulsive test.

Data are from Shank *et al.* (1994), Borowicz *et al.* (2000c, 2002b), and Swiader *et al.* (2000). See text for the adverse potential of these combinations.

0, no interaction; ↑, positive or additive interaction; ↑↑, very potent (or supra-additive) interaction. [a] Pharmacokinetic interaction was found. [b] Isobolographic analysis was performed.

the results were not as remarkable as in the case of gabapentin combined with diazepam, phenobarbital, and valproate. Topiramate co-administered with felbamate or tiagabine demonstrated convincing efficacy against pentylenetetrazol in mice. Combinations of topiramate with gabapentin, vigabatrin, lamotrigine, or remacemide were completely without effect in this seizure model (Sills *et al.*, 1999). Stephen *et al.* (1998) tested the intriguing hypothesis of whether two drugs ineffective against pentylenetetrazol might be effective when combined. Actually, lamotrigine and topiramate, fulfilling these criteria, provided a strong protection in the pentylenetetrazol test.

Interactions of antiepileptic drugs with excitatory amino acid antagonists

N-methyl-D-aspartate receptor antagonists

Endogenous excitatory amino acids, mainly glutamate or aspartate, have been shown to play an important role in the induction of seizure activity (Meldrum, 1984). Also, clinical data indicate that a number of cases of human epilepsy are accompanied by elevated concentrations of excitatory amino acids in plasma (Huxtable *et al.*, 1983; Janjua *et al.*, 1992). In the early 1980s, intensive experimental studies were initiated on the possible anticonvulsant activity of ionotropic glutamate receptor antagonists. Results from various models of experimental epilepsy provided a good deal of data confirming this hypothesis (Czuczwar and Meldrum,

Table 11.3 Antiepileptic drugs and receptors for excitatory amino acids

Antiepileptic drug	NMDA receptor	AMPA/KA receptor	mGluR
Benzodiazepines	0	0	ND
Carbamazepine	+	0	ND
Ethosuximide	0	0	ND
Felbamate	+	0	ND
Lamotrigine	0*	0*	ND
Phenobarbital	0	+	ND
Phenytoin	+	0	ND
Tiagabine	ND	ND	ND
Topiramate	0	+	ND
Valproate	+	0	ND
Vigabatrin	ND	ND	ND

For review see Löscher (1998), Urbañska *et al.* (1998), Deckers *et al.* (2000), and Czuczwar and Patsalos (2001).

0, no effect; +, inhibition of receptor-mediated events; ND, not determined.

*Inhibition of glutamate release was found in vitro but not in vivo.

1982; Croucher *et al.*, 1982; Czuczwar *et al.*, 1985; Smith *et al.*, 1991; Turski *et al.*, 1990, 1992). Ionotropic glutamate receptor antagonists block two major groups of receptors: those sensitive to N-methyl-D-aspartate (NMDA receptors) and those sensitive to α-amino-3-hydroxy-5-methyl-isoxazole-4-propionate/kainate (AMPA/KA or non-NMDA receptors; Watkins *et al.*, 1990). Both groups of receptors control different ion currents – excitation of NMDA receptors is associated with an influx of calcium and sodium ions into a neuron whilst non-NMDA receptors preferentially affect sodium-gated channels (Monaghan *et al.*, 1989). Moreover, it has been suggested that some antiepileptic drugs interact with glutamate receptors (see Table 11.3).

Utilizing the method of Litchfield and Wilcoxon (1949), a number of NMDA or non-NMDA receptor antagonists were tested for their ability to interact with conventional antiepileptic drugs (Table 11.4). D-3-(2-carboxypiperazine-4-yl)-1-propenyl-1-phosphonic acid (D-CPP-ene; a competitive NMDA receptor antagonist – 1 mg/kg) considerably enhanced the protective activity of carbamazepine, diazepam, phenytoin, phenobarbital, or valproate against maximal electroshock-induced seizures in mice without any effect upon their plasma concentrations (Zarnowski *et al.*, 1994a). Except for carbamazepine, combinations of other antiepileptic drugs with D-CPP-ene resulted in serious impairment of motor coordination and long-term memory. A very good correlation between the experimental studies and clinical data needs to be emphasized. D-CPP-ene (as an adjuvant

Table 11.4 Influence of NMDA or AMPA/KA receptor antagonists on the anticonvulsant activity of conventional antiepileptic drugs against maximal electroshock-induced seizures in mice

Excitatory amino acid receptor antagonist (mg/kg)	Phenobarbital	Diphenylhydantoin	Carbamazepine	Valproate
CGP 37849 (0.25)	NT	NT	NT	43
CGP 37849 (1.0)	53	53	66	NT
D-CPP-ene (1.0)	58	50	63	60
GYKI 52466 (5)	91(NS)	51	36	32
LY 300164 (2)	65	70	68	41
Memantine (0.5)	NT	NT	NT	55
NBQX (10)	59	53	74	59
Procyclidine (10)	75	69	75	75

Table data indicate reductions of the ED_{50} values of antiepileptic drugs (in %) after combinations with excitatory amino acid receptor antagonists. ED_{50}s of antiepileptic drugs alone are ascribed to 100%. Excitatory amino acid receptor antagonists were given at doses ineffective upon the convulsive threshold. Data are from Czechowska *et al.* (1993), Pietrasiewicz *et al.* (1993), Zarnowski *et al.* (1993; 1994a, b), Borowicz *et al.* (1995), and Czuczwar *et al.* (1998c).
NS, not significant; NT, not tested.

antiepileptic drug) was also given to patients with complex partial seizures (Sveinbjornsdottir *et al.*, 1993). This combined therapy induced a number of severe adverse reactions in epileptic patients, including poor concentration, ataxia, amnesia, and sedation. Interestingly, no therapeutic improvement with D-CPP-ene was noted, in contrast to findings in the animal study (Zarnowski *et al.*, 1994a). A possible explanation for this discrepancy is that an experimental animal model for complex partial seizures in man is the amygdala-kindled seizure model in rats (Löscher *et al.*, 1986). NMDA receptor antagonists are not very potent in this experimental model, which may result in the poor anticonvulsive effects of D-CPP-ene in patients with complex partial seizures. Memantine or procyclidine, when combined with conventional antiepileptic drugs, considerably disturbed motor coordination and long-term memory in mice, although the protection offered by the antiepileptic drugs was potentiated (Urbañska *et al.*, 1992; Zarnowski *et al.*, 1994b). Some other NMDA receptor antagonists possessed much better profile of activity in this regard. For instance, D,L-(*E*)-2-amino-4-methyl-5-phosphono-3-pentenoate (CGP 37849) and its ethylester (CGP 39551) increased the protective action of valproate against maximal electroshock in mice, maximally by 57% and 55%, respectively. It is remarkable that the combinations with valproate were free from adverse effects upon motor performance and long-term memory, which was not the case with valproate alone at its ED_{50} against maximal electroshock. Again, no pharmacokinetic factor, at least in terms of the plasma concentration of valproate, seems to be involved (Czechowska *et al.*, 1993). Similar results were observed, in terms of the anticonvulsant activity, when these NMDA receptor antagonists were combined with carbamazepine, phenytoin, and phenobarbital (Pietrasiewicz *et al.*, 1993). Only combinations with phenytoin were devoid of adverse effects. The recently studied NMDA receptor antagonist CPP and its active D($-$) isomer potentiated the anti-electroshock efficacy of all four conventional antiepileptic drugs with no adverse potential being observed for carbamazepine, phenytoin, and phenobarbital (Borowicz *et al.*, 2000a). Also, the combinations with valproate were superior to valproate alone in this respect, since valproate alone at its ED_{50} against maximal electroshock-induced seizures produced impairment of motor coordination and long-term memory. Combination with CPP revealed only motor impairment (Borowicz *et al.*, 2000a). It seems reasonable to state that any future therapy of seizures with NMDA receptor antagonists may result in a problem of serious side effects. This was studied in detail by Löscher and Hönack (1991) who showed that amygdala-kindled rats were much more susceptible to adverse activity of NMDA receptor antagonists than naive (non-epileptic) rats. Combined treatment with antiepileptic drugs together with NMDA receptor antagonists may help to partially overcome this problem, especially when there is a potent interaction in terms of anticonvulsant activity. Usually, the adjuvant antiepileptic drugs are used in lower doses than those necessary to produce a protective effect per se. This procedure also leads to reductions of the ED_{50} values of conventional antiepileptic drugs. Some of the experimental data cited above indicate that a number of combinations may be actually free from undesired adverse reactions. Moreover, low-affinity NMDA receptor antagonists possess a lower-adverse effect potential. A good example is remacemide, effective against both experimental and human seizures and well tolerated by epileptic patients (Bialer *et al.*, 1999).

AMPA/KA receptor antagonists

1-(4-Aminophenyl)-4-methyl-7,8-methylenedioxy-5H-2,3-benzodiazepine hydrochloride (GYKI 52466; a non-competitive antagonist of AMPA/KA receptors), at the sub-effective dose of 5 mg/kg potentiated the anticonvulsant action of carbamazepine, phenytoin, and valproate, but not that of phenobarbital, against maximal electroshock-induced seizures in mice (Borowicz *et al.*, 1995). The GYKI 52466-induced enhancement was very significant, the respective ED_{50} values of these antiepileptic drugs being diminished by 64%, 59%, and 68%, respectively. The non-NMDA receptor antagonist did not affect the free-plasma concentration of the affected antiepileptic drugs. No effective combination of GYKI 52466 with the antiepileptic drugs resulted in undesirable effects. Combination of GYKI 52466 (up to 10 mg/kg) with conventional antiepileptic drugs in the pentylenetetrazol test was much less remarkable. This non-NMDA receptor antagonist proved ineffective when combined with clonazepam, ethosuximide, and phenobarbital. Only a combination with valproate was quite effective (Czuczwar *et al.*, 1998a). However, this combination resulted in a mnemonic effect. Promising effects were obtained with the competitive antagonist of AMPA/KA receptors, 2,3-dihydroxy-6-nitro-7-sulfamoylbenzo(*F*)-quinoxaline (NBQX) at 10 mg/kg against maximal electroshock-induced seizures. This excitatory amino acid receptor antagonist potentiated the protective activity of conventional antiepileptic drugs, including phenobarbital. A pharmacokinetic interaction was considered unlikely. Practically, combinations of NBQX with antiepileptic drugs did not produce side effects, the only exception being one with valproate (Zarnowski *et al.*, 1993). A very promising substance among AMPA/KA receptor antagonists is 7-acetyl-5-(4-aminophenyl)-8,9-dihydro-8-methyl-7H-1,3-dioxolo(4,5H)-2,3-benzodiazepine (LY 300164) which was studied in combination with conventional antiepileptic drugs against maximal electroshock, pentylenetetrazol, and amygdala-kindled seizures. In a sub-protective dose of 2 mg/kg, LY 300164 reduced the ED_{50} values of carbamazepine, clonazepam, phenytoin, phenobarbital, and valproate against maximal electroshock in mice very significantly (Czuczwar *et al.*, 1998c; Borowicz *et al.*, 1999). Side effects of clonazepam, phenobarbital, and valproate alone were more pronounced than those of the respective combinations of these antiepileptic drugs with LY 300164 (Czuczwar *et al.*, 1998c; Borowicz *et al.*, 1999). In the pentylenetetrazol test, LY 300164 increased the anticonvulsant-protective potential of valproate and ethosuximide, and these combinations were free from adverse effects (Czuczwar *et al.*, 1998b). A very potent interaction was found for LY 300164 and benzodiazepine derivatives, clonazepam and diazepam in amygdala-kindled rats. The combination of clonazepam (in a non-protective dose of 0.001 mg/kg) with LY 300164 (in a sub-protective dose of 2 mg/kg) resulted in an anticonvulsant effect comparable to that provided by clonazepam alone at 0.1 mg/kg (Borowicz *et al.*, 1999). Similar effects were observed when LY 300164 was combined with diazepam (Borowicz *et al.*, 2000b). The combination of this benzodiazepine (at 1.25 mg/kg) with LY 300164 (at 2 mg/kg) provided a protection against seizures comparable to that of diazepam alone at 10–20 mg/kg. Also, the combinations were devoid of adverse effects whilst diazepam alone very potently disturbed motor coordination and long-term memory in amygdala-kindled rats (Borowicz *et al.*, 2000b). Among the remaining conventional antiepileptic drugs, only a combination of valproate with LY 300164 (at 2 mg/kg) resulted in protective activity against amygdala kindling (Borowicz *et al.*, 2001). In no instance did LY 300164 affect the free-plasma concentration of antiepileptic drugs. The interactions of LY 300164 with conventional antiepileptic drugs in the kindling model

Table 11.5 Combined treatment of selective antagonists of NMDA and AMPA/KA receptors, LY 235959 and LY 300164, with conventional antiepileptic drugs in amygdala-kindled seizures in rats

Antiepileptic drug (mg/kg)	Protective activity		Adverse effects	
	LY 235959	LY 300164	LY 235959	LY 300164
Diazepam (1.25)	0	↑↑	NT	0
Phenobarbital (15)	0	0	NT	NT
Phenytoin (40)	↑	0	↑↑	NT
Carbamazepine (15)	0	0	NT	NT
Clonazepam (0.001)	0	↑↑	NT	0
Valproate (75)	0	↑↑	NT	0

LY 235959 and LY 300164 were administered intraperitoneally (i.p.) in a sub-protective dose of 2 mg/kg, 15 min prior to the convulsive test. Antiepileptic drugs were also given i.p. in sub-effective doses, diazepam, clonazepam, carbamazepine, valproate – 30 min; phenobarbital – 60 min; phenytoin – 120 min before the test.

Data are from Borowicz *et al.* (1999, 2000b, 2001).

0, no interaction or side-effect; ↑, positive interaction; ↑↑, very potent interaction; NT, not tested.

of epilepsy are shown in Table 11.5. Generally, AMPA/KA receptor antagonists display less adverse potential than NMDA receptor antagonists (Parada *et al.*, 1992; Danysz *et al.*, 1994). This may be relevant in terms of their possible clinical use as adjuvant antiepileptic drugs in cases where monotherapy fails.

Ligands of metabotropic glutamate receptors

In the early 1990s, experimental evidence indicated that metabotropic glutamate (mGlu) receptors (mGluRs) participate in the generation of seizure activity (Sacaan and Schoepp, 1992; McDonald *et al.*, 1993; Tizzano *et al.*, 1993). It was later elucidated that different ligands of mGluRs were effective anticonvulsant agents. For example, (*S*)-4-carboxy-3-hydroxyphenylglycine (an antagonist of mGlu1a and agonist of mGlu2 receptors), administered intracerebrally, inhibited sound-induced seizures in mice. This effect could be probably ascribed to a reduced release of glutamate because this process seems to be controlled by mGluRs (Thomsen *et al.*, 1994). This mGluR ligand was also effective in other experimental seizure types, including pentylenetetrazol-induced and electrically-induced convulsions. However, at effective anticonvulsant doses, the substance significantly impaired motor coordination (Dalby and Thomsen, 1996). A number of other agents interacting with mGluRs proved to exert anticonvulsant effects (for review see Urbañska *et al.*, 1998). Recently, an agonist of mGlu2 receptors has been available. 2-Aminobicyclo-(3,1,0)hexane-2,6-dicarboxylate (LY 354740) has a unique property among the mGluR ligands – it can easily enter the brain after peripheral administration. The substance proved effective against pentylenetetrazol- and picrotoxin-induced convulsions and potentiated the anticonvulsant efficacy of diazepam (but not that of ethosuximide or valproate) against pentylenetetrazol. Interestingly, apart from the potentiation of the activity of diazepam, LY 354740 reduced the free-plasma concentration of this antiepileptic drug (Klodzińska *et al.*, 2000).

Blockade of all ionotropic receptors for glutamate – a new therapeutic possibility?

Löscher *et al.* (1993) were first to report on a clearly synergistic effect of NBQX combined with an NMDA receptor antagonist against amygdala-kindled seizures in rats. Also, Czuczwar *et al.* (1995) examined NMDA receptor antagonists (dizocilpine and D-CPP-ene) and AMPA/KA receptor antagonists (NBQX and GYKI 52466) in this regard, finding a strong interaction in terms of anticonvulsant activity. Some combinations were devoid of adverse effects (Czuczwar *et al.*, 1995).

Interaction of antiepileptic drugs with voltage-dependent calcium channel inhibitors

There is no doubt that calcium channels are involved in the generation of seizure activity (Pumain *et al.*, 1984; Speckmann *et al.*, 1993). A hypothesis that voltage-dependent calcium channel inhibitors may be effective anticonvulsants was challenged by Desmedt in the 1970s but it was later confirmed (Desmedt *et al.*, 1976; De Sarro *et al.*, 1988; Jagiello-Wójtowicz *et al.*, 1991). This was followed by attempts to test the combinations of calcium channel inhibitors with antiepileptic drugs. Flunarizine (at a sub-protective dose of 20 mg/kg) considerably decreased the ED_{50}s of carbamazepine (by 51%) and valproate (by 54%) against electrically induced convulsions in mice. The ED_{50} value for phenytoin was reduced by 24%. Nimodipine was considerably weaker in this regard. None of these calcium channel blockers affected the plasma concentrations of these antiepileptic drugs and, generally, no adverse effects were observed (Czuczwar *et al.*, 1992). Also, the anti-electroshock activity of phenytoin and carbamazepine was potentiated by nifedipine and diltiazem, but the activity of phenobarbital and valproate was not influenced (Czuczwar *et al.*, 1990a). Interestingly, verapamil was completely inactive in this respect, both in the maximal electroshock and pentylenetetrazol test (Czuczwar *et al.*, 1990a, b). This clearly indicates that the calcium channel inhibitor-induced hypotension is probably not involved in their interaction with antiepileptic drugs. The lack of effect of verapamil to modulate the anticonvulsant potential of antiepileptic drugs may be associated with its poor penetration through the blood–brain barrier (Hamann *et al.*, 1983). Some conventional antiepileptic drugs were also affected by calcium channel inhibitors in the pentylenetetrazol test in mice. These were ethosuximide and, to a lesser degree, valproate and phenobarbital (Czuczwar *et al.*, 1990b; Gasior *et al.*, 1996). The combination of nimodipine with ethosuximide or valproate, however, resulted in motor impairment (Gasior *et al.*, 1996). It is noteworthy that flunarizine, although potently increasing the protective efficacy of conventional antiepileptic drugs against electrically induced convulsions (Czuczwar *et al.*, 1992), was completely ineffective in the pentylenetetrazol test in mice (Gasior *et al.*, 1996). Amlodipine reduced the ED_{50} values of carbamazepine, phenobarbital, and valproate against maximal electroshock in mice, but the protective activity of phenytoin was not affected. Since amlodipine elevated the free-plasma concentration of carbamazepine, this effect is the consequence of a pharmacokinetic interaction. Combinations of amlodipine with conventional antiepileptic drugs caused a strong motor impairment. Also, co-administration of amlodipine with phenobarbital or valproate resulted in a potent mnemonic effect (Kamiński *et al.*, 1999). In the pentylenetetrazol test, this calcium channel inhibitor enhanced the protective action of ethosuximide, phenobarbital, and valproate without affecting their plasma concentrations. Again, the combined treatment produced a considerable impairment of motor coordination in mice (Kamiñski *et al.*, 2001).

Although many calcium channel inhibitors actually potentiated the anticonvulsant activity of conventional antiepileptic drugs, in many cases significant side effects were evident. In this context, experimental data may help to choose an appropriate calcium channel inhibitor for the treatment of cardiovascular diseases in epileptic patients. One has to consider that there are even certain calcium channel inhibitors, for instance niguldipine, which were shown to impair the anticonvulsant activity of carbamazepine and phenobarbital against maximal electroshock in mice or amygdala-kindled seizures in rats (Borowicz *et al.*, 1997; 2002a). Consequently, some calcium channel inhibitors may be counteracted in epileptic patients.

Recent data by Swiader *et al.* (2002) indicated that flunarizine potentiated the protective activity of LY 300164 against maximal electroshock-induced convulsions in mice, presumably via a pharmacodymanic mechanism. This combination was also free of adverse effects. Among other calcium channel inhibitors, nifedipine did not modify the anticonvulsant activity of LY 300164, while nicardipine significantly raised its free-plasma concentration. Also, flunarizine was the only calcium channel inhibitor that could be shown to enhance the anticonvulsant action of another AMPA/KA receptor antagonist, GYKI 52466 (Gasior *et al.*, 1997).

Concluding remarks

Experimental data may provide a good background for the add-on treatment of epilepsy. It is evident from the data presented above that some combinations of antiepileptic drugs are promising, although the results of experimental studies can only be extrapolated with caution to the clinical setting. A considerable amount of experimental data are in agreement with what is observed in epileptic patients. A good example is D-CPP-ene and its adverse potential in rodents and epileptic patients, already discussed above (Sveinbjornsdottir *et al.*, 1993; Zarnowski *et al.*, 1994a). It is also worth stressing that the psychotomimetic activity of dizocilpine (a non-competitive antagonist of NMDA receptors) found in epileptic patients (Porter, 1990) was also evident in amygdala-kindled rats (Löscher and Hönack, 1991). However, it needs to be taken into consideration that antiepileptic drugs may undergo different metabolism in experimental animals and epileptic patients. For instance, topiramate was documented to increase the free-plasma concentration of carbamazepine in mice (Swiader *et al.*, 2000) while this effect was apparently not confirmed in epileptic patients (Bourgeois, 1996). However, most studies on the use of antiepileptic drugs are carried out acutely in rodents while epileptic patients receive a chronic antiepileptic therapy. It is widely known that carbamazepine and phenytoin are cytochrome P450 inducers when administered chronically, and this may be a reason for some discrepancies. Consequently, all experimental suggestions require careful clinical verification.

According to Majkowski (1994) and Deckers *et al.* (2000), the new antiepileptic drugs are currently used mainly as add-on therapy. Nevertheless, rational polytherapy with new antiepileptic drugs is likely to become increasingly widespread. It will remain a challenge for pharmacologists to provide experimental data on interactions between newer antiepileptic drugs. So far, such evidence is only fragmentary. Detailed interactions between antiepileptic drugs in both experimental and clinical conditions were also reviewed by Fröscher (1994) and Deckers *et al.* (2000). The experimental background for the evaluation of synergistic and additive effects of antiepileptic drugs given in combination was discussed by Czuczwar (1998) and Deckers *et al.* (2000).

In summary, monotherapy is recommended for the treatment of epilepsy, preferentially among newly diagnosed patients. However, in patients who are resistant to monotherapy, combination therapy may be beneficial. Experimental studies provide evidence that a combination of two antiepileptic drugs may produce antagonistic, additive, and supra-additive (synergistic) anticonvulsant effects. A drug combination producing a supra-additive seizure protection should be of clinical interest. However, if in addition to the enhanced protective efficacy against seizures there is also supra-additive toxicity, the protective index (and hence the effectiveness of the drug combination) may be equal or even inferior, when compared with each drug alone.

Two main experimental approaches for studying drug interactions exist. The isobolographic analysis may be employed when antiepileptic drugs are used at active doses against seizures. A shift of the dose–response curve for an antiepileptic drug in the presence of an adjuvant (usually in sub-protective doses) may also indicate which combinations to choose for clinical evaluation. Existing experimental evidence points to a favorable synergistic interaction between valproate and phenytoin (or ethosuximide) or topiramate and carbamazepine (or phenobarbital), or felbamate and all major antiepileptic drugs. However, the anticonvulsant potency of carbamazepine, phenytoin, phenobarbital, and valproate was not affected by felbamate at sub-protective doses against maximal electroshock in mice. This may indicate that synergism is encountered at only some drug concentration ratios. Considerable enhancement of the protective activity of conventional antiepileptic drugs by some calcium channel inhibitors and excitatory amino acid antagonists has also been demonstrated. The experimental data may be helpful for choosing drug combinations potentially beneficial in epileptic patients. However, final conclusions have to be based on appropriate clinical trials.

REFERENCES

Bialer M, Johanessen SI, Kupferberg HJ, *et al.* Progress report on new antiepileptic drugs: a summary of the fourth Eilat conference (EILAT IV). *Epilepsy Res* 1999; **34**: 1–41.

Borowicz KK, Gasior M, Kleinrok Z, *et al.* The non-competitive AMPA/kainate receptor antagonist, GYKI 52466, potentiates the anticonvulsant activity of conventional antiepileptics. *Eur J Pharmacol* 1995; **281**: 319–325.

Borowicz KK, Gasior M, Kleinrok Z, *et al.* Influence of isradipine, niguldipine and dantrolene on the anticonvulsive action of conventional antiepileptics in mice. *Eur J Pharmacol* 1997; **323**: 45–51.

Borowicz KK, Luszczki J, Szadkowski M, *et al.* Influence of LY 300164, an antagonist of AMPA/kainate receptors, on the anticonvulsant activity of clonazepam. *Eur J Pharmacol* 1999; **380**: 67–72.

Borowicz KK, Kleinrok Z, Czuczwar SJ. Influence of D(−)CPP and (±)CPP upon the protective action of conventional antiepileptic drugs against electroconvulsions in mice. *Pol J Pharmacol* 2000a; **52**: 431–439.

Borowicz KK, Kleinrok Z, Czuczwar SJ. The AMPA/kainate receptor antagonist, LY 300164, increases the anticonvulsant effects of diazepam. *Naunyn-Schmiedebergs Arch Pharmacol* 2000b; **361**: 629–635.

Borowicz KK, Stasiuk G, Teter J, *et al.* Low propensity of conventional antiepileptic drugs for interaction with felbamate against maximal electroshock-induced seizures in mice. *J Neural Transm* 2000c; **107**: 733–743.

Borowicz KK, Kleinrok Z, Czuczwar SJ. Glutamate antagonists differentially affect the protective activity of conventional antiepileptics against amygdala-kindled seizures in rats. *Eur Neuropsychopharmacol* 2001; **11**: 61–68.

Borowicz KK, Kleinrok Z, Czuczwar SJ. Niguldipine impairs the protective activity of carbamazepine and phenobarbital against amygdala-kindled seizures in rats. *Eur Neuropsychopharmacol* 2002a; **12**: 225–233.

Borowicz KK, Swiader M, Luszczki J, *et al.* Effect of gabapentin on the anticonvulsant activity of antiepileptic drugs against maximal electroshock in mice – an isobolographic analysis. *Epilepsia* 2002b; **43**: 956–963.

Bourgeois BFD. Antiepileptic drug combinations and experimental background: the case of phenobarbital and phenytoin. *Naunyn-Schmiedebergs Arch Pharmacol* 1986; **333**: 406–411.

Bourgeois BFD. Anticonvulsant potency and neurotoxicity of valproate alone and in combination with carbamazepine or phenobarbital. *Clin Neuropharmacol* 1988a; **11**: 348–359.

Bourgeois BFD. Combination of valproate and ethosuximide: antiepileptic and neurotoxic interaction. *J Pharmacol Exp Ther* 1988b; **247**: 1128–1132.

Bourgeois BFD. Drug interaction profile of topiramate. *Epilepsia* 1996; **37**(Suppl. 2): S14–S17.

Bourgeois BFD, Wad N. Individual and combined antiepileptic and neurotoxic activity of carbamazepine and carbamazepine-10,11-epoxide in mice. *J Pharmacol Exp Ther* 1984; **231**: 411–415.

Chen G, Ensor CR. A study of the anticonvulsant properties of phenobarbital and dilantin. *Arch Int Pharmacodyn Ther* 1954; **100**: 234–238.

Chez MG, Bourgeois BFD, Pippenger E, *et al.* Pharmacodynamic interactions between phenytoin and valproate: individual and combined antiepileptic and neurotoxic actions in mice. *Clin Neuropharmacol* 1994; **17**: 32–37.

Croucher MJ, Collins JF, Meldrum BS. Anticonvulsant action of excitatory amino acid antagonists. *Science* 1982; **216**: 899–901.

Czechowska G, Dziki M, Pietrasiewicz T, *et al.* Competitive antagonists of NMDA receptors, CGP 37849 and CGP 39551, enhance the anticonvulsant activity of valproate against electroconvulsions in mice. *Eur J Pharmacol* 1993; **232**: 59–64.

Czuczwar SJ. Experimental background for synergistic and additive effects of antiepileptic drugs. *Epileptologia* 1998; **6**(suppl. 2): 21–29.

Czuczwar SJ, Meldrum BS. Protection against chemically induced seizures by 2-amino-7-phosphono-heptanoic acid. *Eur J Pharmacol* 1982; **83**: 335–338.

Czuczwar SJ, Patsalos PN. The new generation of GABA enhancers. *CNS Drugs* 2001; **15**: 339–350.

Czuczwar SJ, Turski L, Kleinrok Z. Diphenylhydantoin potentiates the protective effect of diazepam against pentylenetetrazol but not against bicuculline and isoniazid-induced seizures in mice. *Neuropharmacology* 1981; **20**: 675–679.

Czuczwar SJ, Cavalheiro EA, Turski L, *et al.* Phosphonic analogues of excitatory amino acids raise the threshold for maximal electroconvulsions in mice. *Neurosci Res* 1985; **3**: 86–90.

Czuczwar SJ, Chodkowska A, Kleinrok Z, *et al.* Effects of calcium channel inhibitors upon the efficacy of common antiepileptic drugs. *Eur J Pharmacol* 1990a; **176**: 75–83.

Czuczwar SJ, Malek U, Kleinrok Z. Influence of calcium channel inhibitors upon the anticonvulsant efficacy of common antiepileptics against pentylenetetrazol-induced convulsions in mice. *Neuropharmacology* 1990b; **29**: 943–948.

Czuczwar SJ, Gasior M, Janusz W, *et al.* Influence of flunarizine, nicardipine and nimodipine on the anticonvulsant activity of different antiepileptic drugs in mice. *Neuropharmacology* 1992; **31**: 1179–1183.

Czuczwar SJ, Borowicz KK, Kleinrok Z, *et al.* Influence of combined treatment with NMDA and non-NMDA receptor antagonists on electroconvulsions in mice. *Eur J Pharmacol* 1995; **281**: 327–333.

Czuczwar SJ, Gasior M, Kamiński R, *et al.* GYKI 52466 (1-(4-aminophenyl)-4-methyl-7,8-methylenedioxy-5H-2,3-benzodiazepine hydrochloride) and the anticonvulsive activity of conventional antiepileptics against pentetrazol in mice. *Mol Chem Neuropathol* 1998a; **33**: 149–162.

Czuczwar SJ, Kamiński R, Gasior M, *et al.* LY 300164, a novel non-NMDA receptor antagonist, potentiates the anticonvulsive activity of antiepileptic drugs. In *4th Congress of the European Society for Clinical Neuropharmacology.* A. D. Korczyn, ed. Bologna: Monduzzi Editore, 1998b: 35–39.

Czuczwar SJ, Swiader M, Kuzniar H, *et al.* LY 300164, a novel antagonist of AMPA/kainate receptors, potentiates the anticonvulsive activity of antiepileptic drugs. *Eur J Pharmacol* 1998c; **359**: 103–109.

Czuczwar SJ, Kamiński R, Kleinrok Z, *et al.* Influence of gabapentin on the anticonvulsive activity of conventional antiepileptic drugs in mice. *Epilepsia* 1999; **40**(suppl. 2): 125.

Dalby NO, Thomsen C. Modulation of seizure activity in mice by metabotropic glutomate receptor ligands. *J Pharmocol Exp Ther* 1996; **276**: 516–522.

Danysz W, Essman U, Bresink I, *et al.* Glutamate antagonists have different effects on spontaneous locomotor activity in rats. *Pharmacol Biochem Behav* 1994; **48**: 111–118.

Deckers CL, Czuczwar SJ, Hekster YA, *et al.* Selection of antiepileptic drug polytherapy based on mechanisms of action; the evidence reviewed. *Epilepsia* 2000; **41**: 1364–1374.

De Sarro GB, Meldrum BS, Nistico G. Anticonvulsant effects of some calcium entry blockers in DBA/2 mice. *Br J Pharmacol* 1988; **93**: 247–256.

De Sarro GB, Spagnolo C, Gareri P, *et al.* Gabapentin potentiates the antiseizure activity of certain anticonvulsants in DBA/2 mice. *Eur J Pharmacol* 1998; **349**: 179–185.

Desmedt LKC, Niemegeers CJE, Janssen PAJ. Anticonvulsant properties of cinnarizine and flunarizine in mice. *Arzneim Forsch* 1976; **25**: 1408–1413.

Fröscher W. Synergistic effects of drug combinations. *Epileptologia* 1994; **2**(suppl. 1): 23–32.

Gasior M, Kamiński R, Brudniak T, *et al.* Influence of nicardipine, nimodipine and flunarizine on the anticonvulsant efficacy of antiepileptics against pentylenetetrazol in mice. *J Neural Transm* 1996; **103**: 819–831.

Gasior M, Borowicz K, Kleinrok Z, *et al.* Anticonvulsant and adverse effects of MK-801, LY 235959, and GYKI 52466 in combination with Ca^{2+} channel inhibitors in mice. *Pharmacol Biochem Behav* 1997; **56**: 629–635.

Gordon R, Gels M, Wichmann J, *et al.* Interaction of felbamate with several other antiepileptic drugs against seizures induced by maximal electroshock in mice. *Epilepsia* 1993; **34**: 367–371.

Hamann SR, Todd GD, McAllister RG. The pharmacology of verapamil. Tissue distribution of verapamil and norverapamil in rat and dog. *Pharmacology* 1983; **27**: 1–8.

Huxtable RJ, Laird H, Lippincott SE, *et al.* Epilepsy and the concentration of plasma amino acids in humans. *Neurochem Int* 1983; **5**: 125–135.

Jagiello-Wójtowicz E, Czuczwar SJ, Chodkowska E, *et al.* Influence of calcium channel blockers on pentylenetetrazol and electroshock-induced convulsions in mice. *Pol J Pharmacol* 1991; **43**: 95–101.

Janjua NA, Itano T, Kugoh T, *et al.* Familial increase in plasma glutamic acid in epilepsy. *Epilepsy Res* 1992; **11**: 37–44.

Kamiñski R, Jasiñski M, Jagiello-Wójtowicz E, *et al.* Effect of amlodipine upon the protective activity of antiepileptic drugs against maximal electroshock-induced seizures in mice. *Pharmacol Res* 1999; **40**: 319–325.

Kamiñski R, Mazurek M, Turski WA, *et al.* Amlodipine enhances the activity of antiepileptic drugs against pentylenetetrazole-induced seizures. *Pharmacol Biochem Behav* 2001; **68**: 661–668.

Klodziñska A, Bijak M, Chojnacka-Wójcik E, *et al.* Roles of group II metabotropic glutamate receptors in modulation of seizure activity. *Naunyn-Schmiedebergs Arch Pharmacol* 2000; **361**: 283–288.

Leppik IE, Sherwin AL. Anticonvulsant activity of phenobarbital and phenytoin in combination. *J Pharmacol Exp Ther* 1977; **200**: 570–575.

Litchfield JT, Wilcoxon F. A simplified method of evaluating dose–effect experiments. *J Pharmacol Exp Ther* 1949; **96**: 99–113.

Löscher W, Jäckel R, Czuczwar SJ. Is amygdala kindling in rats a model for drug-resistant partial epilepsy? *Exp Neurol* 1986; **93**: 211–226.

Löscher W, Schmidt D. Which animal models should be used in the search for new antiepileptic drugs? A proposal based on experimental and clinical considerations. *Epilepsy Res* 1988; **2**: 145–181.

Löscher W, Hönack D. Anticonvulsant and behavioral effects of two novel competitive N-methyl-D-aspartic acid receptor antagonists, CGP 37849 and CGP 39551, in the kindling model of epilepsy. Comparison with MK-801 and carbamazepine. *J Pharmacol Exp Ther* 1991; **256**: 432–440.

Löscher W, Rundfeldt C, Hönack D. Low doses of NMDA receptor antagonists synergistically increase the anticonvulsant effect of the AMPA receptor antagonist NBQX in the kindling model of epilepsy. *Eur J Neurosci* 1993; **5**: 1545–1550.

Löscher W. New visions in the pharmocology of anticonvulsion. *Eur J Pharmacology* 1998; **342**: 1–13.

Majkowski J. Interactions between new and old generations of antiepileptic drugs. *Epileptologia* 1994; **2**(suppl. 1): 33–42.

Masuda Y, Utsui Y, Shiraishi Y, *et al.* Evidence for a synergistic interaction between phenytoin and phenobarbital in experimental animals. *J Pharmacol Exp Ther* 1981; **217**: 805–811.

McDonald JW, Fix AS, Tizzano JP, *et al.* Seizures and brain injury in neonatal rats induced by 1S,3R-ACPD, a metabotropic glutamate receptor agonist. *J Neurosci* 1993; **13**: 4445–4455.

Meldrum B. Amino acid neurotransmitters and new approaches to anticonvulsant drug action. *Epilepsia* 1984; **25**: S140–S149.

Monaco F, Sechi GP, Russo A, *et al.* Comparison of carbamazepine and phenobarbital given in combination in experimental epilepsy. *Epilepsia* 1985; **26**: 103–108.

Monaghan DT, Bridges RJ, Cotman CW. The excitatory amino-acid receptors: their classes, pharmacology and distinct properties in the function of the central nervous system. *Ann Rev Pharmacol Toxicol* 1989; **29**: 365–402.

Parada J, Czuczwar SJ, Turski WA. NBQX does not affect learning and memory tasks in mice: a comparison with D-CPP-ene and ifenprodil. *Cognitive Brain Res* 1992; **1**: 67–71.

Pietrasiewicz T, Czechowska G, Dziki M, *et al.* Competitive NMDA receptor antagonists enhance the antielectroshock activity of various antiepileptics. *Eur J Pharmacol* 1993; **250**: 1–7.

Porter RJ. New antiepileptic agents: strategies for drug development. *Lancet* 1990; **336**: 423–424.

Pumain R, Kurcewicz I, Louvel J. Fast extracellular calcium transients: involvement in epileptic processes. *Science* 1984; **222**: 177–179.

Sacaan AI, Schoepp DD. Activation of hippocampal metabotropic excitatory amino acid receptors leads to seizures and neuronal damage. *Neurosci Lett* 1992; **139**: 77–82.

Sander JW. Some aspects of prognosis in the epilepsies: a review. *Epilepsia* 1993; **34**: 1007–1016.

Shank RP, Gardocki JF, Vaught JL, *et al.* Topiramate: preclinical evaluation of a structurally novel anticonvulsant. *Epilepsia* 1994; **35**: 450–460.

Sills GJ, Butler E, Forrest C, *et al.* Combination studies with the novel anticonvulsant topiramate in the pentylenetetrazol seizure model. *Epilepsia* 1999; **40**(Suppl. 2): 128.

Smith SE, Durmuller N, Meldrum BS. The non-*N*-methyl-D-aspartate receptor antagonists, GYKI 52466 and NBQX are anticonvulsant in two animal models of reflex epilepsy. *Eur J Pharmacol* 1991; **201**: 179–183.

Speckmann EJ, Stroub H, Köhling R. Contribution of calcium ions to the generation of epileptic activity and antiepileptic calcium antagonism. *Neuropsychobiology* 1993; **27**: 122–126.

Stephen LJ, Sills GJ, Brodie MJ. Lamotrigine and topiramate may be a useful combination. *Lancet* 1998; **351**: 958–959.

Sveinbjornsdottir S, Sander JWAS, Upton D, *et al.* The excitatory amino acid antagonist D-CPP-ene (SDZ EAA-494) in patients with epilepsy. *Epilepsy Res* 1993; **16**: 165–174.

Swiader M, Kotowski J, Gasior M, *et al.* Interaction of topiramate with conventional antiepileptic drugs in mice. *Eur J Pharmacol* 2000; **399**: 35–41.

Swiader M, Borowicz KK, Porebiak J, *et al.* Influence of agents affecting voltage-dependent calcium channels and dantrolene on the anticonvulsant action of the AMPA/kainate receptor antagonist LY 300164 in mice. *Eur Neuropsychopharmacol* 2002; **12**: 311–319.

Tallarida RJ. Statistical analysis of drug combinations for synergism. *Pain* 1992; **49**: 93–97.

Tallarida RJ, Porecca F, Cowan A. Statistical analysis of drug–drug and site–site interactions with isobolograms. *Life Sci* 1989; **45**: 947–961.

Thomsen C, Klitgaard H, Sheardown M, *et al.* (*S*)-4-carboxy-3-hydroxyphenylglycine, an antagonist of metabotropic glutamate receptor (mGluR)1a and an agonist of mGluR2, protects against audiogenic seizures in DBA/2 mice. *J Neurochem* 1994; **62**: 2492–2495.

Tizzano JP, Griffey KI, Johnson JA, *et al.* Intracerebral 1*S*,3*R*-1-aminocyclopentane-1,3-dicarboxylic acid ((1*S*,3*R*)-ACPD) produces limbic seizures that are not blocked by ionotropic glutamate receptor antagonists. *Neurosci Lett* 1993; **162**: 12–16.

Turski WA, Urbañska E, Dziki M, *et al.* Excitatory amino acid antagonists protect mice against seizures induced by bicuculline. *Brain Res* 1990; **514**: 131–134.

Turski L, Jacobsen P, Honoré T, *et al.* Relief of experimental spasticity and anxiolytic/anticonvulsant actions of the α-amino-3-hydroxy-5-methyl-4-isoxazole-propionate antagonist 2,3-dihydroxy-6-nitro-7-sulfamoyl-benzo(*F*)-quinoxaline. *J Pharmacol Exp Ther* 1992; **260**: 742–747.

Urbañska E, Dziki M, Czuczwar SJ, *et al.* Antiparkinsonian drugs memantine and trihexyphenidyl potentiate the anticonvulsant activity of valproate against maximal electroshock-induced seizures. *Neuropharmacology* 1992; **31**: 1021–1026.

Urbañska EM, Czuczwar SJ, Kleinrok Z, *et al.* Excitatory amino acids in epilepsy (invited review). *Restor Neurol Neurosci* 1998; **13**: 25–39.

Watkins JC, Krogsgaard-Larsen P, Honoré T. Structure–activity relationships in the development of excitatory amino acid receptor agonists and competitive antagonists. *Trend Pharmacol Sci* 1990; **11**: 25–33.

Weaver LC, Swinyard EA, Woodbury LA, *et al.* Studied on the anticonvulsant drug combinations: phenobarbital and diphenylhydantoin. *J Pharmacol Exp Ther* 1955; **113**: 359–370.

Zarnowski T, Kleinrok Z, Turski WA, *et al.* 2,3-Dihydroxy-6-nitro-7-sulfamoyl-benzo(*F*)quinoxaline enhances the protective activity of common antiepileptic drugs against maximal electroshock-induced seizures in mice. *Neuropharmacology* 1993; **32**: 895–900.

Zarnowski T, Kleinrok Z, Turski WA, *et al.* The competitive NMDA antagonist, D-CPP-ene, potentiates the anticonvulsant activity of conventional antiepileptics against maximal electroshock-induced seizures in mice. *Neuropharmacology* 1994a; **33**: 619–624.

Zarnowski T, Kleinrok Z, Turski WA, *et al.* The NMDA antagonist procyclidine, but not ifenprodil, enhances the protective efficacy of common antiepileptics against maximal electroshock-induced seizures in mice. *J Neural Transm* 1994b; **97**: 1–12.

12

Clinical studies of pharmacodynamic interactions

John R. Pollard and Jacqueline French

Department of Neurology, University of Pennsylvania, Philadelphia, PA

Introduction

This chapter addresses the clinical impact of pharmacodynamic (PD) interactions of antiepileptic drugs (AEDs) and the strategies that have been used to discover these interactions. Particular attention is paid to the limitations of available studies and the chapter concludes with a summary of expert opinion about optimal study design for identifying PD interactions. For the purposes of this chapter, the definition of a PD interaction is the interaction of two drugs causing a greater or less than expected effect or side-effect in the absence of a pharmacokinetic interaction.

Polypharmacy has undergone a renaissance since the early 1980s (Goldsmith and de Bittencourt, 1995). The old arguments against combination therapy were predicated upon the observation that refractory patients placed in polytherapy were experiencing increased adverse events without better efficacy (Schmidt, 1982). Since then, the advent of monitoring AED levels and a deeper understanding of the mechanisms of AED action have led to more effective use of rational polypharmacy. A combination of drugs can now be used which suppress excitation, enhance inhibition, and work by other novel mechanisms, thus providing a previously lacking theoretical construct for the assertion that the efficacy of combinations of drugs can be additive or supra-additive. In addition, monitoring of AED levels can limit pharmacokinetic variation that often used to cause adverse events when drugs were combined. The clinician's goal is to identify combinations that improve effectiveness, a goal that could be achieved more often if natural synergies could be identified.

For any given effect or side effect, there are four possible outcomes of PD interactions. The first is additivity, which indicates that there is no change in the effect expected from each drug. The second is supra-additivity, a state in which a given combination results in an effect which is greater than that expected from simple additivity. The third possibility is antagonism, which is a combination that does not have at least the total effect that each medicine would be expected to have on its own. Lastly, there is aberrancy, in which a combination results in completely different effects. Alternative nomenclature of *positive-* or *negative-*PD interactions has been used in some literature. These terms imply a deviation in one direction or the other away from the additive state.

Deckers *et al.* (2000) define effectiveness as 'a measure encompassing both efficacy and tolerability', and PD interactions can affect both. This chapter will address the evidence for additivity, supra-additivity, antagonism and aberrancy for various combinations as they relate to both efficacy and tolerability. Also, an attempt will be made to summarize the experiences to date with trial design quantifying PD interactions and to highlight the designs that have the best chance of providing clinically useful knowledge. Of note, the works of Deckers *et al.* (2000, 2003) and Bourgeois (2002) are excellent recent reviews that summarize the results of studies relevant to PD interactions.

Positive-PD interactions: efficacy

The following section will outline trials that have provided, or have attempted to provide, relevant data on PD interactions that impact on efficacy. In assessing the validity of these studies, several issues should be considered.

Should trials be sequential or parallel?

Many of the studies discussed below have been sequential – each patient must 'fail' on monotherapy of one or two drugs, which are then combined, to determine whether the combination succeeds where monotherapy failed. The advantage to this approach is that each patient can be pushed to individual maximal tolerated dose. This ensures that the monotherapy was a true failure, rather than a failure to achieve the proper dose. The disadvantage is that studies designed in this way are long, leading to dropouts, which may bias the outcome.

What is the impact of drug load on PD interactions?

One major problem with many studies of AED combinations is that drug load is not taken into account. Clearly, the same adverse events would not occur when two drugs are given at high doses, as when they are combined in lower doses. Deckers has suggested that toxicity may be a result of total drug load, rather than the combination of two drugs per se. He uses a prescribed daily dose/defined daily dose (PDD/DDD) calculation to determine drug load. In a review, he points out that most studies of add-on therapy do not provide information about doses of background drugs, making it difficult to determine total drug load (Deckers *et al.*, 1997a). However, this concept of total drug load toxicity may not be true for all drugs. A drug that was pharmacodynamically benign might be able to be added to any existing drug combination without causing problems. If a drug proves particularly tolerable, this concept can be used to evaluate combinations that would allow the average patient to exceed normal drug loads (Deckers *et al.*, 1997b).

Is the goal of the study improved efficacy or lowering of toxicity?

In most of the trials discussed below, two drugs are combined at standard doses, to produce additive efficacy. In some cases, however, the goal of combination therapy may be a reduction in toxicity rather than improved efficacy. Most AEDs demonstrate both increase in efficacy as well as toxicity as dosage increases. Even standard dosages may produce undesirable dose-related side effects. Therefore, it may be useful to demonstrate that lower than standard doses of two drugs can be combined to produce the efficacy of either drug at higher (and presumably less well-tolerated) doses in monotherapy. This approach would only be useful if reduced toxicity could be demonstrated, since efficacy presumably is no better than monotherapy.

What type of outcome analysis should be employed?

Seizure freedom is the ultimate goal of any epilepsy therapy. Many studies have focused on this outcome measure in combination trials. Often, seizure freedom is the only outcome measure provided. While this is useful, it may be misleading. For example, by random chance, some patients may improve while others deteriorate. In this case, reporting seizure freedom only might give an appearance of benefit, where none exists.

Definitive data supporting the presence of additive or supra-additive PD interactions are difficult to find and several obstacles will be illustrated in the examples below. A caveat to the following presentation of the available data concerning additivity comes from Patsalos who suggests that there is a possibility that 'some of these therapeutic enhancements result from pharmacokinetic interactions taking place in the central brain compartment, rather than as a result of PD interactions…' (Patsalos *et al.*, 2002). Nevertheless, for clinical purposes, any synergistic result is still important.

Add-on placebo-controlled trials

The most common studies of additive effects of AEDs are the randomized placebo-controlled add-on studies of the new AEDs. The design timeline is shown in Figure 12.1. The patients enter these trials on a variety of baseline drugs, typically with a maximum of two allowed. Increasing doses of the study drugs are employed, often leading to an incremental decrease in seizure frequency (see Figure 12.2) (Cramer *et al.*, 1999). These studies suggest that the study drug does indeed have at least an additive effect on efficacy. Thus the entire generation of newer AEDs that were all

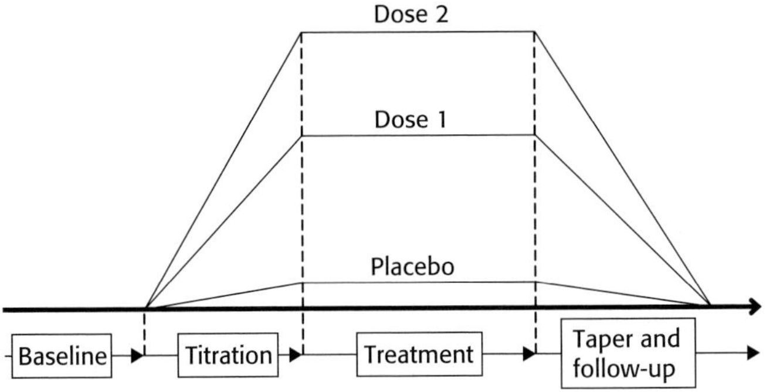

Figure 12.1   Double-blind placebo-controlled trial schema

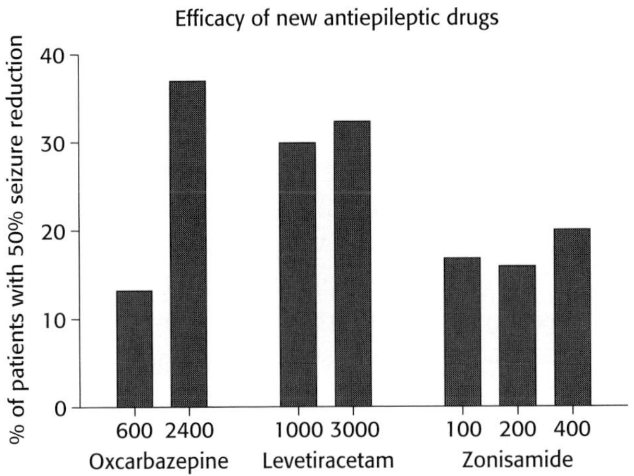

Figure 12.2   Fifty per cent seizure reduction in placebo-controlled add-on trials of three new AEDs
(with placebo rate subtracted) (after Cramer *et al.*, 1999)

tested using this type of study design probably have at least an additive effect on efficacy. Unfortunately, one cannot glean specific information about which combinations were most effective, because of the small number of patients on each baseline AED. It is also difficult to establish definitively that the effect is truly additive, because of problems establishing the efficacy of a baseline drug a study patient received. A very conservative interpretation of these types of study would question whether these add-on studies simply show that the new drug was effective while the older baseline drug was not.

Other studies

Dean and Penry (1998) studied the combination of carbamazepine (CBZ) and valproate (VPA) using 100 patients who had failed monotherapy with CBZ. This study showed good success. However, it is possible that VPA monotherapy would have worked just as well, thus complicating the interpretation of these data as being supportive of an additive effect on efficacy. Of note, Harden *et al.* (1993) presented a smaller number of patients with a similar study design and result.

A trial of phenobarbital (PB) compared to phenytoin (PHT) and the PHT/PB combination was done in a non-randomized fashion in neonates with refractory seizures (Painter *et al.*, 1999). This study suggested that the combination therapy made an additional 12–17% seizure free. As with the aforementioned studies, a monotherapy of the second drug was not tried, so it is not clear what the result would have been with just substituted monotherapy. A similar study design was used by Murri and Iudice (1995) in an add-on study of vigabatrin added to CBZ. There was a dropout rate of 30% but a substantial number of patients became seizure free.

Tanganelli and Regesta (1996) performed a study that used patients with newly diagnosed epilepsy, a good way to avoid the difficulties with establishing the baseline efficacy of each drug. Vigabatrin and CBZ were studied separately and in combination. The patients were randomly assigned to either drug and then titrated until they were either seizure free or experienced toxicity. Patients who became toxic before achieving adequate control were switched to the other medication. Combination therapy was attempted only for those patients who failed monotherapy. A total of 51/58 patients completed the study, and no data is available for the ones who did not complete. Approximately half of the patients responded well to their initial therapy. Of the non-responders 45% had good control with the cross over drug. The combination therapy had good results as well, with 5/14 patients (35%) becoming seizure free. There was no statistically significant difference between the efficacy of the two drugs, but the study was not powered to necessarily detect a small difference in efficacy between the drugs. This study shows an additive effect for efficacy when these two drugs are combined, because many patients who did not respond to either drug separately became seizure free with the combination. This study design was also used by Hakkaraninen (1980) using CBZ and PHT. In this study of 100 patients, presented in abstract form only, 5/33 patients (15%) who failed sequential monotherapy became seizure free on combination therapy.

Walker and Koon (1988) tried a slightly different study design. They compared CBZ, VPA and the combination in series, dropping those patients who responded well from the next study arm. Again some patients became seizure free on the combination. This is relatively good evidence for an additive effect of the two drugs, but the data may be challenged because of the sequential study design.

In another classic add-on study, ethosuximide was added to VPA for control of absence seizures (Rowan *et al.*, 1983). Five patients were involved in the study, and

Latin square design

E. PB group: 3/8 and Diphenylhydantoin (DPH) group: 3/8
F. PB group: 3/4
G. DPH group: 3/4
H. Blank

	Week ⟶			
Group	1st	2nd	3rd	4th
1	E	F	G	H
2	F	H	E	G
3	G	E	H	F
4	H	G	F	E

Figure 12.3   Comparison of PB and DPH (after Gruber *et al.*, 1956)

all became seizure free. Two of these patients had been refractory to ethosuximide monotherapy, so these results also support at least additivity for efficacy.

The issue of using sub-toxic doses of two drugs to reduce side effects was explored in several interesting studies. An oft-cited study by Gruber *et al.* (1956) compared PB and PHT in what today would be considered an unusual design, a latin square (see Figure 12.3). Patients were on their own baseline medication for 3 days of the week and then were given the study drug for 4 days. Given the long half-lives of both study drugs, it is not clear if adequate washout time was given. The study results suggested that 50 mg of either drug daily was just as efficacious as 25 mg of both drugs in combination. This study design is similar to the isobolograms done when studying PD interactions in animals (Chapter XI).

In patients with newly diagnosed epilepsy, Deckers *et al.* (2001) compared full dose CBZ, full dose VPA, and a half drug load of both. No difference was found in overall neurotoxicity or efficacy as measured by seizure frequency. It should be kept in mind, however, that newly diagnosed patients are not as sensitive to efficacy differences between regimens, and are usually responsive to lower doses of medication. No study arm was included with half dose of either drug alone. If we assume that half dose of either AED would translate into less effectiveness than the full dose of either, this study supports the notion that these two AEDs have an additive PD effect with respect to efficacy. This type of study using the concept of drug load may be invaluable for future studies.

Using a latin square design similar to the Gruber study mentioned above, Cereghino *et al.* (1975) compared CBZ, PHT and PB alone and in various combinations. The groups were not assigned randomly, but instead were divided into groups the authors thought were equivalent. As in the Gruber study, the PB arms probably were not given adequate washout time. In addition one criterion for inclusion in the study was that each patient had to be refractory to CBZ treatment, thus complicating the interpretation by raising the possibility that the CBZ was not working at all in some patients. Nonetheless, in terms of total seizure frequency, the combination of all the three drugs was the superior condition for controlling seizures, while the group on combination PB and PHT had the most frequent seizures. Despite many limitations, this study may show an additive effect.

Kwan and Brodie (2000) compared add-on therapy to substitution therapy in refractory patients. In this prospective chart review, patients had similar rates of effectiveness when converted to a sequential therapy or an add-on. The authors observed 'more patients became seizure free when the combination involved a sodium channel blocker and a drug with multiple mechanisms of action compared to other combinations.' These data, while relatively underpowered, would support the theory that PD interaction that results in increased efficacy will likely be a result of targeting multiple points along the pathways of excitatory and inhibitory action (Goldsmith and de Bittencourt, 1995).

Certain specific combinations have been suggested as being more successful than others. Stephen *et al.* (1998) presented three cases where topiramate was added to lamotrigine and the patients became seizure free. There are several studies of the lamotrigine and VPA combination, and these provide the best evidence that there is a supra-additive effect from certain combinations of AEDs. The first notable study was by Brodie and Yuen (1997) (see Figure 12.4). Three hundred and forty-seven patients with any type of refractory epilepsy on monotherapy (VPA, CBZ, PHT) received add-on lamotrigine in addition to their previous drug. If patients had a >50% reduction in seizures, then the first drug was withdrawn. The lamotrigine produced seizure reduction in a proportion of patients when it was added to each of the tested baseline medications. When the primary drug was withdrawn, seizure frequency declined slightly in the PHT and CBZ groups, possibly as a result

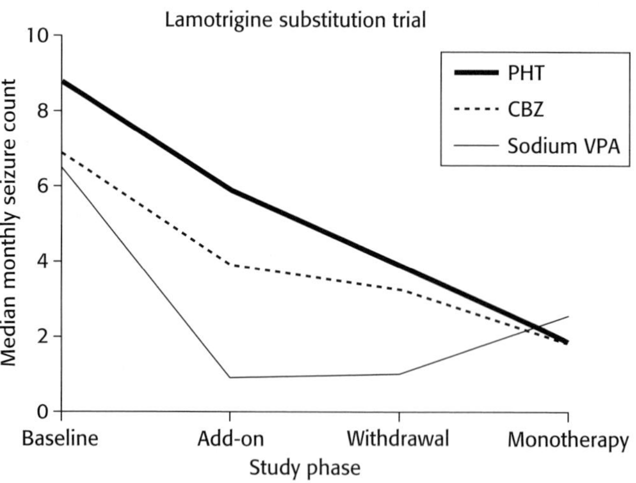

Figure 12.4 Results of lamotrigine substitution for each of the above AEDs (after Brodie *et al.*, 1997)

of removal of the hepatic enzyme-inducing effect of these medications, and a resulting rise in lamotrigine levels. In contrast, when the VPA was withdrawn, there was an increase in seizure frequency, despite the fact that the lamotrigine serum levels were higher as a result of dosage adjustments. This effect suggests that there may be at least an additive effect of these two drugs and possibly even PD supra-additivity. Unfortunately, this part of the study had relatively few subjects due to substantial numbers of patients who dropped out. Of course, this dropout effect may account for the apparent improvement, as those who were doing better would be more likely to remain. Another weakness of this study is the possible selection bias of the primary treatment drug.

Kanner and Frey (2000) specifically studied the combination of lamotrigine and VPA and controlled for pharmacokinetic interactions. The study evaluated 27 patients with partial epilepsy and one with generalized epilepsy who were refractory to treatment on at least three AED. All patients were on lamotrigine monotherapy at sub-toxic doses and then had VPA added. The average seizure free duration was 6.2 months on combination but only 2.1 months on monotherapy. One limitation is that the enrolled patients were selected specifically because they were refractory to lamotrigine monotherapy. These results, from a well-controlled study, again indicate the possibility that an additive or even a supra-additive PD interaction may exist between these two drugs both in efficacy and side effects.

Negative-PD interactions: efficacy

Antagonistic PD interactions for efficacy exist when a combination of two medicines does not have the efficacy that each would be expected to have on its own. In the study by Brodie and Yuen (1997) described above, a group of refractory patients who were taking CBZ or PHT as primary drugs had lamotrigine added on and then the primary drug withdrawn. As noted, during the combination period, patients had more seizures than during lamotrigine monotherapy. Although this result may reflect antagonism for efficacy, it is plausible that pharmacokinetic, rather than PD interactions resulted in a spurious result. However, had pharmacokinetic interactions not been a factor, this study design would have been ideal for identifying PD antagonism.

A few case reports have suggested that the combination of VPA and clonazepam can induce status epilepticus, a result that could be defined as the worst case scenario for antagonistic PD interaction for efficacy. However, other studies with larger numbers of patients showed no episodes of status (Rosenberry *et al.*, 1979; Mireles and Leppik, 1985). It is possible the surprising dearth of data showing antagonistic effects of AED on efficacy may reflect a certain reality. Some have maintained that 'PD interactions (regarding efficacy) … are probably unidirectional and lead only to increased effects' (Reife, 1998). However, another possibility is that the proper studies to look for this type of interaction have not been done. Even drug combinations that produce improvement in many patients may produce worsening in some. Somerville *et al.* (2002) looked at seizure worsening in pooled data from randomized adjunctive trials. He found that more patients worsened when tiagabine was added than when placebo was added, even though tiagabine caused a greater overall seizure reduction than placebo. This would indicate a bimodal distribution, with some patients improving, and others worsening. This indicates that PD interactions are not always unidirectional.

PD interactions: side effects

As noted above, side effects are often dose-related. Negative-PD interactions, also called supra-additivity for side effects, may occur when two drugs with similar side-effect profiles exceed the threshold for that side effect in combination but not individually. The possibility exists of discovering combinations of drugs that have additivity for efficacy permitting the use of doses below the threshold for side effects. A study by Lammers *et al.* (1995) used a quantitative assessment of adverse effects for patients on monotherapy vs. polytherapy. Interestingly, the study showed that as an aggregate measure, adverse events were no more frequent in either group. This suggests that it is possible that specific combinations of medications may offer extra efficacy without producing extra side effects. An alternative explanation for these results is that measuring the percentage of people who suffer from a given side effect may not be the best measure. Some subjects may have experienced worsening of side effects with the combination of medicines, but this would not have been detected by the measurements used in this study.

Several studies of specific AED combinations have demonstrated an increase in side effects. In the study by Kanner and Frey (2000) described above, the combination of VPA and lamotrigine caused an increase in the number of patients complaining of tremor to 55%. This combination of VPA and lamotrigine also caused a notable increase in the fraction of patients experiencing tremor in a study by Pisani *et al.* (1999). It is unclear whether the increase was additive or supra-additive. Another example is the studies by Tanganelli and Regesta (1996) and Murri and Iudice (1995) discussed above, in which the combination of vigabatrin and CBZ led to increase in side effects such as weight gain and ataxia. As another example of a possible combination-specific interaction, in a small case series, four patients on polytherapy that included CBZ were started on levetiracetam and experienced side effects characteristic of CBZ toxicity. All the patients responded to decreasing the dose of one of the drugs, but no levels were drawn (Sisodiya *et al.*, 2002). This interaction has not been confirmed by other investigators.

PD interactions may also increase the likelihood of non-dose-related side effects and serious idiosyncratic reactions. Osteopenia has been reported to occur in highest incidence among patients taking more than one enzyme-inducing AED (Farhat *et al.*, 2002). Hepatic toxicity is significantly more common in patients taking valproic acid in combination therapy than in monotherapy, and this effect becomes even more pronounced in the young. The incidence of VPA-induced hepatic failure increases from 1/2000 in children under 2 years old on monotherapy, to 1/200 in those on polytherapy. The cause of this interaction is unknown (Dreifuss *et al.*, 1987).

Another dramatic PD interaction is the development of side effects that are not described for either drug in isolation. In one descriptive paper, three patients developed new-onset chorea, and all were on a combination of PHT and lamotrigine (Zaatreh *et al.*, 2001). The chorea resolved in all these patients with tapering of one medication. Although this side effect has been described for AEDs, it was unusual that this combination appeared in all three cases of chorea seen at an epilepsy clinic and represents an aberrant PD interaction for side effects.

Trial designs

The problem of designing the ideal trial to assess PD interactions has been addressed by several authors. Pledger (1989) suggests that the most straightforward and ethical design would involve a baseline medication that had no interactions with the two drugs to be studied (X and Y). All patients would be on the baseline drug and then groups would receive X, Y or X + Y as add-on therapy. However, even the author notes that this study design would probably be prohibitively large. Deckers *et al.* (2003) suggest another paradigm that might be less costly. Patients would be evaluated on polytherapy while in the midst of switching monotherapies. He argues that this would provide useful clinical information, and provide information about PD interactions. Additionally since there is very little evidence for negative-PD interactions for efficacy, if a given combination is evaluated and proved not to have higher efficacy than the primary monotherapy, then the secondary therapy likely does not work. This would save the patient from an ineffective second monotherapy. Bourgeois (2002) suggests the optimal model would be to give drug X to maximally tolerated dose, then give drug Y to maximally tolerated dose as monotherapy, then a combination of both. While potentially valid, one must consider the likelihood of spontaneous regression/remission when analyzing such a trial.

Bourgeois has also discussed the impact of drug load, as it relates to PD interactions. He states that while drug load can be used in an isobologram fashion to give half doses of each drug, he considers this option suboptimal. A patient who is not tolerating maximal doses of drug X may be tried randomly in two arms of a trial: half dose X + half dose Y; or convert to drug Y titrated up from half dose. This type of trial was attempted by Deckers *et al.* (2001) but no attempt was made to discover if half dose of drug Y was as effective as the combination.

Bourgeois lists other designs as most likely valid such as: failure of drug X, improvement after addition of drug Y, and then worsening after elimination of drug X; or adding drug D to drugs X, Y, or Z and obtaining significantly better results with one of the combinations.

In summary, the total database of proven PD interactions is far from complete. To date, the best data for a potentially supra-additive effect on efficacy are for the combination of lamotrigine and VPA. Studies undertaken in the future should ideally address many of the difficulties identified above. These include: using universally accepted measures of efficacy, inefficacy, and side effects; accounting for dropouts; using the concept of drug load; and performing well-controlled studies that rule out pharmacokinetic interactions. For many reasons, whether cost or ethics or unavailability of patients, we are unlikely to gain the insights into PD interactions that the perfect studies would afford.

REFERENCES

Bourgeois, BFD. Antiepileptic drug combinations: when two are better than one. *Epilepsy Network News* 2002; **9**(1): 1–3, 6.

Brodie MJ, Yuen AWC, 105 Study Group. Lamotrigine substitution study: evidence for synergism with sodium valproate. *Epilepsy Res* 1997; **26**: 423–432.

Cereghino JJ, Brock JT, Van Meter JC, *et al.* The efficacy of carbamazepine combinations in epilepsy. *Clin Pharmacol Ther* 1975; **18**: 733–741.

Cramer JA, Fisher R, Ben-Menachem E, *et al.* New antiepileptic drugs: comparison of key clinical trials. *Epilepsia* 1999; **40**(5): 590–600.

Dean JC, Penry JK. Carbamazepine/valproate therapy in 100 patients with partial seizures failing carbamazepine monotherapy: long term follow up. *Epilepsia* 1988; **29**: 687.

Deckers CL, Hekster YA, Keyser A, *et al.* Reappraisal of polytherapy in epilepsy: a critical review of drug load and adverse effects. *Epilepsia.* 1997a; **38**(5): 570–575.

Deckers CL, Hekster YA, Keyser A, *et al.* Drug load in clinical trials: a neglected factor. *Clin Pharm Ther* 1997b; **62**: 592–595.

Deckers CLP, Czuczwar SJ, Hekster YA, *et al.* Selection of antiepileptic drug polytherapy based on mechanisms of action: The evidence reviewed. *Epilepsia* 2000; **41**(11): 1364–1374.

Deckers CLP, Hekster YA, Keyser A, *et al.* Monotherapy versus polytherapy for epilepsy: a multicenter double-blind randomized study. *Epilepsia* 2001; **42**(11): 1387–1394.

Deckers CLP, Genton P, Sills GJ, Schmidt D. Current limitations of antiepileptic drug therapy; a conference review. *Epilepsy Res* 2003; **53**: 1–17.

Dreifuss FE, Santilli N, Langer DH, *et al.* Valproic acid hepatic fatalities: a retrospective review. *Neurology* 1987; **37**(3): 379–385.

Farhat G, Yamout B, Mikati MA, *et al.* Effect of antiepileptic drugs on bone density in ambulatory patients. *Neurology* 2002; **58**(9): 1348–1353.

Goldsmith P, de Bittencourt PRM. Rationalized polytherapy for epilepsy. *Acta Neurol Scand Suppl* 1995; **162**: 35–39.

Gruber Cm, Mosier JM, Grant P, *et al.* Objective comparison of phenobarbital and diphenylhydantoin in epileptic patients. *Neurology* 1956; **6**: 640–645.

Hakkaraninen H. Carbamazepine vs. diphenylhydantoin vs their combination in adult epilepsy. *Neurology* 1980; **30**: 354.

Harden CL, Zisfein J, Atos-Radzion EC, *et al.* Combination valproate-carbamazepine therapy in partial epilepsies resistant to carbamazepine monotherapy. *J Epilepsy* 1993; **6**(2): 91–94.

Kanner AM, Frey M. Adding valproate to lamotrigine: a study of the pharmacokinetic interaction. *Neurology* 2000; **55**: 588–591.

Kwan P, Brodie MJ. Epilepsy after the first drug fails: substitution or add-on? *Seizure* 2000; **9**(7): 464–468.

Lammers MW, Hekster YA, Keyser A, *et al.* Monotherapy of polytherapy for epilepsy revisited: a quantitative assessment. *Epilepsia* 1995; **36**(5): 440–446.

Mireles R, Leppik IE. Valproate and clonazepam comedication in patients with intractable epilepsy. *Epilepsia* 1985; **26**(2): 122–126.

Murri L, Iudice A. Vigabatrin as first add-on treatment in carbamazepine-resistant epilepsy patients. *Acta Neurol Scand Suppl* 1995; **162**: 40–42.

Painter MJ, Scher MS, Stein AD, A*et al.* Phenobarbital compared with phenytoin for the treatment of neonatal seizures. *New Engl J Med* 1999; **341**(7): 485–489.

Patsalos PN, Froscher W, Pisani F, *et al.* The importance of drug interactions in epilepsy therapy. *Epilepsia* 2002; **43**(4): 365–385.

Pisani F, Oteri G, Russo MF, *et al.* The efficacy of valproate-lamotrigine comedication in refractory complex partial seizures: evidence for a pharmacodynamic interaction. *Epilepsia* 1999; **40**(8): 1141–1146.

Pledger GW. Drug interactions in clinical trials: statistical considerations. In *Antiepileptic Drug Interactions*, Pitlick, WH. cd. New York: Demos, 1989.

Reife RA. Assessing pharmacokinetic and pharmacodynamic interactions in clinical trials of antiepileptic drugs. In *Antiepileptic Drug Development. Advances in Neurology*, Vol. 76. J. French, M. A. Dichter, eds. Philadelphia: Lippincott-Raven, 1998.

Rosenberry KR, Korberly BH, Graziani LJ. Combination of clonazepam and sodium valproate in the treatment of refractory epileptic seizures in 12 children. *Am J Hosp Pharm* 1979; **36**(6): 736, 738.

Rowan AJ, Meijer JWA, de Beer-Pawlikowski N, *et al.* Valproate-ethosuximide combination therapy for refractory absence seizures. *Arch Neurol* 1983; **40**: 797–802.

Schmidt D. Two antiepileptic drugs for intractable epilepsy with complex-partial seizures. *J Neurol Neurosur Psychiat* 1982; **45**: 1119–1124.

Sisodiya SM, Sander JWAS, Patsolos PN. Carbamazepine toxicity during combination therapy with levetiracetam: a pharmacodynamic interaction. *Epilepsy Res* 2002; **48**: 217–219.

Somerville ER. Aggravation of partial seizures by antiepileptic drugs: is there evidence from clinical trials? *Neurology* 2002; **59**(1): 79–83.

Stephen LJ, Sills GJ, Brodie MJ. Lamotrigine and topiramate may be a useful combination. *Lancet* 1998; **351**: 958–959.

Tanganelli P, Regesta G. Vigabatrin vs. carbamazepine monotherapy in newly diagnosed focal epilepsy: a randomized response conditional cross-over study. *Epilepsy Res* 1996; **25**: 257–262.

Walker JE, Koon R. Carbamazepine versus valproate versus combined therapy for refractory partial complex seizures with secondary generalization. *Epilepsia* 1988; **32**(5): 693.

Zaatreh M, Tennison M, D'Cruz O, *et al.* Anticonvulsants-induced chorea: a role for pharmaco-dynamic drug interaction? *Seizure* 2001; **10**(8): 596–599.

Clinical studies of pharmacodynamic interactions between antiepileptic drugs and other drugs

Gaetano Zaccara[1], Andrea Messori[2] and Massimo Cincotta[1]

[1] Unit of Neurology, Santa Maria Nuova Hospital, Florence, Italy
[2] Drug Information Centre, Careggi Hospital, Florence, Italy

Introduction

Pharmacodynamic (PD) drug–drug interactions can occur when a patient receives concomitant treatment with two or more drugs. In general, the clinical effect resulting from PD interactions can be either advantageous or disadvantageous. A few studies in animal models have addressed the therapeutic or adverse synergistic effects of antiepileptic drugs (AEDs) (Meinardi, 1995). In humans, formal studies aiming to prove PD interactions between AEDs and other drugs are rare.

In this field, one of the most studied PD interactions is that occurring between flumazenil and benzodiazepines (BZD). Flumazenil is a specific and competitive antagonist of central BZD receptors, reversing all effects of BZD agonists. For this reason, incremental intravenous bolus injections of flumazenil are effective and well tolerated in the diagnosis and treatment of BZD overdose; treatment with flumazenil results in complete awakening with restoration of upper airway protective reflexes (Weinbroum *et al.*, 1997). However, withdrawal symptoms and even seizures can be observed after administration of flumazenil in long-term BZD users; these symptoms may be avoided by a slow titration of flumazenil dose.

Alcohol is another substance whose PD interactions with sedative drugs have often been studied. Sedation, which is a typical adverse effect of many AEDs, is increased by the concomitant administration of alcohol in a way that has been described in different studies as either synergistic or additive (Kastberg *et al.*, 1998).

In this chapter, we discuss in more detail the clinical data concerning PD interactions of AEDs with antidepressants (ADs), antipsychotics (APs), central nervous system (CNS) stimulants, anesthetic agents, analgesics and anti-inflammatory drugs.

PD interactions with ADs

AEDs and ADs are often co-administered. In fact, the lifetime prevalence of major depression reported in epileptic patients is remarkably higher than in the general population (8–48% vs. 6–17%, respectively) (Lambert and Robertson, 1999). It has been hypothesized that common pathogenetic mechanisms may predispose to depression in some patients with certain types of epilepsy (Jobe *et al.*, 1999).

Experimental and clinical data suggest that AEDs and ADs have similar mechanisms of action which could result in favorable and/or unfavorable PD interactions depending on the particular agents involved. Recently, biological psychiatrists have assessed the potential usefulness of AEDs in the treatment of affective disorders. Furthermore, some data suggest that ADs can have anticonvulsant and proconvulsant properties. Finally, many drugs of these two classes share similar adverse effects which are worsened by the concomitant administration.

AEDs and affective disorders

In some patients, AEDs may precipitate mood disorders. The probability of developing such adverse events is highest with the combination of barbiturates and vigabatrin (VGB) and very low with the combination of carbamazepine (CBZ) and valproate (VPA). Brent *et al.* (1987) found that the prevalence of depression and suicidal ideation was higher in adolescents and children taking phenobarbital (PB) than in age-matched subjects treated with CBZ. Furthermore, a meta-analysis of clinical studies performed with new AEDs shows that, in patients taking GB, the percentage of withdrawal due to depression was significantly higher than in patients treated with placebo (Marson *et al.*, 1997).

However, the psychiatric prognosis of patients affected by epilepsy is likely to be improved by the use of AEDs. In fact, a better seizure control can have an indirect positive effect on the predisposition to mood disorders. In addition, the established positive psychotropic effects of some AEDs in non-epileptic psychiatric conditions suggest that AEDs could also directly improve the mood of epileptic patients (beyond their influence on seizure activity). In this context, the choice of the appropriate AED in individual patients should not merely be guided by the efficacy of the drug, but also by its AD properties and by its adverse effect profile.

Combination of AEDs and AD in the treatment of affective disorders

In an open, pivotal study, the effect of low doses of CBZ combined with low doses of amitriptyline has been evaluated in patients with major depression (Dietrich and Emrich, 1998). The particularly good results of this drug association have been postulated as a typical example of PD interaction. The authors hypothesize that the mood is regulated by two distinct groups of functional subsystems in the CNS.

While ADs affect the most important neurotransmitter systems (which are assumed to be directly involved in endogenous depression), CBZ would affect some regulatory mechanisms between temporal cortex and amygdala which couple cognition and perception with emotions. Simultaneous targeting of these two functional subsystems would cause a favorable PD interaction and a potentiation of the AD effect of these drugs.

Various new AEDs have been also used in the treatment of mood disorders. Lamotrigine (LTG) is the most widely studied and has proven efficacy in acute bipolar depression and in the long-term treatment of bipolar depression (Yatham *et al.*, 2002). Recently, in a placebo-controlled double-blind study, LTG was added to paroxetine in depressed patients and appeared to accelerate the onset of action of the AD (Normann *et al.*, 2002). One can therefore speculate that LTG also has favorable PD interactions with some ADs. CBZ and VPA are used for the prophylaxis of bipolar disorders in combination with lithium. It is known that in these disorders, monotherapy is associated with a high failure rate. In contrast, the combination of lithium with CBZ or VPA has been reported to be highly effective (Post *et al.*, 1996). Some double-blind and open studies have revealed that lithium and CBZ have additive effects (Kramlinger and Post, 1989). Similar results have been observed for the combination of lithium plus VPA and, in this case, a synergistic effect has been proposed (Salomon *et al.*, 1998). These results are of particular interest because the combination of lithium and ADs gave different results. In fact, in a multi-center study which compared the efficacy of lithium, imipramine and the combination of lithium plus imipramine, the failure rate was similar for treatments with lithium and with lithium plus imipramine (Prien *et al.*, 1984). Some experimental data suggest that lithium and VPA have a true positive PD interaction; they are thought to down-regulate the expression of a protein involved in synaptic transmission which seems to be involved in stabilizing recurrent mood episodes. These two drugs act at different biochemical levels and they can therefore be synergistic (Lenox *et al.*, 1996).

ADs effects on seizure threshold

Shortly after the introduction to the market of the tricyclic antidepressants (TCAs), seizures were reported in people taking these drugs. The most clear-cut situation in which ADs show an effect on seizure activity is overdose; in such a condition the incidence of seizures ranges from 4 to 20% with a mean overall incidence of 8.4% (Pisani *et al.*, 1999). Maprotiline and amoxapine appear to be more frequently associated with seizures. With TCAs, seizures are reported in 3–8% of cases. Finally, the cumulative evidence from published reports shows that selective serotonin-reuptake inhibitors (SSRIs) are much less likely to cause seizures in overdose and that trazodone is the safest agent in this respect (Alldredge, 1999).

Table 13.1 Incidence of seizures induced by AD drugs

Drug	Dose (mg/day)	Seizure incidence (%)
Imipramine	High (>200)	0.6
	Moderate (50–600)	0.3
	Low (≤200)	0.1
Amitriptyline	High (≥200)	0.06
	Moderate–low (<200)	0.00
Bupropion	High (>450)	2.19
	Moderate–low (≤450)	0.44
Clomipramine	Wide range	0.5
Maprotiline	Wide range	0.4
Fluoxetine	20–60	0.2
Fluvoxamine	<100	0.2
Viloxazine	150–800	0.13

Source: From Pisani *et al.* (1999), with some modifications.

The incidence of seizures occurring with therapeutic doses of ADs varies from 0.1 to 4% (Pisani *et al.*, 1999). This incidence differs slightly from the annual incidence of first seizures in the general population (which has been estimated to be from 0.073 to 0.086%). However, under these circumstances, a clear dose-related effect has been observed for some ADs. For example, Peck *et al.* (1983), through the analysis of almost one hundred studies on imipramine, found that the overall incidence of seizures was 0.33%. However, seizures occurred in 0.10% of patients when the drug was prescribed at doses of 200 mg/day or less and in 0.63% of patients treated with doses greater than 200 mg/day. The incidence of AD-related seizures for some ADs is reported in Table 13.1.

Interestingly, some AEDs may also have similar proconvulsant characteristics, particularly in overdose. For example, an increased frequency of partial seizures can be the primary manifestation of intoxication with CBZ or phenytoin (PHT) (Perucca *et al.*, 1998). CBZ, which has the chemical structure of a TCA, may worsen epilepsy in several conditions even at therapeutic dosages. In particular, this agent may precipitate or exacerbate a variety of seizures in patients with generalized epilepsies. Similar paradoxical proconvulsant effects have also been described, although less frequently, with other traditional and new AEDs (Perucca *et al.*, 1998).

In spite of frequent observations of seizures induced by ADs in non-epileptic patients, the few studies in which an AD has been administered to epileptic patients show that the seizure control was improved in most cases (Alldredge, 1999). This effect might be secondary to an attenuation of emotional triggers for seizures or to enhancing the effectiveness of concomitant AED therapy through pharmacokinetic interactions. However, direct anticonvulsant effects of ADs have been shown in animal as well as in some human studies (Alldredge, 1999). In a small double-blind cross-over study, imipramine at a dose of 25 mg/day was effective in the treatment of absences and myoclonic–astatic seizures (Hurst, 1984). In a more recent add-on open-label study, 17 non-depressed patients with drug-resistant complex partial seizures were treated with fluoxetine (Favale *et al.*, 1995). Six patients became seizure free for 8 months, while the remaining patients experienced an average 30% reduction in seizure frequency. An effect against partial seizures has also been reported with doxepin (Pisani *et al.*, 1999). For a more detailed review, see Alldredge (Alldredge, 1999). All of these data suggest that some TCAs and some SSRIs, at a certain dose, may exert an inhibitory action on neural excitability. It seems that the most important factor in determining the direction of a given AD in terms of inhibition or excitation is drug dosage. It would be interesting to explore possible favorable interactions between AEDs and ADs on different epileptic syndromes.

Adverse effects

PD interactions can also cause the appearance or the worsening of some adverse effects. Sedation may be particularly troublesome in patients taking AEDs, particularly barbiturates or BZD. This adverse effect can be aggravated by the co-administration of most of the older ADs, especially TCAs, mianserin, trazodone and mirtazapine (Lambert and Robertson, 1999). Patients with epilepsy often complain of memory disturbances and some AEDs, such as barbiturates and topiramate (TPM) are known to have deleterious effects on memory. The association of these drugs with older TCAs (especially amitriptyline, which has strong anticholinergic effects), mianserin, and trazodone has been found to produce cognitive impairment and therefore should be avoided (Lambert and Robertson, 1999).

Theoretically, monoamine oxidase (MAO) inhibitors should not be co-administered with CBZ because this may precipitate a hypertensive crisis. However, this event has not been observed in practice. In contrast, a case has been described of a toxic serotonin syndrome attributed to the concomitant use of fluoxetine and CBZ in a patient with an affective disorder (Lambert and Robertson, 1999). Finally, CBZ and, more frequently, oxcarbazepine have been associated with hyponatremia. This metabolic effect has also been documented in patients taking SSRI (Bouman *et al.*, 1998). Therefore, attention should be paid when SSRI are co-administered with CBZ or oxcarbazepine, particularly in elderly patients also treated with diuretic drugs.

In summary ADs and AEDs share several clinical effects. The factors which determine the direction of the effect (pro- or anticonvulsant) may be the dosage of drugs and the epileptic syndrome. PD and also pharmacokinetic interactions (some AEDs induce the metabolism of ADs and in turn are inhibited by these drugs) might potentiate or change the direction of these effects and therefore should be investigated.

PD interactions with AP drugs

AP and AEDs are frequently co-administered and PD interactions concerning their effects on psychosis and seizure threshold are possible. Epidemiological studies have identified a variety of psychoses in about 7–8% of patients with epilepsy. The risk for this adverse effect seems to be higher in patients with temporal lobe epilepsy. In a prospective study of psychosis and epilepsy, children with temporal lobe epilepsy had a 10% chance of developing interictal psychoses during a 30-year follow-up compared with a mean incidence of psychosis of 0.8% in the general population. On the other hand, patients with schizophrenia appear to be more prone to seizures than the general population. This vulnerability can be related both to neuropathologic substrate of schizophrenia and to the exposure to psychotropic medications that lower the seizure threshold (Torta and Keller, 1999).

AEDs and psychosis

Neurobiological hypotheses of epileptic psychoses are focused on the neuropathologic alterations observed in epilepsy and on the neurophysiologic modifications of various neurotransmitter systems (particularly 3,4-dihydroxyphenylalanine, DOPA) induced by the epileptic discharge (Torta and Keller, 1999). In general, the overall psychiatric prognosis of epilepsy is thought to be improved by the use of AEDs. However, in many situations, interictal psychoses can be induced or aggravated by some AEDs. Mechanisms related to these adverse events are represented by forced normalization[1], folate deficency, drug toxicity and abrupt withdrawal of a drug. Ethosuximide is associated with forced normalization and psychosis both in children and in adults (Torta and Keller, 1999). Psychoses are also described with PHT when serum level is above 35 mg/l (McDanal and Bolman, 1975). Among the new AEDs, VGB and TPM are more frequently responsible for psychotic disturbances. In patients included in controlled clinical studies, the incidence of this complication was 3.4% with VGB (Ferrie *et al.*, 1996) (which is higher than the incidence of psychosis in patients treated with placebo: 0.6%) and 3% with TPM (Shorvon, 1996).

APs effects on seizure threshold

As far as convulsant effects of APs are concerned, a report of seizures induced by chlorpromazine appeared in the literature within the first year of the introduction

[1] The term forced normalization (Landolt, 1958) indicates the appearance of a psychosis in an epileptic patient in whom the abnormal EEG became normal as a result of anticonvulsant treatment.

Table 13.2 Incidence of seizures induced by APs

Drug	Dose	Seizure incidence (%)
Phenothiazines	High ($\geqslant$1 mg/day)	9.0
	Moderate	0.7
	Low ($\leqslant$200 mg/day)	0.3
Clozapine	High (600–900 mg/day)	4.4
	Moderate (300–599 mg/day)	2.7
	Low ($\leqslant$299 mg/day)	1.0
Olanzapine	Wide range	0.9
Quietapine	Wide range	0.9
Risperidone	Wide range	0.3

Source: Data from Logothetis (1967) and Alldredge (1999).

of this drug in clinical practice (Zaccara *et al.*, 1990). Subsequent studies showed that phenothiazines were able to produce convulsions. In a study of hospitalized psychiatric patients, Logothetis (1967) found that the incidence of spontaneous seizures was 1.2% among 859 patients under treatment with phenothiazines. The incidence increased to 9% among patients receiving large therapeutic doses of these agents, while only 0.5% of patients treated with low or moderate doses had seizures. Patients with organic brain diseases were at higher risk. Seizures were generally observed at the onset of therapy or after a sudden increase in the dose.

To date, almost all of the APs introduced in clinical practice are known to induce seizures in predisposed subjects. In this respect, the aliphatic phenothiazines (e.g. chlorpromazine, promazine and triflupromazine) imply a higher risk of this adverse event than the phenothiazines bearing a piperazine or piperidine moiety (Zaccara *et al.*, 1990). The degree of the epileptogenic power of a neuroleptic seems to be related to the ratio between the blockage of D2 dopaminergic receptor (which is convulsant) and the blockage of D1 receptor (anticonvulsant). It seems also to be associated with the agent's antihistaminergic activity. In general, the more prominent the sedative properties of an individual AP, the higher its epileptic potential. However, as with ADs, the low incidence of reported cases does not allow an accurate assessment of the relative seizure risk. It has been suggested that, among traditional APs, haloperidol, fluphenazine, molindone, pimozide and trifluoperazine have a lower rate of seizures during therapeutic use and should be preferred in patients with epilepsy (Alldredge, 1999).

Convulsant effect of atypical APs (clozapine, olanzapine, quetiapine and risperidone)

Among the atypical APs (AAPs), clozapine carries the highest seizure risk (see Table 13.2). The occurrence of seizures appears to be dose-related, possibly occurring at a dosage rate of 0.7% per 100 mg. At higher doses, seizure risk rises and reaches 5% at doses of 600–900 mg/day (Alldredge, 1999). In schizophrenic patients, the drug causes electroencephalographic (EEG) abnormalities typically characterized by background slowing in the theta and often the delta range. Bilateral spike, polyspike and slow wave discharges have also been described (Malow *et al.*, 1994). Antiepileptic treatment is indicated in patients experiencing seizures with clozapine. Olanzapine has a binding profile similar to that of clozapine but, despite their similarity, the two drugs demonstrate a strong clinical difference concerning induction of seizures (Table 13.2). As far as quietapine is concerned, no difference in the incidence of seizures was observed between patients treated with this drug and those given placebo (incidence of 0.4% and 0.5%, respectively). Finally, as far as risperidone and sertindole are concerned, only a few patients with seizures have been reported (Alldredge, 1999; Torta and Keller, 1999).

In summary, with the exception of clozapine, the new APs are less prone to induce seizures than the traditional ones. Nevertheless, caution is recommended in using these drugs in patients with a history of seizures or with a lowered seizure threshold.

Adverse effects

Clozapine causes agranulocytosis in about 0.4% of patients (Lader, 1999). Similar figures have also been reported with some AEDs. Incidence values for aplastic anemia have been published for CBZ (39 cases per million) and felbamate (FBM) (127 cases per million) (Kaufman *et al.*, 1997). These values are consistently higher than the overall incidence in the general population which is two cases per million per year (Kaufman *et al.*, 1997). Therefore, concomitant administration of clozapine and other AEDs to patients at high risk of developing aplastic anemia (particularly FBM) should be avoided.

The association of low-potency sedative APs and sedative AEDs (e.g. barbiturates, BZD) may precipitate or aggravate sedation. All neuroleptics cause weight gain and this adverse effect is more evident for AAPs olanzapine and clozapine. Some AEDs (VPA and VGB) cause weight gain too. Therefore, the choice of the appropriate association between AEDs and APs should also take into account this aspect. Finally, one case has been described, in the literature, of catatonia-like events apparently induced by the association of VPA, sertraline and risperidone. A complex PD interaction has been advocated to explain this rare adverse effect (Lauterbach, 1998).

PD interactions with stimulants of the CNS

All CNS stimulants produce a dose-related excitation of the CNS which can lower seizure threshold (Zagnoni and Albano, 2002). In fact, seizures are frequently observed during overdose with these drugs. In a retrospective study of seizures associated with poisoning or drug intoxication, CNS stimulants were involved in 29% of the cases (Olson *et al.*, 1994). However, in some patients, amphetamines (whose effect is to increase dopaminergic transmission) may reduce seizure activity and improve EEG (Zaccara *et al.*, 1990).

A reduced level of vigilance, which can be induced by AEDs and particularly by barbiturates, can worsen seizure frequency in some types of epilepsy (Papini *et al.*, 1984). In addition, sedative effects of traditional AEDs can exacerbate the overactivity and aggressiveness of some epileptic patients (Viani *et al.*, 1977). Based on these considerations, the use of amphetamines, which improve vigilance and contrast sedation, was proposed as a comedication in some epileptic disorders. According to this hypothesis, a propylhexedrine salt of PB (barbexaclone, an amphetamine-like molecule) has been used in the treatment of epilepsy. The aim of this association was to determine a favorable PD interaction characterized by potentiation of the anticonvulsant effects and antagonism of the sedative effects of PB. The safety of the use of barbexaclone in epileptic patients has been documented only by a few open studies conducted in small patient groups (Visintini *et al.*, 1981) even though more studies document that amphetamines have beneficial effects on attention deficits in epileptic patients (Gross-Tsur *et al.*, 1997). However, even at low doses, CNS stimulants can have proconvulsant activities. In 234 non-epileptic children with attention deficit and hyperactive disorders, seizures occurred in 2% of the stimulant-treated group (a rate higher but not particularly alarming given that an estimated 1% of unselected children have seizures). Instead, in a subgroup of patients with epileptiform discharges in the EEG, seizures were observed in 20% of cases (Hemmera *et al.*, 2001).

Adverse effects

Dyskinesia is a rare adverse effect of many AEDs. Choreoathetosis, dystonia and orofacial dyskinesias have been described. PHT is the AED most frequently implicated although cases have also been described with CBZ, gabapentin (GBP), FBM, VPA and LTG (Zaatreh *et al.*, 2001). Young subjects with organic brain abnormalities are at higher risk. It has been postulated that PHT may cause chorea through enhancement of central dopaminergic pathways in the basal ganglia. Since amphetamines increase dopaminergic transmission and may cause dyskinesias, the association of amphetamine-like stimulants with some AEDs in high-risk patients can increase the risk of this adverse effect (personal unpublished observation).

In conclusion, at low doses, stimulants are co-administered with AEDs in the epileptic patient and seem to have beneficial PD interactions. However, in some patients with a lower seizure threshold or exposed to high doses, these substances have proconvulsant effects.

PD interactions with anesthetic agents

Some anesthetic agents are used in the treatment of status epilepticus and therefore have strong anticonvulsant properties. However, selected agents used during general anesthesia are reported to be epileptogenic (Zaccara *et al.*, 1990). For example, etomidate and enflurane enhance epileptiform activity in the EEG and have been exploited for their ability to elucidate epileptogenic regions during seizure surgery. Methohexital, a short acting barbiturate, has also been used to enhance epileptiform activity on the EEG, although it paradoxically functions as an anticonvulsant.

Among anesthetic agents, lidocaine is of particular interest. This agent has a concentration-dependent effect on seizures. At concentrations between 0.5 and 5.0 mg/l, lidocaine can effectively suppress seizures in animal models of epilepsy and in clinical practice (DeToledo, 2000). In fact, it has been used in the treatment of convulsive status epilepticus and epilepsia partialis continua. Levels above 8–9 mg/l, however, selectively block inhibitory mechanisms and may induce seizures. This bimodal response has been clearly demonstrated in experimental models of epilepsy and in healthy volunteers (DeToledo, 2000).

Treatment of anesthetic-induced convulsions can be particularly difficult because of many possible unfavorable PD interactions. AEDs (particularly barbiturates) may seriously exacerbate circulatory and respiratory depression caused by anesthetics. Particular attention should be paid to depressive effects on the myocardium which are potentiated by co-administration of anesthetics and barbiturates. Since severe hypoxia, hypercapnia and lactic acidosis occur concomitantly with anesthetic-induced convulsions and may be aggravated by many AEDs, treatment with succinylcholine and simultaneous ventilation should be the immediate treatment of choice to stop convulsions rapidly. However, because this procedure has no effect on cortical electric seizure activity, a co-treatment with BZD is also required (Zaccara *et al.*, 1990).

PD interactions with analgesic and anti-inflammatory agents

AEDs, analgesics and anti-inflammatory drugs can often be co-administered for the treatment of some forms of pain. Neuropathic pain is not a specific entity, but comprises a variety of pain states with differing sensitivities to varying pharmacological interventions (MacPherson, 2000).

AEDs in the treatment of pain

Abnormal ectopic impulse generation represents an important pathophysiologic mechanism of neuropathic pain. This abnormal impulse generation in injured nerves may depend on changes in the cell membrane Na^+ channels. Furthermore, hypofunction of GABA-ergic inhibitory mechanisms and/or hyperfunction of glutamatergic excitatory mechanisms has been hypothesized to explain the diffusion of pain from the peripheral pain generator into the CNS (Bonezzi and Demartini, 1999). It has been observed that CBZ is effective in reducing acute pain but seems ineffective for continuous pain (Bonezzi and Demartini, 1999). GBP is now considered a first-line medication in the treatment of several neuropathic syndromes. VPA and, more recently, LTG have given encouraging results (MacPherson, 2000).

However, several pain mechanisms may be operant in the same neuropathic disorder and, therefore, it is often useful to associate drugs with different mechanisms of action. AEDs may be associated with opioids, ADs, alfa2-adrenergic agonists and non-steroidal anti-inflammatory drugs (MacPherson, 2000).

Effect of analgesic and anti-inflammatory drugs on seizure threshold

When administered in the CNS, both morphine and other opioid peptides can evoke an epileptiform activity in the EEG. These abnormalities are probably mediated by specific opioid receptors and are antagonised by opiate antagonists, such as naloxone (Tortella *et al.*, 1979). However, in some experimental models, morphine has an anticonvulsant effect (Nowack *et al.*, 1987). In the current practice, opioids have a low potency to induce seizures. This does not apply to pethidine. This drug may cause agitation, restlessness and seizures which have been postulated to be due to accumulation of the N-demethylated metabolite norpethidine. However, opioid-induced neurotoxicity, which comprises cognitive failure, organic hallucinations and seizure activity, can result from therapy with any of the opioids, including morphine, fentanyl and hydromorphone (MacPherson, 2000). Seizures can also be observed after salicylate intoxication (Zaccara *et al.*, 1990). In this circumstance, intravenous diazepam is considered the drug of choice. The proconvulsant effect of ADs has already been described.

Opioids in valproic acid overdose

Recently, a few cases have been described in which naloxone has been successfully used to reverse CNS depression associated with acute VPA overdose (Roberge and Francis, 2002). In conclusion, co-administration of AEDs with analgesics and/or anti-inflammatory drugs and/or ADs can be useful in the treatment of neuropathic pain. Since this condition has different pathogenetic mechanisms, it is often necessary to administer drugs with different actions to target pain generation mechanisms at many levels and minimize adverse effects.

Conclusions

Although many AEDs are widely used in combination with other drugs (ADs, analgesics) to treat various diseases, a scarce knowledge has been gained on the PD interactions of these drugs. There are hints that a true synergistic effect between some AEDs and ADs or analgesics can take place in the treatment or prophylaxis of mood disorders and in the treatment of neuropathic pain, respectively. In the field of epilepsy one can speculate that, in particular cases, the combination of AEDs with other drugs might improve seizure control. In addition, the association of stimulants with AEDs could be useful to antagonize some adverse effects (i.e. sedation). Further clinical studies are needed to verify these hypotheses.

REFERENCES

Alldredge BK. Seizure risk associated with psychotropic drugs: clinical and pharmacokinetic considerations. *Neurology* 1999; **53**(Suppl. 2): S68–S75.

Bonezzi C, Demartini L. Treatment options in postherpetic neuralgia. *Acta Neurol Scand* 1999; **173**: 25–35.

Bouman WP, Pinner G, Johnson H. Incidence of selective serotonin reuptake inhibitor (SSRI) induced hyponatremia due to the syndrome of inappropriate antidiuretic hormone (SIADH) secretion in the elderly. *Int J Geriatr Psychiatry* 1998; **13**: 12–15.

Brent DA, Crumrine PK, Varma RR. Phenobarbital treatment and major depressive disorder in children with epilepsy. *Pediatrics* 1987; **80**: 909–917.

DeToledo JC. Lidocaine and seizures. *Ther Drug Monit* 2000; **2**: 320–322.

Dietrich DE, Emrich HM. The use of anticonvulsants to augment antidepressant medication. *J Clin Psychiatry* 1998; **59**(Suppl. 5): 51–58.

Favale E, Rubino V, Mainardi P, *et al.* Anticonvulsant effect of fluoxetine in humans. *Neurology* 1995; **45**:1926–1927.

Ferrie CD, Robinson RO, Panayiotopoulos CP. Psychotic and severe behavioural reactions with vigabatrin: a review. *Acta Neurol Scand* 1996; **93**: 1–8.

Gross-Tsur V, Manor O, van der Meere J, *et al.* Epilepsy and attention deficit hyperactivity disorder: is methylphenidate safe and effective? *J Pediatr* 1997; **130**: 40–44.

Hemmera SA, Pasternak JF, Zecker SG, *et al.* Stimulant therapy and seizure risk in children with ADHD. *Pediatric Neurology* 2001; **24**: 99–102.

Hurst DL. The use of imipramine as an anticonvulsant for minor motor seizures. *Ann Neurol* 1984; **18**: 394.

Jobe PC, Dailey JW, Wernicke JF. A noradrenergic and serotonergic hypothesis of the linkage between epilepsy and affective disorders. *Crit Rev Neurobiol* 1999; **13**: 317–356.

Kastberg H, Jansen JA, Cole G, *et al.* Tiagabine: absence of kinetic or dynamic interactions with ethanol. *Drug Metabol Drug Interact* 1998; **14**: 259–273.

Kaufman DW, Kelly JP, Anderson T, *et al.* Evaluation of case reports of aplastic anaemia among patients treated with felbamate. *Epilepsia* 1997; **38**: 1265–1269.

Kramlinger KG, Post RM. The addition of lithium carbonate to carbamazepine: antimanic efficacy in treatment resistant mania. *Acta Psychiatr Scand* 1989; **79**: 378–385.

Lader M. Some adverse effects of antipsychotics: prevention and treatment. *J Clin Psychiatry* 1999; **60**(Suppl. 12): 18–21.

Lambert MV, Robertson MM. Depression in epilepsy: etiology, phenomenology, and treatment. *Epilepsia* 1999; **40**(Suppl. 10): S21–S47.

Landolt H. In *Lectures on Epilepsy*. L. de Haas, ed. Asterdam: Elsevier, 1958: 91.

Lauterbach EC. Catatonia-like events after valproic acid with risperidone and sertraline. *Neuropsy Neuropsychol Behav Neurol* 1998; **11**: 157–163.

Lenox RH, McNamara RK, Waterson JM, *et al.* Myristoylated alanine-rich C kinase substrate (MARKS): a molecular target for the therapeutic action of mood stabilizers in the brain? *J Clin Psychiatry* 1996; **57**(Suppl. 13): 23–31.

Logothetis J. Spontaneous epileptic seizures and electroencephalographic changes in the course of phenothiazine therapy. *Neurology* 1967; **17**: 869–877.

MacPherson. The pharmacological basis of contemporary pain management. *Pharmacol Ther* 2000; **88**: 163–185.

Malow BA, Reese KB, Sato S, *et al.* Spectrum of EEG abnormalities during clozapine treatment. *Electroencephalogr Clin Neurophysiol* 1994; **91**: 205–211.

Marson AG, Kadir ZA, Hutton JL, *et al.* The new antiepileptic drugs: a systematic review of their efficacy and tolerability. *Epilepsia* 1997; **38**: 859–880.

McDanal CE, Bolman WM. Delayed idiosyncratic psychosis with diphenylhydantoin. *J Am Med Assoc* 1975; **231**: 1063.

Meinardi H. General principles. Use of combined antiepileptic drug therapy. In *Antiepileptic Drugs*, 4th edn. R. H. Levy, R. H. Mattson, S. Meldrum, eds. New York: Raven Press, 1995: 91–97.

Normann C, Hummel B, Scharer LO, *et al.* Lamotrigine as adjunct to paroxetine in acute depression: a placebo-controlled study. *J Clin Psychiatry* 2002; **63**: 337–344.

Nowack WJ, Johnson RN, Hanna GR. Observations of the effect of morphine on thalamo-cortical excitability in the cat. *Epilepsia* 1987; **28**: 457–462.

Olson KR, Kearney TE, Dyer JF, *et al.* Seizures associated with poisoning and drug overdose. *Am J Emerg Med* 1994; **12**: 392–395.

Papini M, Pasquinelli A, Armellini M, *et al.* Alertness and incidence of seizures in patients with Lennox-Gastaut syndrome. *Epilepsia* 1984; **25**: 161–167.

Peck AW, Stern WC, Watckinson C. Incidence of seizures during treatment with tricyclic antidepressant drugs and bupropion. *J Clin Psichiatry* 1983; **44**: 197–201.

Perucca E, Gram L, Avanzini G, *et al.* Antiepileptic drugs as a cause of worsening seizures. *Epilepsia* 1998; **39**: 5–17.

Pisani F, Spina E, Oteri G. Antidepressant drugs and seizure susceptibility: from in vitro data to clinical practice. *Epilepsia* 1999; **40**(Suppl. 10): S48–S56.

Post RM, Ketter TA, Pazzaglia PJ, *et al.* Rational polypharmacy in the bipolar affective disorders. In *Rational Polypharmacy*. J. E. Leppik, ed. Philadelphia: Elsevier Science, 1996: 153–180.

Prien RF, Kupfer DJ, Mansky PA, *et al.* Drug therapy in the prevention of recurrences in unipolar and bipolar affective disorders: report of the NIMH collaborative study group comparing lithium carbonate, imipramine, and lithium carbonate–imipramine combination. *Arch Gen Psychiatry* 1984; **41**: 1096–1104.

Roberge RJ, Francis EH. Use of naloxone in valproic acid overdose: case report and review. *J Emerg Med* 2002; **22**: 67–70.

Salomon DA, Keitner GI, Ryan C, *et al.* Lithium plus valproate as mainteinance polypharmacy for patients with bipolar I disorders: a review. *J Clin Psychopharmacol* 1998; **18**: 38–49.

Shorvon SD. Safety of topiramate: adverse events and relationships to dosing. *Epilepsia* 1996; **37**(Suppl. 2): S18–S22.

Torta R, Keller R. Behavioral, psychotic, and anxiety disorders in epilepsy: etiology, clinical features, and therapeutic implications. *Epilepsia* 1999; **40**(Suppl. 10): S2–S20.

Tortella FC, Moreton J, Khazan N. Electroencephalographic and behavioral effects of D-ala-methionine-enkephalinamide and morphine in rat. *J Pharmacol Exp Therap* 1979; **206**: 636–646.

Viani F, Avanzini G, Baruzzi A, *et al.* Long-term monitoring of antiepileptic drugs in patients with the Lennox-Gastaut syndrome In *Epilepsy: The VIIIth International Symposium.* J. K Penry, ed. New York: Raven Press, 1977: 131–138.

Visintini D, Calzetti S, Mancia D. Barbexaclone in the treatment of the epilepsies. *Riv Patol Nerv Ment* 1981; **102**: 29–37.

Weinbroum AA, Flaishon R, Sorkine P, *et al.* A risk-benefit assessment of flumazenil in the management of benzodiazepine overdose. *Drug Saf* 1997; **17**: 181–196.

Yatham LN, Kusumakar V, Calabrese JR, *et al.* Third generation anticonvulsants in bipolar disorder: a review of efficacy and summary of clinical recommendations. *J Clin Psychiatry* 2002; **63**: 275–283.

Zaatreh M, Tennison M, D'Cruz N, *et al.* Anticonvulsants-induced chorea: a role for pharmacodynamic drug interaction? *Seizure* 2001; **10**: 596–599.

Zaccara G, Muscas GC, Messori A. Clinical features, pathogenesis and management of drug-induced seizures. *Drug Safety* 1990; **5**: 109–151.

Zagnoni PG, Albano C. Psychostimulants and epilepsy. *Epilepsia* 2002; **43**(Suppl. 2): 28–31.

Drug interactions in specific patient populations and special conditions

14

Antiepileptic drug interactions in children

Olivier Dulac[1], Elizabeth Rey[2] and Catherine Chiron[1]

[1] Hôpital Necker-Enfants Malades, Paris, France
[2] Hôpital Saint Vincent de Paul, Paris, France

Introduction

Many clinical practitioners are of the opinion that the optimal treatment of epilepsy is best achieved by use of antiepileptic drugs (AEDs) that have several modes of action, and therefore the drugs that are the most effective in this regard are AEDs such as carbamazepine (CBZ), valproate (VPA) or topiramate (TPM) whose efficacy relates to several modes of action. Thus, from the pharmacodynamic point of view, these AEDs when prescribed as monotherapy in fact comprise polytherapy regimens. On the other hand, because of metabolism, many AEDs reach the brain as combinations of the parent drug and their metabolite(s) and this too can be considered a form of polytherapy. For example, CBZ, which is metabolized to a pharmacologically active metabolite CBZ-epoxide, readily enters the brain where it exerts pharmacological effects. Thus polytherapy at the brain level can in fact be distinguished from polytherapy at the oral level. The same applies to clobazam (CLB) whose metabolism is inhibited by stiripentol leading to significant increase of CLB and norCLB with far better tolerability (Perez *et al.*, 1999; Chiron *et al.*, 2000). This is also observed with VPA for which the proportion of toxic 4-ene-VPA is decreased (Levy *et al.*, 1987). A further consideration is that the metabolic pathway may vary according to age. Therefore, in infants, the hydroxylation of both diazepam and nordiazepam is very limited, combined with low glucoronidation capacity which generates major hypotonia (Morselli *et al.*, 1973).

In clinical practice, access to plasma level monitoring has demonstrated that metabolic interactions are very complex, and contribute to frequent and often insidious side effects including paradoxical increases in seizure frequency (Reynolds and Shorvon, 1981). Thus, insidious occurrence of increased plasma concentration may generate severe toxicity. This is the case for the combination of phenytoin (PHT) with phenobarbital (PB) in children, a combination that results in unpredictable plasma concentrations and carries a risk of increased toxicity to PHT with cerebellar atrophy, due to progressive accumulation of PHT. Another example of the increased toxicity of combined drugs compared to monotherapy is the combination of lamotrigine (LTG) with VPA that produces the highest incidence of skin rash, although this combination is, from the therapeutic point of view, particularly efficacious (Brodie and Yuen, 1997). On the other hand, a supra-additive effect has been observed with LTG and VPA in combination, that could be the consequence of a pharmacokinetic, due to metabolic interaction in the liver, or a pharmacodynamic, due to some modification of the action of the molecules inside the brain, interaction, or both (Pisani *et al.*, 1999).

Therefore, the issue of mono- versus polytherapy covers a wide range of concepts, and proper analysis requires us to take into account the whole pathway from oral administration, through liver metabolism, to the mode of action within the brain, and also pharmacokinetic differences according to age. However, because of to the lack of insight into the mechanism of action of most AEDs, it is not possible to predict the benefit versus negative effects of the various combinations.

Few studies have been performed to address this issue, primarily because of its complexity and the significant number of factors that are involved. Animal studies have provided evidence of some specific AED combinations that are indeed additive, whilst others were supra-additive and still others infra-additive (Bourgeois, 1988). However, these studies were based on acute AED administration and could not take in account the effect of chronic administration, which may modify the supply of drug to the brain because of metabolic interactions in the liver that need at least several days, often a few weeks, to take place after onset of therapy. Pragmatic clinical studies have been performed, but the results obtained could be misleading if not interpreted properly. Thus, no significant difference was found between VPA mono- and polytherapy (Deckers *et al.*, 2001). Clinical experience shows that mono- and polytherapy do not have the same value according to the type of epilepsy, and to the type of polytherapy. Thus, the type of epilepsy needs to be taken in account, and also the type of drug.

Specificity of epilepsy in pediatrics is its considerable heterogeneity with a growing number of epilepsy syndromes identified. The latter is combined with more or less specific response to drugs or to drug combinations for each given syndrome (Luna *et al.*, 1989; Roger, 1992; Schlumberger *et al.*, 1994). This variable response to drugs includes a risk for worsening of seizure frequency and severity that needs to be taken in account, even when addressing the issue of drug combinations (Perucca *et al.*, 1998). The situation is complicated by the fact that a patient may switch over time from one syndrome to another as an effect of age or as a consequence of treatment. Infantile spasms in a patient with focal malformation respond to vigabatrin (VGB), but in approximately 50% of cases the child is left with focal seizures (Lortie *et al.*, 1993). The addition of CBZ raises the risk of relapse of spasms that again disappear with cessation of CBZ (Talwar *et al.*, 1994; unpublished data).

A very particular aspect that impacts on our knowledge of AEDs and the best use we can make of them, relates to the strategy of their development by the pharmaceutical industry, which is guided by registration body requirements, and both ethical and marketing considerations. Drugs are first developed for adults that suffer from partial epilepsy. Then, if it appears useful to adults, the drug is tested in children, with a clear preference for what is considered as the most intractable conditions, partial epilepsy and Lennox–Gastaut syndrome. However, compounds are tested first as add-on because it is given to patients with resistant epilepsy for which it is not possible to withdraw the previous treatment. For this reason the drug reaches the market with an indication restricted to polytherapy. It is only later, and with major methodological difficulties, that studies permit the efficacy in monotherapy to be demonstrated. Often, a few years later, it appears that the AED is much better tolerated in mono- than in polytherapy. The best example is VPA for which several years were needed before the compound was widely and legally used in monotherapy, whereas is was clear that polytherapy had contributed to fatal hepatic toxicity (Dreifuss *et al.*, 1987, 1989; Bryant and Dreifuss, 1996). Such drawbacks of polytherapy also apply to the therapeutic aspect itself: in one open study performed soon after the launch of VPA in polytherapy, patients with idiopathic generalized epilepsy still suffering from tonic–clonic seizures when treated with the combination of VPA with PB, experienced disappearance of seizures just by withdrawing PB, without any modification of the dose of VPA (Dulac *et al.*, 1982). The growing interest for evidenced-based medicine and restrictions given to the use of drugs out of the strict legal indications may therefore contribute to a somewhat vicious use of medication because it is paradoxically only legal to use the compound in its most hazardous condition, polytherapy, before studies demonstrate efficacy in monotherapy. In the present state of knowledge, it is therefore reasonable with drugs that have no monotherapy claim, to start the medication as add-on therapy, as legally required, but then to go to monotherapy as soon as a clear benefit has been obtained. Nevertheless, there are individual cases in which the combination is more effective than monotherapy.

Interactions between AEDs

In this chapter we will review the characteristics of the various interactions between the various AEDs, including those that are in development, and what is presently known regarding their mechanism; we will then highlight the benefits this knowledge can offer to optimize the treatment for each type of epilepsy in children.

Clinically relevant metabolic and pharmacodynamic interactions

Phenobarbital, phenytoin and carbamazepine

PB, PHT and CBZ are potent inducers of hepatic metabolizing enzymes and consequently any comedication compound that undergoes hepatic metabolism will need to be administered at a higher dose so as to achieve an adequate therapeutic response. PHT generates particular difficulties since it follows a similar metabolic pathway to that of PB and may therefore compete on the catabolism enzymatic activity, with unpredictable results. In particular, accumulation of PHT with toxic effects in the cerebellum and in peripheral nerves may occur insidiously. Because of the metabolism of CBZ to a pharmacologically active metabolite, CBZ-epoxide, the administration of CBZ in effect represents two compounds. Thus a CBZ-epoxide plasma level of over 2.2 mg/l combined with CBZ may be toxic in children, whereas each single component seems to be better tolerated; no major side effect was observed when patients achieved similar plasma concentrations of CBZ-epoxide when administered alone (Schoeman *et al.*, 1984). Based on these observations, CBZ was administered in combination with the experimental compound stiripentol, a compound that inhibits the metabolism of CBZ in the liver, thus decreasing the formation of CBZ-epoxide and increasing the plasma concentration of CBZ. This rational polytherapy results in better tolerability and better therapeutic effect (Tran *et al.*, 1996; Perez *et al.*, 1999).

Valproate

VPA being a metabolic inhibitor requires that drugs administered in combination are administered at lower doses. This applies particularly to PB, PHT, CBZ, LTG and ethosuximide (ESM). For PHT, the total plasma concentration is reduced but the free fraction is not affected, and therefore the dose should not be altered. For CBZ, the clearance of CBZ-epoxide is reduced resulting in poor tolerability particularly in relation to cognitive function, thus necessitating CBZ dose reduction. The combination of VPA with PB results in a decrease of VPA and an increase of PB plasma concentrations. This does have some clinical relevance since it could explain the disappearance of tonic–clonic seizures that occurs upon PB withdrawal and without modification of VPA dose (Dulac *et al.*, 1982). For the combination of VPA with LTG, the risk is that of skin rash, when this combination is introduced too rapidly. However, this combination has the advantage that lower LTG doses are needed and therefore treatment costs are reduced. In addition, this combination has been associated with a positive pharmacodynamic interaction (Pisani *et al.*, 1999) as well as a therapeutic synergism (Brodie and Yuen, 1997). With clonazepam, reduced wakefulness may contribute to the precipitation of status epilepticus in intractable epilepsy with myoclonic seizures (Covanis *et al.*, 1982). VPA also has intrinsic metabolites; 2-ene-VPA that has been shown to be more effective than VPA (Loscher and Nau, 1985), and 4-ene-VPA that may be involved in hepatic toxicity (Nau *et al.*, 1984).

Most new compounds have reduced metabolic interactions with comedication. However, VGB does reduce the clearance of PHT, and thus PHT plasma concentrations may become toxic when removing VGB (Luna *et al.*, 1989).

Oxcarbazepine

Oxcarbazepine (OXC) is associated with few metabolic interactions; with PHT, plasma PHT concentration can be increased by 40% (Sallas *et al.*, 2003) and with LTG, plasma LTG concentration is decreased by 33% (May *et al.*, 1999). OXC may induce the metabolism of other non-antiepileptic comedication.

Gabapentin

Gabapentin (GBP) is not metabolized, and does not affect liver enzymes and consequently GBP does not affect the metabolism of drug comedication. However, there may be an interaction with felbamate (FBM) at the level of kidney excretion, resulting in 50% increase in felbamate half-life values (Hussein *et al.*, 1996).

Felbamate

FBM is, from the pharmacokinetic point of view, a particularly complex compound since it increases the clearance of CBZ and CBZ-epoxide, and reduces that of VPA, PB and PHT. This could lead to toxic plasma PHT concentrations. The metabolism of FBM is enhanced by enzyme-inducing drugs. The combination of FBM with VPA is useful in the treatment of Lennox–Gastaut since in one series the frequency of drop attacks was reduced by 40% (Siegel *et al.*, 1999).

Although topiramate (TPM) is mainly excreted through the kidney, this compound is sensitive to the enzyme-inducing AEDs which enhance its hepatic metabolism two-fold (Dooley *et al.*, 1999). The increase in behavioral disorders that have been associated with LTG comedication, are likely to be the consequence of a pharmaco-dynamic interaction (Gerber *et al.*, 2000). Also, TPM may inhibit PHT metabolism. Overall, the tolerability of TPM is clearly far better as a monotherapy regimen compared to when administered in combination, particularly in combination with CBZ or VPA.

Lamotrigine

LTG is particularly sensitive to the metabolic effect of comedication, both of inducer and inhibitor compounds: its elimination half-life is reduced by PB and CBZ but increased by VPA. When starting LTG in combination with VPA, the plasma concentration tends to rise more quickly than when it is given alone, and this increases the risk for skin rash. Indeed, before this pharmacokinetic effect was identified, we experienced a 10% rate of skin rash when adding LTG to VPA (Schlumberger *et al.*, 1994), that decreased to 1% when the dose was titrated more slowly (Besag *et al.*, 1995). The combination of LTG with CBZ is poorly tolerated in terms of vigilance, and produces the effects of overdosage with CBZ (Besag *et al.*, 1995).

Pragmatic aspects of treatment

First-line treatment

At this stage, there is no longer any place for polytherapy. A number of AEDs have now been shown to be effective as monotherapy for various types of epilepsy, in which they may therefore be administered as first-line drug. This is the case for CBZ (Glauser, 2000), VPA (Dulac *et al.*, 1982), OXC (Serdaroglu *et al.*, 2003), and LTG (Ueberall, 2001) which are effective in partial epilepsy. This similarly applies to VGB in infantile spasms, not only those due to tuberous sclerosis (Chiron *et al.*, 1997) but whatever the etiology (Appleton *et al.*, 1999; Elterman *et al.*, 2001). For childhood absence epilepsy, the effects of VPA and ESM seem to be interchangeable (Sato *et al.*, 1982). For juvenile absence epilepsy, the risk of generalized tonic–clonic seizures in combination with absences is an indication not to restrict to ESM monotherapy and, for LTG, no controlled trial has confirmed the effect as monotherapy in absence epilepsy. For idiopathic generalized epilepsy with tonic–clonic and/or myoclonic seizures, controlled trials with VPA monotherapy are only available in adults (Turnbull *et al.*, 1982). The occurrence of repeat tonic–clonic seizures between 2 and 5 years of age in a previously normal child is most likely to be the first expression of myoclonic–astatic epilepsy, that contra-indicates the use of CBZ, and indicates VPA, although VPA is likely to soon prove to be insufficient in monotherapy (Dulac *et al.*, 1998).

Epilepsy resistant to a first-line monotherapy

Epilepsy resistant to a first-line monotherapy requires a switch to a second monotherapy. However, it remains unclear whether there should be an immediate switch with withdrawal of the previous AED, or a progressive addition of a second AED followed by removal of the first as soon as benefit from the second AED is confirmed. In practice, before new data are available, it seems reasonable to decide according to each specific condition: for epilepsy syndromes or seizure types for which the presently administered drug is determined to be worsening, or does not seem appropriate because it is known to comprise a sizeable risk of worsening; for those for which a given AED seems more appropriate; and for the conditions in which the first AED did not give any clear benefit; a simple switch over a couple of weeks should be undertaken. In cases with apparently partial effects, the addition of the second AED should be chosen before returning to monotherapy, because removing the previous AED could generate withdrawal effects if the new AED is not sufficiently effective. In addition, one needs to take into account the potential metabolic interactions between the first and second AED and therefore adapt the dose of the previous drug, and one needs also to adapt the pharmacokinetics of drug withdrawal to the type of AED and to the duration of previous treatment: even if ineffective; a previous treatment with PB, VGB, PHT or CBZ lasting several months could generate dependency, and therefore require very slow withdrawal.

Epilepsy resistant to a second AED

The use of a third AED in the treatment of epilepsy resistant to a second AED in adults is known to be associated with little benefit. Therefore, for partial epilepsy, provided that the diagnosis of the type of epilepsy is correct, that the treatment is properly given and at a proper dose and that there is no underlying progressive disease (Aicardi, 1988), it seems reasonable to consider surgery at this point (Kwan and Brodie, 2000). In children, no such data are available. Typically, controlled add-on trials for partial epilepsy with a new AED report rates of seizure freedom of approximately 5–15%: 10% for VGB (Luna *et al.*, 1989), 14% for TPM (Ritter *et al.*, 2000), and 14% for OXC (Rey *et al.*, 2004), but only 3% for gabapentin (Appleton *et al.*, 2001). However, for generalized epilepsy, the potential benefit depends on the type of syndrome. In absence epilepsy, combining LTG with VPA was associated with significant benefit (Pisani *et al.*, 1999), and the same applies to myoclonic–astatic epilepsy (Dulac *et al.*, 1998).

Treatment according to the type of epilepsy or epilepsy syndrome

Cryptogenic or symptomatic partial epilepsy

In cryptogenic or symptomatic partial epilepsy, whatever the age, monotherapy has a place of choice, with no significant difference of benefit with VPA or CBZ in terms of efficacy following a first seizure (Verity *et al.*, 1995) . However, tolerability seems to be slightly better with the former (Chaigne and Dulac, 2003). In addition, there is a mild restriction about the use of CBZ according to age and the type of epilepsy. In infancy, the risk of secondary development of infantile spasms, following partial epilepsy, is such that unless there is focal lesion usually not combined with infantile spasms, such as Sturge–Weber disease, the use of CBZ should be avoided. When, in childhood, cryptogenic or symptomatic focal epilepsy is combined with major spike wave activity, CBZ could contribute to the generation of continuous spike waves in slow sleep (Corda *et al.*, 2001). Nevertheless, in the chronic condition, CBZ is more efficacious than VPA in preventing the recurrence of focal seizures. Lack of response to this first AED indicates the need to switch to the alternate AED. However, the indication could depend the topography of the epilepsy focus. Thus, OXC may be more efficacious in temporal lobe epilepsy, TPM seems more efficacious in motor seizures generated by the motor strip, whereas LTG seems useful in frontal lobe seizures, namely when combined with VPA.

For patients with transient effect of CBZ, the addition of stiripentol may produce remarkable effects (unpublished data).

Infancy

Dravet syndrome

In infancy, Dravet syndrome may worsen with the addition of CBZ, PB (Thanh *et al.*, 2002), LTG (Guerrini *et al.*, 1998), or VGB (Lortie *et al.*, 1993). Bromide is widely used in Germany and in Japan. Treatment strategy for this disorder clearly improved with the introduction of a new concept of polymedication. Indeed, neither VPA nor PB succeed in preventing status epilepticus that contributes largely to worsening of the condition (Casse-Perrot *et al.*, 2001). The combination of CLB with stiripentol has been shown to prevent the occurrence of status epilepticus in young children, and to significantly reduce seizure frequency (Chiron *et al.*, 2000). A pragmatic study has shown that this combination should be administered as soon as possible in the course of the disease (Thanh *et al.*, 2002). The addition of TPM also reduces seizure frequency, although the occurrence of status epilepticus cannot be prevented, and although in many instances this drug does not permit withdrawal of VPA (Coppola *et al.*, 2002). Nevertheless, it would become possible to withdraw stiripentol and CLB in the second decade, thus reducing the polytherapy to a combination of VPA and TPM.

Infantile spasms

In infantile spasms, monotherapy either with VGB or steroids seems to be the treatment of choice. When the first drug is not efficient, the alternate may prove effective. No controlled study has questioned an eventual benefit from the combination of both. Patients with previous psychomotor retardation but no neuroradiological abnormality were found not to respond to VGB or steroids alone, although half these patients became spasm-free with the combination of both over several months (Villeneuve *et al.*, 1998). In intractable cases, low doses of LTG combined with VPA seem to be of benefit in a small proportion of patients (Cianchetti *et al.*, 2002). In contrast, this is not observed when LTG is combined with CBZ Veggiotti *et al.*, 1994). Clinical practice shows that felbamate may be effective, but no data could show specific benefit of a combination of this compound compared to its administration as monotherapy. However, since for regulatory purposes initial studies were performed as add-on, the AED is registered for add-on administration. A number of patients with infantile spasms exhibit focal seizures, either in combination with the spasms or as residual phenomena after the disappearance of the spasms with the therapy. In these cases, not only is the combination of CBZ ineffective, but it could also precipitate the relapse of spasms (Talwar *et al.*, 1994). LTG could be helpful in these cases, after the age of 2 years (Veggiotti *et al.*, 1994).

Benign partial seizures in infancy and benign myoclonic epilepsy in infancy

Benign partial seizures in infancy and benign myoclonic epilepsy in infancy are easily controlled by monotherapy with, respectively, VPA or either VPA, ESM or a benzodiazepine, primarily CLB.

Childhood

Absences

In childhood, absences usually respond to monotherapy with either VPA or ESM. The older concept that PB should be added because of the risk of occurrence of tonic–clonic seizures is no longer valid since it is clear that very few patients with childhood absence epilepsy do exhibit tonic–clonic seizures and PB may worsen the absences. A majority of patients non-responsive to either VPA or ESM may respond to add-on LTG. Whether they would respond to monotherapy LTG remains to be determined, and usually it is after a few months of the combination with VPA that a progressive reduction to monotherapy could be attempted. However, because the dose required for duotherapy with VPA is lower, one tends to maintain the combination. The dose of both ESM and LTG should be halved, and the introduction of LTG should be undertaken slowly because of VPA comedication. A combination of all three AEDs, VPA, ESM and LTG may occasionally be helpful.

Benign partial epilepsy

Benign partial epilepsy responds well to various monotherapies. The real need with this condition is to make a clear diagnosis in order to reduce, as much as possible, the indication for any AED medication which, in practice, is required in less than one-third of such patients (Ambrosetto and Tassinari, 1990). It is clear that when a treatment is needed, VPA, sulthiame, CBZ and CLB are all very efficacious. The only restriction is that associated with CBZ, which has a small risk of contributing to the occurrence of continuous spike waves during slow sleep (Corda *et al.*, 2001), as has also been reported with LTG (Battaglia *et al.*, 2001).

Myoclonic–astatic epilepsy

Myoclonic–astatic epilepsy is resistant to any monotherapy. VPA is usually administered when the first, tonic–clonic seizure presents between 2 and 5 years of age (Kaminska *et al.*, 1999). Seizure recurrence or the additional occurrence of myoclonic seizures would necessitate the addition of LTG, with the restrictions and cautions mentioned earlier. Because of the long time lag to reaching proper dosage, it is preferable to start adding this compound as soon as the diagnosis becomes likely, based on the recurrence of tonic–clonic seizures with generalized spike waves in this age range, before myoclonic–astatic seizures do occur. The addition of ESM may be useful, in case of very rapid increase of seizure frequency, before the dose of LTG can reach sufficient levels, and when myoclonic seizures or absences persist. In this setting, LTG dosage needs to be reduced by half because of VPA comedication. TPM may be useful in some cases, but the combination with VPA should be avoided because of potential side effects. Indeed speech, which is often affected in this type of epilepsy, is sensitive to TPM, and this is a very specific effect of this AED (Aldenkamp *et al.*, 2000). The addition of clonazepam to VPA may eventually precipitate status epilepticus (Covanis *et al.*, 1982). CLB does not seem to carry this risk. Thus, many patients end up being treated with three AEDs.

Lennox–Gastaut syndrome

Lennox–Gastaut syndrome is rarely controlled with a single AED. As soon as the syndrome is suspected, LTG should be added to VPA. Indeed, LTG has been shown to be effective in this condition, as add-on therapy, with a sizeable number of patients becoming seizure-free (Motte *et al.*, 1997). Since absences are one component of the syndrome, there is likely a pharmacodynamic interaction of both AEDs as in absence epilepsy (Perucca *et al.*, 1998). Persistent seizures are then an indication to add FBM, with the usual biological, hepatic and hematological follow-up monitoring constraints. Although TPM was also shown to significantly reduce seizure frequency in this condition (Sachdeo *et al.*, 1999), no patient became seizure-free, thus polytherapy with this AED would come later in the treatment algorithm. The use of PHT in the polytherapy is more rare, with the aim of reducing the frequency of generalized, namely tonic seizures.

Continuous spike waves in slow sleep

Continuous spike waves in slow sleep are rarely controlled by benzodiazepine or sulthiame monotherapy (Rating *et al.*, 2000). Adding ESM may occasionally be useful. The addition of other conventional AEDs, namely CBZ, PB or PHT is more often deleterious than useful. Even the occurrence of additional focal seizures is not an indication for this type of medication, since it may aggravate the condition (Perucca *et al.*, 1998). Few patients have benefited from TPM (Mikaeloff *et al.*, 2003). At this point, steroids are the most helpful. Whether a benzodiazepine should then be maintained in combination with steroids is not clear.

Combining AEDs with non-AED drugs

Combining AEDs with non-AED drugs needs special attention. In infants treated with VPA, the administration of acetylsalicylic acid should be limited to situations in which there is absolute need. Indeed, this combination is associated with a high risk of liver failure (Dreifuss *et al.*, 1989). Macrolides should not be given with CBZ, because they reduce its clearance and may produce insidious toxicity (Mesdjian *et al.*, 1980). Among old generation AEDs, CBZ, PHT and PB induce the activity of several enzymes involved in drug metabolism leading to decreased plasma concentration and reduced pharmacological effect of drugs, which are substrates of the same enzymes. This occurs with immunosuppressive drugs including cyclosporine (Yusof 1988; Baciewicz and Baciewicz, 1989; Wasfi and Tanira, 1993; Cooney *et al.*, 1995), tacrolimus (Thompson and Mosley, 1996), sirolimus (Fridell *et al.*, 2003), glucocorticoids, tricyclic antidepressants such as imipramine, amitriptyline, some antipsychotic agents such as haloperidol, chlorpromazine, clozapine (Facciola *et al.*, 1998; Lane *et al.*, 1998), antiarrhythmic agents including disopyramide, lidocaine, propranolol (Vu *et al.*, 1983), doxycycline and acetaminophen (Douidar and Ahmed, 1987). In contrast, the new AEDs OXC, GBP, LTG, levetiracetam, and TPM are not hepatic enzyme-inducing drugs and are not reported to be involved in such drug interaction. However, an interaction between cyclosporine and OXC (Rosche *et al.*, 2001) was suspected in a single case study with decrease of the cyclosporine plasma concentration. Regarding enzyme inhibition the clearance of CBZ was decreased by clozapine (Langbehn and Alexander, 2000), and that of PHT was decreased by cimetidine (Rafi *et al.*, 1999) leading in both cases to increase in the plasma concentration of the AED. Similarly, the plasma concentration of PHT is significantly increased by fluconazole (Cadle *et al.*, 1994). Prediction of drug interaction is difficult because enzyme induction or inhibition may coexist and many other factors are involved in determining whether a clinically significant drug interaction will occur or not. Furthermore most of these data are only case reports. Thus, available data should not be regarded as exhaustive.

Interactions with AEDs and chemotherapeutic drugs (CTDs), although poorly documented, do also occur. The coadministration of AED and a CTD may lead either to reduced activity or increased toxicity of an AED. Lowered plasma concentrations of PHT were reported with seizure recurrence during administration of cisplatin or vinca alkaloid, and a 25% decrease in VPA plasma concentration was observed with high-dose infusion of methotrexate in children. Increased toxicity due to higher plasma-PHT concentration was reported when this AED was coadministered with 5-fluouracil. Although this comedication may not be relevant in children, it points out that one should be cautious when CTDs and AEDs have to be administered concomitantly. The effect of drug interaction may also lead to a reduced activity or an increased toxicity of a CTD: the clearance of vincristine was increased by 63% with the coadministration of enzyme-inducing AEDs, however, the impact on the efficacy of vincristine was not investigated. A faster clearance was observed for teniposide with a lower efficacy in children who received PHT, PB or CBZ. Increased toxicity was reported with the coadministration of VPA, cisplatin and etoposide. Pharmacokinetic interactions may be suspected when AED and CTD drugs share a common metabolic pathway (Vecht *et al.*, 2003).

Conclusion

Although the rule of monotherapy as the strategy of choice clearly applies to the majority of pediatric patients suffering from epilepsy, it remains difficult to maintain it for patients with pharmacoresistant epilepsy. In addition, there is clear advantage of comedication in a restricted number of specific types of epilepsy. This may be the strict rational polytherapy. However, too few structured studies have been performed to validate this concept. In all cases, any study design of this type should take into account the epilepsy syndrome. Finally, there is a sizeable number of patients for whom polytherapy is by no means rationally designed, but imposed by the story of the epilepsy, because there can be a significant increase in seizure frequency at any attempt to reduce the polytherapy. Furthermore, episodes of status epilepticus may even occur, if a vigorous reduction of AEDs is attempted. In these patients, polytherapy can be considered a failure, and its reduction should be tried at regular intervals in order to diminish the risk of insidious side effects of the combination.

REFERENCES

Aicardi J. Clinical approach to the management of intractable epilepsy. *Dev Med Child Neurol* 1988; **30**: 429–440.

Aldenkamp AP, Baker G, Mulder OG, *et al.* A multicenter, randomized clinical study to evaluate the effect on cognitive function of topiramate compared with valproate as add-on therapy to carbamazepine in patients with partial-onset seizures. *Epilepsia* 2000; **41**: 1167–1178.

Ambrosetto G, Tassinari CA. Antiepileptic drug treatment of benign childhood epilepsy with rolandic spikes: is it necessary? *Epilepsia* 1990; **31**: 802–805.

Appleton RE, Peters AC, Mumford JP, *et al.* Randomised, placebo-controlled study of vigabatrin as first-line treatment of infantile spasms. *Epilepsia* 1999; **40**: 1627–1633.

Appleton R, Fichtner K, LaMoreaux L, *et al.* Gabapentin as add-on therapy in children with refractory partial seizures: a 24-week, multicentre, open-label study. *Dev Med Child Neurol* 2001; **43**: 269–273.

Baciewicz AM, Baciewicz Jr FA. Cyclosporine pharmacokinetic drug interactions. *Am J Surg* 1989; **157**: 264–271.

Battaglia D, Iuvone L, Stefanini MC, *et al.* Reversible aphasic disorder induced by lamotrigine in atypical benign childhood epilepsy. *Epileptic Disord* 2001; **3**: 217–222.

Besag FM, Wallace SJ, Dulac O, *et al.* Lamotrigine for the treatment of epilepsy in childhood. *J Pediatr* 1995; **127**: 991–997.

Bourgeois BF. Problems of combination drug therapy in children. *Epilepsia* 1988; **29**(Suppl. 3): S20–S24.

Brodie MJ, Yuen AW. Lamotrigine substitution study: evidence for synergism with sodium valproate? 105 Study Group. *Epilepsy Res* 1997; **26**: 423–32.

Bryant III AE, Dreifuss FE. Valproic acid hepatic fatalities. III. U.S. experience since 1986. *Neurology* 1996; **46**: 465–469.

Cadle RM, Zenon III GJ, Rodriguez-Barradas MC, *et al.* Fluconazole-induced symptomatic phenytoin toxicity. *Ann Pharmacother* 1994; **28**: 191–195.

Casse-Perrot C, Wolf P, Dravet C. Neuropsychological aspects of severe myoclonic epilepsy in infancy. In I. Jambaque, M. Lassonde, O. Dulac, eds. *Neuropsychology of Childhood Epilepsy.* New York: Kluwer Academic/Plenum Press, 2001: 131–140.

Chaigne D, Dulac O. Carbamazepine versus valproate in partial epilepsies of childhood. *Advances in Epileptology.* New York: Raven Press, 2003: 17.

Chiron C, Dumas C, Jambaque I, *et al.* Randomized trial comparing vigabatrin and hydrocortisone in infantile spasms due to tuberous sclerosis. *Epilepsy Res* 1997; **26**: 389–395.

Chiron C, Marchand MC, Tran A, *et al.* Stiripentol in severe myoclonic epilepsy in infancy: a randomised placebo-controlled syndrome-dedicated trial. STICLO study group. *Lancet* 2000; **356**: 1638–1642.

Cianchetti C, Pruna D, Coppola G, *et al.* Low-dose lamotrigine in West syndrome. *Epilepsy Res* **2002**; 51: 199–200.

Cooney GF, Mochon M, Kaiser B, *et al.* Effects of carbamazepine on cyclosporine metabolism in pediatric renal transplant recipients. *Pharmacotherapy* 1995; **15**: 353–356.

Coppola G, Capovilla G, Montagnini A, *et al.* Topiramate as add-on drug in severe myoclonic epilepsy in infancy: an Italian multicenter open trial. *Epilepsy Res* 2002; **49**: 45–48.

Corda D, Gelisse P, Genton P, *et al.* Incidence of drug-induced aggravation in benign epilepsy with centrotemporal spikes. *Epilepsia* 2001; **42**: 754–759.

Covanis A, Gupta AK, Jeavons PM. Sodium valproate: monotherapy and polytherapy. *Epilepsia* 1982; **23**: 693–720.

Deckers CL, Hekster YA, Keyser A, *et al.* Monotherapy versus polytherapy for epilepsy: a multicenter double-blind randomized study. *Epilepsia* 2001; **42**: 1387–1394.

Dooley JM, Camfield PR, Smith E, *et al.* Topiramate in intractable childhood onset epilepsy – a cautionary note. *Can J Neurol Sci* 1999; **26**: 271–273.

Douidar SM, Ahmed AE. A novel mechanism for the enhancement of acetaminophen hepatotoxicity by phenobarbital. *J Pharmacol Exp Ther* 1987; **240**: 578–583.

Dreifuss FE, Santilli N, Langer DH, *et al.* Valproic acid hepatic fatalities: a retrospective review. *Neurology* 1987; **37**: 379–385.

Dreifuss FE, Langer DH, Moline KA, *et al.* Valproic acid hepatic fatalities. II. US experience since 1984. *Neurology* 1989; **39**: 201–217.

Dulac O, Steru D, Rey E, *et al.* Sodium valproate (Na VPa) monotherapy in childhood epilepsy. *Arch Fr Pediatr* 1982; **39**: 347–352.

Dulac O, Plouin P, Shewmon A. Myoclonus and epilepsy in childhood: 1996 Royaumont meeting. *Epilepsy Res* 1998; **30**: 91–106.

Elterman RD, Shields WD, Mansfield KA, *et al.* Randomized trial of vigabatrin in patients with infantile spasms. *Neurology* 2001; **57**: 1416–1421.

Facciola G, Avenoso A, Spina E, *et al.* Inducing effect of phenobarbital on clozapine metabolism in patients with chronic schizophrenia. *Ther Drug Monit* 1998; **20**: 628–630.

Fridell JA, Jain AK, Patel K, *et al.* Phenytoin decreases the blood concentrations of sirolimus in a liver transplant recipient: a case report. *Ther Drug Monit* 2003; **25**: 117–119.

Gerber PE, Hamiwka L, Connolly MB, *et al.* Factors associated with behavioral and cognitive abnormalities in children receiving topiramate. *Pediatr Neurol* 2000; **22**: 200–203.

Glauser TA. Expanding first-line therapy options for children with partial seizures. *Neurology* 2000; **55**: S30–S37.

Guerrini R, Dravet C, Genton P, *et al.* Lamotrigine and seizure aggravation in severe myoclonic epilepsy. *Epilepsia* 1998; **39**: 508–512.

Hussein G, Troupin AS, Montouris G. Gabapentin interaction with felbamate. *Neurology* 1996; **47**: 1106.

Kaminska A, Ickowicz A, Plouin P, *et al.* Delineation of cryptogenic Lennox–Gastaut syndrome and myoclonic astatic epilepsy using multiple correspondence analysis. *Epilepsy Res* 1999; **36**: 15–29.

Kwan P, Brodie MJ. Early identification of refractory epilepsy. *New Engl J Med* 2000; **342**: 314–319.

Lane HY, Su KP, Chang WH, *et al.* Elevated plasma clozapine concentrations after phenobarbital discontinuation. *J Clin Psychiatr* 1998; **59**: 131–133.

Langbehn DR, Alexander B. Increased risk of side-effects in psychiatric patients treated with clozapine and carbamazepine: a reanalysis. *Pharmacopsychiatry* 2000; **33**: 196.

Levy R, Loiseau P, Guyot A, *et al.* Effects of stiripentol on valproate plasma level and metabolism. *Epilepsia* 1987; **28**(5): 605.

Lortie A, Chiron C, Mumford J, *et al.* The potential for increasing seizure frequency, relapse, and appearance of new seizure types with vigabatrin. *Neurology* 1993; **43**: S24–S27.

Loscher W, Nau H. Pharmacological evaluation of various metabolites and analogues of valproic acid. Anticonvulsant and toxic potencies in mice. *Neuropharmacology* 1985; **24**: 427–435.

Luna D, Dulac O, Pajot N, *et al.* Vigabatrin in the treatment of childhood epilepsies: a single-blind placebo-controlled study. *Epilepsia* 1989; **30**: 430–437.

May TW, Rambeck B, Jurgens U. Influence of oxcarbazepine and methsuximide on lamotrigine concentrations in epileptic patients with and without valproic acid comedication: results of a retrospective study. *Ther Drug Monit* 1999; **21**: 175–181.

Mesdjian E, Dravet C, Cenraud B, *et al.* Carbamazepine intoxication due to triacetyloleandomycin administration in epileptic patients. *Epilepsia* 1980; **21**: 489–496.

Mikaeloff Y, Saint-Martin A, Mancini J, *et al.* Topiramate: efficacy and tolerability in children according to epilepsy syndromes. *Epilepsy Res* 2003; **53**: 225–232.

Morselli PL, Principi N, Tognoni G, *et al.* Diazepam elimination in premature and full term infants, and children. *J Perinat Med* 1973; **1**: 133–141.

Motte J, Trevathan E, Arvidsson JF, *et al.* Lamotrigine for generalized seizures associated with the Lennox–Gastaut syndrome. Lamictal Lennox–Gastaut Study Group. *New Engl J Med* 1997; **337**: 1807–1812.

Nau H, Loscher W, Schafer H. Anticonvulsant activity and embryotoxicity of valproic acid. *Neurology* 1984; **34**: 400–401.

Perez J, Chiron C, Musial C, *et al.* Stiripentol: efficacy and tolerability in children with epilepsy. *Epilepsia* 1999; **40**: 1618–1626.

Perucca E, Gram L, Avanzini G, *et al.* Antiepileptic drugs as a cause of worsening seizures. *Epilepsia* 1998; **39**: 5–17.

Pisani F, Oteri G, Russo MF, *et al.* The efficacy of valproate–lamotrigine comedication in refractory complex partial seizures: evidence for a pharmacodynamic interaction. *Epilepsia* 1999; **40**: 1141–1146.

Rafi JA, Frazier LM, Driscoll-Bannister SM, *et al.* Effect of over-the-counter cimetidine on phenytoin concentrations in patients with seizures. *Ann Pharmacother* 1999; **33**: 769–774.

Rating D, Wolf C, Bast T. Sulthiame as monotherapy in children with benign childhood epilepsy with centrotemporal spikes: a 6-month randomized, double-blind, placebo-controlled study. Sulthiame Study Group. *Epilepsia* 2000; **41**: 1284–1288.

Rey E, Bulteau C, Motte J, *et al.* Multicenter study of oxcarbazepine pharmacokinetics and long-term tolerability as open-label, add-on therapy in children with refractory epilepsy. *J Clin Pharmacol* 2004; **44**: 1290–1300.

Reynolds EH, Shorvon SD. Monotherapy or polytherapy for epilepsy? *Epilepsia* 1981; **22**: 1–10.

Ritter F, Glauser TA, Elterman RD, *et al.* Effectiveness, tolerability, and safety of topiramate in children with partial-onset seizures. Topiramate YP Study Group. *Epilepsia* 2000; **41**(Suppl. 1): S82–S85.

Roger J. *Epileptic Syndromes in Infancy, Childhood and Adolescence.* M. Bureau, C. Dravet, F. Dreifuss, A. Perret, P. Wolf, eds. London: John Libbey, 1992.

Rosche J, Froscher W, Abendroth D, *et al.* Possible oxcarbazepine interaction with cyclosporine serum levels: a single case study. *Clin Neuropharmacol* 2001; **24**: 113–116.

Sachdeo RC, Glauser TA, Ritter F, *et al.* A double-blind, randomized trial of topiramate in Lennox–Gastaut syndrome. Topiramate YL Study Group. *Neurology* 1999; **52**: 1882–1887.

Sallas WM, Milosavljev S, D'Souza J, *et al.* Pharmacokinetic drug interactions in children taking oxcarbazepine. *Clin Pharmacol Ther* 2003; **74**: 138–149.

Sato S, White BG, Penry JK, *et al.* Valproic acid versus ethosuximide in the treatment of absence seizures. *Neurology* 1982; **32**: 157–163.

Schlumberger E, Chavez F, Palacios L, *et al.* Lamotrigine in treatment of 120 children with epilepsy. *Epilepsia* 1994; **35**: 359–367.

Schoeman JF, Elyas AA, Brett EM, *et al.* Correlation between plasma carbamazepine-10, 11-epoxide concentration and drug side-effects in children with epilepsy. *Dev Med Child Neurol* 1984; **26**: 756–764.

Serdaroglu G, Kurul S, Tutuncuoglu S, *et al.* Oxcarbazepine in the treatment of childhood epilepsy. *Pediatr Neurol* 2003; **28**: 37–41.

Siegel H, Kelley K, Stertz B, *et al.* The efficacy of felbamate as add-on therapy to valproic acid in the Lennox–Gastaut syndrome. *Epilepsy Res* 1999; **34**: 91–97.

Talwar D, Arora MS, Sher PK. EEG changes and seizure exacerbation in young children treated with carbamazepine. *Epilepsia* 1994; **35**: 1154–1159.

Thanh TN, Chiron C, Dellatolas G, *et al.* Long-term efficacy and tolerance of stiripentol in severe myoclonic epilepsy of infancy (Dravet's syndrome). *Arch Pediatr* 2002; **9**: 1120–1127.

Thompson PA, Mosley CA. Tacrolimus–phenytoin interaction. *Ann Pharmacother* 1996; **30**: 544.

Tran A, Vauzelle-Kervroedan F, Rey E, *et al.* Effect of stiripentol on carbamazepine plasma concentration and metabolism in epileptic children. *Eur J Clin Pharmacol* 1996; **50**: 497–500.

Turnbull DM, Rawlins MD, Weightman D, *et al.* A comparison of phenytoin and valproate in previously untreated adult epileptic patients. *J Neurol Neurosurg Psychiatr* 1982; **45**: 55–59.

Ueberall MA. Normal growth during lamotrigine monotherapy in pediatric epilepsy patients – a prospective evaluation of 103 children and adolescents. *Epilepsy Res* 2001; **46**: 63–67.

Vecht CJ, Wagner GL, Wilms EB. Interactions between antiepileptic and chemotherapeutic drugs. *Lancet Neurol* 2003; **2**: 404–409.

Veggiotti P, Cieuta C, Rex E, *et al.* Lamotrigine in infantile spasms. *Lancet* 1994; **344**: 1375–1376.

Verity CM, Hosking G, Easter DJ. A multicentre comparative trial of sodium valproate and carbamazepine in paediatric epilepsy. The Paediatric EPITEG Collaborative Group. *Dev Med Child Neurol* 1995; **37**: 97–108.

Villeneuve N, Soufflet C, Plouin P, *et al.* Treatment of infantile spasms with vigabatrin as first-line therapy and in monotherapy: apropos of 70 infants. *Arch Pediatr* 1998; **5**: 731–738.

Vu VT, Bai SA, Abramson FP. Interactions of phenobarbital with propranolol in the dog. 2. Bioavailability, metabolism and pharmacokinetics. *J Pharmacol Exp Ther* 1983; **224**: 55–61.

Wasfi IA, Tanira MO. The effect of chronic administration of cyclosporin A on phenytoin pharmacokinetic parameters in the rat. *Life Sci* 1993; **52**: 199–204.

Yusof WZ. Gingival hyperplasia: an intra-oral side effect of phenytoin, nifedipine and cyclosporine therapies. *Singapore Med J* 1988; **29**: 498–503.

15

Antiepileptic drug interactions in the elderly

Jeannine M. Conway and James C. Cloyd

Epilepsy Research and Education Program, College of Pharmacy, University of Minnesota, Minneapolis, MN, USA
Department of Experimental and Clinical Pharmacology, University of Minnesota, Minneapolis, MN, USA

Introduction

The elderly ($\geq$65 years) are the fastest growing segment of the population in developed countries. In the USA, older adults presently comprise 13% of the population and are projected to increase to 20% within the next 20 years. Similar demographics exist for many European countries. With advancing age comes increasing morbidity, medication use, and adverse drug reactions. Over two-thirds of older adults have one or more chronic medical problems (Hoffman *et al.*, 1996). As a consequence more elderly take medications than others and the elderly take more drugs per person. In the USA, almost 90% of community-dwelling elderly take one or more medications (Guay *et al.*, 2003). Antiepileptic drugs (AEDs) are frequently prescribed in the elderly due to the high prevalence of AED-treatable neuropsychiatric disorders in this age group. For example, epilepsy is twice as common in those $\geq$65 years (1.5%) than in younger adults (Hauser, 1997). An estimated 1.6% of community-dwelling elderly take one or more AEDs (Nitz *et al.*, 2000).

AED use is even greater among elderly nursing home residents. Based on two national surveys, approximately 10–11% of elderly nursing home residents take at least one AED and within this group 14–19% are on two or more AEDs including combinations known to interact (Schachter *et al.*, 1998; Garrard *et al.*, 2000).

Factors contributing to AED interactions in the elderly

There are several factors associated with AED therapy in the elderly that substantially increase the risk of clinically significant drug interactions. These include multiple medication use including many drugs with a high potential for interactions, altered sensitivity to drug action, and age-related changes in drug disposition.

Pharmacoepidemiology

The probability of an interaction increases significantly with the number of medications a person takes (Nolan and O'Malley, 1989). Community-dwelling elderly take

3.1–7.9 prescription and non-prescription medications whereas nursing home residents take an average of 7.2 maintenance and pro re nata (PRN) medications (Beers *et al.*, 1993; Stewart, 2001). The most common types of medication used include cardiovascular, gastrointestinal, central nervous system (CNS), analgesic, and vitamin agents, all of which have the potential to interact with other medications (Guay *et al.*, 2003).

The AEDs most commonly prescribed for older patients also have the greatest potential for drug interactions. In a survey based on 1995 data, the vast majority of community-dwelling elders on an AED were on one or more of the following: phenytoin (PHT), carbamazepine (CBZ), phenobarbital (PB), and valproic acid (VPA) (Nitz *et al.*, 2000). More recent studies in nursing home residents reveal a similar pattern although there is greater use of gabapentin (GBP) and clonazepam (Schachter *et al.*, 1998; Garrard *et al.*, 2003). Between 14% and 19% of nursing home elderly, who receive at least one AED, receive two or more AEDs, with the most frequently occuring combinations being PHT and CBZ, PB or VPA (Schachter *et al.*, 1998; Garrard *et al.*, 2000). All these AED combinations are known to interact with each other.

The types of co-medication used by community-dwelling elderly taking AEDs have not been characterized, but AED use in nursing home elderly has been extensively studied. Elderly nursing home residents on an AED take more medications than other elderly residents. In one study, those receiving an AED were on 5.6 maintenance medications versus 4.6 for all other elderly residents (Lackner *et al.*, 1998). The most commonly prescribed co-medications in this study included CNS drugs, cardiovascular agents, and anticoagulants, all of which have the potential to interact with AEDs (Figure 15.1).

Age-related alterations in pharmacodynamics

The elderly exhibit altered pharmacodynamics resulting in greater sensitivity to both pharmacological and toxicological drug effects. This can produce either a more narrow therapeutic range or a shift downward in the lower and upper limits of the range. Older persons on AEDs appear to be more sensitive to drug effects even when concentrations are controlled. Ramsay *et al.* analyzed the effect of advancing age on occurrence of adverse effects in a controlled clinical trial comparing the safety and efficacy of CBZ and VPA (Ramsay *et al.*, 1994). They found that patients over 65 years of age experienced side effects at CBZ and VPA concentrations of 50% and 20%, respectively, lower than in younger patients. In the face of increased sensitivity to pharmacological and toxicological effects, elderly patients are more likely to experience a clinically significant pharmacodynamic drug interaction with certain drug combinations. For example, elderly taking both PB for epilepsy and a benzodiazepine for sleep are more likely to have cognitive impairment than with either drug taken alone (Michelucci and

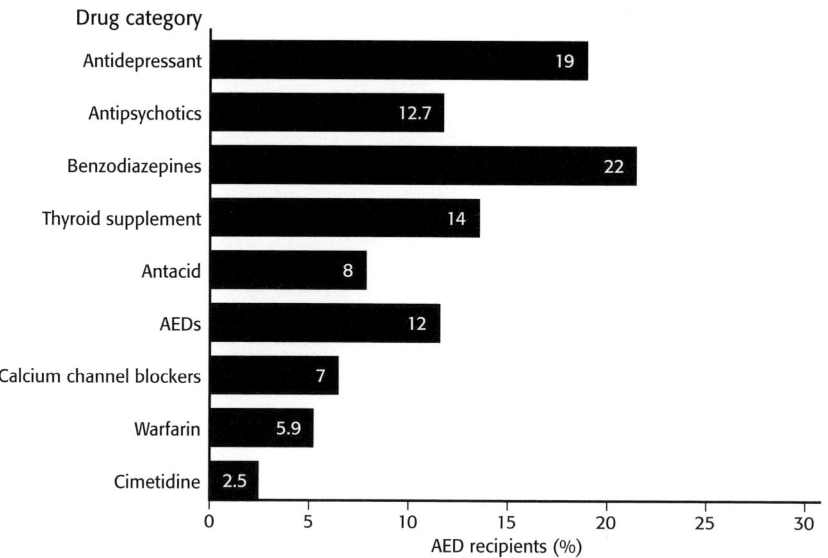

Figure 15.1 Medication use in elderly nursing home residents on AEDs (adapted from Lackner *et al.*, 1998)

Tassinari, 2002). A pharmacodynamic interaction resulting in decreased effectiveness of AED therapy occurs when medications that lower seizure threshold are added to a patient's regimen, as may occur with antipsychotics (Lader, 1999).

Age-related alterations in pharmacokinetics

The most common AED interactions in older patients are associated with either an increase or decrease in one or both interacting drugs. The elderly are particularly susceptible to pharmacokinetic interactions due to age-related changes in drug disposition (Mayersohn, 1992) (Table 15.1). Medical conditions common in the elderly such as cardiovascular, renal or gastrointestinal diseases further alter drug disposition. Advanced age is associated with increased gastric pH, diminished gastrointestinal fluids, slower intestinal transit, and reduced absorptive area. Each of these changes can affect either or both the rate and extent of absorption. Age-related reduction in intestinal and hepatic blood flow, intestinal drug transport and metabolism, and hepatic metabolism can also affect the systemic bioavailability of some drugs. Gastric pH and intestinal transit time may exhibit intra-patient day-to-day variability while other processes tend to slowly decline. Transporter proteins, such as P-glycoprotein, which are located in intestinal enterocytes, facilitate efflux of certain drugs thereby reducing bioavailability. It is not known if advancing age alters the activity of transporter enzymes. Age-related alterations in absorption are most likely to affect slowly absorbed AEDs, particularly those administered as solid dosage

Table 15.1 Age-related changes in physiology

Absorption	
Gastrointestinal blood flow	Decreased
Gastric pH	Decreased
Gastric emptying	Decreased
Intestinal motility	Decreased
Distribuition	
Lean body mass	Decreased
Body fat	Increased
Plasma albumin	Unchanged or decreased
Metabolism	
Liver mass	Decreased
Hepatic blood flow	Decreased
Oxidative metabolism	Decreased by 1%/year; age: >40 years
Conjugation metabolism	Unchanged or decreased
Induction of microsomal enzymes	Decreased?
Excretion	
Kidney mass	Decreased
Renal blood flow	Decreased
Glomerular filtration	Decreased by 1%/year; age: >40 years
Filtration fraction	Decreased

Adapted from Cloyd and Conway (2002).

forms, extended release formulations, or drugs absorbed by active transport (GBP). A recent report described highly variable PHT concentrations collected from 56 elderly nursing home residents on constant maintenance doses of PHT with no changes in interacting co-medication. Although there is no direct evidence, an alteration in bioavailability is the most likely explanation for this phenomenon (Birnbaum *et al.*, 2003). The addition of drugs that affect AED absorption can compound the effects of age-related changes in gastrointestinal function. For example, calcium-containing products are commonly used in elderly patients, particularly women. These products can chelate with PHT resulting in decreased bioavailability (Cacek, 1986).

Older persons undergo a gradual reduction in serum albumin: by age 65 years, many individuals have low normal albumin concentrations or are frankly hypoalbuminemic (Wallace and Verbeeck, 1987). Albumin concentration may be further reduced by conditions such as malnutrition, renal insufficiency, and rheumatoid arthritis. As serum albumin levels decline, the greater the likelihood that drug binding will decrease. This has the effect of lowering the total serum drug concentration while unbound serum drug concentration remains unchanged. The elderly are more susceptible to protein-binding interactions due to lower serum albumin levels and the use of multiple medications, many of which are highly bound to serum proteins. Protein-binding competitive displacement interactions, which are the most common, occur when the unbound concentration of the displacer drug or its binding affinity is greater than that of the displaced drug (MacKichan, 1992). Displacer drug concentrations are often higher in elderly patients due to reduced clearance. Hence elderly patients are likely to have a displacement interaction and the extent of displacement will be greater than in younger patients. Protein-binding interactions complicate interpretation of total serum AED concentrations. Measurement of unbound AED concentrations may be useful in assessing the clinical significance of this type of interaction.

Several studies have shown that both hepatic and renal drug clearances decline at a rate of 10% per decade of life beginning at the age 40 years (Mayersohn, 1992). Age-related decreases in clearance result in higher drug concentrations when standard doses are used in older persons. Most interactions with drugs that inhibit clearance are concentration dependent. When a standard dose of an inhibiting drug is given to an elderly patient, its concentration will be higher and, hence, its inhibition of the affected drug's clearance will be greater than in a younger adult. If the elderly patient is also taking a standard dose of the affected drug, the greater decrease in its clearance results in a further increase in concentration that was already elevated as compared to a younger adult on the same dose. As a result drug interactions that are clinically important in younger adults will have an even greater impact in the elderly; and drug combinations not known to interact in younger adults may be clinically important in older patients. Even when dosage adjustments are made to the inhibitor and the affected drug, the concentration of the latter can still increase if the inhibitor concentration approaches or exceeds its K_i. In this situation, the increased pharmacodynamic sensitivity in the elderly can result in an adverse drug interaction although the rise in the concentration of the affected drug is limited.

Drug interactions occurring as a result of induction of hepatic metabolism follow a similar pattern. In most cases, induction of hepatic metabolism is concentration dependent although there is some controversy as to whether the elderly respond to inducers to the same extent as younger adults (Mayersohn, 1992). Consequently, standard doses of the inducer may result in higher concentrations that, in turn, may cause a greater extent of induction.

Finally, management of pharmacokinetic interactions must consider both initiation and discontinuation of drug therapy. If appropriate dosage adjustments have been made to control drug concentrations in the presence of an interaction, the concentration of the affected drug will fall or rise once the inhibitor or inducer is withdrawn. As the elderly are likely to have a more narrow therapeutic range for many medications, the clinical impact of withdrawing an interacting drug can also be significant.

AEDs versus other drug combinations

The elderly frequently take numerous medications for a variety of medical conditions. The use of polypharmacotherapy leaves the elderly patient at an increased risk for adverse events. There are many medications that are frequently prescribed for ailments that the elderly experience and unfortunately this chapter cannot address every possible drug interaction.

Antihypertensives

Carbamazepine

Diltiazem and verapamil are inhibitors of cytochrome P450 (CYP) 3A4, which is the major metabolic elimination pathway for CBZ (Ma *et al.*, 2000). This inhibition may lead to increased CBZ blood concentrations and neurotoxicity (Macphee *et al.*, 1986; Eimer and Carter, 1987; Beattie *et al.*, 1988; Bahls *et al.*, 1991; Shaughnessy and Mosley, 1992). CBZ is a potent inducer of CYP3A4 (Luo *et al.*, 2002). As a result, any medications that are metabolized via that pathway are likely to be affected. CBZ also induces CYP1A2, CYP2C9, and to a variable degree CYP2C19. Patients will likely require increased doses of affected antihypertensives to decrease blood pressure adequately.

Phenorbital

PB is a significant enzyme inducer of CYP3A4, CYP2C8, CYP2C9, and CYP2C19 (Gerbal-Chaloin *et al.*, 2001; Raucy *et al.*, 2002; Edwards *et al.*, 2003). Any antihypertensive medication that is metabolized via these metabolic enzymes is likely to fall victim to increased metabolism. Hence, if an elderly patient is on PB they may require higher doses of their antihypertensive to get a therapeutic response. Conversely, if PB therapy is initiated, the existing antihypertensive medication may lose its efficacy.

Phenytoin

Diltiazem has been demonstrated to cause PHT toxicity, most likely due to enzyme inhibition although the exact mechanism is unclear (Bahls *et al.*, 1991; Clarke *et al.*, 1993). Careful monitoring for PHT toxicity is recommended if diltiazem is prescribed. As PHT may cause an induction in metabolism, antihypertensives that are metabolized by CYP P450 may be affected.

Other

There are no known drug interactions with antihypertensives with the following AEDs: felbamate (FBM), GBP, lamotrigine (LTG), levetiracetam (LEV), oxcarbazepine (OXC), tiagabine (TGB), topiramate (TPM), VPA, and zonisamide (ZNS).

Antihyperlipidemics

Carbamazepine

CBZ is a substrate and inducer of CYP3A4 (Luo *et al.*, 2002). A recent study demonstrated that CBZ significantly increases the clearance of simvastatin. This resulted in an 80% decrease in patient exposure to simvastatin (Veor *et al.*, 2004). While there are no published reports of drug interactions with other antihyperlipidemics it may be inferred depending on their metabolic pathway including atorvastatin and lovastatin (Wang *et al.*, 1991; Mazzu *et al.*, 2000; Paoletti *et al.*, 2002). CBZ co-medication may increase a patient's dose requirement in order to get an adequate therapeutic response.

Phenobarbital

Atorvastatin, lovastatin, and simvastatin are substrates of CYP3A4 (Wang *et al.*, 1991; Mazzu *et al.*, 2000; Paoletti *et al.*, 2002). PB co-medication may increase a patient's dose requirement in order to get an adequate therapeutic response.

Phenytoin

Atorvastatin, lovastatin, and simvastatin are substrates of CYP3A4 (Wang *et al.*, 1991; Mazzu *et al.*, 2000; Paoletti *et al.*, 2002). PHT co-medication may increase a patient's dose requirement in order to get an adequate therapeutic response.

Other

There are no known drug interactions with antihyperlipidemics with the following AEDs: FBM, GBP, LTG, LEV, OXC, TGB, TPM, VPA, and ZNS.

Anticoagulants/antiplatelets

Carbamazepine

Warfarin is metabolized via several CYP P450 enzymes (Kaminsky and Zhang, 1997). If a patient is stabilized on CBZ and warfarin therapy is initiated, the patient will require a larger warfarin dose than patients not receiving CBZ will require (Ross and Beeley, 1980; Kendall and Boivin, 1981; Massey, 1983). If a patient is stabilized on both CBZ and warfarin and the CBZ is discontinued, the patient is very likely to experience an increase in their internationalized normalized ratio (INR) that would place the patient at an increased risk of bleeding (Denbow and Fraser, 1990).

Felbamate

There are no known documented drug interactions between anticoagulants and FBM, but FBM inhibits CYP2C19, which may increase the effect of warfarin, resulting in an increased risk of bleeding (Glue *et al.*, 1997).

Oxcarbazepine

There are no known documented drug interactions with anticoagulants or antiplatelets, but OXC inhibits CYP2C19 and induces CYP3A4, which may alter the metabolism of warfarin (Trileptal, 2001). Caution should be taken if adding OXC to a medication regimen that includes warfarin.

Phenobarbital

The clearance of warfarin is increased when a patient is also on PB (Udall, 1975; Mungall *et al.*, 1985). Management of this interaction is similar to the interaction of warfarin with CBZ. If PB is added to a medication regimen including warfarin, the practitioner needs to monitor for a decrease in INR and efficacy. If PB is removed from a stable medication regimen including warfarin, the practitioner needs to monitor for an increased INR and an increased risk of bleeding. The dose of warfarin will need to be appropriately decreased.

Phenytoin

The interaction between PHT and warfarin is unpredictable, with reports of increased and decreased effects of warfarin (Nappi, 1979; Levine and Sheppard, 1984; Panegyres and Rischbieth, 1991). The initiation of PHT may cause warfarin to be displaced from protein-binding sites, followed by an increase in the metabolism of warfarin (Levine and Sheppard, 1984). Caution must be used when managing a patient on warfarin and PHT. Ticlopidine inhibits CYP2C19 that may cause inhibition of the metabolism of PHT, resulting in toxicity (Klaassen, 1998; Donahue *et al.*, 1999). Aspirin may cause protein-binding displacement of PHT at doses that exceed 650 mg every 4 h (Leonard *et al.*, 1981). There is no evidence that aspirin dosed at 81–325 mg per day should cause a clinically significant interaction.

Topiramate

There are no known drug interactions between TPM and anticoagulants or antiplatelets. TPM is a weak inhibitor of CYP2C19 and an inducer of CYP3A4 (Benedetti, 2000). Caution should be taken when prescribing TPM with clopidogrel, ticlopidine, and warfarin, as the presence or absence of drug interactions is not established.

Valproate

Aspirin may displace VPA from protein-binding sites and inhibit metabolism (Goulden *et al.*, 1987). Patients should be monitored for VPA toxicity while taking aspirin. VPA may displace warfarin from protein-binding sites in vitro (Depakote, 2002). Caution should be taken when prescribing VPA with warfarin.

Other

There are no known drug interactions between anticoagulants/antiplatelets and the following AEDs: GBP, LTG, LEV, TGB, or ZNS.

Analgesics

Carbamazepine

Fentanyl is a substrate of CYP3A4 and the addition of CBZ may reduce its effectiveness (Labroo *et al.*, 1997; Duragesic, 2001). There is no documented interaction between CBZ and valdecoxib. Valdecoxib is metabolized via CYP3A4, CYP2C9, and glucuronidation (Bextra, 2002). It is an inhibitor of CYP2C19 and a weak inhibitor of CYP3A4 and CYPC9 (Bextra, 2002). It may be hypothesized that CBZ may induce the metabolism of valdecoxib, reducing its effectiveness, or valdecoxib may inhibit the metabolism of CBZ, resulting in toxicity. The drug interaction between propoxyphene and CBZ has been reported numerous times in the literature (Kubacka and Ferrante, 1983; Yu *et al.*, 1986; Oles *et al.*, 1989; Allen, 1994; Bergendal *et al.*, 1997). Propoxyphene appears to inhibit the metabolism of CBZ resulting in toxicity. This combination should be cautiously used. CBZ increases the metabolism of tramadol that may decrease its efficacy at usual doses (Ultram, 2000).

Lamotrigine

Only one interaction with analgesics has been reported with LTG. One study examined the pharmacokinetics of a single dose of LTG following multiple doses of acetaminophen. The investigators found that it appears that acetaminophen increases the clearance of LTG (Depot *et al.*, 1990). It is not clear if this interaction is clinically significant.

Phenobarbital

There is no documented drug interaction between celecoxib and PB. Celecoxib is metabolized via CYP2C9 and PB induces CYP2C9 (Tang *et al.*, 2000; Raucy *et al.*, 2002). It is possible that PB will reduce the efficacy of celecoxib. There is no documented drug interaction between valdecoxib and PB. Valdecoxib is metabolized via CYP3A4, CYP2C9, and glucuronidation (Bextra, 2002). It is an inhibitor of CYP2C19 and a weak inhibitor of CYP3A4 and CYP2C9 (Bextra, 2002). PB may induce the metabolism of valdecoxib, reducing its effectiveness, or valdecoxib may inhibit the metabolism of PB resulting in toxicity. Propoxyphene may cause up to a 20% increase in PB blood concentrations (Hansen *et al.*, 1980). Patients should be monitored for toxicity.

Phenytoin

PHT induces the metabolism of acetaminophen, resulting in increased clearance and a decrease in the duration of analgesia (Miners *et al.*, 1984). Aspirin may cause displacement of PHT from its protein-binding sites at high doses (>650 mg every 4 h), however lower-dose aspirin (<650 mg every 4 h) should not be very problematic (Leonard *et al.*, 1981). There is no documented drug interaction between valdecoxib and PHT. Valdecoxib is metabolized via CYP3A4, CYP2C9, and glucuronidation (Bextra, 2002). It is an inhibitor of CYP2C19 and a weak inhibitor of CYP3A4 and CYP2C9 (Bextra, 2002). PHT may induce the metabolism of valdecoxib, reducing its effectiveness, or valdecoxib may inhibit the metabolism of PHT resulting in toxicity. Propoxyphene inhibits CYP2C9 and may increase PHT serum concentrations resulting in increased toxicity (Levy, 1995).

Valproate

Aspirin may displace VPA from protein-binding sites and inhibit metabolism (Goulden *et al.*, 1987). Patients should be monitored for VPA toxicity while taking aspirin.

Other

There are no known drug interactions between analgesics with the following AEDs: FBM, GBP, LEV, OXC, TGB, TPM, and ZNS.

Gastrointestinal agents

Carbamazepine

Cimetidine is a modest inhibitor of CYP3A4 (Martinez *et al.*, 1999). The addition of cimetidine may result in CBZ toxicity.

Gabapentin

Concomitant use of antacids (Maalox®) has been shown to decrease the absorption of GBP by 20% (Neurontin, 2002). The manufacturer recommends taking antacids and GBP at least 2 h apart.

Phenobarbital

There are no known drug interactions between gastrointestinal agents and PB. Interactions may be possible depending on the metabolism of the gastrointestinal agents and the pathways that PB induces.

Phenytoin

Antacids, when taken simultaneously with PHT, may create an insoluble complex resulting in decreased or erratic absorption of PHT (Carter *et al.*, 1981; McElnay *et al.*, 1982). To avoid any potential interaction, it is recommended that patients take antacids and PHT at least 2 h apart. Cimetidine appears to cause a decrease in the clearance of PHT resulting in toxicity (Algozzine *et al.*, 1981; Hetzel *et al.*, 1981; Bartle *et al.*, 1983; Frigo *et al.*, 1983). The mechanism of the drug interaction is likely to be the inhibition of CYP2C19 (Furuta *et al.*, 2001). Caution should be taken when prescribing cimetidine with PHT. There is potential for a drug interaction between omeprazole and PHT (Prichard *et al.*, 1987). Omeprazole is a potent inhibitor of CYP2C19 that may cause inhibition of PHT metabolism resulting in toxicity (Furuta *et al.*, 2001). Careful monitoring is warranted.

Valproate

One study, of six subjects, demonstrated decreased clearance of a single dose of VPA when cimetidine was also administered (Webster *et al.*, 1984). It is not known if cimetidine interacts with multiple doses of VPA, but caution should be taken if prescribing cimetidine and VPA.

Other

There are no known drug interactions with gastrointestinal agents and the following AEDs: FBM, LTG, LEV, OXC, TGB, TPM, and ZNS.

Endocrine/metabolic agents

Carbamazepine

There is no documented interaction between hormone replacement therapy and CBZ but it is well known that CBZ increases the metabolism of hormones (Ramsay and Slater, 1991). It would be expected that women who choose hormone replacement therapy might require higher doses of hormones for control of menopausal symptoms. There is no documented interaction with pioglitazone and CBZ. Pioglitazone is metabolized via CYP3A4 and may undergo increased metabolism secondary to CBZ induction (Actos, 2002).

Felbamate

There is no documented interaction between hormone replacement therapy and FBM. There was one study that examined the effect of FBM on oral contraceptives and it was found that FBM decreases hormone blood levels (Saano *et al.*, 1995). It is unknown if FBM would also adversely affect blood levels of hormone replacement therapy.

Lamotrigine

There is no documented interaction between hormone replacement therapy and LTG but it has been demonstrated that oral contraceptives increase the clearance of LTG by as much as 50% (Jaben *et al.*, 2003). LTG clearance may be increased by hormone replacement therapy.

Oxcarbazepine

There is no documented interaction between hormone replacement therapy and OXC. There is one study that examined the effect of OXC on oral contraceptives that found OXC decreases hormone blood levels (Fattore *et al.*, 1999). It is unknown if OXC would also adversely affect blood levels of hormone replacement therapy.

Phenobarbital

Both glypizide and tolbutamide are CYP2C9 substrates (Kidd *et al.*, 1999; Kirchheiner *et al.*, 2002). There is no documented interaction with PB and glypizide or tolbutamide. PB may cause some enzyme induction altering the metabolism of both agents (Gerbal-Chaloin *et al.*, 2001). Close monitoring of therapeutic response and glucose levels is warranted. There is no documented interaction between hormone replacement therapy and PB. There is evidence that PB induces the metabolism of hormones and monitoring of therapy is recommended (Ramsay and Slater, 1991). There is no documented drug interaction between pioglitazone and PB. Pioglitazone is metabolized via CYP3A4 and may be susceptible to increased metabolism secondary to PB co-medication (Actos, 2002; Luo *et al.*, 2002; Edwards *et al.*, 2003). There is no documented drug interaction between rosiglitazone and PB. Rosiglitazone is metabolized via CYP2C8, a metabolic pathway induced by PB (Baldwin *et al.*, 1999; Gerbal-Chaloin *et al.*, 2001).

Phenytoin

There is no documented interaction between PHT and glypizide or tolbutamide. Both glypizide and tolbutamide are CYP2C9 substrates (Kidd *et al.*, 1999; Kirchheiner *et al.*, 2002). PHT may cause some enzyme induction altering the metabolism of both agents. Close monitoring of therapeutic response and glucose levels is warranted. There is no documented drug interaction between hormone replacement therapy and PHT. However, there is evidence that PHT increases the clearance of oral contraceptives (Coulam and Annegers, 1979; Mattson *et al.*, 1986). It may be extrapolated that PHT will increase the clearance of other hormone replacement therapy. There is no documented drug interaction between pioglitazone and PHT. Pioglitazone is metabolized via CYP3A4 and may be susceptible to increased metabolism secondary to PHT co-medication (Actos, 2002; Luo *et al.*, 2002).

Topiramate

There is no documented drug interaction between hormone replacement therapy and TPM. There is one study that documented a 14–33% increase in clearance of ethinyl estradiol when administered with TPM (Rosenfeld *et al.*, 1997). The formulation ethinyl estradiol used in this study is an oral contraceptive. It may be extrapolated that TPM may increase the clearance of other estrogen supplements.

Other

There are no known drug interactions between endocrine/metabolic agents and the following AEDs: GBP, LEV, TGB, VPA, and ZNS.

Respiratory agents

There are no established interactions between inhaled respiratory medications and the AEDs.

Phenobarbital

There is a study of six adults that demonstrated an increased clearance of theophylline when they were also receiving PB (Landay *et al.*, 1978). It is unknown what the significance of this drug interaction is in the elderly. It may be inferred that they would require larger doses of theophylline while being treated with PB.

Phenytoin

There are several case reports and studies that have demonstrated that PHT increases the clearance of theophylline (Miller *et al.*, 1984; Sklar and Wagner, 1985; Adebayo, 1988). Patients on PHT may require increased doses of theophylline to get an adequate response.

CNS agents

Carbamazepine

There are numerous antidepressants whose metabolism is increased by CBZ, including tricyclic antidepressants, bupropion, mirtazepine, and sertraline (Leinonen *et al.*, 1991; Wellbutrin, 1999; Sitsen *et al.*, 2001; Pihlsgard and Eliasson, 2002). Several antidepressants may cause an elevation of CBZ blood concentrations including fluoxetine, fluvoxamine, and nefazodone. Fluoxetine has been shown to cause inhibition of CBZ in one study of six subjects (Grimsley *et al.*, 1991), while another study of eight subjects showed no change in CBZ pharmacokinetics (Spina *et al.*, 1993). Fluvoxamine was hypothesized to cause inhibition of metabolism of CBZ in three cases (Fritze *et al.*, 1991), while a study of seven subjects showed no change in CBZ pharmacokinetics when fluvoxamine was added (Spina *et al.*, 1993). Nefazodone is a CYP3A4 inhibitor (Rotzinger and Baker, 2002). The metabolism of CBZ is decreased when nefazodone is added to a patient's regimen (Laroudie *et al.*, 2000). Patients should be monitored for signs of CBZ toxicity and increased blood concentrations if nefazodone is prescribed to a patient also on CBZ. The metabolism of olanzapine, an atypical antipsychotic, is increased by CBZ by approximately 40%, which may not be clinically significant since olanzapine has a wide therapeutic range (Lucas *et al.*, 1998; Olesen and Linnet, 1999; Linnet and Olesen, 2002). When CBZ was added to a regimen containing haloperidol, the clearance of haloperidol increased by 60% (Jann *et al.*, 1985). The resulting increase in clearance may lead to treatment failure due to insufficient efficacy (Hesslinger *et al.*, 1999). The metabolism of risperidone may be increased by CBZ (Ono *et al.*, 2002). Alternatively risperidone may modestly increase plasma concentrations of CBZ and its metabolite CBZ-epoxide (CBZ-E) (Mula and Monaco, 2002). Monitoring the efficacy of both agents is warranted. There are two case reports of quetiapine being added to a CBZ regimen that was thought to cause toxicity secondary to an increase in CBZ-E (Fitzgerald and Okos, 2002). The metabolism of quetiapine may be increased by CBZ (DeVane and Nemeroff, 2001). CBZ increases the metabolism of ziprasidone but it is not clear if the increase is clinically significant (Miceli *et al.*, 2000).

Donepezil, a reversible inhibitor of acetylcholinesterase, used to treat dementia, is metabolized by CYPZD6, CYP3A4 and glucuronidation (Aricept, 2002). Galantamine, also a reversible inhibitor of acetylcholinesterase used to treat dementia, is metabolized via CYP2D6 and CYP3A4 (Reminyl, 2003). It is expected that CBZ may increase their clearance.

Lamotrigine

There are two case reports of patients receiving LTG to which sertraline was added to therapy resulting in toxicity secondary to increased LTG blood concentrations (Kaufman and Gerner, 1998). It was hypothesized that a glucuronidation pathway interaction may be the cause of the reaction, but further research is needed. Patients on LTG and sertraline should be monitored for signs of toxicity secondary to LTG.

Phenobarbital

There are no well-documented drug interaction studies done between antidepressants and PB. Since it is established that PB induces CYP2C9, CYP2C19, and CYP3A4, interactions may be inferred by looking at the metabolic pathway of the antidepressant being prescribed (Glue *et al.*, 1997; Raucy *et al.*, 2002; Edwards *et al.*, 2003). The metabolism of clozapine is increased by co-medication with PB (Facciola *et al.*, 1998). It has also been reported that PB may increase the metabolism of haloperidol (Linnoila *et al.*, 1980). An increase in metabolism may result in a loss of efficacy without adequate dose adjustments. It is expected that PB may increase the clearance of donepezil and galantamine (Aricept, 2002; Reminyl, 2003).

Phenytoin

There are several case reports of the addition of fluoxetine to a regimen with PHT resulting in PHT toxicity (Jalil, 1992; Woods *et al.*, 1994). An in vitro study examining the effect of fluoxetine on PHT metabolism demonstrated that fluoxetine inhibited CYP2C9 resulting in impaired metabolism of PHT (Nelson *et al.*, 2001). Fluvoxamine inhibits CYP2C19, which may result in PHT toxicity, and doses may need to be appropriately adjusted (Schmider *et al.*, 1997; Hemeryck and Belpaire, 2002). Tricyclic antidepressants may cause inhibition of CYP2C9 and CP2C19 resulting in an increased risk of PHT toxicity (Shin *et al.*, 2002). Monitoring of blood concentrations and dose adjustments of PHT may be necessary. Sertraline has been associated with increased PHT toxicity in a report of two elderly patients (Haselberger *et al.*, 1997). In vitro data also demonstrated that sertraline has the potential to inhibit CYP2C9 (Schmider *et al.*, 1997; Nelson *et al.*, 2001). The addition of PHT to quetiapine resulted in a five-fold increase in the metabolism of quetiapine (Wong *et al.*, 2001). Patients should be monitored for a loss of efficacy if PHT is added to a regimen containing quetiapine. It is expected that PHT may increase the clearance of donepezil and galantamine (Aricept, 2002; Reminyl, 2003). It has been reported that PHT decreases the efficacy of levodopa therapy in patients with Parkinson's; as a result, larger doses of levodopa may be necessary (Mendez *et al.*, 1975).

Valproate

There are no well-documented clinically significant drug interactions between CNS medications and VPA.

Other

There are no documented drug interactions between CNS agents and the following AEDs: FBM, GBP, LEV, OXC, TGB, TPM, and ZNS.

Conclusion

AED interactions in the elderly are common and often lead to serious adverse events. A growing number of elderly are taking AEDs, usually in combination with other medications. Older patients appear to be more sensitive to adverse effects even when drug concentrations are controlled. Age-related changes in drug disposition and the use of multiple medications greatly increase the risk of clinically significant interactions in older patients. A number of AEDs either induce or inhibit drug metabolizing enzymes and, in turn, their metabolism is affected by many co-medications. Clinicians and older patients need to recognize that the addition or discontinuation of medications can place the patient at risk of an adverse event due to a drug interaction. An understanding of the principles that determine interactions and the pharmacokinetics of specific AEDs and other medications permits prospective assessment of the risk of an interaction when a drug is added or stopped. This allows clinicians to avoid interactions by selecting an alternate medication or rationally managing an interaction when it cannot be avoided. Several of the newer AEDs do not appear to interact with other medications, while others are affected by enzyme induction of inhibition but do not appear to alter the disposition of co-medications. Thus, the newer AEDs may be particularly useful in older patients.

REFERENCES

Actos (2002). Package Insert. *Takeda Pharmaceuticals America, Inc.*

Adebayo GI. Interaction between phenytoin and theophylline in healthy volunteers. *Clin Exp Pharmacol Physiol* 1988; 15(11): 883–887.

Algozzine GJ, Stewart RB, Springer PK. Decreased clearance of phenytoin with cimetidine. *Ann Intern Med* 1981; **95**(2): 244–245.

Allen S. Cerebellar dysfunction following dextropropoxyphene-induced carbamazepine toxicity. *Postgrad Med J* 1994; **70**(828): 764.

Aricept (2002). Package Insert. *Eisai Co, Ltd.*

Bahls FH, Ozuna J, Ritchie DE. Interactions between calcium channel blockers and the anticonvulsants carbamazepine and phenytoin. *Neurology* 1991; **41**(5): 740–742.

Baldwin SJ, Clarke SE, Chenery RJ. Characterization of the cytochrome P450 enzymes involved in the in vitro metabolism of rosiglitazone. *Br J Clin Pharmacol* 1999; **48**(3): 424–432.

Bartle WR, Walker SE, Shapero T. Dose-dependent effect of cimetidine on phenytoin kinetics. *Clin Pharmacol Ther* 1983; **33**(5): 649–655.

Beattie B, Biller J, Mehlhous B, *et al.* Verapamil-induced carbamazepine neurotoxicity. A report of two cases. *Eur Neurol* 1988; **28**(2): 104–105.

Beers MH, Fingold SF, Ouslander JG, *et al.* Characteristics and quality of prescribing by doctors practicing in nursing homes. *J Am Geriatr Soc* 1993; **41**(8): 802–807.

Benedetti MS. Enzyme induction and inhibition by new antiepileptic drugs: a review of human studies. *Fundam Clin Pharmacol* 2000; **14**(4): 301–319.

Bergendal L, Friberg A, Schaffrath AM, *et al.* The clinical relevance of the interaction between carbamazepine and dextropropoxyphene in elderly patients in Gothenburg, Sweden. *Eur J Clin Pharmacol* 1997; **53**(3–4): 203–206.

Bextra (2002). Package Insert. *Pfizer.*

Birnbaum A, Hardie NA, Leppik IE, *et al.* Variability of total phenytoin serum concentrations within elderly nursing home residents. *Neurology* 2003; **60**: 555–559.

Cacek AT. Review of alterations in oral phenytoin bioavailability associated with formulation, antacids, and food. *Ther Drug Monit* 1986; **8**(2): 166–171.

Carter BL, Garnett WR, Pellock JM, *et al.* Effect of antacids on phenytoin bioavailability. *Ther Drug Monit* 1981; **3**(4): 333–340.

Clarke TA, Waskell LA. The metabolism of clopidogrel is catalyzed by human cytochrome P450 3A and is inhibited by atorvastatin. *Drug Metab Dispos* 2003; **31**(1): 53–59.

Clarke WR, Horn JR, Kawabori I, *et al.* Potentially serious drug interactions secondary to high-dose diltiazem used in the treatment of pulmonary hypertension. *Pharmacotherapy* 1993; **13**(4): 402–405.

Cloyd J, Conway J. Age-related changes in pharmacokinetics, drug interactions, and adverse effects. In *Clinical Neurology of the Older Adult.* J. Sirven, B. Malamut, eds. Philadelphia, PA: Lippincott Williams & Wilkins, 2002: 29–44.

Coulam CB, Annegers JF. Do anticonvulsants reduce the efficacy of oral contraceptives? *Epilepsia* 1979; **20**(5): 519–525.

Denbow CE, Fraser HS. Clinically significant hemorrhage due to warfarin–carbamazepine interaction. *South Med J* 1990; **83**(8): 981.

Depakote (2002). Package Insert. *Abbott Laboratories.*

Depot M, Powell JR, Messenheimer JA, *et al.* Kinetic effects of multiple oral doses of acetaminophen on a single oral dose of lamotrigine. *Clin Pharmacol Ther* 1990; **48**(4): 346–355.

DeVane CL, Nemeroff CB. Clinical pharmacokinetics of quetiapine: an atypical antipsychotic. *Clin Pharmacokinet* 2001; **40**(7): 509–522.

Donahue S, Flockhart DA, Abernethy DR, *et al.* Ticlopidine inhibits phenytoin clearance. *Clin Pharmacol Ther* 1999; **66**(6): 563–568.

Duragesic (2001). Package Insert. *Janssen.*

Edwards RJ, Price RJ, Walts PS, *et al.* Induction of cytochrome P450 enzymes in cultured precision-cut human liver slices. *Drug Metab Dispos* 2003; **31**(3): 282–288.

Eimer M, Carter BL. Elevated serum carbamazepine concentrations following diltiazem initiation. *Drug Intell Clin Pharm* 1987; **21**(4): 340–342.

Facciola G, Avenoso A, Spina E, *et al.* Inducing effect of phenobarbital on clozapine metabolism in patients with chronic schizophrenia. *Ther Drug Monit* 1998; **20**(6): 628–630.

Fattore C, Cipolla G, Gatti G, *et al.* Induction of ethinylestradiol and levonorgestrel metabolism by oxcarbazepine in healthy women. *Epilepsia* 1999; **40**(6): 783–787.

Fitzgerald BJ, Okos AJ. Elevation of carbamazepine-10,11-epoxide by quetiapine. *Pharmacotherapy* 2002; **22**(11): 1500–1503.

Frigo GM, Lecchini S, Caranaggi M, *et al.* Reduction of phenytoin clearance caused by cimetidine. *Eur J Clin Pharmacol* 1983; **25**(1): 135–137.

Fritze J, Unsorg B, Lanczik M, *et al.* Interaction between carbamazepine and fluvoxamine. *Acta Psychiatr Scand* 1991; **84**(6): 583–584.

Furuta S, Kamada E, Suzuki T, *et al.* Inhibition of drug metabolism in human liver microsomes by nizatidine, cimetidine and omeprazole. *Xenobiotica* 2001; **31**(1): 1–10.

Garrard J, Cloyd J, Gross C, *et al.* Factors associated with antiepileptic drug use among elderly nursing home residents. *J Gerontol A Biol Sci Med Sci* 2000; **55**(7): M384–M392.

Garrard J, Harms S, Hardie N, *et al.* Antiepileptic drug use in nursing home admissions. *Annals of Neurology* 2003; **54**: 75–85.

Gerbal-Chaloin S, Pascussi JM, Pichard-Garcia L, *et al.* Induction of CYP2C genes in human hepatocytes in primary culture. *Drug Metab Dispos* 2001; **29**(3): 242–251.

Glue P, Banfield CR, Perhach JL, *et al.* Pharmacokinetic interactions with felbamate. In vitro–in vivo correlation. *Clin Pharmacokinet* 1997; **33**(3): 214–224.

Goulden KJ, Dooley JM, Camfield PR, *et al.* Clinical valproate toxicity induced by acetylsalicylic acid. *Neurology* 1987; **37**(8): 1392–1394.

Grimsley SR, Jann MW, Carter JG, *et al.* Increased carbamazepine plasma concentrations after fluoxetine coadministration. *Clin Pharmacol Ther* 1991; **50**(1): 10–15.

Guay D, Artz M, Hanlon J, *et al.* The pharmacology of aging. In *Brocklehurst's Textbook of Geriatric Medicine.* R. Tallis, H. Fillit, eds. London, UK: Churchill Livingstone, 2003: 155–161.

Hansen BS, Dam M, Brandt J, *et al.* Influence of dextropropoxyphene on steady state serum levels and protein binding of three anti-epileptic drugs in man. *Acta Neurol Scand* 1980; **61**(6): 357–367.

Haselberger MB, Freedman LS, Tolbert S. Elevated serum phenytoin concentrations associated with coadministration of sertraline. *J Clin Psychopharmacol* 1997; **17**(2): 107–109.

Hauser W. Epidemiology of seizures in the elderly. In *Seizures and Epilepsy in the Elderly.* A. Rowan, R. Ramsay, eds. Boston, MA: Butterworth-Heinemann, 1997: 7–20.

Hemeryck A, Belpaire FM. Selective serotonin reuptake inhibitors and cytochrome P-450 mediated drug–drug interactions: an update. *Curr Drug Metab* 2002; **3**(1): 13–37.

Hesslinger B, Normann C, Langosch JM, *et al.* Effects of carbamazepine and valproate on haloperidol plasma levels and on psychopathologic outcome in schizophrenic patients. *J Clin Psychopharmacol* 1999; **19**(4): 310–315.

Hetzel DJ, Bochner F, Hallike JF, *et al.* Cimetidine interaction with phenytoin. *Br Med J (Clin Res Ed)* 1981; **282**(6275): 1512.

Hoffman C, Rice D, Jung HY. Persons with chronic conditions. Their prevalence and costs. *J Am Med Assoc* 1996; **276**(18): 1473–1479.

Jalil P. Toxic reaction following the combined administration of fluoxetine and phenytoin: two case reports. *J Neurol Neurosurg Psychiatry* 1992; **55**(5): 412–413.

Jann MW, Ereshefsky L, Jaklod SR, *et al.* Effects of carbamazepine on plasma haloperidol levels. *J Clin Psychopharmacol* 1985; **5**(2): 106–109.

Kaminsky LS, Zhang ZY. Human P450 metabolism of warfarin. *Pharmacol Ther* 1997; **73**(1): 67–74.

Kaufman KR, Gerner R. Lamotrigine toxicity secondary to sertraline. *Seizure* 1998; **7**(2): 163–165.

Kendall AG, Boivin M. Warfarin-carbamazepine interaction. *Ann Intern Med* 1981; **94**(2): 280.

Kidd RS, Straughn AB, Mayer MC, *et al.* Pharmacokinetics of chlorpheniramine, phenytoin, glipizide and nifedipine in an individual homozygous for the CYP2C9*3 allele. *Pharmacogenetics* 1999; **9**(1): 71–80.

Kirchheiner J, Bauer S, Meineke I, *et al.* Impact of CYP2C9 and CYP2C19 polymorphisms on tolbutamide kinetics and the insulin and glucose response in healthy volunteers. *Pharmacogenetics* 2002; **12**(2): 101–109.

Klaassen SL. Ticlopidine-induced phenytoin toxicity. *Ann Pharmacother* 1998; **32**(12): 1295–1298.

Kubacka RT, Ferrante JA. Carbamazepine–propoxyphene interaction. *Clin Pharm* 1983; **2**(2): 104.

Labroo RB, Paine MF, Thummel KE, *et al.* Fentanyl metabolism by human hepatic and intestinal cytochrome P450 3A4: implications for interindividual variability in disposition, efficacy, and drug interactions. *Drug Metab Dispos* 1997; **25**(9): 1072–1080.

Lackner TE, Cloyd JC, Thomas LW, *et al.* Antiepileptic drug use in nursing home residents: effect of age, gender, and comedication on patterns of use. *Epilepsia* 1998; **39**(10): 1083–1087.

Lader M. Some adverse effects of antipsychotics: prevention and treatment. *J Clin Psychiatry* 1999; **60**(Suppl. 12): S18–S21.

Landay RA, Gonzalez MA, Taylor JC. Effect of phenobarbital on theophylline disposition. *J Allergy Clin Immunol* 1978; **62**(1): 27–29.

Laroudie C, Salazar DE, Cosson JP, *et al.* Carbamazepine–nefazodone interaction in healthy subjects. *J Clin Psychopharmacol* 2000; **20**(1): 46–53.

Leinonen E, Lillsunde P, Laukkanen V, *et al.* Effects of carbamazepine on serum antidepressant concentrations in psychiatric patients. *J Clin Psychopharmacol* 1991; **11**(5): 313–318.

Leonard RF, Knott PJ, Rankin GO, *et al.* Phenytoin–salicylate interaction. *Clin Pharmacol Ther* 1981; **29**(1): 56–60.

Levine M, Sheppard I. Biphasic interaction of phenytoin with warfarin. *Clin Pharm* 1984; **3**(2): 200–203.

Levy RH. Cytochrome P450 isozymes and antiepileptic drug interactions. *Epilepsia* 1995; **36**(Suppl. 5): S8–S13.

Linnet K, Olesen OV. Free and glucuronidated olanzapine serum concentrations in psychiatric patients: influence of carbamazepine comedication. *Ther Drug Monit* 2002; **24**(4): 512–517.

Linnoila M, Viukari M, Vaisanen K, *et al.* Effect of anticonvulsants on plasma haloperidol and thioridazine levels. *Am J Psychiatry* 1980; **137**(7): 819–821.

Lucas RA, Gilfillan DJ, Bergstrom RF. A pharmacokinetic interaction between carbamazepine and olanzapine: observations on possible mechanism. *Eur J Clin Pharmacol* 1998; **54**(8): 639–643.

Luo G, Cunningham M, Kim S, *et al.* CYP3A4 induction by drugs: correlation between a pregnane X receptor reporter gene assay and CYP3A4 expression in human hepatocytes. *Drug Metab Dispos* 2002; **30**(7): 795–804.

Ma B, Prueksaritanont T, Lin JH. Drug interactions with calcium channel blockers: possible involvement of metabolite-intermediate complexation with CYP3A. *Drug Metab Dispos* 2000; **28**(2): 125–130.

MacKichan J. Influence of protein binding and use of unbound (free) drug concentrations. In *Applied Pharmacokinetics.* W. Evans, J. Schentag, W. Jusko, eds. Vancouver, WA: Applied Therapeutics, Inc., 1992.

Macphee GJ, McInnes GT, Thompson GG, *et al.* Verapamil potentiates carbamazepine neuro-toxicity: a clinically important inhibitory interaction. *Lancet* 1986; **1**(8483): 700–703.

Martinez C, Albet C, Agundez JA, *et al.* Comparative in vitro and in vivo inhibition of cytochrome P450 CYP1A2, CYP2D6, and CYP3A by H2-receptor antagonists. *Clin Pharmacol Ther* 1999; **65**(4): 369–376.

Massey EW. Effect of carbamazepine on Coumadin metabolism. *Ann Neurol* 1983; **13**(6): 691–692.

Mattson RH, Cramer JA, Dorney PD, *et al.* Use of oral contraceptives by women with epilepsy. *J Am Med Assoc* 1986; **256**(2): 238–240.

Mayersohn M. Special Pharmacokinetic Considerations in the Elderly. In *Applied Pharmacokinetics.* W. Evans, J. Schentag and W. Jusko, eds. Vancouver, WA: Applied Therapeutics, Inc., 1992.

Mazzu AL, Lasseter KC, Shamblen EC, *et al.* Itraconazole alters the pharmacokinetics of atorvas-tatin to a greater extent than either cerivastatin or pravastatin. *Clin Pharmacol Ther* 2000; **68**(4): 391–400.

McElnay JC, Uprichard G, Collier PS. The effect of activated dimethicone and a proprietary antacid preparation containing this agent on the absorption of phenytoin. *Br J Clin Pharmacol* 1982; **13**(4): 501–505.

Mendez JS, Cotzias GC, Mena I, *et al.* Diphenylhydantoin. Blocking of levodopa effects. *Arch Neurol* 1975; **32**(1): 44–46.

Miceli JJ, Anziano RJ, Roberge L, *et al.* The effect of carbamazepine on the steady-state pharmaco-kinetics of ziprasidone in healthy volunteers. *Br J Clin Pharmacol* 2000; **49**(Suppl. 1): S65–S70.

Michelucci R, Tassinari C. Benzodiazepines-adverse effects. In *Antiepileptic Drugs.* R. Levy, R. Mattson, B. Meldrun, E. Percucca, eds. Philadelphia, PA: Lippincott Williams & Wilkins, 2002.

Miller M, Cosgriff J, Kwong T, *et al.* Influence of phenytoin on theophylline clearance. *Clin Pharmacol Ther* 1984; **35**(5): 666–669.

Miners JO, Attwood J, Birkett DJ. Determinants of acetaminophen metabolism: effect of induc-ers and inhibitors of drug metabolism on acetaminophen's metabolic pathways. *Clin Pharmacol Ther* 1984; **35**(4): 480–486.

Mula M, Monaco F. Carbamazepine–risperidone interactions in patients with epilepsy. *Clin Neuropharmacol* 2002; **25**(2): 97–100.

Mungall DR, Ludden TM, Marshall J, *et al.* Population pharmacokinetics of racemic warfarin in adult patients. *J Pharmacokinet Biopharm* 1985; **13**(3): 213–227.

Nappi JM. Warfarin and phenytoin interaction. *Ann Intern Med* 1979; **90**(5): 852.

Nelson MH, Birnbaum AK, Remmel RP. Inhibition of phenytoin hydroxylation in human liver microsomes by several selective serotonin re-uptake inhibitors. *Epilepsy Res* 2001; **44**(1): 71–82.

Neurontin (2002). Package Insert. *Pfizer, Inc.*

Nitz N, Garrard J, Harms S, *et al.* Prevalence of antiepileptic drug use among medicare beneficiaries. *Epilepsia* 2000; **41**(Suppl. 7): S251.

Nolan L, O'Malley K. Adverse drug reactions in the elderly. *Br J Hosp Med* 1989; **41**(5): 446, 448, 452–457.

Oles KS, Mirza W, Penry JK. Catastrophic neurologic signs due to drug interaction: Tegretol and Darvon. *Surg Neurol* 1989; **32**(2): 144–151.

Olesen OV, Linnet K. Olanzapine serum concentrations in psychiatric patients given standard doses: the influence of comedication. *Ther Drug Monit* 1999; **21**(1): 87–90.

Ono S, Mihara K, Suzuki A, *et al.* Significant pharmacokinetic interaction between risperidone and carbamazepine: its relationship with CYP2D6 genotypes. *Psychopharmacology (Berl)* 2002; **162**(1): 50–54.

Panegyres PK, Rischbieth RH. Fatal phenytoin warfarin interaction. *Postgrad Med J* 1991; **67**(783): 98.

Paoletti R, Corsini A, Bellosta S. Pharmacological interactions of statins. *Atheroscler Suppl* 2002; **3**(1): 35–40.

Pihlsgard M, Eliasson E. Significant reduction of sertraline plasma levels by carbamazepine and phenytoin. *Eur J Clin Pharmacol* 2002; **57**(12): 915–916.

Prichard PJ, Walt RP, Kitchingman GK, *et al.* Oral phenytoin pharmacokinetics during omeprazole therapy. *BrJ Clin Pharmacol* 1987; **24**(4): 543–545.

Ramsay RE, Slater JD. Effects of antiepileptic drugs on hormones. *Epilepsia* 1991; **32**(Suppl. 6): S60–S67.

Ramsay R, Rowan A, Slater J, *et al.* Effect of age on epilepsy and its treatment: results of the VA cooperative study. *Epilepsia* 1994; **35**(Suppl. 8): 91A.

Raucy JL, Mueller L, Duan K, *et al.* Expression and induction of CYP2C P450 enzymes in primary cultures of human hepatocytes. *J Pharmacol Exp Ther* 2002; **302**(2): 475–482.

Reminyl (2003). Package Insert. *Janssen Pharmaceutical Products.* L.P., Titusville, NJ.

Rosenfeld WE, Doose DR, Walker JA, *et al.* Effect of topiramate on the pharmacokinetics of an oral contraceptive containing norethindrone and ethinyl estradiol in patients with epilepsy. *Epilepsia* 1997; **38**(3): 317–323.

Ross JR, Beeley L. Interaction between carbamazepine and warfarin. *Br Med J* 1980; **280**(6229): 1415–1416.

Rotzinger S, Baker GB. Human CYP3A4 and the metabolism of nefazodone and hydroxynefazodone by human liver microsomes and heterologously expressed enzymes. *Eur Neuropsychopharmacol* 2002; **12**(2): 91–100.

Saano V, Glue P, Banfield CR, *et al.* Effects of felbamate on the pharmacokinetics of a low-dose combination oral contraceptive. *Clin Pharmacol Ther* 1995; **58**(5): 523–531.

Schachter SC, Cramer GW, Thompson GD, *et al.* An evaluation of antiepileptic drug therapy in nursing facilities. *J Am Geriatr Soc* 1998; 46(9): 1137–1141.

Schmider J, Greenblatt DJ, Von Moltke LL, *et al.* Inhibition of CYP2C9 by selective serotonin reuptake inhibitors in vitro: studies of phenytoin p-hydroxylation. *Br J Clin Pharmacol* 1997; 44(5): 495–498.

Shaughnessy AF, Mosley MR. Elevated carbamazepine levels associated with diltiazem use. *Neurology* 1992; 42(4): 937–938.

Shin JG, Park JY, Kim MJ, *et al.* Inhibitory effects of tricyclic antidepressants (TCAs) on human cytochrome P450 enzymes in vitro: mechanism of drug interaction between TCAs and phenytoin. *Drug Metab Dispos* 2002; 30(10): 1102–1107.

Sitsen J, Maris F, Timmer C. Drug–drug interaction studies with mirtazapine and carbamazepine in healthy male subjects. *Eur J Drug Metab Pharmacokinet* 2001; 26(1–2): 109–121.

Sklar SJ, Wagner JC. Enhanced theophylline clearance secondary to phenytoin therapy. *Drug Intell Clin Pharm* 1985; 19(1): 34–36.

Spina E, Avenoso A, Pollicino AM, *et al.* Carbamazepine coadministration with fluoxetine or fluvoxamine. *Ther Drug Monit* 1993; 15(3): 247–250.

Stewart RB. Drug use in the elderly. In *Therapeutics in the Elderly*. J. Delafuente, R. Stewart, eds. Cincinnati: Harvey Whitney, 2001: 235–256.

Tang C, Shou M, Mei Q, *et al.* Major role of human liver microsomal cytochrome P450 2C9 (CYP2C9) in the oxidative metabolism of celecoxib, a novel cyclooxygenase-II inhibitor. *J Pharmacol Exp Ther* 2000; 293(2): 453–459.

Trileptal (2001). Package Insert. *Novartis.*

Ucar M, Neuronen M, Luurila H, *et al.* Carbamazepine markedly reduces serum concentrations of simvastatin and simvastatin acid. *Eur J Pharmacol* 2004; 59: 879–882.

Udall JA. Clinical implications of warfarin interactions with five sedatives. *Am J Cardiol* 1975; 35(1): 67–71.

Ultram (2000). Package Insert. *Ortho-McNeil Pharmaceutical, Inc.*

Wallace SM, Verbeeck RK. Plasma protein binding of drugs in the elderly. *Clin Pharmacokinet* 1987; 12(1): 41–72.

Wang RW, Kari PH, Lu AY, *et al.* Biotransformation of lovastatin. IV. Identification of cytochrome P450 3A proteins as the major enzymes responsible for the oxidative metabolism of lovastatin in rat and human liver microsomes. *Arch Biochem Biophys* 1991; 290(2): 355–361.

Webster LK, Mihaly GW, Jones DB, *et al.* Effect of cimetidine and ranitidine on carbamazepine and sodium valproate pharmacokinetics. *Eur J Clin Pharmacol* 1984; 27(3): 341–343.

Wellbutrin (1999). Package Insert. *Glaxo Smith-Kline.*

Wen X, Wary JS, Bockman JT, *et al.* Genfibrozil is a potent inhibitor of human cytochrome P4502C9. *Drug Metab Dispos* 2001; 29: 1354–1361.

Wong YW, Yeh C, Thyrum PT. The effects of concomitant phenytoin administration on the steady-state pharmacokinetics of quetiapine. *J Clin Psychopharmacol* 2001; 21(1): 89–93.

Woods DJ, Coulter DM, Pillans P. Interaction of phenytoin and fluoxetine. *NZ Med J* 1994; 107(970): 19.

Yu YL, Huang CY, Chin D, *et al.* Interaction between carbamazepine and dextropropoxyphene. *Postgrad Med J* 1986; 62(725): 231–233.

16

Antiepileptic drug interactions in pregnancy

Mark S. Yerby

North Pacific Epilepsy Research, Oregon Health Sciences University, Portland, Oregon, USA

Scope of the problem

Women with epilepsy require chronic antiepilepsy drugs (AEDs) to prevent seizures, maintain their function and health. Unlike most young women they are unable to discontinue their medications if they become pregnant, for to do so increases their risk of seizures, personal injury, miscarriage and developmental delay in the offspring. With a prevalence of between 0.6% and 1.0% and an estimated 40% of those with epilepsy being women of childbearing years one can see that the potential public health impact is significant. Most women with epilepsy have healthy children but there is an increased risk for congenital malformations, fetal loss, developmental delay and neonatal hemorrhage. Maternal epilepsy is a contributor but the use of AEDs is a significant confounder. To make matters more complicated 86% of pregnant women take medications during pregnancy. A survey by the World Health Organization of 14778 women in 22 countries reported that of the 86% of women taking medications during pregnancy the average number of prescriptions was 2.9 (range of 1–15). This study did not evaluate over-the-counter medications. The preponderance of prescriptions, 73%, were written by obstetricians (Collaborative Drug Use in Pregnancy, 1991).

When evaluating AED use in pregnancy one is hampered by the lack of knowledge of specific co-medications, even though it is clear that this is a common event. While monotherapy with AEDs is a goal of epilepsy management, it is not always an obtainable one. Polytherapy is also more common with the "newer" post-1993 introduction AEDs, because all were initially approved for use as adjunctive therapy. The pregnancy outcome of greatest interest is congenital malformations. While there are substantial data on this outcome, most are in the form of case series and case reports, and accurate rates and risks cannot be determined. Other adverse outcomes are at least as common in terms of incidence (developmental delay, fetal loss), but have received significantly less attention.

Let us review some of the clinically important issues surrounding pregnancy and AED exposure.

Antiepileptic drugs and hormonal contraceptives

A discussion of pregnancy needs to be preceded by reviewing the problems of contraception. Oral contraceptives have not been associated with exacerbation of epilepsy (Mattson *et al.*, 1986). The effectiveness of hormonal contraceptives can, however, be reduced by enzyme-inducing AED (carbamazepine, phenytoin, phenobarbital, felbamate, topiramate). Hormonal contraceptives come in three formulations:

- oral (estrogen–progesterone combinations or progesterone only);
- subcutaneous (levonorgestrel) or intrauterine (progestasert) implants;
- injectable (depoprovera).

All three forms can be adversely impacted by enzyme-inducing AED.

AEDs may lower concentrations of estrogens by 40–50%. They also increase sex hormone-binding globulin (SHBG), which increases the binding of progesterone and reduces the unbound fraction. The result is that hormonal contraception is less reliable with enzyme-inducing AEDs.

The low- or mini-dose oral contraceptives are therefore to be used with caution. As it is the progesterone not the estrogen that inhibits ovulation, using higher-dose estrogens alone may not be effective. The more rapid clearance of the oral contraceptive when used in conjunction with an enzyme-inducing AED will reduce the likelihood of unwanted side effects from higher-dose tablets.

Failure of implantable hormonal contraceptives has also occurred (Shane-McWhorter *et al.*, 1998). Mid-cycle spotting or bleeding is a sign that ovulation is not suppressed. If this occurs alternative or supplementary methods of contraception are required. Contraceptive failure may not always be predictable, even when mid-cycle spotting does not occur. Failure of basal body temperature to rise at mid-cycle can be used to document ovulatory suppression.

Medroxyprogesterone injections should be given every 10 instead of 12 weeks to women on enzyme-inducing AED. This shorter cycle is less likely to result in unintended pregnancy (Crawford, 2002a).

For multiparous women with epilepsy, intrauterine devices may be an excellent contraceptive choice. Alternatively non-enzyme-inducing AEDs may need to be considered (valproate, lamotrigine, gabapentin or zonisamide). A recent report suggests that topiramate at doses of <200 mg a day lacks enough enzyme induction to effect hormonal contraceptives. Higher doses however do reduce ethinyl estradiol concentrations by 18% on 200 mg, 21% with 400 mg and 30% with 800 mg of topiramate a day (Doose *et al.*, 2002).

The importance of the potential impact of enzyme-inducing AEDs cannot be underestimated. In a survey of 294 general practices in the General Practice Research Database, 16.7% of women aged 15–45 with epilepsy were taking an oral contraceptive. Two hundred were on an enzyme-inducing AED and 56% on low estrogen ($<$50 μg) hormonal contraceptives (Shorvon *et al.*, 2002).

There has been at least one circumstance in which oral contraceptives effect AED concentration. Sabers and colleagues (2003) have demonstrated a marked reduction in lamotrigine concentrations when oral contraceptives are also taken. The average plasma concentration in 22 women on lamotrigine monotherapy and an oral contraceptive was 13 μmol/l. In a similar group of women on lamotrigine monotherapy with no oral contraceptive use, the plasma concentrations averaged 28 μmol/l: a significant reduction in AED concentration of over 50%. It has been suggested that oral contraceptives may induce the metabolism of glucuronidated drugs such as lamotrigine.

Maternal complications associated with AED

Seizures not infrequently worsen during pregnancy. One-quarter to one-third of woman with epilepsy (WWE) will have an increase in seizure frequency during pregnancy. This increase is unrelated to seizure type, duration of epilepsy, or seizure frequency in a previous pregnancy. In a recent series of 215 pregnancies in WWE an increase in seizures during the first trimester occurred in 30% of monotherapy- and 43% of polytherapy-treated women. One in 8 or 12.5% had to be hospitalized for their seizures during the pregnancy (Cahill *et al.*, 2002).

Plasma concentrations of anticonvulsant drugs decline as pregnancy progresses, even in the face of constant and in some instances increasing doses (Tomson *et al.*, 1994; Rodriguez-Palomares *et al.*, 1995; Tomson *et al.*, 1997). Although reduction of plasma drug concentration is not always accompanied by an increase in seizure frequency, virtually all women with increased seizures in pregnancy have subtherapeutic drug levels (Dansky *et al.*, 1982; Janz, 1982; Schmidt, 1982; Schmidt *et al.*, 1983; Otani, 1985). The decline of anticonvulsant levels during pregnancy is largely a consequence of decreased plasma protein binding (Perruca, 1982; Yerby *et al.*, 1985; Tomson *et al.*, 1994), reduced concentration of albumin and increased drug clearance (Dam *et al.*, 1979; Nau *et al.*, 1981; Janz, 1982; Philbert and Dam, 1982). The clearance rates are greatest during the third trimester.

Kaarkuzhali and colleagues (2002) found that a majority of their pregnant patients on carbamazepine, phenytoin or phenobarbital required numerous dose adjustments during pregnancy to maintain therapeutic levels. Fifty percent of the pregnancies had breakthrough seizures when the levels fell below the therapeutic range. It is therefore imperative to monitor AED levels at least monthly and adjust dosage to maintain therapeutic levels (Levy and Yerby, 1985). Table 16.1 summarizes some of the pharmacokinetics of anticonvulsant drugs during pregnancy.

Less is known about the kinetics of the newer AEDs in pregnancy. A report demonstrates that lamotrigine clearance increases by $>$50% during pregnancy

Table 16.1 Pharmacokinetic data for first generation AEDs

Anticonvulsant	Percent decrease Total level by third trimester	Percent free fraction		
		Normal	Maternal	Neonatal
Carbamazepine	40	22	25	35
Ethosuximide	?	90	?	?
Phenobarbital	55	51	58	66
Phenytoin	56	9	11	13
Primidone	55	?	?	?
Derived phenobarbital	70	75	80	?
VPA	50	9	15	19

and that the clearance changes occur relatively early in pregnancy. Eleven of 12 pregnancies required increased doses of lamotrigine to maintain therapeutic levels during pregnancy (Tran *et al.*, 2002).

Polycystic ovaries

A great deal of confusing literature has been written about the effect of AEDs on the development of polycystic ovaries (PCO). Ovarian cysts are found in approximately 6.6% of women of childbearing age. Most of these cysts (over 80%) will disappear within 3 months (Borgfeldt and Andolf, 1999). Multiple or PCO are more commonly found in women taking hormonal contraceptives with progesterone, and women who are infertile. The rates vary but average between 10% and 20% (Borgfeldt and Andolf, 1999).

The polycystic ovarian syndrome (PCOS) is a specific disturbance of neuroendocrine function defined as no or irregular menses (oligomenorrhea), elevated levels of male sex steroid hormones (hyperandrogenism) without evidence of other disturbances such as hyperprolactinemia, thyroid dysfunction or 21-hydroxylase deficiency. It is uncommon as occurs in approximately 6.5% of women of reproductive age (Asuncion *et al.*, 2000). It is associated with sustained release of gonadotropic-releasing hormone (GnRH) and lutenizing hormone (LH), and affected women are often overweight, have elevated serum lipids and are less sensitive to insulin. PCOS is also seen in higher than expected rates in mothers (24–52%) and sisters (32–66%) of women with this disorder leading some to believe that it is a genetic disorder (Govind *et al.*, 1999; Kahsar-Miller *et al.*, 2001).

Isojarvi and colleagues (1993) demonstrated an excess of menstrual abnormalities in WWE taking valproic acid (VPA) compared to other AEDs. They also stated that

80% of women taking valproate before the age of 20 developed PCO. Despite this observation other researchers have not found a consistent association between specific AED or epilepsy types and PCOS (Chappell *et al.*, 1999; Bilo *et al.*, 2001; Genton *et al.*, 2001). Women with bipolar disorder are often treated with valproate and do not have an increase in PCOS (Rasgon *et al.*, 2000).

Fetal complications associated with AED

A number of adverse outcomes of pregnancy are known to occur more often in infants of mothers with epilepsy (IME). Of the three major variables – maternal epilepsy, maternal seizures during gestation, and AEDs – it is not always possible to determine which is the most significant. For the outcome congenital malformations, AEDs appear to be a significant risk factor. A recent epidemiological study in Iceland suggests that untreated women with epilepsy have approximately the same rate of malformations in their offspring as do treated mothers, 4.8 vs. 5.9%, respectively. This suggests that a portion of the increased risk is secondary to maternal epilepsy itself (Olafsson *et al.*, 1998). On balance however, malformation rates are twice that seen in the general population, and the proportion of women with epilepsy who are untreated is so small that it is clinically insignificant.

Congenital malformations are defined as a physical defect requiring medical or surgical intervention, and resulting in a major functional disturbance. Congenital anomalies in contrast are defined as deviations from normal morphology that do not require intervention. It is uncertain whether these aberrations represent distinct entities or a spectrum of physiological responses to insult to the developing fetus: malformations at one extreme and anomalies at the other. For the purposes of this review, congenital malformations and anomalies will be discussed separately.

IME, exposed to anticonvulsant drugs in utero, are twice as likely to develop malformations as infants not exposed to these drugs. Malformation rates in the general population range from 2% to 3%. Reports of malformation rates in various populations of exposed infants range from 1.25% to 11.5% (Fedrick, 1973; Nakane *et al.*, 1980; Philbert and Dam, 1982; Kelly, 1984a; Steegers-Theunissen *et al.*, 1994; Jick and Terris, 1997; Olafsson *et al.*, 1998; Kaneko *et al.*, 1999; Vajda *et al.*, 2002). These combined estimates yield a risk of malformations in a pregnancy of a WWE of 4–6%. Cleft lip, cleft palate, or both, and congenital heart disease account for many of the reported cases. Orofacial clefts are responsible for 30% of the increased risk of malformations in these infants (Kelly, 1984a; Friis *et al.*, 1986; Abrishamchian *et al.*, 1994).

The increased rate of malformations in the offspring of mothers with epilepsy appears to be related to AED exposure in utero. Evidence to support this association comes from four observations.

1 Comparisons of the malformation rates in the offspring of mothers with epilepsy treated with AEDs as opposed to those with no AED treatment reveal consistently higher rates in the children of the treated women (South, 1972; Speidel and Meadow, 1972; Lowe, 1973; Monson *et al.*, 1973; Annegers *et al.*, 1978; Nakane *et al.*, 1980).

2 Mean plasma AED concentrations are higher in mothers with malformed infants than mothers with healthy children (Dansky *et al.*, 1980).

3 Infants of mothers taking multiple AEDs have higher malformation rates than those exposed to monotherapy (Nakane, 1979; Lindhout *et al.*, 1984).

4 Maternal seizures during pregnancy do not appear to increase the risk of congenital malformations (Fedrick, 1973).

Majewski and co-workers (1980) described increased malformation rates and central nervous system injury in IMEs exposed to maternal seizures. More recently, Lindhout and co-workers (1992) described a marked increase in malformations amongst infants exposed to first trimester seizures (12.3%) compared to fetuses that were not subject to any maternal seizures (4.0%). Malformations were more often observed in infants exposed to partial seizures than to generalized tonic–clonic seizures. Nonetheless, most investigators have found that maternal seizures during pregnancy had no impact on the frequency of malformations, development of epilepsy or febrile convulsions (Annegers *et al.*, 1978; Nakane *et al.*, 1980).

A variety of congenital malformations have been reported in children of mothers with epilepsy, and every anticonvulsant medication has been implicated in their development. Cleft lip and/or palate, and congenital heart disease account for a majority of reported cases (Elshove and Van Eck, 1971; Anderson, 1976; Annegers *et al.*, 1978). Orofacial clefts are relatively common malformations in the general population, occurring with a frequency of 1.5 per 1000 live births. IME have a rate of orofacial clefting of 13.8 per 1000, a nine-fold increase in risk (Kelly, 1984a; Kallen, 1986a). Early observations that persons with clefting of the lip or palate were twice as likely to have family members with epilepsy as controls suggested that orofacial clefts were associated with epilepsy (Friis *et al.*, 1981). Subsequent studies of the prevalence of facial clefts in the siblings and children of 2072 persons with epilepsy found observed or expected ratios increased only for maternal epilepsy. The risk was greater if AEDs were taken during pregnancy (4.7) than if no AED treatment was used (2.7). The authors concluded that there was no evidence that epilepsy itself contributed to the development of orofacial clefts (Friis *et al.*, 1986). Israeli researchers have found that children with cleft lip or palate are four times as likely to have a mother with epilepsy as the general population, and mothers with epilepsy are six times as likely to bear a child with an orofacial cleft as non-epileptic women (Gatoh *et al.*, 1987). Orofacial clefts account for 30% of the excess of congenital malformations in IMEs.

Congenital heart defects are the second most frequently reported teratogenic abnormality associated with AEDs. IME have a 1.5–2% prevalence of congenital heart disease, a relative risk (RR) of three-fold over the general population (Kallen, 1986b). Anderson (1976) prospectively studied maternal epilepsy and AED use in 3000 children with heart defects at the University of Minnesota. Eighteen IMEs were identified. Twelve of these had ventricular septal defects; 9 of the 18 children had additional non-cardiac defects, 8 of which were orofacial clefts.

No AED can be considered absolutely safe in pregnancy, but for the vast majority of drugs no specific pattern of major malformations has been identified (Kallen, 1986b). This lack of a particular or characteristic pattern of defects has been cited as evidence that AEDs are not teratogenic. When phenobarbital is given during pregnancy for conditions other than epilepsy, no increase in malformation rates has been demonstrated (Shapiro *et al.*, 1976). Phenobarbital has been demonstrated to be relatively teratogenic in mono- and polytherapy. Five of 79 phenobarbital monotherapy-exposed pregnancies were associated with major malformations (proportion 6.3%; 95% confidence interval (CI): 2.1–14.2%). When compared to the background rate (1.62%), there was a significantly increased risk for major malformations, with a RR of 3.8 (95% CI: 1.7–9.0%). A two-fold increase in risk was found when phenobarbital was compared to three other frequently used AED monotherapies (RR 2.2; 95% CI: 0.9–5.2%) (Holmes *et al.*, in press).

Mechanisms of teratogenicity

A hypothesis that metabolites of AEDs are responsible for malformations has been developed on the basis of the following observations:

1 an arene oxide metabolite of phenytoin or other AED is the ultimate teratogen;
2 a genetic defect in epoxide hydrolase (arene oxide detoxifying enzyme) system increases the risk of fetal toxicity;
3 free radicals produced by AED metabolism are cytotoxic;
4 a genetic defect in free radical scavenging enzyme activity (FRSEA) increases the risk of fetal toxicity.

Epoxides

A large number of drugs can be converted into epoxides, in reactions that are catalyzed by the microsomal monoxygenase system (Jerina and Daly, 1974; Sims and Grover, 1974). Arene oxides are unstable epoxides formed by aromatic compounds. Various epoxides are electrophilic and may elicit carcinogenic, mutagenic and other toxic effects by covalent binding to cell macromolecules (Nebert and Jensen, 1979; Shum *et al.*, 1979). Epoxides are detoxified by two processes:

1 conversion to dihydrodiols catalyzed by epoxide hydrolase in the cytoplasm,
2 conjugation with glutathione (GSH) in the microsomes.

Epoxide hydrolase activity has been found in the cytosol and the microsomal sub-cellular fraction of adult and fetal human hepatocytes. Epoxide hydrolase activity in fetal liver is lower than that of adults (Pacifici *et al.*, 1983). One-third to one-half of fetal circulation bypasses the liver, resulting in higher direct exposure of extra-hepatic fetal organs to potential toxic metabolites (Pacifici and Rane, 1982).

Phenytoin teratogenicity

Formation of arene oxides by phenytoin

Arene oxides are obligatory intermediates in the metabolism of aromatic compounds to transdihydrodiols. Phenytoin forms a transdihydrodiol metabolite (Chang *et al.*, 1970). This metabolite is also formed by neonates exposed to phenytoin in utero (Horning *et al.*, 1974). In vitro studies have shown that an oxidative (NADPH/02 dependent) metabolite of phenytoin binds irreversibly to rat liver microsomes (Martz *et al.*, 1977). This binding is increased by an inhibitor of epoxide hydrolase (trichloroponene oxide, TCPO) and decreased by GSH (Martz *et al.*, 1977; Pantarotto *et al.*, 1982; Wells and Harbison, 1985). Using human lymphocytes to assess cell defense mechanisms against toxicity, Spielberg *et al.* (1981) showed that cytotoxicity was enhanced by inhibitors of epoxide hydrolase.

Phenytoin birth defects and lymphocyte cytotoxicity

Strickler *et al.* (1985) examined lymphocytes of 24 children exposed to phenytoin during gestation and lymphocytes from their families using the Spielberg test of cytotoxicity (Spielberg *et al.*, 1981). Lymphocytes were incubated with phenytoin in a mouse microsomal system. A positive response was defined as increase in cell death over baseline. Cells from 15 children gave a positive response. Each positive child had a positive parent (as many mothers as fathers), and a positive response was highly correlated with major birth defects. The authors concluded that a genetic defect in arene oxide detoxification increased the risk of the child having major birth defects (Strickler *et al.*, 1985).

Phenytoin birth defects and epoxide hydrolase activity

In 1985, Buchler reported epoxide hydrolase activity in skin fibroblasts of a pair of dizygotic twins exposed to phenytoin in utero. The infant who had more features of the fetal hydantoin syndrome (FHS) showed lower epoxide hydrolase activity. Although this finding supports the epoxide hydrolase hypothesis, it should be noted that a full report of the experimental details has not yet appeared.

The evidence that epoxide metabolites of phenytoin are teratogenic can be summarized as follows. Phenytoin has an epoxide metabolite that binds to tissues.

Inhibition of the detoxifying enzyme epoxide hydrolase increases the rate of orofacial clefts in experimental animals, lymphocyte cytotoxicity, and the binding of epoxide metabolite to liver microsomes.

These facts cannot completely explain the teratogenicity seen in phenytoin or other AEDs. The lymphocyte cytotoxicity seen with epoxide metabolites correlates with major but not minor malformations (Dansky *et al.*, 1987). Dysmorphic abnormalities have been described in siblings exposed to ethotoin in utero. Ethotoin is not metabolized through an arene oxide intermediate (Finnell and DiLiberti, 1983). Embryopathies have been described with exposure to mephenytoin, which also does not form an arene oxide intermediate (Wells *et al.*, 1982). Trimethadione is clearly teratogenic but has no phenyl rings and thus cannot form an arene oxide metabolite. Therefore, an alternate mechanism must exist.

Free radical intermediates of AEDs and teratogenicity

Some drugs are metabolized or bioactivated by co-oxidation during prostaglandin synthetase (PGS)-catalyzed synthesis of prostaglandins. Such drugs serve as electron donors to peroxidases, resulting in an electron-deficient drug molecule, which by definition, is called a free radical. In the search for additional electrons to complete their outer ring, free radicals can covalently bind to cell macromolecules, including nucleic acids (DNA, RNA), proteins, cell membranes and lipoproteins to produce cytotoxicity.

Phenytoin is co-oxidized by PGS, thyroid peroxidase and horseradish peroxidase producing reactive free radical intermediates that bind to proteins (Kubow and Wells, 1989). Phenytoin teratogenicity can be modulated by substances that reduce the formation of phenytoin-free radicals. Acetylsalicylic acid (ASA) irreversibly inhibits PGS, caffeic acid is an antioxidant, alpha-phenyl-*N*-*t*-butylnitrone (PBN) is a free radical spin-trapping agent. Pretreatment of pregnant mice with these compounds reduces the number of cleft lip or pathies secondary to phenytoin in their offspring (Wells *et al.*, 1989).

GSH is believed to detoxify free radical intermediates by forming a non-reactive conjugate. *N*-acetylcysteine (NACl) a GSH precursor, decreases phenytoin-induced orofacial clefts and fetal weight loss in rodents (Wong and Wells, 1988). 1,3-bis(2-chloroethyl)-1-nitrosourea (BCNU) inhibits GSH reductase, an enzyme necessary to maintain adequate cellular GSH concentrations, and increases phenytoin embryopathy at doses at which BCNU alone has no embryopathic effect (Wong and Wells, 1989). The metabolism of phenytoin or other AEDs to free radical intermediates may be responsible for the teratogenicity seen in IMEs. Twenty-six children with myelomeningocele and their parents were studied by Graf and colleagues (1995). They were found to have significantly lower antioxidant enzymes, particularly GSH peroxidase, than controls.

Neural tube defects and AEDs

Antiepileptic drugs as a group do not produce any specific pattern of major malformations. A possible exception to this is the association of sodium valproate and carbamazepine with neural tube defects (NTDs). Robert and Guibaud (1982) were the first to make this association while working in a birth defects registry in the Rhone Alps region of France. They reported NTDs in IME exposed to VPA. Other studies have revealed an association between carbamazepine exposure in utero and NTDs (Rosa, 1991; Little *et al.*, 1993). Subsequent evaluations of these exposures identify spina bifida aperta (SB) as the specific NTD associated with the VPA or carbamazepine exposure (Lindhout *et al.*, 1992). Methodologic problems make frequency estimates imprecise since most published data are case reports, case series or very small cohorts from registries that were not designed to evaluate pregnancy outcomes. The prevalence of SB with valproate exposure is approximately 1–2% (Lindhout and Schmidt, 1986) and with carbamazepine 0.5% (Rosa, 1991; Hiilesmaa, 1992). A recent prospective study in the Netherlands, however, found IME exposed to valproate had a 5.4% prevalence rate of SB. Average daily valproate doses were higher in the IME with SB (1640 $\pm$ 136 mg/day) than in the unaffected IME (941 $\pm$ 48 mg/day). Another group of investigators has found that valproate doses of 1000 mg/day or plasma concentrations of $<$70 μg/ml are unlikely to cause malformations (Kaneko *et al.*, 1999). Both groups recommend that valproate dose be reduced whenever valproate must be used in pregnancy (Omtzigt *et al.*, 1992; Kaneko *et al.*, 1999). It has also been suggested that multiple daily doses or the use of extended release formulations may reduce the peak plasma concentrations and thus reduce the risk of malformations.

NTDs are uncommon malformations occurring in 6/10 000 pregnancies. Spina bifida and anencephaly are the most commonly reported NTD and affect approximately 4000 pregnancies annually resulting in 2500–3000 births in the US each year (Mullinare and Erickson, 1997; Honein *et al.*, 2001). The types of NTD associated with AED exposure are primarily myelomeningocele and anencephaly, which are the result of abnormal neural tube closure between the third and fourth weeks of gestational age.

Previous thinking about NTD visualized the fusion of the neural tube as one in which the lateral edges met in the middle and fused both rostrally and caudally similar to a bi-directional zipper. Recent studies have suggested there are multiple sites for neural tube closure (Van Allen *et al.*, 1993; Golden and Chenroff, 1995) and that different etiologies may result in different types of abnormality.

There are differences in specific sites and timing of each individual closure region. The majority of human NTD can be explained by failure of one or more closure sites. Anencephaly with frontal and parietal defects is due to failure at closure site two. Holocrania which also involves defects of the posterior cranium to the foramen magnum is due to failure of closure of areas two and four. Lumbar spina bifida results from failure of closure one. The development of closure sites appears to be under genetic control and also affected by environmental factors. In twins, concordance rates are only 56% for anencephaly and 71% for spina bifida. In Great Britain there is a male preponderance of lumbar spina bifida and female preponderance of holocrania and anencephaly. Even VPA appears to have species differential effects being associated with spina bifida in humans and exencephaly in mice (Seller, 1995).

A number of risk factors are associated with NTDs. A previous pregnancy with NTD is the strongest association, with a RR of 10. There are strong ethnic or geographic associations with NTDs. Rates per 1000 are 0.22 for Whites, 0.58 for persons of Hispanic descent and 0.08 for persons of African descent. The incidence of NTDs in Mexico is 3.26/1000, for Mexican-born persons living in California 1.6/1000 and for US-born persons of Mexican descent 0.68/1000 (Harris and Shaw, 1995). Diabetic mothers have 7.9 times the rates of NTDs in their offspring (Becerra *et al.*, 1990). Deficiencies of GSH, folate, vitamin C, riboflavin, zinc, cyancobalamin, selenium and excessive exposure to vitamin A have been associated with NTD. Higher rates are seen in children of farmers, cleaning women and nurses (Matte *et al.*, 1993; Blatter *et al.*, 1996). Pre-pregnancy weight has also been demonstrated to be a factor. Werler and colleagues (1996) compared RR for NTD in control women weighing 50–59 kg and found the RR increased to 1.9 in women weighing 80–89 kg and 4.0 for those weighing over 110 kg. AEDs may be a necessary but not sufficient risk factor for the development of NTDs.

Folate deficiency as a potential mechanism of AED teratogenicity

Folate is a coenzyme necessary for the development of white and red blood cells, and proper function of the central nervous system. Normal concentrations are typically measured in the serum (plasma folate = 6–20 ng/ml) and erythrocytes (red blood cell folate, RBCF = 160–640 ng/ml). Low levels of folate are associated with hyperhomocysteinemia and concentrations required to prevent this are 6.6 ng/ml for SF and 140 ng/ml for RBCF.

Deficiencies of folate have been implicated in the development of birth defects. Dansky *et al.* (1987) found significantly lower blood folate concentrations in women with epilepsy with abnormal pregnancy outcomes. Co-treatment of mice with folic acid, with or without vitamins and amino acids, reduced malformation rates, and increased fetal weight and length in mice pups exposed to phenytoin in utero (Zhu and Zhou, 1989). Biale and Lewenthal (1984) reported a 15% malformation rate in IMEs with no folate supplementation, whereas none of 33 folate-supplemented children had congenital abnormalities. Eight trials have demonstrated that preconceptual folate reduces the risk of recurrence of neural tube defects in women with a previous affected pregnancy (Table 16.2).

Table 16.2 Pre-conceptual folate, after Lewis *et al.* (in press)

Authors	Study type	N	Dose of folate	Results
Smithells *et al.*, 1983	Non-randomized, controlled	Fully supplemented = 454 Partially supplemented = 519 Unsupplemented = 114	0.36 mg	86% risk reduction
Seller and Nevin, 1984	Non-randomized	Unsupplemented = 543 Supplemented = 421	0.36 mg	Risk reduction
Mulinare *et al.*, 1988	Case–control	Case = 181 Control = 1480	Multivitamins with folate	60% risk reduction
Milinsky *et al.*, 1989	Cohort	23 491	Multivitamins with folate	71% risk reduction
MRC, 1991	Randomized, double blind, controlled	1195	4.0 mg	72% risk reduction
Czeizel and Dudas, 1992	Randomized, controlled	Case = 2420 Control = 2333	0.8 mg	No defects with folate supplementation
Werler *et al.*, 1993	Case–control	Case = 436 Control = 2615	?	60% risk reduction
Werler *et al.*, 1996	Case–control	Case = 604 Control = 1658	Folate supplements	Folate did not decrease rates in women >70 kg

Unfortunately pre-conceptual folate supplementation may not be protective for women with epilepsy. Craig and colleagues (1999) reported a young woman whose seizures were controlled for 4 years by 2000 mg of VPA a day. Though she took 4.0 mg of folic acid a day for 18 months prior to her pregnancy she delivered a child with a lumbosacral NTD, a ventricular and atrial septal defect, cleft palate and bilateral talipes. Two Canadian women delivered children with NTD despite folate supplementation. One taking 3.5 mg folic acid for 3 months prior to conception and 1250 mg of VPA aborted a child with lumbosacral spina bifida, Arnold Chiari malformation and hydrocephalus. A second woman who took 5.0 mg of folic acid had one spontaneous abortion of a fetus with an encephalocele and two therapeutic abortions of fetuses with lumbosacral spina bifida (Duncan *et al.*, 2001). These cases might have been predicted given the demonstrated failure of folate to reduce

NTD and embryotoxicity in vitro and in vivo in rodent models (Hansen and Grafton, 1991; Hansen *et al.*, 1995). In fact not all research supports the association with folate deficiency and malformations. Mills *et al.* (1992) found no difference between serum folate levels in mothers of children with NTD and controls. A number of other studies also failed to demonstrate a protective effect of pre-conceptual folate (Laurence *et al.*, 1981; Winship *et al.*, 1984; Vergel *et al.*, 1990; Bower and Stanley, 1992; Kirke *et al.*, 1992; Friel *et al.*, 1995). These studies are problematic due to small sample sizes, failure to document folate supplementation and recall bias in the retrospective investigation.

There is evidence to suggest that women with similar folate intake may have difference serum concentrations due to differences in folate metabolism. Absorption does not account for the difference in plasma concentration between cases and controls (Davis *et al.*, 1995).

New AED in pregnancy

A number of new AEDs have been marketed since 1993. Gabapentin, felbamate, lamotrigine, levetiracetam, oxcarbazepine, tiagabine, topiramate and zonisamide are all now available in the US. The numbers of reported exposed pregnancies with these drugs is very low, and unfortunately not large enough for one to determine if there is an increased risk of adverse outcome with fetal exposure to these compounds. We know that lamotrigine and levetiracetam concentrations decline during pregnancy and expect that this is also true for the other new AEDs (Tomson *et al.*, 1997). This is what we know to date.

Gabapentin

Despite its extensive use for a variety of conditions little has been published about its effect on pregnancy outcomes. A large post-marketing surveillance study of 3100 English patients taking this drug identified 11 pregnancies and no malformations (Wilton and Shakir, 2002). Dr. Georgia Montouris (2002) has collected 51 pregnancies from 39 women with epilepsy. The malformation rate was 4.5%. Eighty-seven percent of the pregnancies were live births, there were 11.3% miscarriages and 2% therapeutic abortions.

Lamotrigine

The International Lamotrigine Pregnancy Registry has identified 334 pregnancies reported in women taking lamotrigine in the first trimester. One hundred and sixty eight of these were with monotherapy, 166 with polytherapy. There is a significant difference in malformation rates when lamotrigine is used in monotherapy (1.8%), polytherapy with VPA (10%) and polytherapy without VPA (4.3%) (Tennis and Eldridge, 2002).

Lamotrigine clearance increases early in pregnancy and continues to accelerate through all three trimesters in most women taking this medication. In at least one case report the apparent clearance increased by <700% (Pennell *et al.*, 2002).

Lamotrigine crosses the placenta and at delivery fetus and mother have similar plasma concentrations. Elimination in infants appears to be rather slow. Seventy-two hours postpartum infant plasma levels are 75% that of the mother. Median milk/plasma (M/P) ratios are 0.61 (Ohman *et al.*, 2000).

Oxcarbazepine

In the first 12 reported cases of pregnancy with oxcarbazepine there have been nine live births and three spontaneous abortions (Friis *et al.*, 1993). In a prospective study of 11 pregnancies one child with spina bifida exposed to oxcarbazepine in polytherapy was reported. The manufacturer has been notified of five cases of fetal malformations in the post-marketing period. One was a cardiac defect and there were three cleft palates and one facial dysmorphism. Three of the five were exposed to AED polytherapy. The drug has been available in Europe for 10 years, but an accurate denominator is not available thus we are unable to calculate rates. In a recent prospective report of 42 pregnant women taking oxcarbazepine, 25 on monotherapy and 17 on polytherapy, no malformations were seen in the monotherapy group. A child with a ventricular septal defect was exposed to oxcarbazepine and phenobarbital (Rabinowicz *et al.*, 2002). Oxcarbazepine crosses the placenta with equivalent maternal and fetal cord levels (Myllynen *et al.*, 2001).

Topiramate

We have little information of the number of pregnancies with topiramate exposure. In the clinical trials there were 28 reported pregnancies with one malformation and two children with anomalies. All of these were polytherapy cases. Post-marketing surveillance has collected 139 reports of pregnancy. These included 87 live births, 23 therapeutic abortions, 29 cases lost to follow-up and five cases of hypospadias. Topiramate crosses the placenta with cord and maternal plasma levels being equivalent at delivery. M/P concentration ratios average 0.86. Infant elimination appears to be substantial with little measurable drug found in plasma of breast fed infants 2–3 weeks postpartum (Ohman *et al.*, 2002).

Zonisamide

There have been 26 reported pregnancies with zonisamide exposure. Two of the 26 (7.7%) had congenital malformations. One child was also exposed to phenytoin and the other to both phenytoin and VPA (Kondo *et al.*, 1996).

Zonisamide also freely crosses the placenta with transfer rates of 92%. Though data is available from only two children M/P ratios are 0.8 and elimination half-life ranges from 61 to 102 h (Kawada *et al.*, 2002).

Syndromes of anomalies

In distinction to malformations, which are deformities of anatomy requiring medical or surgical intervention to maintain a functionally healthy person, anomalies are abnormalities of structure, which, while varying from the norm, do not constitute a threat to health. Patterns of anomalies in IMEs have been noted with certain AED exposure. Five clinical syndromes have been reported in IMEs: fetal trimethadione syndrome, FHS, a primidone embryopathy, a fetal valproate syndrome and a fetal carbamazepine syndrome.

Fetal trimethadione syndrome

In 1970, German and colleagues described a case of a WWE treated with trimethadione who had had four unsuccessful pregnancies. After trimethadione was discontinued, she went on to have two healthy children. Her physician then surveyed trimethadione-exposed infants delivered at New York Hospital between 1946 and 1968. The records of 278 women with epilepsy were reviewed and, of these, 14 had taken trimethadione during pregnancy. Only 2 of these 14 children were normal. One had multiple hernias and diabetes; 8 had developmental defects; 3 were spontaneously aborted and only 3 of the 14 actually survived infancy.

The peculiar facial characteristics of these children were delineated by Zackai *et al.* (1975), who noted that not only were these children short in stature and suffering from microcephaly, they had V-shaped eyebrows epicanthal folds, low set ears, anteriorly folded helices, and irregular teeth. Other abnormalities were often frequent: inguinal hernias, hypospadias and simian creases. Feldman *et al.* (1977) reviewed 53 pregnancies in which trimethadione was used. In 46 of these (87%), there was fetal loss or the development of a congenital malformation. Follow-up studies of the surviving children have reported significant rates of mental retardation (Goldman *et al.*, 1986).

FHS

The most famous and controversial of the dysmorphic syndromes associated with AEDs is the FHS. It was first reported by Loughnan *et al.* (1973), who described seven infants exposed to hydantoin in combination with a barbiturate, in utero. The children displayed hypoplasia and irregular ossification of the distal phalanges. In 1974, Barr and co-workers reported distal digital hypoplasia (DDH) in eight children exposed to phenytoin and phenobarbital. The syndrome was given its name by Hanson and Smith (1975), who reported five IMEs who had been exposed to hydantoin in utero. The infants had multiple systemic abnormalities of the face, cranium, and nails, DDH, intrauterine growth retardation, and mental deficiencies. Only one of the five was exposed to phenytoin monotherapy. Of the others, three were exposed to phenobarbital, one to mephobarbital and one to a combination of phenobarbital, phensuximide and mephenytoin. Despite the multiplicity of exposures, the authors noted the resemblance to the fetal alcohol syndrome and described their cases as suffering from FHS.

Subsequent work by Hanson's group found that approximately 11% of infants exposed to hydantoin in utero demonstrated the complete syndrome, and an additional 30% would have some anomalous components (Hanson *et al.*, 1976). Many of the features of the syndrome appear to be subjective, but some investigators believe that DDH is a unique and relatively constant feature (Kelly *et al.*, 1984b).

The prevalence and significance of the dysmorphic features of FHS remain unclear. Researchers at the University of Virginia followed 98 women with epilepsy who took phenytoin during pregnancy and found that 30% of their offspring had DDH with no other features of FHS (Kelly *et al.*, 1984b). Gaily *et al.* (1988a) reported a prospective study of 121 IMEs at the University of Helsinki, 82 of whom were exposed to phenytoin. None of the children had FHS. Hypertelorism and DDH were the only dysmorphic features associated with phenytoin exposure. In our own experience following 64 IMEs, no children with FHS were seen. Dysmorphic features could be seen with any drug exposure (Yerby *et al.*, 1992).

Hanson (1986) feels that there are three components to the syndrome:

1 abnormal growth,
2 abnormal performance,
3 dysmorphic cranial facial features.

An unexpected sequela of the syndrome may be an increased risk of cancer. Four cases of neuroblastoma associated with the FHS have been described since 1976, although all children were also exposed in utero to primidone or phenobarbital. There have also been reports of carcinoma, ganglioneuroblastoma, Wilms' tumor, a melanotic neuroectodermal tumor and a malignant mesenchymona in children with FHS (Ehrenband and Chaganti, 1981).

The contention that FHS results in abnormal performance or mental deficiency is not supported by subsequent research. Of 103 IMEs exposed to phenytoin, only 1.4% displayed mental deficiency on the Wechsler Preschool and Primary Scale of Intelligence or Leiter International Performance Scale, not significantly different from the general population (Gaily *et al.*, 1988b).

Gaily's work suggests that there is a genetic component that permits expression of the FHS. Children of mothers with epilepsy who are not exposed to AEDs in utero have frequencies of dysmorphic abnormalities intermediate to those children exposed to AEDs and controls. Dizygotic twins exposed to hydantoins in utero have been shown to display discordant dysmorphism (Phelan *et al.*, 1982; Buchler, 1985). If the first child in a family has FHS, the chance of a second such child is 90%, compared to the 2% chance of having a second child with FHS if the first is normal (Van Dyke *et al.*, 1988). Such observations suggest that hydantoin exposure may be a necessary but not sufficient cause of infant dysmorphism.

Krauss and co-workers (1984) described four siblings with features of FHS. The first two were exposed to both phenytoin and primidone in utero. In an attempt to prevent further fetal injury, Krauss discontinued the phenytoin and the patient was treated with primidone monotherapy. Two subsequent pregnancies resulted in children with similar dysmorphic features to their elder siblings.

Primidone embryopathy

Five years before Krauss' report, Rudd and Freedom (1979) had described craniofacial abnormalities in children exposed to primidone in utero. These children had hirsute foreheads, thick nasal roots, antiverted nostrils, long philtrum, straight thin upper lips and hypoplastic nails. These children were also likely to be small for their gestational age and have psychomotor retardation and heart defects (Gustavson and Chen, 1985).

Fetal valproate syndrome

Reports of dysmorphic children exposed to valproate in utero had previously been made by other investigators (Dalens *et al.*, 1980; Clay *et al.*, 1981), but it was DiLiberti *et al.* (1984) who described a specific fetal valproate syndrome. They reported seven infants exposed to VPA in utero who had facial abnormalities characterized by interiorepicanthal folds, a net nasal bridge, an upturned nose, a long upper lip, a thin vermillion border, a shallow philtrum and downturned mouth. These children also had abnormalities of their distal digits, and they tended to have long thin overlapping fingers, toes and hyperconvex nails. Subsequent reports of valproate-exposed infants having radial ray aplasia have also been made.

The prevalence of this syndrome has not yet been established. Jaeger-Roman *et al.* (1986) described it in 5 of 14 children exposed to valproate monotherapy. In this same group, 43% of the children were distressed at labor, and 28% had low Apgar scores and other major malformations. High doses of valproate were associated with drug withdrawal, hypotonia, and motor and language delay. In a review of 344 women who took valproate during the first trimester of pregnancy, Jeavons (1984) described a 19.8% rate of abnormal deliveries, but no evidence of a dose–response effect with valproate exposure.

Felding and Rane (1984) described an infant with severe congenital liver disease after in utero exposure to VPA and phenytoin. Ardinger and co-workers (1988) reported craniofacial dysmorphism in 19 children exposed to valproate in utero and confirmed the features described by DiLiberti. They also found a large proportion of these infants had postnatal growth deficiency and microcephaly, particularly if the children were exposed to polytherapy. The association of valproate with spina bifida is discussed further on.

Benzodiazepine syndrome

Infants exposed to benzodiazepines in utero are at greater risk for intrauterine growth retardation, dysmorphic features and neurological dysfunction. Seven of 37 infants exposed to benzodiazepine drugs in utero were described as hypotonic and hyperexcitable, with dystonic postures and choreoathetotic movements (Laegreid *et al.*, 1987). Delayed hand–eye coordination, psychomotor slowing and a learning disability were also noted. Four infants had major malformations and dysmorphic faces with wide-set eyes, epicanthal folds, upturned noses, dysplastic oracles, high-arched palates, webbed necks and wide-spaced nipples (Laegreid *et al.*, 1987). In a survey of 278 women whose infants had congenital malformations, children with a history of diazepam exposure in the first trimester had a four-fold increase in cleft lip and/or palate (Safra and Oakley, 1975).

Carbamazepine syndrome

The most recently described syndrome of anomalies associated with AED exposure is the carbamazepine syndrome. One group of investigators has described cranio-facial defects (upslanting palpebral fissures, epicanthal folds, short nose, long philtrum), hypoplastic nails, and microcephaly, in 37 IMEs exposed to carbamazepine monotherapy (Jones *et al.*, 1989). The authors used the Bayley Scale of Infant Development, the Stanford-Binet IV, and the Wechsler Scale of Preschool and Primary Intelligence in their evaluations and found a 20% rate of developmental delay in 25 children of mothers taking carbamazepine monotherapy. They used an unconventional one standard deviation from the mean to define delay, however.

A case of DDH in an IME exposed to carbamazepine monotherapy had been described earlier (Niesen and Froscher, 1985), but that child was otherwise normal.

Low birth weight has been reported with in utero exposure to carbamazepine monotherapy (Kallen, 1986b). A reduction in fetal head circumference has been noted in IMEs exposed to carbamazepine (Hiilesmaa *et al.*, 1981). While smaller than control children, the head sizes were still within the normal range. Subsequent studies on the same clinical population failed to find differences in head circumference as the children matured (Granstrom, 1987).

Newer AED and anomalies

There have been case reports of anomalies associated with exposure to the newer (introduced after 1993), AEDs, but no drug-specific syndrome of anomalies described. Three children exposed to lamotrigine and VPA have been reported to have dysmorphic facial features of broad nasal bridge, low set ears and hyper-telorism. One child was karyotyped as 47, XXX and another simply had epicanthal folds (GlaxoSmithKline, 2002).

Clinical and laboratory evidence clearly supports the association of certain anticonvulsants with teratogenic effects, especially facial and distal digital anomalies. However, the existence of drug-specific syndromes is doubtful. Facial dysmorphism is difficult to quantify and clearly is not drug specific. Infants of epileptic mothers with similar dysmorphic features have been described in the pre-anticonvulsant era (Baptist, 1938; Philbert and Dam, 1982). Follow-up of these infants into adult life has yet to be accomplished, and therefore the significance of these anomalies is unclear. Gaily *et al.* (1988a) followed a cohort of IMEs to 5½ years of age. These children had more minor anomalies characteristic of FHS than control children but so did their mothers. Only hypertelorism and digital hypoplasia were associated with phenytoin exposure. Certain anomalies, particularly epicanthal folds, appeared to be associated with maternal epilepsy, not with AED exposure.

The hypothesized association of dysmorphic features with mental retardation (Kelly, 1984a) has not been confirmed (Hutch *et al.*, 1975; Granstrom, 1982). In the few cases that have been followed into early childhood, the dysmorphic features tend to disappear as the child grows older (Janz, 1982). Mental deficiency was found in only 1.4% of IMEs followed to 5½ years of age (Gaily *et al.*, 1988b). Exposure to AEDs below toxic concentrations or to maternal seizures did not increase the risk of lower intelligence. No association between features of FHS and mental retardation could be demonstrated.

The primary abnormalities in these syndromes involve the midface and distal digits. A retrospective study spanning 10 years of deliveries in Israel found hypertelorism to be the only anomaly seen more often in IME than in controls (Neri *et al.*, 1983). This was associated with all AEDs except primidone. A prospective study of 172 deliveries of IMEs evaluated eight specific AEDs and other potential confounding factors and found no dose-dependent increase in the incidence of malformations associated with any individual AED. Furthermore, no specific defect could be associated with individual AED exposure (Kaneko *et al.*, 1988). It has been suggested that, since a variety of similar anomalies of the midface and distal digits are seen in a small proportion of children exposed to anticonvulsants in utero, a better term for the entire group of abnormalities would be fetal anticonvulsant syndrome or AED embryopathy (Dieterich *et al.*, 1980; Vorhees, 1986; Huot *et al.*, 1987).

Neonatal complications associated with AED

A unique neonatal hemorrhagic phenomenon has been described in the IME. It differs from other hemorrhagic disorders in infancy in that the bleeding tends to occur internally during the first 24 h of life. It was initially associated with exposure to phenobarbital or primidone, but has subsequently also been described in children exposed to phenytoin, carbamazepine, diazepam, mephobarbital, amobarbital and ethosuximide (Van Creveld, 1957; Mountain *et al.*, 1970). One group of investigators suggests that vigabatrin may also increase the risk of neonatal hemorrhage (Howe *et al.*, 1999). Prevalence figures are as high as 30% but appear to average 10%. Mortality is high, over 30%, because bleeding occurs within internal cavities and is often not noticed until the child is in shock.

The hemorrhage is the result of a deficiency of vitamin K-dependent clotting factors II, VII, IX and X. Anticonvulsants can act like warfarin, and inhibit vitamin K transport across the placenta. This results in the increase in an abnormal pro-thrombin induced by vitamin K absence of factor II (PIVKA-II). Maternal coagulation parameters are invariably normal. The fetus, however, will demonstrate increased levels of PIVKA, diminished clotting factors, and prolonged prothrombin and partial thromboplastin times. PIVKA-II has been demonstrated in 54% of infants exposed to AEDs in utero compared to 20% of controls ($P = 0.01$), and maternal vitamin K concentrations are lower in WWE than those untreated though PIVKA is rarely detectable in mothers (Cornelissen *et al.*, 1993).

This phenomenon can be prevented by maternal ingestion of oral vitamin K in the last month of gestation (Deblay *et al.*, 1982; Crawford, 2002b). I use 10 mg/day of oral vitamin K. Routine intramuscular administration of vitamin K at birth is not adequate to prevent hemorrhage within the first 24 h of life.

The prevalence of AED-associated neonatal hemorrhage is unclear. One report states it is 1.6 times as common in IME as controls (Speidel and Meadow, 1972). A more recent prospective study followed 667 IME and 1334 controls and found neonatal bleeding in 5 of 667 (0.7%) IME and 5 of 1334 (0.4%) of controls. While more prevalent there was no statistical difference between the groups. The authors concluded that there was no increased risk for neonatal bleeding in the IME (Kaaja *et al.*, 2002). I would point out that the sample size for a low frequency outcome such as this may need to be larger and there was clearly a trend for more bleeding in the IME.

Developmental complications associated with AED

Developmental delay

IME have been reported to have higher rates of mental retardation than controls. This risk is increased by a factor of two- to seven-fold according to various authors (Speidel and Meadow, 1972; Hill *et al.*, 1974). None of these studies controlled for parental intelligence, although differences in IQ scores at age 7 between groups of children exposed (full-scale IQ, FSIQ = 91.7) or not exposed (FSIQ = 96.8) to phenytoin reached statistical significance, the clinical significance of such difference is unknown (Hill and Tennyson, 1982).

We have found that IME display lower scores in measures of verbal acquisition at both 2 and 3 years of age. Though there was no difference in physical growth parameters between IME and controls, IME scored significantly lower in the Bailey Scale of Infant Development's mental developmental index (MDI) at 2 and 3 years. They also performed significantly less well on the Bates Bretherton early language inventory ($P \le 0.02$) and in the Peabody Picture Vocabulary's scales of verbal reasoning ($P \le 0.001$) and composite IQ ($P \le 0.01$), and they displayed significantly shorter mean lengths of utterance ($P \le 0.001$) (Leavitt *et al.*, 1992).

Polytherapy-exposed infants performed significantly less well on neuropsychometric testing than those exposed to monotherapy. Socioeconomic status had the strongest association with poor test scores, but maternal seizures during pregnancy was also a significant risk factor (Losche *et al.*, 1994).

Leonard *et al.* (1997) has in part addressed the question of whether maternal seizures or in utero exposure to AEDs are responsible for the developmental delay seen. A group of children of mothers with epilepsy followed to school age were found to have a rate of intellectual deficiency of 8.6%. The Wechsler Intelligence Scale for Children revealed significantly lower scores for children exposed to seizures during gestation (100.3), than for children whose mother's seizures were controlled (104.1) or controls (112.9). All AEDs are clearly not created equal and Koch and co-workers (1999) have demonstrated that primidone, particularly when used in polytherapy, is associated with lower Wechsler score of intelligence.

Conclusion

The potential interactions of AEDs in pregnant women with epilepsy can be characterized by those effecting the mother, and those effecting the fetus. While pregnancy, maternal seizures and AEDs pose risks for successful pregnancy outcome, the majority of patients can and do have healthy children. Physicians cannot eliminate risk, but can reduce it. Pre-conceptual folic acid is an approved intervention but may not prevent all malformations. Though there are no head to head studies of the safety of AEDs in pregnancy some principles have been clearly established. Monotherapy is safer than polytherapy. Phenobarbital is no safer than, and probably more hazardous than, other AEDs in monotherapy. VPA has in addition to the underlying increased risk for malformations an additional risk for development of NTDs. The newer AEDs have theoretical advantages over older ones in terms of malformations but the sample sizes collected to date are not adequate to determine relative safety. Malformations are not the only adverse outcome that one should be concerned about. Developmental delay is, in terms of magnitude, as significant as birth defects. There is no drug-specific syndrome of anomalies but a tendency for all AEDs to cause facial dysmorphism, which is a relatively transient condition.

Given the nature of the data available to date clinical judgement in determining the most effective AED for the seizure type and using the lowest effective dose is still the best approach.

REFERENCES

Abrishamchian AR, Khoury MJ, Calle EE. The contribution of maternal epilepsy and its treatment to the etiology of oral clefts: a population based case–control study. *Genet Epidemiol* 1994; 11(4): 343–351.

Anderson RC. Cardiac defects in children of mothers receiving anticonvulsant therapy during pregnancy. *J Pediatr* 1976; 89: 318–319.

Annegers JF, Hauser WA, Elveback LR, *et al.* Congenital malformations and seizure disorders in the offspring of parents with epilepsy. *Int J Epidemiol* 1978; 7: 241–247.

Ardinger HH, Atkin JF, Blackston RD, *et al.* Verification of the fetal valproate syndrome phenotype. *Am J Med Genet* 1988; 29: 171–185.

Asuncion M, Calvo RM, San Millan JL, *et al.* A prospective study of the prevalence of the polycystic ovary syndrome in unselected Caucasian women from Spain. *J Clin Endocrinol Metab* 2000; 85: 2434–2438.

Barr M, Pozanski AK, Schmickel RD. Digital hypoplasia and anticonvulsant during gestation: a teratogenic syndrome? *J Pediatr* 1974; 84: 254–256.

Becerra JE, Khoury MJ, Cordero JF, *et al.* Diabetes mellitus during pregnancy and the risks for specific birth defects: a population based case control study. *Pediatrics* 1990; 85: 1–9.

Biale Y, Lewenthal H. Effect of folic acid supplementation on congenital malformations due to anticonvulsant drugs. *Eur J Obstet Gynecol Reprod Biol* 1984; 18: 211–216.

Bilo L, Meo R, Valentino R, *et al.* Characterization of reproductive endocrine disorders in women with epilepsy. *J Clin Endocrinol Metab* 2001; 86: 2950–2956.

Blatter BM, Roeleveld N, Zielhuis GA, *et al.* Spina bifida and prenatal occupation. *Epidemiology* 1996; 7: 188–193.

Borgfeldt C, Andolf E. Transvaginal sonographic ovarian findings in a random sample of women 25–40 years old. *Ultrasound Obstet Gynecol* 1999; 13(5): 345–350.

Bower C, Stanley FJ. Periconceptual vitamin supplementation and neural tube defects: evidence from a case control study in Western Australia and a review of recent publications. *J Epidemiol Commun Health* 1992; 46: 157–161.

Buchler BA. Epoxide hydrolase activity and the fetal hydantoin syndrome. *Clin Res* 1985; 33: A129.

Cahill, WT, Kovilam OP, Pastor D, *et al.* Neurologic and fetal outcomes of pregnancies of mothers with epilepsy. *Epilepsia* 2002; 43(Suppl. 7): 289.

Chang T, Savory A, Glazko AJ. A new metabolite of 5,5-diphenylhydantoin (Dilantin). *Biochem Biophys Res Commun* 1970; 38: 444–449.

Chappell KA, Markowitz JS, Jackson CW. Is valproate pharmacotherapy associated with polycystic ovaries? *Ann Pharmacother* 1999; 33: 1211–1216.

Clay SA, McVie R, Chen HC. Possible teratogenic effect of valproic acid. *J Pediatr* 1981; **98**: 828.

Collaborative Drug Use in Pregnancy: an international survey on drug use in pregnancy. *Int J Risk Safety Med* 1991; **1**: 1.

Cornelissen M, Steegers-Theunissen R, Kollee L, *et al.* Increased incidence of neonatal vitamin K deficiency resulting from maternal anticonvulsant therapy. *Am J Obstet Gynecol* 1993; **168** (3 Pt 1): 923–928.

Craig J, Morrison P, Morrow J, *et al.* Failure of preconceptual folic acid to prevent a neural tube defect in the offspring of a mother taking sodium valproate. *Seizure* 1999; **8**: 253–254.

Crawford P. Epilepsy and pregnancy. *Seizure* 2002a; **11**(Suppl. A): 212–219.

Crawford P. Interactions between antiepileptic drugs and hormonal contraception. *CNS Drug* 2002b; **16**(4): 263–272.

Czeizel AE, Dudas I. Prevention of the first occurrence of neural tube defects by preconceptional vitamin supplementation. *New Engl J Med* 1992; **327**: 1832–1835.

Dalens B, Raynaud EJ, Gaulme J. Teratogenicity of valproic acid. *J Pediatr* 1980; **97**: 332–333.

Dam M, Christiansen J, Munck O, *et al.* Antiepileptic drugs: Metabolism in pregnancy. *Clinical Pharmacokinetics* 1979; **4**: 53–62.

Dansky LV, Andermann E, Sherwin AL, *et al.* Maternal epilepsy and congenital malformations: a prospective study with monitoring of plasma anticonvulsant levels during pregnancy. *Neurology* 1980; **3**: 15.

Dansky LV, Andermann E, Andermann F, *et al.* Maternal epilepsy and congenital malformations: Correlation with maternal plasma anticonvulsants levels during pregnancy. In Janz D, Dam M, Richens A, Bossi L, Helge H, Schmidt D, eds. *Epilepsy, Pregnancy and the Child.* New York: Raven Press, 1982: 251–258.

Dansky LV, Strickler SM, Andermann E, *et al.* Pharmacogenetic susceptibility to phenytoin teratogenesis. In *The XIth Epilepsy International Symposium. Advances in Epileptology*, vol. 16. P. Wolf, M. Dam, D. Janz, F. E. Dreifuss, eds. New York: Raven Press, 1987: 555–559.

Davis BA, Bailey LB, Gregory JF, *et al.* Folic acid absorption in women with a history of pregnancy with neural tube defect. *Am J Clin Nutr* 1995; **62**: 782–784.

Deblay MF, Vert P, Andre M, *et al.* Transplacental vitamin K prevents hemorrhagic disease of infants of epileptic mothers. *Lancet* 1982; **1**: 1247.

Dieterich E, Steveling A, Lukas A, *et al.* Congenital anomalies in children of epileptic mothers and fathers. *Neuropediatrics* 1980; **11**: 274–283.

DiLiberti JH, Farndon PA, Dennis NR, *et al.* The fetal valproate syndrome. *Am J Med Genet* 1984; **19**: 473–481.

Doose DR, Jacobs D, Squires L, *et al.* Oral contraceptive-AED interactions: no effect of topiramate as monotherapy at clinically effective dosages of 200 mg or less. *Epilepsia* 2002; **34**(Suppl. 7): 235.

Duncan S, Mercho S, Lopes-Cendes I, *et al.* Repeated neural tube defects and valproate monotherapy suggest a pharmacogenetic abnormality. *Epilepsia* 2001; **42**(6): 750–753.

Ehrenband LT, Chaganti RSK. Cancer in the fetal hydantoin syndrome. *Lancet* 1981; **1**: 97.

Elshove J, Van Eck JHM. Aangeboren misvorminge, met name gespleten lipmet zonder gespleten verhemelte, bij kinderen van moeders met epilepsie. *Nederland T Geneesk* 1971; **115**(33): 1371–1375.

Fedrick J. Epilepsy and pregnancy: a report from the Oxford record linkage study. *Br Med J* 1973; 2: 442–448.

Felding I, Rane A. Congenital liver damage after treatment of mother with valproic acid and phenytoin? *Acta Pediatr Scand* 1984; 73: 565–568.

Feldman GL, Weaver DD, Lovrien EW. The fetal trimethadione syndrome: report of an additional family and further delineation of this syndrome. *Am J Dis Child* 1977; 131(13): 89–92.

Finnell RH, DiLiberti JH. Hydantoin induced teratogenesis: are arene oxide intermediates really responsible? *Helv Paediatr Acta* 1983; 38: 171–177.

Freil JK, Frecker M, Fraser FC. Nutritional patterns of mothers of children with neural tube defects in Newfoundland. *Am J Med Genet* 1995; 55: 195–199.

Friis ML, Breng-Nielsen B, Sindrup EH, *et al.* Facial clefts among epileptic patients. *Arch Neurol* 1981; 38: 227–229.

Friis ML, Holm NV, Sindrup EH, *et al.* Facial clefts in sibs and children of epileptic patients. *Neurology* 1986; 38: 346–350.

Friis ML, Kristensen O, Boas J, *et al.* Therapeutic experiences with 947 epileptic out-patients in oxcarbazepine treatment. *Acta Neurol Scand* 1993; 87(3): 224–227.

Gaily E, Granstrom ML, Hiilesmaa V, *et al.* Minor anomalies in offspring of epileptic mothers. *J Pediatr* 1988a; 112: 520–529.

Gaily E, Sorsa EK, Granstrom ML. Intelligence of children of epileptic mothers. *J Pediatr* 1988b; 113: 677–684.

Gatoh N, Millo Y, Taube E, *et al.* Epilepsy among parents of children with cleft lip and palate. *Brain Dev* 1987; 9: 296–299.

Genton P, Bauer J, Duncan S, *et al.* On the association between valproate and polycystic ovary syndrome. *Epilepsia* 2001; 42: 295–304.

German J, Kowal A, Ellers KH. Trimethadione and human teratogenesis. *Teratology* 1970; 3: 349–362.

GlaxoSmithKline. *Lamotrigine Pregnancy Registry Interim Report 2002.*

Golden JA, Chenroff GF. Multiple sites of anterior neural tube closure in humans: evidence from anterior neural tube defects (anencephaly). *Pediatrics* 1995; 95: 506–510.

Goldman AS, Zachai EH, Yaffe SJ. Environmentally induced birth defect risks. In *Teratogen Update.* J. L. Sever, R. L. Brent, eds. New York: Liss, 1986: 35–38.

Govind A, Obhrai MS, Clayton RN. Polycystic ovaries are inherited as an autosomal dominant trait: analysis of 29 polycystic ovary syndrome and 10 control families. *J Clin Endocrinol Metab* 1999; 84(1): 38–43.

Graf WD, Pippenger CE, Shurtleff DB. Erythrocyte antioxidant enzyme activities in children with myelomeningocele. *Dev Med Child Neurol* 1995; 37: 900–905.

Granstrom ML. Development of the children of epileptic mothers, preliminary results from the prospective Helsinki study. In Janz D, Dam M, Richens A, Bossi L, Helge H, Schmidt D (eds) *Epilepsy Pregnancy and the Child.* New York: Raven Press, 1982: 403–408.

Granstrom ML. Early postnatal growth of the children of epileptic mothers. In *The XVIth Epilepsy International Symposium. Advances in Epileptology*, vol. 16. P. Wolf, M. Dam, D. Janz, F. E. Dreifuss, eds. New York: Raven Press, 1987: 573–577.

Gustavson EE, Chen H. Goldenhar syndrome, anterior encephalocele and aqueductal stenosis following fetal primidone exposure. *Teratology* 1985.

Hansen DK, Grafton TF. Lack of attenuation of valproic acid induced effects by folinic acid in rat embryos in vitro. *Teratology* 1991; **43**: 575–582.

Hansen DK, Grafton TF, Dial SL, *et al.* Effect of supplemental folic acid on valproic acid induced embryotoxicity and tissue zinc levels in vivo. *Teratology* 1995; **52**: 277–285.

Hanson JW. Teratogen update: fetal hydantoin effects. *Teratology* 1986; **33**: 349–553.

Hanson JW, Smith DW. The fetal hydantoin syndrome. *J Pediatr* 1975; **87**: 285–290.

Hanson JW, Myrianthopoulos NC, Sedgwich MA, *et al.* Risks to the offspring of women treated with hydantoin anticonvulsants with emphasis on the fetal hydantoin syndrome. *J Pediatr* 1976; **89**: 662–668.

Harris JA, Shaw GM. Neural tube defects – why are rates high among population of Mexican descent? *Environ Health Perspect* 1995; **103**(Suppl. 6): 163–164.

Hiilesmaa VK. Pregnancy and birth in WWE. *Neurology* 1992; **42**(Suppl. 5): 8–11.

Hiilesmaa VK, Teramo K, Granstrom ML, *et al.* Fetal head growth retardation associated with maternal antiepileptic drugs. *Lancet* 1981; **2**: 165–167.

Hill RM, Verniaud WM, Horning MG, *et al.* Infants exposed in utero to antiepileptic drugs. A prospective study. *Am J Dis Child.* 1974; **127**: 645–653.

Hill RM, Tennyson L. Premature delivery, gestational age, complications of delivery, vital data at birth on newborn infants of epileptic mothers: review of the literature. In *Epilepsy, Pregnancy and the Child.* D. Janz, L. Bossi, M. Dam, *et al.*, eds. New York: Raven Press, 1982: 167–173.

Hill D, Pond DA, Mitchell W, *et al.* Personality change following temporal lobectomy for epilepsy. *J Ment Sci* 1957; **103**: 18–27.

Holmes LB, Wyszynski DF, Lieberman E. The AED pregnancy registry. A six year experience. *Arch Neurol* 2004; **61**: 673–678.

Honein MA, Paulozzi LJ, Mathews TJ, *et al.* Impact of folic acid fortification of the US food supply on the occurrence of neural tube defects. *J Am Med Assoc* 2001; **285**(23): 2981–2986.

Horning MG, Stratton C, Wilson A, *et al.* Detection of 5-(3-4)-diphenylhydantoin in the newborn human. *Anal Lett* 1974; **4**: 537–582.

Howe AM, Oakes DJ, Woodman PD, *et al.* Prothrombin and PIVKA-II levels in cord blood from newborn exposed to anticonvulsants during pregnancy. *Epilepsia* 1999; **40**(7): 980–984.

Huot C, Gauthier M, Lebel M, *et al.* Congenital malformations associated with maternal use of valproic acid. *Can J Neurol Sci* 1987; **14**: 290–293.

Isojarvi JI, Laatikainen TJ, Pakarinen AJ, *et al.* Polycystic ovaries and hyperandrogenism in women taking valproate for epilepsy. *New Engl J Med* 1993; **329**(19): 1383–1388.

Jaeger-Roman E, Deichl A, Jakob S, *et al.* Fetal growth, major malformations, and minor anomalies in infants born to women receiving valproic acid. *J Pediatr* 1986; **108**: 997–1004.

Janz D. Antiepileptic drugs and pregnancy: altered utilization patterns and teratogenesis. *Epilepsia* 1982; **23**(Suppl. 1): 853–863.

Jeavons PM. Non dose related side effects of valproate. *Epilepsia* 1984; **25**(Suppl. 1): 550–555.

Jerina DM, Daly JW. Arene oxides: a new aspect of drug metabolism. *Science* 1974; **185**: 573.

Jick SS, Terris BZ. Anticonvulsants and congenital malformations. *Pharmacotherapy* 1997; **17**(3): 561–564.

Jones KL, Lacro RV, Johnson KA, *et al.* Pattern of malformations in the children of women treated with carbamazepine during pregnancy. *New Engl J Med* 1989; **320**: 1661–1666.

Kaaja E, Kaaja R, Matila R, *et al.* Enzyme-inducing antiepileptic drugs in pregnancy and the risk of bleeding in the neonate. *Neurology* 2002; **58**(4): 549–553.

Kallen B. A register study of maternal epilepsy and delivery outcome with special reference to drug use. *Acta Neurol Scand* 1986a; **73**(3): 253–259.

Kallen B. Maternal epilepsy, antiepileptic drugs and birth defects. *Pathologia* 1986b; **78**: 757–768.

Kaneko S, Otani K, Fukushima Y, *et al.* Teratogenicity of antiepileptic drugs: analysis of possible risk factors. *Epilepsia* 1988; **29**: 459–467.

Kaneko S, Battino D, Andermann E, *et al.* Congenital malformations due to antiepileptic drugs. *Epilepsy Res* 1999; **33**(2–3): 145–158.

Kahsar-Miller MD, Nixon C, Boots LR, *et al.* Prevalence of polycystic ovary syndrome (PCOS) in first-degree relatives of patients with PCOS. *Fertil Steril* 2001; **75**(1): 53–58.

Kawada K, Itoh S, Kusaka T, *et al.* Pharmacokinetics of zonisamide in perinatal period. *Brain Dev* 2002; **24**: 95–97.

Kelly TE. Teratogenicity of anticonvulsant drugs I. Review of literature. *Am J Med Genet* 1984a; **19**: 413–434.

Kelly TE, Edwards P, Rein M, *et al.* Teratogenicity of anticonvulsant drugs II. A prospective study. *Am J Med Genet* 1984b; **19**: 435–443.

Kirke PN, Daly LE, Elwood JH. A randomized trial of low dose folic acid to prevent neural tube defects. *Arch Dis Child* 1992; **67**: 1442–1446.

Koch S, Titze K, Zimmermann RB, *et al.* Long-term neuropsychological consequences of maternal epilepsy and anticonvulsant treatment during pregnancy for school age children and adolescents. *Epilepsia* 1999; **40**: 1237–1243.

Kondo T, Kaneko S, Amano Y, *et al.* Preliminary report on teratogenic effects of zonisamide in the offspring of treated women with epilepsy. *Epilepsia* 1996; **37**(12): 1242–1244.

Krauss CM, Holmes LB, Van Lang QC, *et al.* Four siblings with similar malformations after exposure to phenytoin and primidone. *J Pediatr* 1984; **105**: 750–755.

Krishnamurthy KB, Sundstrom DT, Beaudoin JM, *et al.* Pregnant women with epilepsy taking older anticonvulsant medications must have drug levels checked frequently to avoid seizures. *Epilepsia* 2002; **43**(Suppl. 7): 232–233.

Kubow S, Wells PG. In vitro bioactivation of phenytoin to a reactive free radical intermediate by prostaglandin synthetase, horseradish peroxidase, and thyroid peroxidase. *Mol Pharmacol* 1989; **35**: 504–511.

Laegreid L, Olegard R, Wahlstrom J, *et al.* Abnormalities in children exposed to benzodiazepines in utero. *Lancet* 1987; **1**: 108–109.

Laurence KM, James J, Miller MH, *et al.* Double blind randomized controlled trial of folate treatment before conception to prevent recurrence of neural tube defects. *Br Med J* 1981; **282**: 1509–1511.

Leavitt AM, Yerby MS, Robinson N, *et al.* Epilepsy and pregnancy: developmental outcomes at 12 months. *Neurology* 1992; **42**(Suppl. 5): 141–143.

Leonard G, Andermann E, Pitno A, *et al.* Cognitive effects of antiepileptic drug therapy during pregnancy on school age offspring. *Epilepsia* 1997; **38**(Suppl. 3): 170.

Levy RH, Yerby MS. Effect of pregnancy on antiepileptic drug utilization. *Epilepsia* 1985; **26**(Suppl. 1): 525–557.

Lindhout D, Schmidt D. In utero exposure to valproate and neural tube defects. *Lancet* 1986; **1**: 1392–1393.

Lindhout D, Hoeppener RJEA, Meinardi H. Teratogenicity of antiepileptic drug combinations with special emphasis on epoxidation (of carbamazepine). *Epilepsia* 1984; **25**: 77–83.

Lindhout D, Omtzigt JG, Cornel MC. Spectrum of neural tube defects in 34 infants prenatally exposed to antiepileptic drugs. *Neurology* 1992; **42**(4 Suppl. 5): 111–118.

Little BB, Santos-Ramos R, Newell JF, *et al.* Megadose carbamazepine during the period of neural tube closure. *Obstet Gynecol* 1993; **82**(4 Pt 2 Suppl.): 705–708.

Losche G, Steinhausen H-C, Koch S, *et al.* The psychological development of children of epileptic parents. II. The differential impact of intrauterine exposure to anticonvulsant drugs and further influential factors. *Acta Paediatr* 1994; **83**(9): 961–966.

Loughnan PM, Gold H, Vance JC. Phenytoin teratogenicity in man. *Lancet* 1973; **1**: 70–72.

Lowe CR. Congenital malformations among infants born to epileptic women. *Lancet* 1973; **1**: 9–10.

Majewski F, Raft W, Fischer P, *et al.* Zur tertogenitat von anticonvulsiva. *Deut Med Wochenschr* 1980; **105**: 719–723.

Martz F, Failinger C, Blake D. Phenytoin teratogenesis: correlation between embryopathic effect and covalent binding of putative arene oxide metabolite in gestational tissue. *J Pharmacol Exp Ther* 1977; **203**: 231–239.

Matte TD, Mulinare J, Erickson JD. Case–control study of congenital defects and parental employment in health care. *Am J Ind Med* 1993; **24**: 11–23.

Mattson RH, Cramer JA, Darney PD, *et al.* The use of oral contraceptives by women with epilepsy. *J Am Med Assoc* 1986; **256**(2): 238–240.

Milinsky A, Jick H, Jick SS, *et al.* Multivitamin/folic acid supplementation in early pregnancy reduces the prevelance of neural tube defects. *J Am Med Assoc* 1989; **262**: 2847–2852.

Mills JL, Tuomileho J, Yu KF, *et al.* Maternal vitamin levels during pregnancies producing infants with neural tube defects. *J Pediatr* 1992; **120**: 863–871.

Monson RR, Rosenberg L, Hartz SC. Diphenylhydantoin and selected congenital malformations. *New Engl J Med* 1973; **289**: 1049–1052.

Montouris G. Safety of gabapentin treatment during pregnancy. *Epilepsia* 2002; **43**(Suppl. 7): 234.

Mountain KR, Hirsh J, Gallus AS. Maternal coagulation defect due to anticonvulsant treatment in pregnancy. *Lancet* 1970; **1**: 265–268.

MRC Vitamin Study Group. Prevention of neural tube defects: Results of the Medical Research Council Vitamin Study. *Lancet* 1991; **338**: 131–137.

Mulinare J, Cordero JF, Erickson JD, *et al.* Periconceptional use of multivitamins and the occurrence of neural tube defects. *J Am Med Assoc* 1988; **260**: 3141–3145.

Myllynen P, Pienimaki P, Jouppila P, *et al.* Transplacental passage of oxcarbazepine and its metabolites in vivo. *Epilepsia* 2001; **42**(11): 1482–1485.

Nakane Y. Congenital malformations among infants of epileptic mothers treated during pregnancy. *Folia Psychiatr Neurol Japon* 1979; **33**: 363–369.

Nakane Y, Okuma T, Takahashi R, *et al.* Multi-institutional study on the teratogenicity and fetal toxicity of antiepileptic drugs: report of a collaborative study group in Japan. *Epilepsia* 1980; **21**: 663–680.

Nau H, Rating D, Koch S, *et al.* Valproic acid and its metabolites: placental transfer, neonatal pharmacokinetics, transfer via mother's milk and clinical status in neonates of epileptic mothers. *J Pharmacol Exp Ther* 1981; **219**: 768–777.

Nebert DW, Jensen NM. The Ah locus: genetic regulation of the metabolism of carcinogens, drugs, and other environmental chemicals by cytochrome P-450 mediated mono-oxygenases. *CRC Crit Rev Biochem* 1979; **6**: 401–437.

Neri A, Heifetz L, Nitke S, *et al.* Neonatal outcomes in infants of epileptic mothers. *Eur J Obstet Gynecol Reproduct Biol* 1983; **16**: 263–268.

Niesen M, Froscher W. Finger and toenail hypoplasia after carbamazepine monotherapy in late pregnancy. *Neuropediatrics* 1985; **16**: 167–168.

Ohman I, Vitols S, Tomson T. Lamotrigine in pregnancy: pharmacokinetics during delivery, in the neonate, and during lactation. *Epilepsia* 2000; **41**(6): 709–713.

Ohman I, Vitols S, Luef G, *et al.* Topiramate kinetics during delivery, lactation, and in the neonate: preliminary observations. *Epilepsia* 2002; **43**(10): 1157–1160.

Olafsson E, Hallgrimsson JT, Hauser WA, *et al.* Pregnancies of women with epilepsy: a population-based study in Iceland. *Epilepsia* 1998; **39**(8): 887–892.

Omtzigt JG, Los FJ, Hagenaars AM, *et al.* Prenatal diagnosis of spina bifida aperta after first trimester valproate exposure. *Prenat Diagn* 1992; **12**(11): 893–897.

Otani K. Risk factors for the increased seizure frequency during pregnancy and the puerpurium. *Fol Psychiar Neurol Japan* 1985; **39**: 33–44.

Pacifici GM, Rane A. Metabolism of styrene oxide in different human fetal tissues. *Drug Metab Dispos* 1982; **10**: 302–305.

Pacifici GM, Colizzi C, Giuliani L, *et al.* Cytosolic epoxide hydrolase in fetal and adult human liver. *Arch Toxicol* 1983; **54**: 331.

Pantarotto C, Arboix M, Sezzano P, *et al.* Studies on 5,5-diphenylhydantoin irreversible binding to rat liver microsomal proteins. *Biochem Pharmacol* 1982; **31**: 1501–1507.

Pennell PB, Montgomery JQ, Clements SD, *et al.* Lamotrigine clearance markedly increases during pregnancy. *Epilepsia* 2002; **43**(Suppl. 7): 234–235.

Perruca E, Crema A. Plasma protein binding of drugs in pregnancy. *Clinical Pharmacokinetics.* 1982; **7**: 336–352.

Phelan MC, Pellock JM, Wance WE. Discordant expression of fetal hydantoin syndrome in heteropaternal dizygotic twins. *New Engl J Med* 1982; **307**: 99–101.

Philbert A, Dam M. The epileptic mother and her child. *Epilepsia* 1982; **23**: 85–99.

Rabinowicz A, Meischenguiser R, Ferraro SM, *et al.* Single-center 7 year experience of oxcarbazepine exposure during pregnancy. *Epilepsia* 2002; **43**(Suppl. 7): 208–209.

Rasgon NL, Altshuler LL, Gudeman D, *et al.* Medication status and polycystic ovary syndrome in women with bipolar disorder: a preliminary report. *J Clin Psychiatr* 2000; **61**: 173–178.

Rodriguez-Palomares C, Belmont-Gomez A, Amancio-Chassin O, *et al*. Phenytoin serum concentration monitoring during pregnancy and puerperium in Mexican epileptic women. *Arch Med Res* 1995; **26**: 371–377.

Robert E, Guibaud P. Maternal valproic acid and congenital neural tube defects. *Lancet* 1982; **11**: 937.

Rosa FW. Spina bifida in infants of women treated with carbamazepine during pregnancy. *New Engl J Med* 1991; **324**: 674–677.

Rudd NL, Freedom RM. A possible primidone embryopathy. *J Pediatr* 1979; **94**: 835–837.

Sabers A, Ohman I, Christensen J, *et al*. Oral contraceptives reduce lamotrigine plasma levels. *Neurology* 2003; **61**(4): 570–571.

Safra MJ, Oakley GP. Association between cleft lip with or without cleft palate and prenatal exposure to diazepam. *Lancet* 1975; **2**: 478–480.

Schmidt D, Canger R, Avanzini G, *et al*. Change of seizure frequency in pregnant epileptic women. *J Neurol Neurosurg Psychiatr* 1983; **46**: 751–755.

Seller MJ, Nevin NC. Periconceptional vitamin supplementation and the prevention of neural tube defects in south-east England and Northern Ireland. *J Med Genet* 1984; **21**(5): 325–330.

Seller MJ. Recent developments in the understanding of the aetiology of neural tube defects. *Clin Dysmorphol* 1995; **4**: 93–104.

Shane-McWhorter L, Cerveny JD, MacFarlane LL, *et al*. Enhanced metabolism of levonorgestrel during phenobarbital treatment and resultant pregnancy. *Pharmacotherapy* 1998; **18**(6): 1360–1364.

Shapiro S, Slone D, Hartz SC, *et al*. Anticonvulsant and parental epilepsy in the development of birth defects. *Lancet* 1976; **1**: 272–275.

Shorvon SD, Tallis RC, Wallace HK. Antiepileptic drugs: coprescription of proconvulsant drugs and oral contraceptives: a national study of antiepileptic drug prescribing practice. *J Neurol Neurosurg Psychiatr* 2002; **72**(1): 114–115.

Shum S, Jensen NM, Nebert DW. The Ah locus: in utero toxicity and teratogenesis associated with genetic differences in B(a)P metabolism. *Teratology* 1979; **20**: 365–376.

Sims P, Grover PL. Epoxides in polycyclic aromatic hydrocarbon metabolism and carcinogenesis. *Adv Cancer Res* 1974; **20**: 165.

Smithells RW, Nevin NC, Seller MJ. Further experience of vitamin supplementation for prevention of neural tube defect recurrences. *Lancet* 1983; **1**: 1027–1031.

South J. Teratogenic effects of anticonvulsants. *Lancet* 1972; **2**: 1154.

Speidel BD, Meadow SR. Maternal epilepsy and abnormalities of the fetus and newborn. *Lancet* 1972; **2**: 839–843.

Spielberg SP, Gordon GB, Blake DA, *et al*. Anticonvulsant toxicity in vitro: possible role of arene oxides. *J Pharmacol Exp Ther* 1981; **217**: 386–389.

Steegers-Theunissen RP, Reiner WO, Borm GF, *et al*. Factors influencing the risk of abnormal pregnancy outcomes in epileptic women: a multicenter prospective study. *Epilepsy Res* 1994; **18**(3): 261–269.

Strickler SM, Dansky LV, Miller MA, *et al*. Genetic predisposition to phenytoin-induced birth defects. *Lancet* 1985; **2**: 746–749.

Tennis P, Eldridge RR. Scientific Advisory Committee. International Lamotrigine Pregnancy Registry. *Epilepsia* 2002; **43**(10): 1161–1167.

Tomson T, Lindbom U, Ekqvist B, *et al.* Epilepsy and pregnancy: a prospective study of seizure control in relation of free and total plasma concentrations of carbamazepine and phenytoin. *Epilepsia* 1994; **35**: 122–130.

Tomson T, Ohman I, Vitols S. Lamotrigine in pregnancy and lactation: a case report. *Epilepsia* 1997; **38**(9): 1039–1041.

Tran TA, Leppik IE, Blesi K, *et al.* Lamotrigine clearance during pregnancy. *Neurology* 2002; **59**(2): 251–255.

Vajda FJ, O'Brien TJ, Hitchcock A, *et al.* The Australian Registry of antiepileptic drugs in pregnancy: multivariate regression analysis demonstrating an increased risk for valproate, with a dose-dependent relation. *Epilepsia* 2002; **43**(Suppl. 7): 211.

Van Allen MI, Kalousek DK, Chernoff GF, *et al.* Evidence for multi-site closure of the neural tube in humans. *Am J Genet* 1993; **47**: 723–743.

Van Creveld S. Nouveaux aspects de la maladie hemorragique du nouveau ne. *Ned Tijdschr Geneeskd* 1957; **101**: 2109–2112.

Van Dyke DC, Hodge SE, Helde F, *et al.* Family studies in fetal phenytoin exposure. *J Pediatr* 1988; **113**: 301–306.

Vergel RG, Sanchez LR, Heredero BL, *et al.* Primary prevention of neural tube defects with folic acid supplementation: Cuban experience. *Prenat Diagn* 1990; **10**: 149–152.

Vorhees CV. Developmental effects of anticonvulsants. *Neurotoxicology* 1986; **7**: 235–244.

Wells PG, Harbison RD. Significance of the phenytoin reactive arene oxide intermediate, its oxepin tautomer, and clinical factors modifying their roles in phenytoin-induced teratology. In T. M. Hassell, M. C. Johnston, K. H. Dudley, eds. *Phenytoin-Induced Teratology and Gingival Pathology.* New York: Raven Press, 1980: 83–108.

Wells PG, Kuper A, Lawson JA, *et al.* Relation of in vivo drug metabolism to stereoselective fetal hydantoin toxicology in mouse: evaluation of mephenytoin and its metabolite, nirvanol. *J Pharmacol Exp Ther* 1982; **221**: 228–234.

Wells PG, Zubovits JT, Wong ST, *et al.* Modulation of phenytoin teratogenicity and embryonic covalent binding by acetylsalicylic acid, and alpha-phenyl-*N-t*-butylnitrone implications for bioactivation by prostaglandin synthetase. *Toxicol Appl Pharmacol* 1989; **97**: 192–202.

Werler MM, Shapiro S, Mitchell AA. Periconceptual folic acid exposure and risk of occurrent neural tube defects. *J Am Med Assoc* 1993; **269**: 1257–1261.

Werler MM, Louik C, Shapiro S, *et al.* Prepregnant weight in relation to risk of neural tube defects. *J Am Med Assoc* 1996; **275**: 1089–1092.

Wells PG, Harbison RD. Significance of the phenytoin reactive arene oxide intermediate, its oxepin tautomer, and clinical factors modifying their roles in phenytoin-induced teratology. In Hassell TM, Johnson MC, Dudley KH, eds. *Phenytoin-induced teratology and gingival pathology.* New York: Raven Press, 1980; 83–108.

Wilton LV, Shakir S. A post-marketing surveillance study of gabapentine as add on therapy for 3,100 patients in England. *Epilepsia* 2002; **43**(9): 983–992.

Winship KA, Cahal DA, Weber JCP, *et al.* Maternal drug histories and central nervous system anomalies. *Arch Dis Child* 1984; **59**: 1052–1060.

Wong M, Wells PG. Effects of N-acetylcysteine on fetal development and on phenytoin teratogenicity in mice. *Teratogenesis Carcinog Mutagen* 1988; **8**: 65–79.

Wong M, Wells PG. Modulation of embryonic glutathione reductase and phenytoin teratogenicity by 1,3-bis(2-chloroethyl)-1-nitrosourea (BCNU). *J Pharmacol Exp Ther* 1989; **250**: 336–342.

Yerby MS, Koepsell T, Daling J. Pregnancy complications and outcomes in a cohort of women with epilepsy. *Epilepsia* 1985; **26**: 631–635.

Yerby MS, Leavitt A, Erickson D, *et al.* Antiepileptics and the development of congenital anomalies. *Neurology* 1992; **42**(Suppl. 5): 132–140.

Zackai EH, Mellman WJ, Neiderer B, *et al.* The fetal trimethadione syndrome. *J Pediatr* 1975; **87**: 280–284.

Zhu M, Zhou S. Reduction of the teratogenic effects of phenytoin by folic acid and a mixture of folic acid, vitamins, and amino acids: a preliminary trial. *Epilepsia* 1989; **30**: 246–251.

17

Antiepileptic drug interactions in handicapped and mentally retarded patients

Matti Sillanpää

Departments of Child Neurology and Public Health, University of Turku, Turku, Finland

Introduction

Epilepsy in the mentally retarded differs from epilepsy in the mentally normal patient in relation to etiology, seizure types, epilepsy syndromes, choice of antiepileptic drugs, identification of their side effects and treatment outcome. Consequently, a successful antiepileptic drug therapy is a demanding task in terms of choice of drug therapy, combinations of drugs and side effects in mentally retarded patients compared with mentally normal people. Adverse effects and interactions between different antiepileptic drugs are a potential risk in the presence of many and difficult-to-treat seizure types, leading to frequent polytherapy. There is also an increased risk of interactions between antiepileptic drugs and other drugs because of the increased incidence of co-morbidity among these patients.

In patients who are handicapped or mentally retarded, there is no evidence that pharmacokinetic drug interactions *per se* are quantitatively or qualitatively different from those seen in otherwise normal epilepsy patients. However, it is the context of the treatment of their epilepsy that puts a different emphasis on the potential for interactions. These patients are characterized by an increased incidence of co-morbidity that may require treatment with other medications. Their epilepsies are generally more refractory to treatment and antiepileptic drug combinations are more likely to be used. Also, central nervous system (CNS) toxicity of drugs may be more prominent in mentally retarded patients, and this may include neurotoxic pharmacodynamic interactions between antiepileptic drugs as well as pharmacodynamic interactions between antiepileptic drugs and other psychotropic drugs. As a group, these patients may be particularly vulnerable to the problems associated with polytherapy. The main purpose of this chapter is not to provide an exhaustive discussion of possible pharmacokinetic interactions that are discussed elsewhere in this book, but to emphasize the context in which pharmacokinetic and pharmacodynamic interactions are likely to occur during the treatment of epilepsy in handicapped and mentally retarded patients.

Epidemiology of epilepsy in the mentally retarded

Epilepsy occurs in approximately 15% of patients with mild mental retardation (IQ 50–69) (Blomquist *et al.*, 1981; Drillien *et al.*, 1966; Hagberg *et al.*, 1981) and 30% of those with severe mental retardation (IQ < 50) (Corbett, 1993; Drillien *et al.*, 1966; Gustavson *et al.*, 1977a, b). In institutionalized patients with mostly severe or profound mental retardation, the prevalence of epilepsy ranges from 35% to 60% (Iivanainen, 1974; Illingworth, 1959; Mariani *et al.*, 1993). The age at the onset of the epilepsy does not differ from that in the general population (Forsgren *et al.*, 1990; Goulden *et al.*, 1991; Richardson *et al.*, 1980). However, children with severe mental retardation were found to have a significantly earlier seizure onset than those with a mild mental retardation (Steffenburg *et al.*, 1996).

Table 17.1 shows several lesional, developmental, chromosomal and metabolic conditions in which epilepsy is associated in up to 100% of the cases. The etiology of severe mental retardation is reportedly prenatal in 55–78%, perinatal in 8–15%,

Table 17.1 Occurrence of epilepsy in certain syndromes with MR

Syndrome	Prevalence (%)	Author(s) and year
Cerebral palsy and MR	28–38	Goulden *et al.* (1991), Sillanpää (1978)
Mitochondrial disorders	96–100	Hirano and Pavlakis (1994)
Polymicrogyria	90	Kuzniecky *et al.* (1993)
Tuberous sclerosis	90	Barkovich and Kjos (1992), Fois *et al.* (1988)
Chromosomal anomalies		
Angelman syndrome	84–90	Cassidy and Schwartz (1998), Viani *et al.* (1995), Zori *et al.* (1992)
Rett syndrome	75–80	Hagberg (1996), Perry (1991)
Wolf–Hirschhorn syndrome	70	Jennings and Bird (1981)
Fragile-X syndrome	25	Wisniewski *et al.* (1991)
Prader–Willi syndrome	15–20	Bray *et al.* (1983)
Down syndrome	6–12	Stafstrom *et al.* (1991), Veall (1974)
Klinefelter syndrome	2–10	Becker *et al.* (1996), Nielsen and Pedersen (1969), Zuppinger *et al.* (1967)
Metabolic disorders		
Peroxisomal diseases	80	Garcia-Alvarez *et al.* (1997)
Krabbe's disease	50–75	
Biotinidase deficiency	50–75	
Disorders of urea cycle	60	

MR, mental retardation.

Table 17.2 Failure to recognize epileptic seizures in the mentally retarded

Seizures with vertigo
Seizures with paresthesias
Seizures with visceral disturbances
Seizures with headache
Seizures with loss of emotional control
Partial seizures with other clinical manifestations
Supplementary sensorimotor area seizures
Simple partial seizures
Absence seizures
Drop attacks
Automatisms

postnatal in 1–12% and unknown in 13–22% (Goulden *et al.*, 1991; Gustavson *et al.*, 1977b; Hagberg and Kyllerman, 1983; Linna, 1989). In patients who have a mild mental handicap, the corresponding figures are 23–43%, 7–18%, 4–5% and 43–55%, respectively. In many patients, the etiology is still unknown but probably prenatal (Blomquist *et al.*, 1981; Hagberg and Kyllerman, 1983).

Problems in diagnosing epilepsy

The diagnosis of epileptic seizures may be difficult in mentally retarded patients, because they cannot in many cases express themselves and therefore fail to tell about their perceived symptoms (Table 17.2). Also, in these patients, motor automatisms are not easily distinguished from stereotypic movements, nor are nocturnal seizures easy to separate from parasomnias. Table 17.3 lists the most important non-epileptic conditions which may lead to a misdiagnosis of epilepsy.

Intractability of seizures

The main groups of reasons for intractability of seizures are related to actions by the physician, to the patient, to the epilepsy itself and to the drugs (Table 17.4). The type of epilepsy may be *a priori* intractable. Epileptic and non-epileptic seizures may be intermingled in the same patient. Certain antiepileptic medications, at therapeutic or at toxic doses, may cause or aggravate seizures. Remote symptomatic etiology, abnormal neurological status, occurrence of status epilepticus and poor short-term effect of drug therapy have been shown to be independent predictors of intractability (Kwan and Brodie, 2000; Sillanpää, 1993).

Table 17.3 Differential diagnosis of non-epileptic seizures in the mentally retarded

Cardiovascular mechanisms
Infantile syncope
- Breath-holding spells
  - Cyanotic infantile syncope
  - Reflex anoxic seizures
- Syncope in older children

Paroxysmal movement disorders
Infantile jitteriness
Benign myoclonus of early infancy
Hyperekplexia
Gastroesophageal reflux
Paroxysmal dystonia/choreoathetosis
Shuddering attacks
Stereotypic movements
Alternating hemiplegia of childhood
Masturbation
Stool withholding activity and constipation

Psychological disorders
Psychogenic or pseudoseizures
Hyperventilation
Münchhausen by proxy

Migraine and migraine equivalents
Recurrent abdominal pain
Basilar migraine

Sleep disorders
Arousal disorders
REM sleep disorders

REM, rapid eye movement.

Drug interactions and adverse effects

Most of the untoward effects are not as readily recognized in mentally retarded as in mentally normal patients. These patients may also be at higher risk for certain adverse effects of antiepileptic therapy, such as reduced bone density (Andress *et al.*, 2002; Tolman *et al.*, 1975). Pharmacokinetics of antiepileptic drugs may be affected in many ways. Administration of the drugs may be complicated by the reluctance of the patient to take the pills, or decreased absorption due to slow bowel movements and constipation. Elimination of drugs metabolized by the liver may also be altered due to changes in genetic capacity, especially in inborn errors of neurometabolism

Table 17.4 Intractability of epilepsy in the mentally retarded

Physician related
Incorrect diagnosis
Misclassification of epilepsy
Failure to recognize all seizure types
Failure in choice of drug
Failure to recognize seizure freedom

Patient related
Non-compliance

Epilepsy related
Severe early infantile encephalopathies
Minor motor seizures
Complex partial seizures
Atonic seizures
Multiple seizure types
Organic etiology of epilepsy
Progressive etiology of seizures
Non-epileptic seizures
Concomitant non-epileptic seizures

Drug related
Problems in ingestion of drug
Lack of good early effect of therapy
Side effects of single drug therapy
Side effects of polytherapy
Drug interactions
Deviating drug kinetics

involving the liver. Epilepsy in mental retardation commonly presents with several seizure types, drug resistance, concomitant psychiatric symptoms and syndromes with various enzyme abnormalities, which increase the risk of interactions. Often, polytherapy in mentally retarded patients with epilepsy can be reduced successfully (Bennett *et al.*, 1983). In a 10-year study in 244 institutionalized patients, the percentage of patients receiving monotherapy could be increased from 36.5% to 58.1% with no observed loss in seizure control (Pellock and Hunt, 1996). Whenever polytherapy is reduced, it is important to keep in mind that existing pharmacokinetic interactions are reversible upon removal of the drug responsible for the interaction.

Phenobarbital

Phenobarbital (and other barbiturates) has been used for almost one century for its good anticonvulsive efficacy. Phenobarbital (and primidone, the main active metabolite of which is phenobarbital) is considered to typically affect cognition, behavior and affect in mentally normal people. Combination of valproate with phenobarbital therapy results in elevated phenobarbital levels, due to inhibition of phenobarbital hydroxylation, with subsequent somnolence and even coma or hyperkinesis, aggressive bursts and insomnia (Bruni *et al.*, 1980). Inversely, phenobarbital accelerates the metabolism of valproate, thus lowering valproate levels in relation to the dose. The metabolism of cimetidine, used against peptic ulcer, which is not so uncommon in the mentally retarded, may be induced by phenobarbital with subsequent decreased blood levels (Somogyi and Gugler, 1982). Because of its potential adverse effects, phenobarbital cannot be recommended as the first or second choice of drug for epileptic seizures associated with mental retardation.

Phenytoin

Along with phenobarbital, phenytoin was for decades the most important tool against seizures in the mentally retarded. Phenytoin therapy is not easily managed because of its saturation kinetics, marked differences in attaining steady-state levels in the blood and in other features of metabolism, and certain pharmacokinetic interactions which may in some cases result in toxic levels of phenytoin. Combined with primidone, phenytoin may cause phenobarbital intoxication by causing a marked rise in the ratio of phenobarbital to primidone (Fincham and Schottelius, 1989).

The most serious groups of side effects include neurological adverse effects. Brain damage, which is commonly associated with mental retardation, and phenytoin in polytherapy further increase the risk for neurological adverse effects at therapeutic or even low levels of plasma phenytoin (Iivanainen, 1998). A chronic and in the mentally retarded often irreversible syndrome of phenytoin encephalopathy was seen in 28% (Iivanainen *et al.*, 1977).

Phenytoin can no longer be recommended as the first or second drug of choice against epileptic seizures associated with mental retardation. This is particularly true when the patient has primary locomotion disorder or evidence of cerebellar disease.

Valproate

Valproate is a major antiepileptic drug with a broad spectrum, which is an advantage because it can cover several types of seizure so typical of the many mentally retarded. Seizure freedom is achieved by 20–70% of children with mental retardation and infantile spasms (Friis, 1998), and one-fifth of those with Lennox–Gastaut syndrome (Covanis *et al.*, 1982; Henriksen and Johannessen, 1982) become seizure-free on a high-dosage valproate monotherapy. Valproate may have a clinically significant displacing effect on phenytoin and can cause phenytoin intoxication due to high free levels of phenytoin, even in the presence of therapeutic total levels (Wilder and

Rangel, 1989). Valproate can significantly elevate levels of phenobarbital (also derived from primidone), ethosuximide and lamotrigine. The risk of death from liver failure is highest in children who are less than 2 years of age, especially among those with mental retardation, genetic metabolic disorders, brain injury or a family history of severe hepatic disease and/or who are receiving valproate in polytherapy (Bryant III and Dreifuss, 1996).

Carbamazepine

Carbamazepine is effective against focal and generalized seizures. It is not effective against atypical absence, atonic and myoclonic seizures, and may even cause or increase these seizures, which are common in mentally retarded patients. Neurotoxicity is for the most part dose related. Though negative behavioral effects are in general fewer on carbamazepine than on phenytoin, phenobarbital or primidone, they may occur in mentally retarded patients and particularly in those with brain damage and those with pre-existing behavioral problems (Alvarez *et al.*, 1998; Friedman *et al.*, 1992; Reid *et al.*, 1981).

Carbamazepine levels are lower but carbamazepine-epoxide concentrations are higher in combination therapy with phenobarbital, phenytoin, primidone and valproate than in monotherapy. But carbamazepine and epoxide levels do not appear to be affected by newer anticonvulsants. Increasing displacement of carbamazepine from plasma proteins increases free fraction of carbamazepine during valproate co-medication (Haidukewych *et al.*, 1989). In case of co-medication with felbamate, lamotrigine, phenobarbitone, phenytoin, primidone, progabide and valnoctamide, carbamazepine-epoxide concentrations may reach toxic levels. Carbamazepine combined with valproate appears to have synergistic effects in frontal and temporal focal seizures (Gupta and Jeavons, 1985).

Oxcarbazepine

Oxcarbazepine is similar to carbamazepine in its mode of action and efficacy against epileptic seizures. Few data are available on its efficacy in people with mental retardation. Given as adjunctive therapy for difficult-to-treat patients with mental retardation, a 50% or greater decrease in seizure frequency has been achieved in 50–60% of patients (Gaily *et al.*, 1997; Sillanpää and Pihlaja, 1988/1989; Singh and Ramani, 2001). The tolerability of oxcarbazepine is better and interactions are less frequent than those observed with carbamazepine, with the exception of higher frequency of hyponatremia. Electrical status epilepticus in sleep may occur during oxcarbazepine therapy in the mentally retarded. Oxcarbazepine has not shown any significant autoinduction or interactions with other drugs (Baruzzi *et al.*, 1994), and may therefore be a useful drug for polytherapy in the treatment of difficult-to-treat seizures.

Benzodiazepines

Benzodiazepines are in most cases used as an adjunctive therapy, for example in children with Lennox–Gastaut syndrome or other epilepsy types with mental retardation. Clinically relevant interactions of benzodiazepines are rare, if any. In some patients, however, adjunctive therapy with clonazepam may cause toxic levels of phenytoin (Isojärvi and Tokola, 1998). The incidence of tolerance is higher in patients with clonazepam-treated West syndrome or Lennox–Gastaut syndrome than in epilepsy with typical absence seizures (Specht *et al.*, 1989). Interactions with other drugs are based on pharmacodynamic influences. A combination with other CNS-depressant drugs may increase depression (Haefely, 1989).

Vigabatrin

Vigabatrin proved to be an efficient drug against difficult-to-treat seizures in people with mental retardation (Pitkänen *et al.*, 1993) and particularly in children with infantile spasms, with a 50% or greater decrease in seizure frequency in two-thirds (Chiron *et al.*, 1991). Vigabatrin does not cause excessive behavioral disturbances in mentally retarded patients (Pitkänen *et al.*, 1993). Hyperactive agitation or aggression, on the other hand, have been observed in up to 15–26% of pediatric patients (Dulac *et al.*, 1991; Uldall *et al.*, 1991). Myoclonic jerks may be provoked by vigabatrin, necessitating discontinuation of the drug (Dean *et al.*, 1999).

The good efficacy of vigabatrin on seizures (Kälviäinen *et al.*, 1995) is shadowed by recent observations of visual field constriction, which occurs in one-third (Kälviäinen and Nousiainen, 2001), is caused by accumulation of vigabatrin in the retina (Sills *et al.*, 2001), and appears irreversible (Nousiainen *et al.*, 2001). The benefits, however, outweigh the risks and the therapy can be continued under strict clinical control (Paul *et al.*, 2001). This is particularly true for infantile spasms due to tuberous sclerosis (Harding, 1998). Vigabatrin has not been found to be involved in any pharmacokinetic interaction.

Lamotrigine

The antiepileptic efficacy of lamotrigine is similar to that of other major antiepileptic drugs in placebo-controlled studies. In a retrospective evaluation of 44 institutionalized patients with mental retardation (Gidal *et al.*, 2000), lamotrigine, added to other antiepileptic drug therapy, decreased seizure frequency by 50% or more in 55% of the patients with mental retardation (Beran and Gibson, 1998). Addition of lamotrigine to carbamazepine may accentuate or cause carbamazepine side effects, such as dizziness, diplopia and sedation which are subjective symptoms, and may present as behavioral disturbances in the mentally retarded (Besag *et al.*, 1998a). The most important effect of other antiepileptic drugs is inhibition of lamotrigine metabolism by valproate and the acceleration of lamotrigine metabolism by enzyme-inducing antiepileptic drugs. Methsuximide lowers lamotrigine to a clinically significant extent and this must be considered in the dosing of lamotrigine (Besag *et al.*, 1998b). Several other papers have reported favorable effects on seizure frequency (Buchanan, 1995), cognition and behavior (Meador and Baker, 1997), and quality of life (Nadarajah and Duggan, 1995) and less successful involvement of behavior (Beran and Gibson, 1998; Davanzo and King, 1996).

Gabapentin

Gabapentin has been shown to be effective as an adjunct on refractory partial-onset seizures. Eleven (42%) of 26 children with mental retardation experienced a 50% or greater decrease in seizure frequency on gabapentin add-on therapy. The response did not differ from that of mentally normal study subjects (Khurana *et al.*, 1993; Mikati *et al.*, 1998). Gabapentin has an effect on focal seizures but not on myoclonic, atonic or absence seizures. With regard to adverse effects, 16% of 110 mentally retarded people showed aggressiveness, 15% had increase in seizure frequency, and 9% had ataxia or lethargy (Mayer *et al.*, 1999). Mikati *et al.* (1998) reported behavioral adverse changes in 58% of 26 mentally retarded children. In one study, gabapentin was shown to extend the elimination half-life of felbamate by a 50% (Hussein *et al.*, 1996). No other interactions involving gabapentin have been described.

Tiagabine

Tiagabine, another GABAergic antiepileptic drug, is in many respects similar to gabapentin. According to a meta-analysis (Marson *et al.*, 1997), the chance for at least 50% reduction in seizure decrease was three-fold with add-on tiagabine than without. No separate data on mentally retarded patients are so far available. Lack of clinically relevant cognitive adverse effects may encourage tiagabine trials in mentally retarded individuals. On the other hand, dizziness, asthenia, nervousness, abnormal thinking, depression, aphasia and abnormal abdominal pain are significantly more common compared with placebo. Three patients with tiagabine-associated encephalopathy have been reported (So *et al.*, 2001). The elimination of tiagabine is accelerated by enzyme-inducing antiepileptic drugs, but tiagabine does not seem to affect the pharmacokinetics of any other drugs.

Topiramate

The meta-analysis of six pooled double-blind, placebo-controlled studies on the effectiveness of topiramate on partial-onset seizures (Reife *et al.*, 2000) showed that the seizure frequency had decreased by at least 50% in 43% of 527 patients, compared with 12% on placebo. In 98 patients with Lennox–Gastaut syndrome, topiramate decreased the frequency of both drop attacks and generalized tonic–clonic seizures in every third patient, whereas the same effect occurred in only every eighth patient on placebo (Glauser *et al.*, 2000). Interactions affecting other drugs are negligible due to predominantly renal excretion and low protein binding, but the half-life of topiramate is shortened by enzyme-inducing antiepileptic drugs such as carbamazepine, phenytoin, phenobarbital and primidone. Side effects during topiramate therapy include dizziness, fatigue, visual disturbance, diplopia, ataxia, psychomotor slowing, weight decrease and, in rare cases, renal stones, and hypohidrosis.

Felbamate

When felbamate was launched, it soon appeared effective in patients with, among other conditions, the Lennox–Gastaut syndrome and infantile spasms (The Felbamate Study Group, 1993). Dangerous adverse effects, mainly aplastic anemia and liver failure, have greatly restricted its use. Felbamate has also several interactions with other drugs. It increases significantly carbamazepine epoxide, phenobarbital, phenytoin and valproate plasma levels and decreases total carbamazepine concentrations. Both carbamazepine and phenytoin induce felbamate metabolism and hence increase its clearance. For the moment, felbamate can only be used in well-selected patients under strict and individualized control.

Zonisamide

Few data are available on the efficacy of zonisamide in patients with mental retardation and refractory seizures. Iinuma *et al.* (1998) reported a more than 50% decrease in seizure frequency in 67% of mentally normal and in 41% of retarded patients. Adverse effects were as common in the retarded as in the mentally normal children (27% vs. 30%). The most common untoward effect was aggravation of seizures, which was more common in the mentally normal than in the retarded (28% vs. 18%), and drowsiness. No data on antiepileptic drug interactions were reported. Zonisamide does not induce or inhibit other drugs but its half-life is shortened in humans by enzyme-inducing drugs such as carbamazepine, phenobarbital, phenytoin and valproate (Sackellares *et al.*, 1985).

Levetiracetam

Levetiracetam, a novel broad-spectrum antiepileptic drug, is effective against focal and generalized seizures. In three multicenter, double-blind, placebo-controlled studies (Ben-Menachem and Falter, 2000; Cereghino *et al.*, 2000; Shorvon *et al.*, 2000), about one-third of 904 patients with partial-onset, drug-refractory seizures achieved an at least 50% overall decrease in seizure frequency. The tolerability was good. According to existing data, no interactions can be anticipated in clinical use (Patsalos, 2000). The place of levetiracetam in the treatment of seizures in the handicapped and mentally retarded patient remains to be established.

Outcome of epilepsy in the mentally retarded

The outcome of drug therapy may be difficult to assess in the mentally retarded, for example in patients with infantile spasms. Video electroencephalograph (EEG) monitoring may be needed for this purpose. Most of the few population-based studies dealing with the prognosis of epilepsy in the mentally retarded show a less favorable seizure outcome (seizure freedom in 38–46%) than in mentally normal patients (65–89%) (Aicardi, 1986; Brorson and Wranne, 1987; Wakamoto *et al.*, 2000). In another recent long-term follow-up prospective study (Sillanpää, to be published), 34% of patients with epilepsy and mental retardation and 67% of patients with uncomplicated epilepsy became seizure-free. The prognosis is better, the higher the intelligence level (Goulden *et al.*, 1991; Rowan *et al.*, 1980; Sillanpää, to be published). Additional predictors of poor outcome are symptomatic etiology, association of cerebral palsy and perinatal brain injury.

Conclusion

Epilepsy is a common concomitant disorder in people with mental retardation. The diagnosis of epilepsy may be more difficult, because epilepsy in the mentally retarded often presents with several seizure types. The differential diagnosis between epileptic and non-epileptic events may also at times cause difficulties. In many patients, epileptic and non-epileptic seizures may co-occur. The effects of medication are difficult to evaluate, not least due to impaired abilities of these individuals to express themselves about perceived side effects. Video EEG monitoring may be needed. The responses to antiepileptic drugs may be different from that in mentally normal individuals. Numerous attempts in individual patients to attain seizure freedom or an acceptable level of seizure frequency mostly result in polytherapy and increasing adverse effects. These side effects may result from a different susceptibility of the brain to the drugs, to pharmacokinetic interactions, or to a greater susceptibility to pharmacodynamic interactions. To avoid or minimize these effects, the drugs should be as few as possible and a conversion to monotherapy with a broad-spectrum drug should be preferred when feasible. This seems to be particularly important in patients with mental retardation. The impact of the newer antiepileptic drugs may consist of a better tolerability with fewer interactions.

REFERENCES

Aicardi J. *Epilepsy in Children.* New York: Raven Press, 1986.

Alvarez N, Besag F, Iivanainen M. Use of antiepileptic drugs in the treatment of epilepsy in people with intellectual disability. *J Intellect Disabil Res* 1998; **42**(Suppl. 1): 1–15.

Andress DL, Ozuna J, Tirschwell D, *et al.* Antiepileptic drug-induced bone loss in young male patients who have seizures. *Arch Neurol* 2002; **59**: 781–786.

Annegers JF, Rocca WA, Hauser WA. Causes of epilepsy: contributions of the Rochester epidemiology project. *Mayo Clin Proc* 1996; **71**: 570–575.

Barkovich AJ, Kjos BO. Gray matter heterotopias: MR characteristics and correlation with developmental and neurologic manifestations. *Radiology* 1992; **182**: 493–499.

Baruzzi A, Albani F, Riva R. Oxcarbazepine: pharmacokinetic interactions and their clinical significance. *Epilepsia* 1994; **35**(Suppl. 3): 14–19.

Becker KL, Hoffman DL, Albert A, *et al.* Klinefelter's syndrome: clinical and laboratory findings in 50 patients. *Arch Int Med* 1996; **118**: 314–321.

Ben-Menachem E, Falter U. Efficacy and tolerability of levetiracetam 3000 mg in patients with refractory partial seizures: a multicenter, double-blind, responder-selected study evaluating monotherapy. *Epilepsia* 2000; **41**: 1276–1283.

Bennett HS, Dunlop T, Ziring P. Reduction of polypharmacy for epilepsy in an institution for the retarded. *Dev Med Child Neurol* 1983; **25**: 735–737.

Beran RG, Gibson RJ. Aggressive behaviour in intellectually challenged patients with epilepsy treated with lamotrigine. *Epilepsia* 1998; **39**: 280–282.

Besag FMC, Berry DJ, Pool F, *et al.* Carbamazepine toxicity with lamotrigine: pharmacokinetic or pharmacodynamic interaction? *Epilepsia* 1998a; **39**: 183–187.

Besag FMC, Berry DJ, Pool F. Methsuximide lowers LTG blood levels: a pharmacokinetic AED interaction (abstract). *Epilepsia* 1998b; **39**(Suppl. 2): 25–26.

Blomquist HK, Gustavson KH, Holmgren G. Mild mental retardation in children in a Northern Swedish county. *J Ment Defic Res* 1981; **25**: 92–109.

Borusiak P, Korn-Merker E, Holert N, *et al.* Hyponatremia induced by oxcarbazepine in children. *Epilepsy Res* 1998; **30**: 241–246.

Bray GA, Dahms WT, Swerdloff RS, *et al.* The Prader–Willi syndrome: a study of 40 patients and a review of the literature. *Medicine (Baltimore)* 1983; **62**: 59–80.

Brorson LO, Wranne L. Long-term prognosis of childhood epilepsy: survival and seizure prognosis. *Epilepsia* 1987; **28**: 324–330.

Bruni J, Wilder BJ, Perchalski RJ, *et al.* Valproic acid and plasma levels of phenobarbital. *Neurology (Minneap)* 1980; **30**: 94–97.

Bryant III AE, Dreifuss FE. Valproic acid hepatic fatalities. III. U.S. experience since 1986. *Neurology* 1996; **46**: 465–469.

Buchanan N. The efficacy of lamotrigine on seizure control in 34 children, adolescents and young adults with intellectual and physical disability. *Seizure* 1995; **4**: 233–236.

Cassidy SB, Schwartz S. *Reviews in Molecular Medicine: Prader–Willi and Angelman Syndromes, Disorders of Genomic Imprinting.* Baltimore: Williams & Wilkins, Medicine, 1998: 140–151.

Cereghino JJ, Briton V, Abou-Khalil B, *et al.* Levetiracetam for partial seizures: results of a double-blind, randomized clinical trial. *Neurology* 2000; **55**: 236–242.

Chiron C, Dulac O, Beaumont D, *et al.* Therapeutic trial of vigabatrin refractory infantile spasms. *J Child Neurol* 1991; **6**: 52–59.

Commission on Classification and Terminology of the ILAE. Proposal for revised clinical and electroencephalographic classification of epileptic seizures. *Epilepsia* 1981; **22**: 489–501.

Corbett J. Epilepsy and mental handicap. In *A Textbook of Epilepsy*. J. Laidlaw, A. Richens, D. Chadwick, eds. Edinburgh: Churchill Livingstone, 1993: 631–636.

Covanis A, Gupta AK, Jeavons PM. Sodium valproate: monotherapy and polytherapy. *Epilepsia* 1982; **23**: 693–720.

Davanzo PA, King BH. Open trial lamotrigine in the treatment of self-injurious behaviour in an adolescent with profound mental retardation. *J Child Adolesc Psychopharmacol* 1996; **6**: 273–279.

Dean C, Mosier M, Penry K. Dose–response study of vigabatrin as add-on therapy in patients with uncontrolled complex partial seizures. *Epilepsia* 1999; **40**: 74–82.

Drillien CM, Jameson S, Wilkinson EM. Studies in mental handicap. Part I: Prevalence and distribution by clinical type and severity of defect. *Arch Dis Childh* 1996; **41**: 528–538.

Dulac O, Chiron C, Luna D, *et al.* Vigabatrin in childhood epilepsy. *J Child Neurol* 1991; **6**(Suppl. 2): 30–37.

The Felbamate Study Group in Lennox–Gastaut Syndrome. Efficacy of felbamate in childhood epileptic encephalopathy (Lennox–Gastaut syndrome). *New Engl J Med* 1993; **328**: 29–33.

Fincham RW, Schottelius DD. Primidone: interactions with other drugs. In *Antiepileptic drugs*, 3rd edn. R. Levy, R. Mattson, B. Meldrum, J. K. Penry, F. E. Dreifuss, eds. New York: Raven Press, 1989: 413–422.

Fois A, Tomaccini D, Balestri P, *et al.* Intractable epilepsy: etiology, risk factors and treatment. *Clin EEG* 1988; **19**: 68–73.

Forsgren L, Edvinsson SO, Blomquist HK, *et al.* Epilepsy in a population of mentally retarded children and adults. *Epilepsy Res* 1990; **6**: 234–248.

Friedman LD, Kastner T, Plummer AT, *et al.* Adverse behavioral effects in individuals with mental retardation and mood disorders treated with carbamazepine. *Am J Mental Defic* 1992; **96**: 541–546.

Friis ML. Valproate in the treatment of epilepsy in people with intellectual disability. *J Intellect Disabil Res* 1998; **42**(Suppl. 1): 32–35.

Gaily E, Granström ML, Liukkonen E. Oxcarbazepine in the treatment of early childhood epilepsy. *J Child Neurol* 1997; **12**: 496–498.

Garcia-Alvarez M, Nordli DR, De Vivo DC. Inherited metabolic diseases. In *Epilepsy: A Comprehensive Textbook*. E. Engel, T. A. Pedley, eds. Philadelphia: Lippincott-Raven Press, 1997: 2547–2562.

Gidal BE, Walker JK, Lott RS, *et al.* Efficacy of lamotrigine in institutionalized, developmentally disabled patients with epilepsy: a retrospective evaluation. *Seizure* 2000; **9**: 131–136.

Glauser TA, Levisohn PM, Ritter F, *et al.* Topiramate in Lennox–Gastaut syndrome: open-label treatment of patients completing a randomized controlled trial. *Epilepsia* 2000; **41**(Suppl. 1): 86–90.

Goulden KJ, Shinnar S, Koller H, *et al.* Epilepsy in children with mental retardation: a cohort study. *Epilepsia* 1991; **32**: 690–697.

Gupta AK, Jeavons PM. Complex partial seizures: EEG foci and response to carbamazepine and sodium valproate. *J Neurol Neurosurg Psychiatr* 1985; **48**: 1010–1014.

Gustavson KH, Hagberg B, Hagberg K, *et al.* Severe mental retardation in a Swedish county. I. Epidemiology, gestational age, birth weight and associated CNS handicaps in children born 1959–70. *Acta Paediatr Scand* 1977a; **66**: 373–379.

Gustavson KH, Holmgren G, Jonsell R, *et al.* Severe mental retardation in children in a Northern Swedish county. *J Ment Defic Res* 1977b; **21**: 161–180.

Haefely W. Benzodiazepines, mechanisms of action. In *Antiepileptic drugs*. R. H. Levy, R. H. Mattson, B. Meldrum, J. K. Penry, F. E. Dreifuss, eds. 3rd edn. New York: Raven Press, 1989; 721–734.

Hagberg B. Rett syndrome: clinical peculiarities and biological mysteries. *Acta Paediatr* 1996; **84**: 971–976.

Hagberg B, Kyllerman M. Epidemiology of mental retardation – a Swedish survey. *Brain Devel* 1983; **5**: 441–449.

Hagberg B, Hagberg G, Lewerth A, *et al.* Mild mental retardation in Swedish school children. II. Etiologic and pathogenetic aspects. *Acta Paediatr Scand* 1981; **70**: 445–452.

Haidukewych D, Zielinski JJ, Rodin EA. Derivation and evaluation of an equation for prediction of free carbamazepine concentration in patients comedicated with valproic acid. *Ther Drug Monit* 1989; **11**: 528–532.

Harding GF. Severe persistent visual field constriction associated with vigabatrin. Benefit risk ratio must be calculated from individual patients. *Br Med J* 1998; **316**: 232–233.

Henriksen O, Johannessen SI. Clinical and pharmacokinetic observations on sodium valproate: a five-year follow-up study of 100 children with epilepsy. *Acta Neurol Scand* 1982; **65**: 504–523.

Hirano M, Pavlakis SG. Mitochondrial myopathy, encephalopathy, lactic acidosis, and strokelike episodes (MELAS): current concepts. *J Child Neurol* 1994; **9**: 4–13.

Hussein G, Troupin AS, Montouris G. Gabapentin interaction with felbamate. *Neurology* 1996; **47**: 1106.

Iinuma K, Minami T, Cho K, *et al.* Long-term effects of zonisamide in the treatment of epilepsy in children with intellectual disability. *J Intellect Disabil Res* 1998; **42**(Suppl. 1): 68–73.

Iivanainen M. *A Study of Origins of Mental Retardation. Clinics in Developmental Medicine No. 51.* Spastics International Publications. London: William Heinemann Medical Books, 1974.

Iivanainen M. Phenytoin: effective but insidious therapy for epilepsy in people with intellectual disability. *J Intellect Disabil Res* 1998; **42**(Suppl. 1): 24–31.

Iivanainen M, Viukari M, Helle EP. Cerebellar atrophy in phenytoin-treated mentally retarded epileptics. *Epilepsia* 1977; **18**: 375–386.

Illingworth RS. Convulsions in mentally retarded children with or without cerebral palsy. *J Ment Defic Res* 1959; **3**: 88–93.

Isojärvi JIT, Tokola RA. Benzodiazepines in the treatment of epilepsy in people with intellectual disability. *J Intellect Disabil Res* 1998; **42**(Suppl. 1): 80–92.

Jennings MT, Bird TD. Genetic influences in the epilepsies. *Am J Dis Child* 1981; **135**: 450–457.

Kälviäinen R, Nousiainen I. Visual field defects with vigabatrin: epidemiology and therapeutic implications. *CNS Drug* 2001; **15**: 217–230.

Kälviäinen R, Äikiä M, Saukkonen AM, *et al.* Vigabatrin vs. carbamazepine monotherapy in patients with newly diagnosed epilepsy. A randomized, controlled study. *Arch Neurol* 1995; **52**: 989–996.

Khurana DS, Riviello JJ, Helmess S, *et al.* Efficacy of gabapentin therapy in children with refractory partial seizures. *J Pediatr* 1993; **128**: 829–833.

Kuzniecky R, Andermann F, Guerrini R. Congenital bilateral perisylvian syndrome: study of 31 cases. *Lancet* 1993; **341**: 608–612.

Kwan P, Brodie MJ. Early identification of refractory epilepsy. *New Engl J Med* 2000; **342**: 314–319.

Linna SL. *Prevalence, Aetiology, Associated Handicaps and Self Care Ability in 5–19-Old Severely Mentally Retarded.* A doctoral thesis. Oulu: University of Oulu Printing Center, 1989.

Mariani E, Ferini-Strambi L, Sala M, *et al.* Epilepsy in institutionalized patients with encephalopathy: clinical aspects and nosological considerations. *Am J Ment Retard* 1993; **98**(Suppl.): 27–33.

Marson AG, Kadir ZA, Hutton JL, *et al.* The new antiepileptic drugs: a systematic review of their efficacy and tolerability. *Epilepsia* 1997; **38**: 859–880.

Mayer T, Schutte W, Wolf P, *et al.* Gabapentin add-on treatment: how many patients become seizure-free? An open-label multicenter study. *Acta Neurol Scand* 1999; **99**: 1–7.

Meador KJ, Baker GA. Behavioral and cognitive effects of lamotrigine. *J Child Neurol* 1997; **12**(Suppl.): 44–47.

Mikati MA, Choueri R, Khurana DS, *et al.* Gabapentin in the treatment of refractory partial epilepsy in children with intellectual disability. *J Intellect Disabil Res* 1998; **42**(Suppl. 1): 57–62.

Nadarajah J, Duggan L. A missed diagnosis. A missed opportunity for community integration. *Seizure* 1995; **4**: 151–153.

Nielsen J, Pedersen E. Electro-encephalographic findings in patients with Klinefelter's syndrome and the XXY-syndrome. *Acta Neurol Scand* 1969; **45**: 87–94.

Nousiainen I, Mäntyjärvi M, Kälviäinen R. No reversion in vigabatrin-associated visual field defects. *Neurology* 2001; **57**: 1916–1917.

Patsalos PN. Pharmacokinetic profile of levetiracetam: toward ideal characteristics. *Pharmacol Therapeut* 2000; **85**: 77–85.

Paul SR, Krauss GL, Miller NR, *et al.* Visual function is stable in patients who continue long-term vigabatrin therapy: implications for clinical decision making. *Epilepsia* 2001; **42**: 525–530.

Pellock JM, Hunt PA. A decade of modern epilepsy therapy in institutionalized mentally retarded patients. *Epilepsy Res* 1996; **25**: 263–268.

Perry A. Rett syndrome: a comprehensive review of the literature. *Am J Ment Retard* 1991; **3**: 275–290.

Pitkänen A, Ylinen A, Matilainen R, *et al.* Long-term antiepileptic efficacy of vigabatrin in drug-refractory epilepsy in mentally retarded patients. A 5-year follow-up study. *Arch Neurol* 1993; **50**: 24–29.

Reid AH, Naylor GJ, Kay DS. A double blind placebo controlled crossover trial of carbamazepine in overactive severely mentally handicapped patients. *Psychol Med* 1981; **11**: 109–113.

Reife R, Pledger G, Wu SC. Topiramate as add-on therapy: pooled analysis of randomized controlled trials in adults. *Epilepsia* 2000; **41**(Suppl. 1): 66–71.

Richardson SA, Koller H, Katz M, *et al.* Seizures and epilepsy in a mentally retarded population over the first 22 years of life. *Appl Res Ment Retard* 1980; **1**: 123–138.

Rowan AJ, Overweg J, Sadikoglu S, *et al.* Seizure prognosis in long-stay mentally subnormal epileptic patients: interrater EEG and clinical studies. *Epilepsia* 1980; **21**: 219–225.

Sackellares JC, Donofrio PD, Wagner JG, *et al.* Pilot study of zonisamide (1,2-benzisoxazole-3-methanesulfonamide) in patients with refractory partial seizures. *Epilepsia* 1985; **26**: 206–211.

Shorvon SD, Lowenthal A, Janz D, *et al.* Multicenter double-blind, randomized, placebo-controlled trial of levetiracetam as add-on therapy in patients with refractory partial seizures. European Levetiracetam Study Group. *Epilepsia* 2000; **41**: 1179–1186.

Sillanpää M. CP-vammaisen ennuste sosiaalilääketieteelliseltä kannalta (Prognosis of cerebral palsies with special reference to socio-medical aspects). *Kansanterveystiet Julk* M33. Turku: Gill OY (in Finnish, with English summary), 1978.

Sillanpää M. Remission of seizures and predictors of intractability in long-term follow-up. *Epilepsia* 1993; **34**: 930–936.

Sillanpää M, Pihlaja T. Oxcarbazepine (GP 47680) in the treatment of intractable seizures. *Acta Paediatr Hung* (1988/1989); **29**: 359–364.

Sills GJ, Patsalos PN, Butler E, *et al.* Visual field constriction: accumulation of vigabatrin but not tiagabine in the retina. *Neurology* 2001; **57**: 196–200.

Singh BK, Ramani V. Oxcarbazepine in adults with developmental disabilities. *Epilepsia* 2001; **42**(Suppl. 7): 186–187.

So EL, Fessler AJ, Cascino GD, *et al.* Tiagabine-associated encephalopathy. *Epilepsia* 2001; **42**(Suppl. 7): 261.

Somogyi A, Gugler R. Drug interaction with cimetidine. *Clin Pharmacokinet* 1982; **7**: 23–41.

Specht U, Boenigk HE, Wolf P. Discontinuation of clonazepam after long-term treatment. *Epilepsia* 1989; **30**: 458–463.

Stafstrom CE, Patxot CE, Gilmore HE, *et al.* Seizures in children with Down syndrome: etiology, characteristics and outcome. *Dev Med Child Neurol* 1991; **33**: 191–200.

Steffenburg U, Hagberg G, Kyllerman M. Characteristics of seizures in a population-based series of mentally retarded children with active epilepsy. *Epilepsia* 1996; **37**: 850–856.

Tolman KG, Jubiz W, Sannella JJ, *et al.* Osteomalacia associated with anticonvulsant drug therapy in mentally retarded children. *Pediatrics* 1975; **56**: 45–51.

Uldall P, Alving J, Gram L, *et al.* Vigabatrin in pediatric epilepsy – an open study. *J Child Neurol* 1991; **6**(Suppl. 2): 38–44.

Veall RM. The prevalence of epilepsy among mongols related to age. *J Ment Def Res* 1974; **18**: 99–106.

Viani F, Romeo A, Viri M, *et al.* Seizure and EEG patterns in Angelman's syndrome. *J Child Neurol* 1995; **10**: 467–471.

Wakamoto H, Nagao H, Hayashi M, *et al.* Long-term medical, educational` social prognoses of childhood-onset epilepsy: a population-based study in a rural district of Japan. *Brain Dev* 2000; **22**: 246–255.

Wilder BJ, Rangel RJ. Clinically relevant antiepileptic drug interactions. In *Antiepileptic Drug Interactions*. W. H. Pitlick, ed. New York: Demos Publications, 1989: 65–75.

Wisniewski KE, Segan SM, Miezejesji CM, *et al.* The Fra(X) syndrome: neurological, electrophysiological and neuropathological abnormalities. *Am J Med Genet* 1991; **38**: 476–480.

Zori RT, Henrickson J, Woolven S, *et al.* Angelman syndrome: clinical profile. *J Child Neurol* 1992; **7**: 270–280.

Zuppinger K, Engel E, Forber AP, *et al.* Klinefelter's syndrome, a clinical and cytogenetic study in 24 cases. *Acta Endocrinol* 1967; **34**(Suppl. 113): 5–48.

18

Antiepileptic drugs and sex steroids

Richard H. Mattson

Department of Neurology, Yale University School of Medicine, New Haven, CT, USA

Background

In 1972 Kenyon sent a letter to the *British Medical Journal* describing a patient with epilepsy treated with phenytoin (PHT) who became pregnant despite taking usual amounts of oral contraceptive (OC) pills (Kenyon, 1972). She astutely attributed the contraceptive failure to an inductive effect of the PHT on the metabolism of the sex steroid hormones. This observation was soon confirmed by others (Coulam and Annegers, 1979; Janz and Schmidt, 1974) and the underlying mechanisms were further elucidated (Back, 1980). All the older antiepileptic drugs (AEDs), carbamazepine (CBZ), phenobarbital (PB), PHT and primidone (PRM) except valproate (VPA) (Crawford 1986; Sonnen, 1983) were found to have similar effects (Mattson *et al.*, 1986; Schmidt, 1981). In contrast most of the new AEDs with the exception of felbamate (FBM), oxcarbazepine (OXC) and topiramate (TPM) do not change the metabolism of the OCs. Parenteral formulations (intramuscular (i.m.) depot, subcutaneous implant and dermal patch) of contraceptive female sex hormones have also been reported to be subject to increased clearance.

The effect of the AEDs on testosterone metabolism has also indicated changes occur although the evidence of clinical effects is less easily assessed than an unplanned pregnancy. Conversely, except for lamotrigine (LTG) the OCs do not appear to change the pharmacokinetics of AEDs.

Frequency and importance of interactions

Following the initial case report by Kenyon, three other cases of OC failure were cited by Janz and Schmidt (1974). By 1983 Sonnen found that 52 cases had been reported. He concluded that the incidence was probably much higher because 12 women in his own small population had experienced an unplanned pregnancy while using OC pills when taking AEDs (Sonnen, 1983). Although the effect of

CBZ, PB and PHT became established, the exact risk of an unplanned likelihood could only be estimated. The probability approximates that of condom use, a five- to ten-fold increase relative to use of OCs in women not receiving enzyme-inducing drugs (Mattson *et al.*, 1986). Considering the very large usage of OCs, the occurrence of an unplanned pregnancy may be relatively low but the consequences can be of great importance.

The increased clearance of LTG by OCs can result in loss of seizure control or conversely, when OCs are discontinued, overdose of LTG may occur. AED-induced clearance and increased sex-hormone-binding globulin (SHBG) may result in lower free testosterone with resultant decrease in libido, potency and spermatogenesis.

Awareness of the issues

On the basis of accumulating reports of OC drug failure the Epilepsy Foundation of America and the American College of Obstetricians and Gynocologists invited us to write a position paper on the problem of unplanned pregnancy associated with the use of AEDs (Mattson *et al.*, 1986). The review with recommendations for management was published in the *Journal of the American Medical Association*, a publication with the widest physician distribution in the USA. It was estimated that failure rates of OC in patients on CBZ, PB, PB and PRM were approximately five-fold the expected numbers. In contrast VPA use, a non-enzyme inducer, was not associated with increased risk of pregnancy (Crawford, 2002; Sonnen, 1983). Breakthrough bleeding, an effect of low estrogen levels, was advised to be a warning sign of insufficient steroid effect. Increasing the strength of the oral steroid was recommended if continuation of an enzyme-inducing AED was deemed clinically advisable. A decade later Krauss *et al.* (1996) conducted a large survey of licensed neurologists and obstetricians and found approximately a quarter of those surveyed had a patient who had an unplanned pregnancy due to presumed OC failure. A majority did not know which specific AEDs were involved in interactions and did not make an effort to change the dose of the OC. Only 4% of neurologists and none of the obstetricians knew the interactions of all of the AEDs available at that time. Four years later Morrell *et al.* (1996) in a survey of health care professionals found only a small majority was aware of increased failure rates of OCs with AED use and only 27% could correctly identify the responsible drugs. At about the same time a survey in the UK revealed about half of women receiving AEDs and OC did not receive education about a possible interaction (Crawford, 2002). It may be that the efforts to educate health care professionals and women about these interactions, the consequences and the options are now being heard. Aggressive marketing and educational efforts have been made by a number of organizations and especially by pharmaceutical companies that have introduced new AEDs not having interactions with sex steroid hormones.

Mechanism of interactions and contraceptive failure

Most pharmacokinetic studies have suggested the estrogens and progestins in the OC pill were cleared approximately twice as rapidly in women patients receiving enzyme-inducing AEDs compared to normal controls.

The primary mechanism of action of the contraceptive sex hormones is thought to be due to inhibition of release of luteinizing hormone (LH) by the progestin and prevention of ovulation. The critical concentration of hormones needed to have this effect is not predictable, but the evidence that doubling of hormone clearance has been associated with contraceptive failure indicates a concentration below which failure is possible or likely.

The concentration of contraceptive sex hormones in the blood and brain is determined by a number of pharmacokinetic factors (Emery, 2000). After oral intake, a significant first-pass effect occurs especially for the estrogen component (usually ethinyl estradiol or mestranol). Some conjugation with sulfates and glucuronides occurs in the gut as well as hepatic hydroxylation to inactive polar metabolites (Back *et al.*, 1980). Enterohepatic recirculation of these products may result in change back to ethinylestradiol and reabsorption into the blood. These multiple variables make uncertain the final quantity reaching the general circulation. The major hepatic biotransformation of the estrogen is by the CYP3A4 isoenzyme system. Mestranol is converted to ethinylestradiol, the active drug, by demethylation thought to involve the CYP2C9 isoenzyme. Even in normal women from different populations bioavailability of ethynylestradiol (ethinyl) was found to vary up to ten-fold (Fotherby *et al.*, 1981). (It is unclear if compliance could be assured.) The synthetic progestins used in older OC combination pills are norethindrone and levonorgestrel. More recent formulations have included other progestins, norgestimate (converted in part to levonorgesterol), degestrel and gestodene. The synthetic progestin, medroxyprogesterone, has been and continues to be used extensively although primarily in parenteral formulations. The progestin metabolism is less well defined than the estrogens but conjugation, oxidation and reduction all occur and can be induced by the AEDs (Emery, 2000).

CBZ, PB, PRM (that is metabolized to PB) and PHT have inductive effects on the CYP isoenzymes as well as conjugation involved in sex steroid metabolism. Although having lesser inductive effect, FBM, OXC and TPM can all increase clearance of sex steroid hormones in contraceptive preparations. In contrast, VPA as well as many of the newer AEDs, gabapentin (GBP), lamotrigine (LTG), levetiracetam (LEV), tiagabine (TGB) and vigabatrin (VGB) have no effect on sex steroid clearance.

The progestins undergo both oxidation and reduction as well as conjugation after entering the circulation. First-pass effect is much more extensive for norethindrone than levonorgesterol. Since the older enzyme-inducing AEDs increase clearance of these sex steroids the amount circulating in the blood and brain may reach levels too low for the progestin to inhibit ovulation, especially in formulations containing 50 μg of ethinylestradiol or less (and comparable but higher doses of the pro-drug, mestranol) and 1 mg of levonorgesterol. After entering the circulation the sex steroids are protein bound. The progestins are extensively bound to SHBG. This is relevant because the enzyme-inducing AEDs increase the amount of SHBG, which in turn effectively reduces the free, pharmacologically active, circulating progestin. This represents a second mechanism for OC failure.

Specific AED interactions with OCs

Among the older AEDs, CBZ, PB, PRM and PHT have specifically been found to increase clearance of the OC sufficiently to reduce sex hormone levels by approximately 50% (Back *et al.*, 1980; Coulam and Annegers, 1979; Crawford *et al.*, 1986; 1990; Janz and Schmidt, 1974; Kenyon, 1972; Mattson, 1985; Schmidt, 1981; Wilbur and Enson, 2000) whereas VPA had no such effect (Crawford, 2002; Sonnen, 1983). Among the new AEDs introduced since the 1990s GBP (Eldon *et al.*, 1998), LTG (Holdich *et al.*, 1991), LEV (Ragueneau-Majlessi *et al.*, 2002), TGB (Mengel *et al.*, 1994) and VGB (Bartoli *et al.*, 1997) have been studied and found to have no significant effect on clearance of the OCs. In addition progesterone levels did not rise during the luteal phase in the studies of LTG, LEV or TGB, a finding that confirmed the prevention of ovulation. FBM administration had modest effect on clearance of ethinylestradiol but lowered the area under the curve (AUC) of gestodene, a newer synthetic progestin, by 42%. However, progesterone levels did not rise during the luteal phase suggesting ovulation had been blocked (Saano *et al.*, 1995). Somewhat surprisingly OXC, a relatively non-CYP-inducing newer AED, had clear effect on clearance of OCs. Even in doses as low as 600 mg/day the AUC of both ethinylestradiol and levonorgestrol were reduced by 47% (Fattore *et al.*, 1999). The risk of contraceptive failure must be considered in view of the interaction.

The interaction between TPM and OCs is more complex. In an initial study Rosenfeld *et al.* (1997) studied the effect of TPM 200, 400 or 800 on the metabolism of OCs containing 35 μg of ethinylestradiol and 1 mg of norethindrone. Although norethindrone was not affected, ethinylestradiol clearance increased 15–33%. A follow up study was done using lower doses that are now more commonly used. Administration of 50, 100 or 200 mg of TPM in women using the same OC did not significantly reduce concentrations of ethinylestradiol in the blood. In contrast a control group given 600 mg of CBZ exhibited an increase of oral clearance of norethindrone by 69% and ethinylestradiol by 127%. It was concluded a clinically

Table 18.1 Effect of AEDs on OC clearance and effectiveness

Increased	Equivocal	No effect
CBZ	FLB[a]	GBP
PB	TPM[b]	LTG
PHT		TGB
PRM		ZNS[c]
OXC		VPA

[a] OC clearance increased but ovulation blocked.

[b] OC clearance not significantly increased at doses of 200 mg or less.

[c] Unpublished data from Elan (Eisai).

significant interaction of TPM with a 'standard' OC did not occur at doses of 200 mg/day or less (Table 18.1).

Specific AED interactions with parenteral sex steroid administration

Parenteral administration of synthetic progestins and in particular, medroxy-progesterone (Depo-Provera-Ortho), has been available for decades. The route of administration has the advantage of steady release of hormone and minimizes the risk of non-compliance. We conducted studies giving medroxyprogesterone 10 mg three times daily in an effort to achieve amenorrhea to adequately assess any antiepileptic effect (Mattson *et al.*, 1984). Blood mycophenolic acid (MPA) levels (determined by Upjohn Co.) were only about one-half (3–15 ng/ml) compared to normal controls (5–30 ng/ml). To assure compliance and avoid first-pass effect six patients were given 120 mg or 150 mg i.m. medroxyprogesterone (Depo-Provera, Upjohn Co.). Again concentrations in the blood ranged from 1–9 ng/ml (mean 2.6 μg/ml) compared to 5–10 μg/ml for controls. This suggested increased clearance secondary to use of enzyme-inducing AEDs. Although these lower MPA blood levels were found, the dose still sufficed to produce amenorrhea and inhibition of a rise in either estrogen or progesterone. A combination of medroxyprogesterone combined with a pro-drug of estradiol cypionate (Lunelle, Upjohn) has recently become available for contraceptive use. A dermal patch containing norelgestromin and ethinylestradiol (Ortho-Evra) has also become available. Although specific reports are not available, it can be inferred that increased clearance will occur with concomitant use of enzyme-inducing AEDs with an increased risk of contraceptive failure. A subcutaneous implant slow-release formulation of levonorgesterol (Norplant) has been used with excellent contraceptive effects but numerous failures have been reported in women on enzyme-inducing AEDs (Haukkamaa, 1986; Krauss *et al.*, 1996; Odlind and Olsson, 1986). Wyeth no longer manufactures this product. It can be predicted that increased clearance of all these parenteral products can be expected along with decreased efficacy despite avoiding first-pass effect.

Testosterone

Testosterone is produced in the Leydig cells of the testis. Testosterone is highly bound to proteins in the circulation primarily to SHBG. Testosterone is metabolized to dihydroxytestosteroe that is physiologically active. Conversion to estrogen occurs in tissues in the body by an aromatase. Many investigators have reported that total and free testosterone levels are below normal in men with epilepsy (Bauer *et al.*, 2004; Isojarvi *et al.*, 1990; 1995; 2004; Macphee, 1988; Mattson and Cramer, 1985). The enzyme-inducing AEDs can not only increase clearance of testosterone, but increase SHBG resulting in lower free testosterone levels (Isojarvi *et al.*, 1990; 1995; 2004). The effect of AED use on testosterone is more difficult to characterize clinically. Testosterone affects libido, potency and spermatogenesis and can lead to disturbances in these functions if amounts are deficient. However, determinants of libido and potency are multi-factorial so attributing dysfunction to low testosterone associated with AED use is more difficult to establish. This is in contrast to the obvious endpoint of unplanned pregnancy with use of OCs. However, Fenwick *et al.* (1986) were able to correlate erectile dysfunction with low testosterone levels using penile tumescence measurements.

OC effect on LTG

In a study of LTG levels during delivery, in the neonate and during lactation, Ohman *et al.* (2000) found that LTG levels at delivery were markedly lower than pre-pregnancy and 2–3 weeks post partum. Although many reasons can be found for a reduction in AED levels during pregnancy, such changes were not seen in patients also taking CBZ or PHT. They concluded that, glucuronidation was induced by the elevated sex steroid hormones present during pregnancy. This finding was confirmed by Tran *et al.* (2002), who did LTG clearance studies before, during and after delivery. They found a 65% increase in clearance during the first trimester of pregnancy. Sabers *et al.* (2001, 2003) reported a marked decrease (mean 49%) in LTG levels after initiating OC treatment in seven epilepsy patients and return after discontinuing the OCs. They concluded that the OCs act on the glucosonyltransferases which catalyzed the conjugation of LTG with glucuronic acid. This initial observation was confirmed in a larger series of 56 women receiving OCs and LTG. A two- to three-fold change in levels, was associated with adding or discontinuing OCs. In these two reports the changes resulting in a drop in LTG levels were sometimes associated with an increase or breakthrough in seizures or adverse effects when LTG levels rose with OC discontinuation.

Management of women on OC

The safest way of dealing with the problem of unwanted loss of OC effectiveness is to avoid AEDs that affect the clearance of sex steroids. Before the introduction of the newer AEDs, VPA was the obvious choice. Unfortunately, if a woman elected to become or accidentally became pregnant, the concern about possible teratogenicity was of critical importance. Knowing the effect of an AED on sex hormone clearance allows some ability to predict the likelihood of success or failure of a contraceptive therapy. A second, but undependable, indicator of inadequate hormone effect is breakthrough bleeding. Sonnen (1983) observed 60–90% of 133 women taking OCs containing 30 or 50 µg of ethinylestradiol had breakthrough bleeding, whereas this bleeding occurred in only 6% of those taking VPA. A better measure of contraceptive effect is the absence of a rise is progesterone above 5 ng/ml during the luteal phase of the menstrual cycle. The limitation to this method of detection of a contraceptive steroid effect is timing of the day of the blood sample for analysis, unless samples are drawn every few days.

A change is the strength of the OC pill may compensate for increased clearance by the enzyme-inducing AEDs and provide a sufficient amount in the blood to allow adequate protection (American Academy of Neurology, 1998).

It is possible that increasing the quantity of ethinylestradiol from 20 or 30 µg to 50 µg (and the combined progestin) is insufficient. Krauss *et al.* (1996) pointed out that two of five unplanned pregnancies they observed were taking an OC containing 50 µg of ethinylestradiol. Sonnen (1983) observed that increasing the dose to 75 µg corrected breakthrough bleeding in his patients on enzyme-inducing AEDs. Since the bioavailability of the OCs is so variable, it may be difficult to predict the dose needed to provide protection and patients need to be advised of this uncertainty.

Summary

Interactions occur between enzyme-inducing AEDs and synthetic sex hormones used for contraception whether given orally or parenterally. The decrease in available hormones is sufficient to lead to contraceptive failure. AEDs also lower free testosterone levels in men and may contribute to problems with libido, potency and fertility. These effects are not seen with use of VPA and the newer AEDs, GBP, LEV, TGB and VGB. Increased clearance and possible loss of contraceptive effect is found with FBM and OXC. No effect is seen with use of TPM at or below 200 mg/day. A reverse interaction is found with use of OCs. These hormones cause increased clearance and loss of effect of LTG. Surveys indicate that a widespread lack of awareness of these issues persists despite original observations made more than three decades ago.

REFERENCES

American Academy of Neurology, Quality Standards Subcommittee. Practice parameter: management issues for women with epilepsy. *Neurology* 1998; **51**: 944–948.

Back DL, Bates M, Bowden A, *et al.* The interaction of phenobarbital and other anticonvulsants with oral contraceptive steroid therapy. *Contraception* 1980; **22**: 495–503.

Bauer J, Blumenthal S, Reuber M, *et al.* Epilepsy syndrome, focus location, and treatment choice affect testicular function in men with epilepsy. *Neurology* 2004; **62**: 243–246.

Bartoli A, Gatti G, Cipolla G, *et al.* A double-blind, placebo controlled study on the effect of vigabatrin on in vivo parameters of hepatic microsomal enzyme induction and on the kinetics of steroid oral contraceptives in healthy female volunteers. *Epilepsia* 1997; **38**: 702–707.

Coulam CB, Annegers JE. Do oral anticonvulsants reduce the efficacy of oral contraceptives? *Epilepsia* 1979; **20**: 519–526.

Crawford P. Interactions between antiepileptic drugs and hormonal contraceptives. *CNS Drugs* 2002; **16**: 265–272.

Crawford P, Chadwick D, Cleland P, *et al.* The lack of effect of sodium valproate on the pharmacokinetics of oral contraceptive steroids. *Contraception* 1986; **33**: 23–29.

Crawford P, Chadwick DJ, Martin C, *et al.* The interaction of phenytoin and carbamazepine with combined oral contraceptive steroids. *Br J Clin Pharmacol* 1990; **30**: 892–896.

Doose DR, Wang S, Padmanabhan M, *et al.* Effect of topiramate or carbamazepine on the pharmacokinetics of an oral contraceptive containing norethidrone and ethynil estradiol in healthy obese and nonobese female subjects. *Epilepsia* 2003; **44**: 540–549.

Eldon MA, Underwood BA, Randinitis EJ, *et al.* Gabapentin does not interact with a contraceptive regimen of norethindrone acetate and ethinyl estradiol. *Neurology* 1998; **50**: 1146–1148.

Emery MG. Estrogens and Progestins. In *Metabolic Drug Interactions*, R. H. Levy, K. E. Thummel, W. F. Trager, *et al.*, eds. Philadelphia: Lippincott Williams and Wilkens, 2000: 511–528.

Fattore C, Cipolla G, Gatti G, *et al.* Induction of ethinylestradiol and levonorgestrol metabolism by oxcarbazepine in healthy women. *Epilepsia* 1999; **40**: 783–787.

Fenwick PBC, Mercer S, Grant R, *et al.* Nocturnal penile tumescense and serum testosterone levels. *Archiv Sexual Behav* 1986; **15**: 13–21.

Fotherby K, Abdel-Rahman HA, deSouza JC, *et al.* Pharmacokinetics of ethynylestradiol in women from different populations. *Contraception* 1981; **23**: 487–496.

Haukkamaa M. Contraception by Norplant subdermal capsules is not reliable in epileptic patients on anticonvulsant treatment. *Contraception* 1986; **33**: 559–565.

Holdich T, Whiteman P, Orme M, *et al.* Effect of lamotrigine on the pharmacology of the combined oral contraceptive pill (abstract). *Epilepsia* 1991; **32**(Suppl. 1): 67.

Isojarvi JIT, Pakarinen AJ, Ylipalosaari, *et al.* Serum hormones in male epileptic patients receiving antiepileptic medication. *Arch Neurol* 1990; **47**: 670–676.

Isojarvi JIT, Repo M, Pakarinen AJ, *et al.* Carbamazepine, phenytoin, sex hormones and sexual function in men with epilepsy. *Epilepsia* 1995; **36**: 366–370.

Isojarvi JIT, Lofgren E, Juntunen KST, *et al.* Effect of epilepsy and antiepileptic drugs on male reproductive health. *Neurology* 2004; **62**: 246–253.

Janz D, Schmidt D. Antiepileptic drugs and failure of oral contraceptives. *Lancet* 1974; 1(1113) (letter).

Kenyon IE. Unplanned pregnancy in an epileptic. *Br Med J* 1972; 1: 686–687.

Krauss GL, Brandt J, Campbell M, *et al*. Antiepileptic medication and oral contraceptive interactions: a national survey of neurologists and obstetricians. *Neurology* 1996; **46**: 1534–1539.

Mattson RH, Cramer JA. Epilepsy, sex hormones and antiepileptic drugs. *Epilepsia* 1985; **26** (Suppl. 1): 540–551.

Mattson RH, Cramer JC, Darney PD, *et al*. Use of oral contraceptives by women with epilepsy. *J Am Med Assoc* 1986; **256**: 238–240.

Mattson RH, Cramer JA, Siconolfi B, *et al*. Medroxyprogesteronee (Provera) in treatment of women with epilepsy. *Neurology* 1984; **34**: 1255–1258.

Macphee GJ, Larkin JG, Butler E, *et al*. Circulating hormones and pituitary responsiveness in young epileptic men receiving long-term antiepileptic medication. *Epilepsia* 1988; **29**: 468–475.

McAuley JW, Anderson GD. Treatment of epilepsy in women of reproductive age: pharmacokinetic considerations. *Clin Pharmacokient* 2004 (in press).

Mengel HB, Houston A, Back DJ. A evaluation of the interaction between tiagabine and oral contraceptives in female volunteers. *J Pharm Med* 1994; **4**: 141–150.

Morrell MJ, Sarro GE, Osborne Schaefer P, *et al*. 1996; Health issues for women with epilepsy: a descriptive survey to access knowledge and awareness among healthcare providers. *J Women Health Gend Base Med* 2000; **9**: 959–965.

Odlind V, Olsson SE. Enhanced metabolism of levonorgesterol during phenytoin treatment in a woman with Norplant implants. *Contraception* 1986; **33**: 257–261.

Ohman I, Vitols S, Tomson T. Lamotrigine in pregnancy: pharmacokinetics during delivery, in the neonate, and during lactation. *Epilepsia* 2000; **41**: 709–713.

Ragueneau-Majlessi I, Levy RH, Janik F. Levetiracetam does not alter the pharmacokinetics of an oral contraceptive in healthy women. *Epilepsia* 2002; **43**: 697–702.

Rosenfeld WE, Doose DR, Walker SA, *et al*. Effect of topiramate on the pharmacokinetics of an oral contraceptive containing norethindrone and ethinyl estradiol in patients with epilepsy. *Epilepsia* 1997; **38**: 317–323.

Saano V, Glue P, Banfield CR, *et al*. Effect of felbamate on the pharmacokinetics of a low-dose combination oral contraceptive. *Clin Pharmacol Ther* 1995; **58**: 523–531.

Sabers I, Buchholt JM, Udall P, *et al*. Lamotrigine plasma levels reduced by oral contraceptives. *Epilepsy Res* 2001; **47**: 151–154.

Sabers A, Ohman I, Christiansen J, *et al*. Oral contraceptives reduce lamotrigine plasma levels. *Neurology* 2003; **61**: 570–571.

Schmidt D. Effect of antiepileptic drugs on estrogen and progesterone metabolism and on oral contraception. In *Advances in Epileptology. Xllth Epilepsy International Symposium*, M. Dam, L. Gram, J. K. Penry, eds New York: Raven Press, 1981: 423–431.

Sonnen AE. Sodium valproate and the contraceptive pill. *Br J Clin Prac Symp Supp* 1983; **27**: 31–36.

Tran TA, Leppik IE, Blesi K, *et al*. Lamotrigine clearance during pregnancy. *Neurology* 2002; **59**: 251–255.

Wilbur K, Enson MHH. Pharmacokinetic drug interactions between oral contraceptives and second-generation anticonvulsants. *Clinl Pharmacokinet* 2000; **38**: 355–365.

19

Antiepileptic drug interactions in patients requiring psychiatric drug treatment

Michael R. Trimble[1] and Marco Mula[2]

[1] The National Hospital for Neurology and Neurosurgery, Institute of Neurology, Queen, Square, London, UK
[2] Amadeo Avogadro University, Novara, Italy

Classification of psychotropic drugs

Antidepressant drugs

Everybody is familiar with the tricyclic antidepressant drugs (TCAs). However, in recent years a number of newer antidepressant drugs have been introduced into clinical practice (Table 19.1). Essentially these are mainly non-tricyclic, earlier variants included mianserin, maprotiline and viloxazine.

The selective serotonin re-uptake inhibitors (SSRIs) are represented by citalopram, fluoxetine, fluvoxamine, sertraline and paroxetine. Of these, citalopram is the most selective on serotonergic uptake, inhibiting serotonin uptake 3000 times more than noradrenaline uptake, and 22 000 times more than that of dopamine. In general, the SSRIs are better tolerated and safer in overdose when compared with tricyclic drugs.

The latest generation of antidepressants has been developed to derive therapeutic benefits from tailor-made actions at specific monoamine receptor and re-uptake sites, in theory providing better efficacy and tolerability.

Reboxetine is a selective noradrenergic re-uptake inhibitor (NARI) with low affinity for histaminergic, cholinergic, dopaminergic and alpha-1 adrenergic receptors. It appears to be equally as effective as the tricyclics in treating depression, and there is a suggestion that it may be more effective than fluoxetine (Montgomery, 1997). Venlafaxine is a serotonin-noradrenergic re-uptake inhibitor (NSRI), which is similar to the earlier generation of antidepressants, but it does not interact with histaminergic or cholinergic receptors, thus diminishing side effects due to those receptor systems. Several studies have indicated equipotentiality or superior effectiveness with this compound compared with tricyclics (Burnett and Dinan, 1994).

Nefadazone is a noradrenaline serotonin re-uptake inhibitor whose most potent action is blockade of 5HT2 post-synaptic receptors, leading to a dual mechanism

Table 19.1 Classification of the psychotropic drugs currently in use

---

Antidepressants

Mono-amino-oxidase inhibitors (IMAOs) – moclobemide

Tricyclic antidepressant drugs (TCAs) – amitryptiline, nortriptyline, clomipramine, imipramine, desipramine

SSRIs – fluoxetine, paroxetine, sertraline, fluvoxamine, citalopram

NARIs – reboxetine

NSRIs – venlafaxine, nefazodone

Noradrenaline-selective serotonin reuptake inhibitors (NASSAs) – mirtazapine

Antipsychotics

Typical

  Phenothiazines – thioridazine, mesoridazine, chlorpromazine, prochlorperazine

  Buthyrophenones – haloperidol

  Others

Atypical

  Benzioxazoles and benzisothiazoles – risperidone, ziprasidone, perospirone

  Thienobenzodiazepine, dibenzothiazepine and dibenzothiazepine derivatives – clozapine, olanzapine, quetiapine

Minor tranquillizers

Barbiturates

Benzodiazepines

Others

Mood stabilizers

Lithium

Psychostimulant drugs

Methylphenidate, dextroamphetamine and permoline

Others (beta blockers, buspirone)

---

of action on the serotonin system at 5HT1 and 5HT3 subsites. Noradrenaline re-uptake inhibition is only minimal, and there is no interaction with histamine or cholinergic receptors.

Mirtazapine, or noradrenaline-specific serotonergic antidepressant has a selective action at alpha-2 adrenoreceptors, and only at some serotonin receptor subtypes. Its actions increase noradrenergic and serotoninergic transmission by blocking the alpha-2 autoreceptors. However, because it also blocks 5HT2 and 5HT3 receptors, the increased serotonin turnover only stimulates 5HT1 receptors. Thus it enhances noradrenergic and 5HT1A mediated serotoninergic neurotransmission. It is free of muscarinic, alpha-1 adrenergic and 5HT2- and 5HT3-related side effects, but its effects on histamine receptors can cause sedation and increased appetite. Several studies have shown equal or superior efficacy of this compound compared with other antidepressants (Bremner, 1995).

Antipsychotic drugs

As with the antidepressant drugs, in recent years there have been several newer agents introduced into clinical practice. These essentially, with some exceptions, fall into the class of atypical antipsychotics.

The classical neuroleptic drugs, such as chlorpromazine and haloperidol, antagonize dopamine D2 receptors. Their clinical efficacy has been shown to correlate with inhibitory activity at these receptor subtypes. However, these drugs block dopamine receptors in the striatum leading to catalepsy in animal models, and unwanted extrapyramidal side effects in patients.

The new generation of antipsychotic drugs essentially fall into two categories; those that are clozapine related, which included olanzapine and quetiapine, and others such as risperidone.

Although clozapine has been available for many years, it was initially not available for clinical use on account of its potential to produce agranulocytosis. However it has been reintroduced into clinical practice as a model of an atypical antipsychotic. The term essentially relates to the low potential of these compounds to cause extrapyramidal problems, and to have minimum effects on serum prolactin levels. The mechanism of atypicality seems to relate to activity at different receptor subtypes.

In general, the atypical antipsychotics occupy lower levels of D2 receptors than the classical antipsychotics, but one reason for their differing profile may be due to the rapid displacement of these agents from receptors by endogenous dopamine, then thus being more loosely bound to the receptor. The newer antipsychotic agents also have lower relative affinity for striatal D2 receptors as opposed to limbic D2 receptors (dorsal vs. ventral striatum).

Others

The minor tranquilizers mainly in use are the benzodiazepines, but their use in epilepsy is limited. Problems with dependency have led to caution with the use of these drugs, and in epilepsy withdrawal seizures can be a problem. Clobazam, a 1-5-benzodiazepine is used in the management of intractable seizures, and has effective anxiolytic properties.

The mood stabilizers include lithium, which is proconvulsant, and several antiepileptic drugs (AEDs). Of the older generation, carbamazepine (CBZ) and valproic acid have been shown to have antimanic properties and they help in the prophylaxis of mood disorders. Topiramate and lamotrigine are under investigation at the present time for their mood regulating properties. The mode of action on mood is unclear, and it may not be directly related to their antiepileptic properties.

Stimulants include amphetamine and methylphenidate. These are used mainly to control attention-deficit-hyperactivity disorders, which are not uncommon in the learning disabled, many of which patients also have epilepsy.

On the use of psychotropic drugs in epilepsy

It seems accepted that many patients with epilepsy have psychiatric syndromes, and recent epidemiologic evidence from selective clinics suggests that over 50% of patients may have a recognizable psychiatric disorder. It is also known that many patients with epilepsy receive psychotropic drugs, sometimes but not always on account of psychiatric symptoms. However, the effect of these drugs on the seizure threshold is variable, some, such as the benzodiazepines, being anticonvulsant, others, including many antidepressant and antipsychotic drugs, in contrast, are pro-convulsant.

It has been known ever since their introduction that tricyclic drugs are proconvulsant, and lead to seizures, which, for example in overdose, is one method of fatality.

Of the non-tricyclic drugs, both maprotiline and mianserin seem to be at the more proconvulsant end of the spectrum. Of the newer generation of drugs, the SSRIs are considered to provoke less in the way of seizures than tricyclics, and there is a possibility that the even newer, more selective drugs provoke even less in the way of seizures than the SSRIs, but more data on these compounds are needed. The reporting of seizures with all of the new drugs in clinical trials is at very low levels, either similar to, or lower than the less convulsant tricyclics (Hensiek and Trimble, 2001).

As with the newer antidepressants, there is little information about the effect of atypical neuroleptic drugs on the seizure threshold with the singular exception of clozapine. The latter was known to be proconvulsant from early studies, the seizures seemed to be a dose-related effect. The incidence of seizures rises to about 5% at doses of 600 mg, although electroencephalograph (EEG) changes may be recorded at lower doses, these results emerging from patients with schizophrenia, and not epilepsy. The seizures are often myoclonic, but can be generalized tonic/clonic, or partial depending on the individual patient.

It is perhaps of no coincidence, and of considerable interest that clozapine is probably the most effective antipsychotic drug available, reinforcing again a link between seizures and psychosis, and an integral part of neuropsychiatric practice.

Pharmacokinetic interactions between psychotropic drugs and anticonvulsants

The role of CYP450 system on metabolism of psychotropic drugs

The role of the CYP450 enzyme system and glucuronosyltransferases (UGTs) in clinical psychopharmacology is being increasingly recognized (Mula and Monaco, 2002b; Green and Tephly, 1998). Among antidepressants, TCAs, such as amitriptyline, clomipramine and imipramine, are extensively metabolized by CYP1A2, 2D6 and 3A4 (Table 19.2). Nortriptyline and desipramine are, respectively, the active metabolites

Table 19.2 CYP enzymes involved in psychotropic drug metabolism

CYP1A2	CYP3A4	CYP2C9/10	CYP2C19	CYP2D6
Antidepressants	**Antidepressants**	**Anticonvulsants**	**Antidepressants**	**Antidepressants**
Amitriptyline	Amitriptyline	Phenytoin	Amitriptyline	Fluoxetine
Clomipramine	Clomipramine	**Antipsychotics**	Citalopram	Paroxetine
Imipramine	Desipramine	Thioridazine	Clomipramine	Mianserin
Trazodone	Imipramine	Olanzapine	Imipramine	Venlafaxine
Fluvoxamine	Norclomipramine		Moclobemide	Trazodone
Antipsychotics	Nortriptyline		**Anticonvulsants**	Nefazodone
Chlorpromazine	Trimipramine		Mephenytoin	Amitriptyline
Haloperidol	Nefazodone		Esobarbital	Clomipramine
Clozapine	Sertraline		Mephobarbital	Desipramine
Olanzapine	Venlafaxine			Imipramine
Ziprasidone	**Antipsychotics**			Norclomipramine
	Haloperidol			Nortryptiline
	Clozapine			Trimipramine
	Risperidone			Maprotiline
	Ziprasidone			**Antipsychotics**
	Iloperidone			Chlorpromazine
	Quetiapine			Thioridazine
	Anticonvulsants			Haloperidol
	Carbamazepine			Olanzapine
				Risperidone
				Iloperidone
				Quetiapine

of amitriptyline and imipramine and are metabolized mainly by CYP2D6.
Moclobemide is primarily metabolized by CYP2C subfamily, of which it is probably
an inhibitor, while the atypical antidepressants mianserin and trazodone are metabolized by CYP2D6.

The SSRIs, fluoxetine and paroxetine are metabolized by CYP2D6, while sertraline, fluvoxamine and citalopram are respectively metabolized by CYP3A4, 1A2
and 2C. Paroxetine and fluvoxamine are, respectively, inhibitors of CYP2D6 and
1A2 (Table 19.3). In vitro and in vivo data demonstrated a moderate inhibition
activity of fluoxetine on CYP2D6 and 3A4, probably mediated by its metabolites.
No clinically significant induction–inhibition properties have been demonstrated
for sertraline and citalopram.

Among the new generation of antidepressant drugs, venlafaxine is primarily
metabolized by CYP2D6, while CYP3A4 metabolizes nefazodone and reboxetine.
Nefazodone is a potent inhibitor of this enzymatic pathway.

Table 19.3 CYP enzymes inhibited by different psychotropic drugs

CYP isoenzyme	Antidepressants	Antipsychotics
CYP1A2	Fluvoxamine	
CYP3A4	Fluoxetine Sertraline Nefazodone	Chlorpromazine Thioridazine Haloperidol Risperidone
CYP2C9/10/19	Fluoxetine Sertraline Fluvoxamine Moclobemide	Thioridazine Clozapine
CYP2D6	Fluoxetine Paroxetine Sertraline	Thioridazine Haloperidol Clozapine Olanzapine Risperidone

Neuroleptics, such as phenothiazines, are metabolized by intestinal sulfoxidases, although CYP2D6 plays an important role in chlorpromazine and thioridazine metabolism. They are also partially metabolized by CYP1A2 and 2C, respectively, and partially inhibit CYP3A4. Haloperidol's metabolism has been studied for more than 30 years. It is metabolized by CYP3A4 and 1A2 and only partially by 2D6.

Among the atypical antipsychotics, clozapine undergoes extensive hepatic metabolism and multiple CYP enzymes are involved, however the two prominent ones are CYP1A2 and CYP3A4.

New antipsychotic drugs usually have better pharmacokinetic profiles. Risperidone is primarily metabolized by CYP2D6, although a correlation study using a panel of human microsomes suggest that CYP3A4 may also be involved. Olanzapine undergoes extensive hepatic metabolism and shares some of its metabolic routes with the structurally and pharmacologically related clozapine, but UGTs appear to be major metabolic pathways. Quetiapine shares some pharmacologic and structural characteristics with clozapine and olanzapine. In vitro studies using human microsomes showed that CYP3A4 is the main isoenzyme involved in quetiapine metabolism.

Interactions between anticonvulsants and antidepressants

SSRI–NSRI

Data about fluoxetine–CBZ interactions are contradictory. Spina *et al.* (1993) found no modification in CBZ plasma levels before and after fluoxetine administration, although in a small group of patients. Grimsley *et al.* (1991) observed a slight increase in CBZ area under curve (AUC) levels and a decrease in 10,11-CBZ-epoxide AUC.

Nelson *et al.* (2001) studied the inhibition properties of several SSRIs on phenytoin (PHT) metabolism in an in vitro study with human liver microsomes. They suggested that the risk for a PHT–SSRI interaction is highest with fluoxetine and less likely with the others (paroxetine and sertraline).

Andersen *et al.* (1991) investigated possible kinetic interaction between paroxetine and CBZ, VPA and PHT in a single-blind, placebo-controlled, crossover trial. Paroxetine caused no change in plasma concentrations and protein binding of the anticonvulsants. Studies of paroxetine plasma concentrations are lacking, but the major enzymatic pathway is a non-inducible enzyme (CYP2D6), therefore modifications in plasma levels are unlikely, when co-administrated with AEDs with inducer properties.

Leinonen *et al.* (1996) observed an increase in citalopram levels when CBZ was substituted with oxcarbazepine in two patients, demonstrating a significant induction effect of CBZ on citalopram metabolism.

Spina *et al.* (1993) studied the potential interaction between CBZ and fluvoxamine in eight epileptic patients in steady state for CBZ. No significant changes in CBZ and CBZ-10,11-epoxide occurred.

Mamiya *et al.* (2001) described a single case of PHT intoxication (from 16.6 to 49.1 µg/ml) after fluvoxamine administration. There are no studies of VPA–fluvoxamine interactions.

Not clear is the possibility of an interaction between sertraline and PHT. Haselberger *et al.* (1997) described an elevation in PHT plasma levels in two elderly patients, but without any symptoms of toxicity, while Rapeport *et al.* (1996a) demonstrated the absence of any pharmacokinetic interaction in a double-blind, randomized, placebo-controlled study with 30 healthy volunteers.

Kaufman and Gerner (1998) reported two cases of lamotrigine–sertraline interaction, leading to high lamotrigine plasma levels (doubled in the first case and 33% increase in the second one). Rapeport *et al.* (1996b), in a double-blind, randomized, placebo-controlled study on 14 healthy volunteers, observed no significant effects of sertraline on CBZ pharmacokinetics. Bonate *et al.* (2000) demonstrated the absence of drug interaction between clonazepam and sertraline in a randomized, double-blind, placebo-controlled, crossover study with 13 subjects.

No clinical studies are available about potential interactions between venlafaxine and AEDs. Toy *et al.* (1995) demonstrated no pharmacokinetic interactions between venlafaxine and diazepam in a randomized, crossover study with 18 male subjects.

Roth and Bertschy (2001) reported three cases of increased CBZ plasma levels (from 20% to 100%) after nefazodone introduction. Laroudie *et al.* (2000) investigated kinetic interactions between nefazodone and CBZ in 12 healthy subjects. They observed a significant decrease in nefazodone AUC and an increase in CBZ AUC, demonstrating a potential inhibition property of nefazodone on CBZ metabolism.

TCA

Generally, phenobarbital (PB), CBZ and PHT stimulate the metabolism of TCAs, while VPA can increase their plasma levels (Monaco and Cicolin, 1999). Wong *et al.* (1996) investigated the effect of VPA on amitriptyline and its active metabolite (nortriptyline) in an open-label study. The mean AUC and the peak plasma concentration, for the sum of nortriptyline and amitriptyline, were 42% and 19% higher. Fehr *et al.* (2000) reported the increase in serum clomipramine levels when coprescribed with VPA.

Szymura *et al.* (2001) investigated the effect of CBZ on imipramine and desipramine serum concentrations in 13 patients with major depression. They demonstrated that CBZ affects not only the metabolism of both TCAs but also their protein binding, leading to a significant increase in the free fraction. Because of this phenomenon, a modification in imipramine dosage regimen does not seem to be necessary in practice. Conversely, Van Belle *et al.* (1995) demonstrated a significant inhibition in CBZ metabolism by clomipramine in rats.

Others

Ketter *et al.* (1995) investigated the safety and efficacy of CBZ-moclobemide cotreatment in a double-blind study. The combination was well tolerated with no modifications in CBZ kinetics, but they did not assess moclobemide plasma concentrations.

Nawishy *et al.* (1981) investigated the presence of kinetic interactions between mianserin and three commonly prescribed anticonvulsants (PHT, CBZ and PB). All of them are inducers of the CYP450 enzyme system. They observed a significant reduction in mianserin plasma concentrations.

The use of bupropion is limited by the high seizure risk. CBZ is a potent inducer of its metabolism, taking the antidepressant plasma concentrations to undetectable levels. On the other hand, bupropion has shown marked inhibition properties, increasing VPA levels when prescribed in cotherapy (Popli *et al.*, 1995), and Tekle and al-Kamis (1990) suggested a potential inhibition property of bupropion on PHT metabolism. Odishaw and Chen (2000) investigated the effect of steady state slow release bupropion on the pharmacokinetics of lamotrigine in a randomized, open-label, crossover study with 12 healthy subjects. The kinetic parameters of a single 100-mg lamotrigine dose were not modified significantly.

Interactions between anticonvulsants and antipsychotic drugs

Phenothiazines–butyrophenones

Thioridazine is metabolized by intestinal sulfoxidases that are induced only partially by AED inducers such as CBZ, PHT and PB but some authors have reported an increased clearance of thioridazine and a relevant decrease of mesoridazine (the active metabolite of thioridazine) in patients taking CBZ and/or PHT (Ellenor *et al.*, 1978; Linnoila *et al.*, 1980). On the other hand, thioridazine, as chlorpromazine and prochlorperazine, inhibits PHT (Vincent, 1980; Kutt, 1984), PB (Gay and Madsen, 1983) and VPA (Guengerich, 1997) metabolism.

Several studies have shown that haloperidol plasma levels decrease by 50–60% after CBZ co-administration, with concomitant worsening of the psychiatric clinical features (Kidron *et al.*, 1985; Jann *et al.*, 1985; Arana *et al.*, 1986). Hirokane *et al.* (1999) evaluated haloperidol levels in patients comedicated with CBZ or PB. In the first group plasma levels were 37% lower; in patients treated with PB they were 22% lower. Interestingly, Iwahashi *et al.* (1995) observed that serum CBZ concentrations in patients treated without haloperidol were significantly decreased (on average 40%), compared to those treated with both CBZ and haloperidol. Hesslinger *et al.* (1999) compared the effects of CBZ and VPA cotreatment on the plasma levels of haloperidol and on the psychopathologic outcome in schizophrenic patients. VPA had no significant effects on haloperidol plasma levels and it was associated with a better psychopathologic outcome. Doose *et al.* (1999) investigated the effect of topiramate on haloperidol pharmacokinetics in healthy volunteers, observing no clinically significant interactions.

Benzisoxazoles and benzisothiazoles

Preliminary evidence from drug monitoring studies and case reports (Bork *et al.*, 1999; Spina *et al.*, 2000) demonstrated that CBZ might cause a prominent decrease in plasma concentrations of risperidone. Spina *et al.* (2000) compared the risperidone total active moiety (risperidone plus its active metabolite – TAM) steady state plasma concentrations in patients treated with risperidone alone and in patients comedicated with CBZ or VPA. Unlike CBZ, VPA (at dosages up to 1200–1500 mg/day) had minimal and clinically insignificant effects on plasma levels of risperidone TAM, suggesting that VPA could be added safely to an existing treatment with risperidone. Ono *et al.* (2002) evaluated the relationship between CYP2D6 genotype and the pharmacokinetic interaction with CBZ, suggesting that the decrease in risperidone concentration is dependent on the CYP2D6 activity. Recently, an open study described a mild increase in CBZ plasma levels in eight patients with epilepsy after addition of risperidone 1 mg, suggesting that the antipsychotic, or more likely its metabolites, could modulate CYP3A4 activity

(Mula and Monaco, 2002a). Interestingly, Furukory *et al.* (2001) demonstrated a different enantioselective 9-hydroxylation of risperidone by CYP2D6 and CYP3A4. In the literature, there is no information about differences in pharmacologic activity of these two enantiomers.

Ziprasidone and perospirone are newly available antipsychotic drugs and there are few clinical studies about their interactions. Miceli *et al.* (2000) studied the effect of CBZ on steady-state ziprasidone in healthy volunteers in an open, randomized, parallel-group study. They observed a clinically insignificant reduction ($<36\%$) in steady-state ziprasidone levels.

Thienobenzodiazepine, dibenzothiazepine and dibenzothiazepine derivatives

Generally, PHT, PB and CBZ (Facciola *et al.*, 1998; Prior *et al.*, 1999) cause a decrease in clozapine plasma concentrations. However, CBZ is rarely used in combination with clozapine because of the high risk of haematologic side effects. Existing data on the effect of VPA co-administration are contradictory (Centorrino *et al.*, 1994; Costello and Suppes, 1995; Longo and Salzman, 1995; Facciola *et al.*, 1999). According to some authors, VPA has a moderate inhibiting effect on the demethylation of clozapine (catalysed by CYP1A2 and 3A4) but, in two small studies (Finley and Warner, 1994; Longo and Salzman, 1995) serum concentrations of clozapine and norclozapine (one of clozapine's metabolites) were found to decrease respectively by 15% and 65%, suggesting induction of clozapine metabolism. Moreover, clozapine disposition is characterized by large interindividual variability, being affected by age, gender, body weight, dose per kg, smoking habits and ethnicity (Chong and Remington, 1998).

Olanzapine plasma concentrations are decreased by CBZ (Lucas *et al.*, 1998), but the authors did not consider this interaction clinically relevant because of the wide therapeutic index of the antipsychotic. In the literature, there are no controlled studies assessing drug interactions between olanzapine and new AEDs in humans.

Quetiapine is a newly introduced atypical antipsychotic, and clinical data about pharmacokinetic interactions are lacking. Wong *et al.* (2001) demonstrated that PHT has a marked effect on the metabolism of quetiapine, suggesting that dosage adjustment of quetiapine may be necessary when quetiapine is coprescribed with other AED inducers such as CBZ or PB.

Interactions between anticonvulsants and anxiolytics

Generally, anxiolytics have a wide therapeutic index; therefore the clinical relevance of pharmacokinetic interactions is very limited. AEDs with enzyme-inducing properties may stimulate the biotrasformation of many benzodiazepines. CBZ has been reported to induce clobazam and diazepam metabolism (Dhillon and Richens, 1981; Levy *et al.*, 1983). CBZ has also been demonstrated to enhance the clearance of clonazepam and alprazolam (Lai *et al.*, 1978; Furukori *et al.*, 1998). A clinically relevant interaction occurs between AED inducers and midazolam (Backman *et al.*, 1996) that is extensively metabolized by CYP3A4.

Pharmacodynamic interactions between antiepileptic and psychotropic agents

Anticonvulsants and antidepressants

Antidepressants have been extensively evaluated in relation to the general problem of their proconvulsant activity. But the definition of pharmacodynamic interaction implies that the typical pharmacologic properties of a drug are modified by another drug, without any change in the drug concentration. This definition comprises also side effects such as sedation, confusion, psychomotor impairment and others.

The risk of antidepressant-induced seizures is well known, particularly in people with epilepsy. Most of the data arise from studies using in vitro technique, animal studies and clinical observations (Torta and Monaco, 2002). Among SSRIs, fluoxetine is the most studied drug. It is interesting to note that several studies emphasized the role of serotoninergic transmission in enhancing the anticonvulsant effects of AEDs (Trimble *et al.*, 1977; Yan *et al.*, 1994). Leander (1992) demonstrated, in an animal model of epilepsy, that the selective inhibition of serotonin uptake by fluoxetine can enhance the anticonvulsant potency of PHT and CBZ. Therefore, a favourable pharmacodynamic interaction may be suggested (Table 19.4).

As far as other interactions are concerned, Dursun *et al.* (1993) reported a single severe case of the serotonin syndrome after fluoxetine was added to carbamazepine. The occurrence of an extrapyramidal syndrome within fluoxetine and AED cotreatment (Gernaat *et al.*, 1991) are described, but clinical studies are lacking.

Two different studies of Rapeport *et al.* (1996a, b) investigated pharmacodynamic interactions between sertraline and PHT or CBZ. Both of them showed no clinically significant interactions.

Anticonvulsants and antipsychotic drugs

Historically, antipsychotic drugs have been considered proconvulsants possibly because of their D2-receptor blocking activity. One of the most important issues in prescribing these two types of drug at the same time is about the effect of antipsychotics on the anticonvulsant effect of AEDs.

To determine the risk for drug-induced seizures we can use different approaches: observational studies (case-control studies and case reports), drug-induced EEG changes, animal models and in vitro techniques in isolated tissue samples. One of the problems of the recent literature is that most of the studies have been

Table 19.4 Pharmacokinetic interactions between antiepileptic and antidepressant drugs (from Mula and Trimble, 2003)

	CBZ	VPA	PHT	LTG	TPM	PB
Fluoxetine	(=↑)	(↓)	(↑)			
Paroxetine	(=)	(=)	(=)			
Citalopram	↓ (=)					
Sertraline	↓ (=)		(↑=)			
Fluvoxamine	(=)		(↑)			
Venlafaxine	(=)					
Reboxetine	↓					
Amitryptiline	↓	↑				
Clomipramine	↓ (↑)	↑	↓			↓
Imipramine	↓*	↑	↓			↓
Desipramine	↓*	↑	↓			↓
Nortriptyline	↓	↑	↓			↓
Moclobemide	(=)					
Mianserin	↓		↓			↓
Trazodone			(↑)			
Mirtazapine	↓ (=)					
Nefazodone	↓ (↑)					
Bupropion	↓	(↑)	(↑)	(=)		
Viloxazine			(↑)	(↑)		

Symbols on the left are referred to antidepressant drug and within brackets to anticonvulsant drug, when prescribed in combination (in blank fields data are not available).

↑, Increased plasma concentration; ↓, decreased plasma concentration; =, unchanged plasma concentration.

*Dosage adjustments are not necessary.

LTG, lamotrigine; TPM, topiramate.

performed on psychiatric patients and, although theoretically correct, it is not known if drug-related seizures in non-epileptic patients predict risk in patients with epilepsy, and if different syndromes of epilepsy have different risks for psychotropic-induced seizures.

Generally chlorpromazine and clozapine are considered proconvulsant in epileptic patients. The former only at high doses (1000 mg/day) and the latter at medium and high doses (>600 mg/day) (Alldredge, 1999). Clozapine frequently causes epileptiform EEG changes and seizures in 3–5% of patients treated, even at therapeutic doses. Devinsky *et al.* (1991) observed a mean prevalence of seizures of 2.9% with clozapine, and considering different doses, the prevalence is respectively 1, 2.7 and 4.4% for doses <300 mg, 300–600 mg or 600–900 mg/daily. Pacia and

Table 19.5 Risk for seizures exhibited by some antidepressant and antipsychotic drugs

High risk	Intermediate risk	Low risk
Antidepressant drugs		
Buproprion	Amitriptyline	SSRIs
Clomipramine	Imipramine	Trazodone
Maprotiline		Venlafaxine
		IMAO
Antipsychotic drugs		
Chlorpromazine (dose related)	Olanzapine	Fluphenazine
Clozapine (titration and dose related)	Quetiapine	Pimozide
	Haloperidol	Trifluoperazine
		Risperidone

Table 19.6 Pharmacokinetic interactions between antiepileptic and antipsychotic drugs (from Mula and Monaco, 2002)

	CBZ	PB	PHT	VPA	LTG	TPM
Chlorpromazine	↓ (↑)	(↑)	(↑)	(↑)		
Thioridazine	↓	↓ (↑)	↓ (↑)	(↑)		
Mesoridazine	↓		↓			
Haloperidol	↓ (↑)	↓	↓	=	=*	=
Clozapine	↓	↓	↓	=↑		
Olanzapine	↓	↓*	↓*	↑*	=*	
Risperidone	↓ (↑)	↓*	↓*	=		
Ziprasidone	↓	↓*	↓*			
Iloperidone	↓* (↑)	↓*	↓*	=*		
Quetiapine	↓	↓*	↓			

Symbols on the left are referred to antipsychotic drug and within brackets to anticonvulsant drug, when prescribed in combination (in blank fields data are not available).

↑, Increased plasma concentration; ↓, Decreased plasma concentration; =, Unchanged plasma concentration;

*Theoretical data, no clinical studies available.

Devinsky (1994) analysed only patients without a previous history of seizures and the prevalence of seizures was respectively 0.9, 0.8 and 1.5% for the same range of doses of the previous study. Thus, with clozapine this seems to be a dose-related phenomenon but probably the role of the titration time and increase of dose is more important (Langosch and Trimble, 2002).

Olanzapine, quetiapine and risperidone demonstrated an extremely low risk of seizures when compared with haloperidol and can be considered safer (Tables 19.5 and 19.6).

Anticonvulsants and lithium

Lithium carbonate is frequently used for manic episodes in bipolar disorder, in association with valproate and carbamazepine. Carbamazepine also demonstrates antimanic properties, and a possible favourable pharmacodynamic interaction could be suggested, but carbamazepine can increase lithium toxicity as well. Shukla *et al.* (1984) suggested that CBZ enhanced the development of a lithium neurotoxic syndrome in patients with underlying central nervous system (CNS) disease or metabolic disease. This syndrome is characterized by symptoms such as confusion, drowsiness, lethargy, tremor and cerebellar signs that are typical of both lithium and CBZ toxicity. Therefore, a pharmacodynamic synergic interaction is probable. Kramlinger and Post (1990) studied the effects of this combination in 23 patients with affective disorders. They observed a significant increase in many haematologic parameters (mainly the mean white blood cell count, probably lithium counteracts the neutropenic properties of carbamazepine) and a significant modification in thyroid function with decrease in T4 and freeT4. Another well-known issue is the opposing effects of CBZ and lithium on electrolyte regulation, with the occurrence of severe hyponatremia when lithium alone is stopped (Vieweg *et al.*, 1991).

The combination of lithium and VPA is widely used in rapid cycling, manic, depressive and mixed episodes in bipolar disorder. This combination has a higher tolerability than the co-administered CBZ and a pharmacodynamic synergistic interaction has been suggested (Freeman and Stoll, 1998).

Chen *et al.* (2000) investigated lithium pharmacokinetics when co-prescribed with lamotrigine in 20 healthy subjects. There were no significant differences in lithium pharmacokinetic parameters.

Conclusions

Several factors must be considered when predicting the outcome of a potential interaction: patient-related (sex, age, ethnicity) and drug-related (the presence of active metabolites, the activity and potency at the enzyme site, the therapeutic window). Clinicians should be aware of these potential interactions especially if the patient shows no response to a psychotropic drug therapy or signs and symptoms of intoxication.

As far as antidepressant drugs are concerned, fluoxetine and nefazodone interactions are probably the most relevant in epilepsy from a clinical point of view. The former for its long half-life and the presence of different enantiomers with different kinetic properties, and the latter for its inhibitory properties on CYP3A4. AED inducers increase the clearance of all the antipsychotic drugs; therefore dosage adjustments are quite often required for antipsychotics.

Careful clinical monitoring and personalized dosages and titration time can usually lower the risk threshold of side effects due to pharmacologic interactions, which is one of the major factors for good clinical practice and patient compliance.

REFERENCES

Andersen BB, Mikkelsen M, Vesterager A, *et al*. No influence of the antidepressant paroxetine on carbamazepine, valproate and phenytoin. *Epilepsy Res* 1991; **10**: 201–204.

Arana GW, Goff DC, Friedman H, *et al*. Does carbamazepine reduction in haloperidol plasma levels worsen psychotic symptoms? *Am J Psychiatry* 1986; **143**: 650–651.

Ascalone V, Ripamonti M, Malavasi B. Stereospecific determination of amisulpride, a new benzamide derivative, in human plasma and urine by automated solid-phase extraction and liquid chromatography on chiral column application to pharmacokinetics. *J Chromatogr B Biomed Appl* 1986; **676**: 95–105.

Backman TJ, Olkkola KT, Ojala M, *et al*. Concentrations and effects of oral midazolam are greatly reduced in patients on carbamazepine or phenytoin. *Epilepsia* 1996; **37**: 253–257.

Bonate PL, Kroboth PD, Smith RB, *et al*. Clonazepam and sertraline: absence of drug interaction in a multiple-dose study. *J Clin Psychopharmacol* 2000; **20**: 19–27.

Bork JA, Rogers T, Wedlund PJ, *et al*. A pilot study on risperidone metabolism: the role of Cytochrome P450 2D6 and 3A. *J Clin Psychiatry* 1999; **60**: 469–476.

Bremner JD. A double blind comparison of ORE 3770, amitriptyline and placebo in major depression. *J Clin Psychiatry* 1995; **56**: 519–526.

Burnett FE, Dinan TG. The clinical effectiveness of venlafaxine in the treatment of depression. *Rev Contemp Pharmacol* 1994; **9**: 303–320.

Centorrino F, Baldessarini RJ, Kando J, *et al*. Serum concentrations of clozapine and its major metabolites: effects of cotreatment with fluoxetine or valproate. *Am J Psychiatry* 1994; **151**: 123–125.

Chen C, Veronese L, Yin Y. The effects of lamotrigine on the pharmacokinetics of lithium. *Br J Clin Pharmacol* 2000; **50**: 193–195.

Chong SA, Remington G. Ethnicity and clozapine metabolism. *Br J Psychiatry* 1998; **172**: 97 [Letter].

Costello LE, Suppes T. A clinically significant interaction between clozapine and valproate. *J Clin Psychopharmacol* 1995; **15**: 139–141.

Coukell AJ, Spencer CM, Benfield P. Amisulpride: a review of its pharmacodynamic and pharmacokinetic properties and therapeutic efficacy in the management of schizophrenia. *CNS Drugs* 1996; **6**: 237–256.

Devinsky O, Honigfeld G, Patin J. Clozapine-related seizures. *Neurology* 1991; **41**(3): 369–371.

Dhillon S, Richens A. Pharmacokinetics of diazepam in epileptic patients and normal volunteers following intravenous administration. *Br J Clin Pharmacol* 1981; **12**: 841–844.

Doose DR, Kohl KA, Desai-Krieger D, *et al*. No clinically significant effect of topiramate on haloperidol plasma concentration. *Eur Neuropsychopharmacol* 1999; **9**: S357 [Abstract].

Dorn JM. A case of phenytoin toxicity possibly precipitated by trazodone. *J Clin Psychiatry* 1986; **47**: 89–90.

Dursun SM, Mathew VM, Reveley MA. Toxic serotonin syndrome after fluoxetine plus carbamazepine. *Lancet* 1993; **342**: 442–443.

Ellenor GL, Musa MN, Beuthin FC. Phenobarbital–thioridazine interaction in man. *Res Commun Chem Pathol Pharmacol* 1978; **21**: 185–188.

Ereshefsky L. Pharmacokinetics and drug interactions: update for new antipsychotics. *J Clin Psychiatry* 1996; **57**(Suppl. 11): 12–25.

Facciola G, Avenoso A, Spina E, *et al.* Inducing effect of phenobarbital on clozapine metabolism in patients with chronic schizophrenia. *Ther Drug Monit* 1998; **20**: 628–630.

Facciola G, Avenoso A, Scordo MG, *et al.* Small effects of valproic acid on the plasma concentrations of clozapine and its major metabolites in patients with schizophrenic or affective disorders. *Ther Drug Monit* 1999; **21**: 341–345.

Fang J, Bourin M, Becher GB. Metabolism of risperidone to 9-hydroxy-risperidone by human cytochromes P450 2D6 and 3A4. *Naunyn Schniedeberg's Arch Pharmacol* 1999; **359**: 147–151.

Fehr C, Grunder G, Hiemke C, *et al.* Increase in serum clomipramine concentrations caused by valproate. *J Clin Psychopharmacol* 2000; **20**: 493–494.

Finley P, Warner D. Potential impact of valproic acid therapy on clozapine disposition. *Biol Psychiatry* 1994; **36**: 487–488.

Freeman MP, Stoll AL. Mood stabilizer combinations: a review of safety and efficacy. *Am J Psychiatry* 1998; **155**: 12–21.

Furukori H, Otani K, Yasui N, *et al.* Effect of carbamazepine on the single oral dose pharmacokinetics of alprazolam. *Neuropsychopharmacology* 1998; **18**: 364–369.

Furukory NY, Hidestrand M, Spina E, *et al.* Different enantioselective 9-hydroxylation of risperidone by the two human CYP2D6 and CYP3A4 enzymes. *Drug Metab Dispos* 2001; **29**: 1263–1268.

Gay PE, Madsen JA. Interaction between phenobarbital and thioridazine. *Neurology* 1983; **33**: 1631–1632.

Gernaat HB, Van de Woude J, Touw DJ. Fluoxetine and parkinsonism in patients taking carbamazepine. *Am J Psychiatry* 1991; **148**: 1604–1605.

Green MD, Tephly TR. Glucuronidation of amine substrates by purified and expressed UDP-glucuronosyltransferase proteins. *Drug Metab Dispos* 1998; **26**: 860–867.

Grimsley SR, Jann MW, Carter JG, *et al.* Increased carbamazepine plasma concentrations after fluoxetine coadministration. *Clin Pharmacol Ther* 1991; **50**: 10–15.

Guengerich FP. Role of cytochrome P450 enzymes in drug–drug interactions. *Adv Pharmacol* 1997; **43**: 7–35.

Hamon-Vilcot B, Chaufour S, Deschamps JT, *et al.* Safety and pharmacokinetics of a single dose of amisulpride in healthy elderly volunteers. *Eur J Clin Pharmacol* 1998; **54**: 405–409.

Haselberger MB, Freedman LS, Tolbert S. Elevated serum phenytoin concentrations associated with coadministration of sertraline. *J Clin Psychopharmacol* 1997; **17**: 107–109.

Hensiek A, Trimble MR. Relevance of new psychotropic drugs for the neurologist. *J Neurol Neurosurg Psychiatry* 2002; **72**: 281–285.

Hesslinger B, Normann C, Langosch JM, *et al.* Effects of carbamazepine and valproate on haloperidol plasma levels and on psychopathologic outcome in schizophrenic patients. *J Clin Psychopharmacol* 1999; **19**: 310–315.

Hirokane G, Someya T, Takahashi S, *et al.* Interindividual variation of plasma haloperidol concentrations and the impact of concomitant medications: the analysis of therapeutic drug monitoring data. *Ther Drug Monit* 1999; **21**: 82–86.

Iwahashi K, Miyatake R, Suwaki H, *et al.* The drug–drug interaction effects of haloperidol on plasma carbamazepine levels. *Clin Neuropharmacol* 1995; **18**: 233–236.

Jann MW, Ereshefsky L, Saklad SR, *et al.* Effects of carbamazepine on plasma haloperidol levels. *J Clin Psychopharmacol* 1985; **5**: 106–109.

Kaufman KR, Gerner R. Lamotrigine toxicity secondary to sertraline. *Seizure* 1998; **7**: 163–165.

Ketter TA, Post RM, Parekh PI, *et al.* Addition of monoamine oxidase inhibitors to carbamazepine: preliminary evidence of safety and antidepressant efficacy in treatment-resistant depression. *J Clin Psychiatry* 1995; **56**: 471–475.

Kidron R, Averbuch I, Klein E, *et al.* Carbamazepine-induced reduction of blood levels of haloperidol in chronic schizophrenia. *Biol Psychiatry* 1985; **20**: 219–222.

Kramlinger KG, Post RM. Addition of lithium carbonate to carbamazepine: haematological and thyroid effects. *Am J Psychiatry* 1990; **147**: 615–620.

Kudo S, Ishizaki T. Pharmacokinetics of haloperidol: an update. *Clin Pharmacokinet* 1999; **37**: 435–456.

Kutt H. Interactions between anticonvulsants and other commonly prescribed drugs. *Epilepsia* 1984; **225**(Suppl. 2): S118–S131.

Lai AA, Levy RH, Cutler RE. Time-course of interaction between carbamazepine and clonazepam in normal man. *Clin Pharmacol Ther* 1978; **24**: 316–323.

Langosch JM, Trimble MR. Epilepsy, psychosis and clozapine. *Human Psychopharmacol: Clin and Exp* 2002; **17**: 115–119.

Laroudie C, Salazar DE, Cosson JP, *et al.* Carbamazepine–nefazodone interaction in healthy subjects. *J Clin Psychopharmacol* 2000; **20**: 46–53.

Leander JD. Fluoxetine, a selective serotonin-uptake inhibitor, enhances the anticonvulsant effects of phenytoin, carbamazepine and ameltolide (LY201116). *Epilepsia* 1992; **33**: 573–576.

Leinonen E, Lepola U, Koponen H. Substituting carbamazepine with oxcarbazepine increases citalopram levels. A report on two cases. *Pharmacopsychiatry* 1996; **29**: 156–158.

Levy RH, Lane EA, Guyot M, *et al.* Analysis of parent drug-metabolite relationship in the presence of an inducer: application to the carbamazepine–clobazam interaction in normal man. *Drug Metab Dispos* 1983; **11**: 286–292.

Linnoila M, Viukari M, Vaisanen K, *et al.* Effect of anticonvulsants in plasma haloperidol and thioridazine levels. *Am J Psychiatry* 1980; **137**: 829–921.

Longo LP, Salzman C. Valproic acid effects on serum concentrations of clozapine and norclozapine. *Am J Psychiatry* 1995; **152**: 650.

Lucas RA, Gilfillan DJ, Bergstrom RF. A pharmacokinetic interaction between carbamazepine and olanzapine: observations on possible mechanism. *Eur J Clin Pharmacol* 1998; **54**: 639–643.

Lucena MI, Blanco E, Corrales MA, *et al.* Interaction of fluoxetine and valproic acid. *Am J Psychiatry* 1998; **155**: 575.

Mamiya K, Kojima K, Yukawa E, *et al.* Phenytoin intoxication induced by fluvoxamine. *Ther Drug Monit* 2001; **23**: 75–77.

Miceli JJ, Anziano RJ, Robarge L, *et al.* The effect of carbamazepine on the steady-state pharmacokinetics of ziprasidone in healthy volunteers. *Br J Clin Pharmacol* 2000; **49**(Suppl. 1): S65–S70.

Monaco F, Cicolin A. Interaction between anticonvulsant and psychoactive drugs. *Epilepsia* 1999; **40**(Suppl. 10): S71–S76.

Montgomery SA. Reboxetine: additional benefits to depressed patients. *J Psychopharmacol* 1997; **11**(Suppl.): S9–S15.

Mula M, Monaco F. Carbamazepine–risperidone interactions in patients with epilepsy. *Clin Neuropharmacol* 2002a; **25**: 97–100.

Mula M, Monaco F. Antiepileptic–antipsychotic drug interactions. A critical review of the evidence. *Clin Neuropharmacol* 2002b (in press).

Mutlib AE, Klein JT. Application of liquid chromatography/mass spectrometry in accelerating the identification of human liver cytochrome P450 isoforms involved in the metabolism of iloperidone. *J Pharmacol Exp Ther* 1998; **286**: 1285–1293.

Nawishy S, Hathaway N, Turner P. Interactions of anticonvulsant drugs with mianserin and nomifensine. *Lancet* 1981; **2**: 871–872.

Nelson MH, Birnbaum AK, Remmel RP. Inhibition of phenytoin hydroxylation in human liver microsomes by several selective serotonin re-uptake inhibitors. *Epilepsy Res* 2001; **44**: 71–82.

Odishaw J, Chen C. Effects of steady state bupropion on the pharmacokinetics of lamotrigine in healthy subjects. *Pharmacotherapy* 2000; **20**: 1448–1453.

Ono S, Mihara K, Suzuki A, *et al.* Significant pharmacokinetic interaction between risperidone and carbamazepine: its relationship with CYP2D6 genotypes. *Psychopharmacology (Berl)* 2002; **162**: 50–54.

Pacia SV, Devinsky O. Clozapine seizures: experience with 5629 patients. *Neurology* 1994; **44**: 2247–2249.

Popli AP, Tanquary J, Lamparella V, *et al.* Bupropion and anticonvulsant drug interactions. *Ann Clin Psychiatry* 1995; **7**: 99–101.

Prior TI, Chue PS, Tibbo P, *et al.* Drug metabolism and atypical antipsychotics. *Eur Neuropsychopharmacol* 1999; **9**: 301–309.

Rapeport WG, Muirhead DC, Williams SA, *et al.* Absence of effect of sertraline on the pharmacokinetics and pharmacodynamics of phenytoin. *J Clin Psychiatry* 1996a; **57**(Suppl. 1): 24–28.

Rapeport WG, Williams SA, Muirhead DC, *et al.* Absence of sertraline-mediated effect on the pharmacokinetics and pharmacodynamics of carbamazepine. *J Clin Psychiatry* 1996b; **57**(Suppl. 1): 20–23.

Ring BJ, Catlow J, Lindsay TJ, *et al.* Identification of the human cytochromes P450 responsible for the in vitro formation of the major oxidative metabolites of the antipsychotic agent olanzapine. *J Pharmacol Exp Ther* 1996; **276**: 658–666.

Roth L, Bertschy G. Nefazodone may inhibit the metabolism of carbamazepine: three case reports. *Eur Psychiatry* 2001; **16**: 320–321.

Shukla S, Godwin CD, Long LEB, *et al.* Lithium–carbamazepine neurotoxicity and risk factors. *Am J Psychiatry* 1984; **141**: 1604–1606.

Spina E, Avenoso A, Pollicino AM, *et al.* Carbamazepine coadministration with fluoxetine or fluvoxamine. *Ther Drug Monit* 1993; **15**: 247–250.

Spina E, Avenoso A, Facciolà G, *et al.* Plasma concentrations of risperidone and 9-hydrox-yrisperidone: effect of comedication with carbamazepine or valproate. *Ther Drug Monit* 2000; **22**: 481–485.

Szymura-Oleksiak J, Wyska E, *et al.* Pharmacokinetic interaction between imipramine and carbamazepine in patients with major depression. *Psychopharmacology (Berl)* 2001; **154**: 38–42.

Tekle A, al-Kamis KI. Phenytoin–bupropion interaction: effect on plasma phenytoin concentration in the rat. *J Pharm Pharmacol* 1990; **42**: 799–801.

Torta R, Monaco F. Atypical antipsychotics and serotoninergic antidepressants in patients with epilepsy: pharmacodynamic considerations. *Epilepsia* 2002; **43**(Suppl. 2): 8–13.

Toy SM, Lucki I, Peirgies AA, *et al.* Pharmacokinetic and pharmacodynamic evaluation of the potential drug interaction between venlafaxine and diazepam. *J Clin Pharmacol* 1995; **35**: 410–419.

Trimble M, Anlezark G, Meldrum B. Seizure activity in photosensitive baboons following antidepressant drugs and the role of serotoninergic mechanisms. *Psychopharmacology* 1977; **51**: 159–164.

Van Belle K, Sarre S, Ebinger G, *et al.* Brain, liver and blood distribution kinetics of carbamazepine and its metabolic interaction with clomipramine in rats: a quantitative microdialysis study. *J Pharmacol Exp Ther* 1995; **272**: 1217–1222.

Vieweg V, Shutty M, Hundley P, *et al.* Combined treatment with lithium and carbamazepine. *Am J Psychiatry* 1991; **148**: 398–399.

Vincent FM. Phenothiazine induced phenytoin intoxication. *Ann Intern Med* 1980; **93**: 56–57.

Wong SL, Cavanaugh J, Shi H, *et al.* Effects of divalproex sodium on amitriptyline and nortriptyline pharmacokinetics. *Clin Pharmacol Ther* 1996; **60**: 48–53.

Wong YW, Yeh C, Thyrum PT. The effects of concomitant phenytoin administration on the steady-state pharmacokinetics of quetiapine. *J Clin Psychopharmacol* 2001; **21**: 89–93.

Yan QS, Jobe PC, Dailey JW. Evidence that a serotonergic mechanism is involved in the anticonvulsant effect of fluoxetine in genetically epilepsy-prone rats. *Eur J Pharmacol* 1994; **252**: 105–112.

20

Antiepileptic drugs in non-epileptic health conditions: possible interactions

Jerzy Majkowski

Center for Epilepsy Diagnosis and Treatment Foundation of Epileptology, Warsaw, Poland

Introduction: AEDs in non-epileptic conditions

Ever since they first appeared, antiepileptic drugs (AEDs) have not infrequently been used to treat patients with conditions other than epilepsy. Some AEDs, e.g. phenytoin (PHT), carbamazepine (CBZ) and valproic acid (VPA), have for long been indicated in a number of neurological and psychiatric disorders. The same is true for some of the new generation AEDs, such as gabapentin (GBP), lamotrigine (LTG), levetiracetam (LEV), oxcarbazepine (O-CBZ), tiagabine (TGB), topiramate (TPM) and pregabalin (PGB). It seems that newer AEDs – compared with the older ones – may be at least equally effective in non-epileptic disorders, but with fewer adverse events, and with minimal or no drug interactions. However, it should be stressed that evidence-based medicine varies broadly as far as the efficacy of particular drugs in given disorders or health conditions is concerned. Moreover, the number of reports and trials, and the extent of usage of these drugs vary greatly.

Epilepsy with its prevalence of about 1% is one of the most common neurological conditions. However, because AEDs have been used in several other neurological and psychiatric conditions with a higher prevalence than epilepsy, altogether they present a large market for AED usage. For example, in the United States LTG, TPM and GBP use – in terms of pharmaceutical market (IMS, 2000, 2001, 2002) – is greater for non-epileptic disorders than for epilepsy; moreover, there is an increasing trend for use of TPM and LTG from 2000 to 2002 (Table 20.1). In European countries (e.g. France, Germany, Italy, Spain and UK) GBP use is also greater in other fields than epilepsy, and as in the USA this trend is increasing. Two other AEDs (TPM and LTG) have been, also, showing an increasing use in non-epileptic disorders in Germany and Spain (IMS, 2000, 2001, 2002).

A national survey in the USA showed that approximately 10% of nursing home residents were taking AEDs, usually with other drugs (Cloyd *et al.*, 1994; Lackner *et al.*, 1998). In 18% of the residents receiving AEDs, indications were other than epilepsy. In Poland in 2002, the number of VPA prescriptions for non-epileptic

Table 20.1 AEDs used in non-epileptic disorders in 2002
(first 9 months of the year)

AED	Country	Pharmaceutical market
LTG[a]	USA	61%
TPM[a]	USA	71%
GBP	USA	85%
GBP	France	
GBP[a]	Germany	
GBP[a]	Italy	56–89%
GBP[a]	Spain	
GBP[a]	UK	

[a] Increasing from 2000 to 2002 (percentages calculated for year
2000–2002, refer to the first 9 months of each year).

disorders was about 21% (IMS, Health Poland, 2002). Thus, the term antiepileptic
does not reflect the whole spectrum of these drugs' potential therapeutic effects.

It is estimated that combination therapy occurs in about 10% of the general
population, and in the elderly and in women the percentage is even higher (Nobili
et al., 1997). Patients over 65 years use 2–6 prescribed medications, and 1–3.4
over-the-counter drugs (Stewart and Cooper, 1994). Therefore, knowledge of possible
drug interactions in non-epileptic patients taking AEDs is just as important as it is
in epileptic patients. Rules for combination therapy and information concerning
possible interactions between AEDs and non-epileptic drugs (non-AEDs) are the
same as those discussed in Chapters 8, 16, 18 and 19.

The purpose of this chapter is to emphasize the spectrum and scale of AED usage
in medical disciplines other than epilepsy, and to increase awareness of unpredicted
drug interactions when combination therapy with two or three drugs is used. As in
the treatment of epilepsy, awareness of possible drug interactions with AEDs is an
important part of the treatment strategy.

Rationale for using AEDs in disorders other than epilepsy

There are a number of pharmacological reasons why AEDs have therapeutic effects
in non-epileptic neurological and psychiatric conditions. With the exception of two
AEDs (TGB and vigabatrine (VGB)) that are thought to have a single mechanism
of pharmacological action, all other AEDs have multiple neurophysiological and
neurochemical actions (Macdonald, 1997; Moshē, 2000). Even when various mechanisms are involved, the primary mechanism of reducing high frequency firing in
neurones is by enhancing sodium channel inactivation. Indeed, this mechanism

may be one of the main reasons for the antineuralgic effects of AEDs in various pain syndromes (Brau *et al.*, 2001; Carter and Galer, 2001). However, AEDs have several other ways of modifying abnormal neuronal activity, presumably involved in a number of neurological and psychiatric disorders, which at first glance are very different from those found in epilepsy. These mechanisms involve: inhibition of the sodium, L-, N-, T-calcium and chloride channels; blockage of the *N*-methyl-D-aspartic acid (NMDA) receptor, decrease of glutamate release, antagonism of alpha-amino-3-hydroxy-5-methyl-4-isoxasole propionate (AMPA) and adenosine receptors, increase in 5-HT release, increase in different modes of operation of gamma-amino butyric acid (GABA) – one of the principal inhibitory neurotransmitters. AEDs have been shown to potentiate GABAergic synaptic transmission either by increasing GABA concentrations through the inhibition of GABA-transaminase (VGB) or GABA up-take (TGB). Other drugs act directly at the synaptic GABA receptor complex (benzodiazepines, PB) or increase GABA concentration in several specific brain regions (VPA) (Löscher, 1999; Macdonald and McLean, 1986). The parallels of the neurochemistry and pathophysiology of epilepsy and chronic pain provide the basis for re-evaluating the use of AEDs in various pain syndromes (Ross, 2000).

Recently, research into the mechanisms of migraine and the progressive recognition that cortical hyperexcitability and an imbalance between neuronal inhibition and excitation (mediated by GABA and amino acids, respectively) may play an important role in migraine pathophysiology, provided rationale for using AEDs in prophylaxis and treatment of migraine and other headaches (Krychmantowski *et al.*, 2002). Quality of evidence-based reviews and guidelines for the efficacy of various AEDs in migraine prophylaxis and in migraine aura therapy have been provided by the American Academy of Neurology (2000) and D'Andrea *et al.* (2003).

There are also physiological reasons for using AEDs in bipolar psychosis or other recurrent disorders. Ever since Kraepelin (1921), it has been postulated that bipolar affective disorders are of a progressive nature, just like seizures, and a kindling mechanism has been proposed (Post and Weiss, 1989).

Drug interactions in various health conditions

In pregnant women serum propranolol concentrations are increased by 50%. However, in hypertensive pregnant women treated with 90 mg of PB, a significant decrease in serum propranolol concentration has been observed, thus suggesting that pregnancy alters the half-life of propranolol therapy associated with PB (Hoffmann-Traeger *et al.*, 1987).

It has also been reported that clearance of LTG in pregnancy may be increased (Tomson *et al.*, 1997). Moreover, in one study LTG plasma concentrations were slightly lower in females (13.7%) than in males (May *et al.*, 1996). However, in another study this difference was not confirmed (Chen, 2000).

Combination of PB and theophylline results in increased theophylline clearance in children and adults but not in premature neonates (Kandrotas *et al.*, 1990).

Serum concentration of tirilazad mesylate (a membrane lipid peroxydation inhibitor), when given with PB in subarachnoid hemorrhage, may increase by 69% (Fleishaker *et al.*, 1996).

Drugs which compete for albumin bindings may increase the risk of kernicterus, e.g. combination of PB with aminophyline, cefotaxime and vancomycin shows that the bilirubin-displacing effect in the drug combinations cannot be predicted from each drug's individual effect in premature infants (Robertson and Brodersen, 1991).

Primidone (PRM) withdrawal in a 14-year-old girl with congenital adrenal dysplasia and epilepsy resulted in a three-fold increase of hypercorticolism and a reduction of plasma testosterone and 17 OH progesterone concentrations (Young and Hughes, 1991), thus showing the need to adjust the dose.

In patients with liver cirrhosis grade A, B and C (Child-Hugh classification), the median oral clearance was 0.31, 0.24 and 0.10 ml/min/kg, respectively, in comparison with 0.34 ml/min/kg in normal healthy subjects. Correspondingly, median $T_{1/2}$ of LTG was 36, 60 and 110 h, whereas for patients with normal liver function it was 32 h (Glaxo Wellcome Inc., 1999). LTG dosage must be downwardly adjusted in patients with liver dysfunction.

LTG clearance in patients with hyperbilirubinemia (Gilbert's syndrome) was 32% lower, and $T_{1/2}$ was 37% longer than in the healthy controls (Posner *et al.*, 1989). Close clinical monitoring of such patients is needed when LTG is administered; possible downward dosage adjustment should be considered.

Clearance of LTG in Asians and non-Whites is lower than in Whites. This difference may have significant clinical relevance for non-Whites if LTG is administered, particularly when it is combined with non-AEDs, which are hepatic enzyme inhibitors.

Renal failure slows down the urinary excretion of prednisone and its metabolites, making dose reduction of corticosteroids necessary. However, combination of prednisone and PB increases excretion of prednisone without any clear change in 17 OH steroids and prednisolone urinary excretion (Perignon *et al.*, 1985). This drug interaction is associated with a decrease of graft tolerance in renal transplant patients.

It is interesting to note that serum VPA concentrations are higher in uremic serum than in normal serum, but there is no further displacement of VPA in the presence of mefenamic acid or fenoprofen. However, when uremic serum is treated with charcoal at pH 3.0, it removes the protecting effect of uremic serum, and VPA displacement from protein binding is higher (Dasgupta and Emerson, 1996).

VPA displacement from albumin binding may depend on concentrations of non-AED, e.g. ketoconazole is an antifungal agent widely used in the management of patients with fungal infections, especially patients with acute acquired immuno-deficiency syndrome (AIDS). Ketoconazole is 99% bound to serum albumin and readily interacts with VPA. Statistically significant displacement of VPA has been observed at normal albumin level but only when ketoconazole concentrations were high (10–20 μg/ml). However, in patients with hypoalbuminemia, significant displacement of VPA was observed with lower ketoconazole concentrations (Dasgupta and Luke, 1997). It is interesting that there is no displacement of VPA by ketoconazole in uremic serum. On the contrary, the free fraction of VPA decreases in the presence of ketoconazole in uremic serum.

Salicylate displaces CBZ from protein binding in normal sera but this effect is significantly reduced in uremic sera (Dasgupta and Thompson, 1995). On the other hand, significant displacement of CBZ from protein binding by tolmetin, ibuprofen and naproxen (non-steroidal inflammatory drugs) has been observed in uremic serum whereas in normal serum significant displacement has been found only with higher concentrations of naproxen (Dasgupta and Volk, 1996).

Renal elimination plays only a minor role in overall elimination of LTG. Thus, even in patients with moderate renal dysfunction and much lower clearance than in healthy people, the difference is not clinically relevant (Wootton *et al.*, 1997). However, in patients with more severe renal failure and particularly if hemodialysis is required, the daily dose of LTG should be downwardly adjusted to the overall renal clearance (Fillastre *et al.*, 1993).

Seizures are a relatively common occurrence in patients with human immuno virus (HIV) infection. Seropositive patients are usually treated with AEDs. In such patients AEDs should be carefully chosen. The ideal AED:

1 should not stimulate viral replication,
2 has limited protein bindings,
3 has no effect on the cytochrome P450 system.

GBP, TPM, TGB and PRG meet these criteria. VPA stimulates HIV replication. Thus combination of AED with antiretrovirals should be carefully considered (Romanelli and Ryan, 2002). Combination of CBZ and ritonavir in patients with HIV infection may result in CBZ intoxication (Mateu-de Antonio *et al.*, 2001) and antiretroviral therapy failure (Hugen *et al.*, 2000).

Unpredicted interactions when more than two drugs are used

Pindolol (beta-adrenergic blocking agent) does not increase serum PHT concentrations when PHT is administered in monotherapy. However, it does increase PHT concentrations when PHT is combined with other AEDs (Greendyke and Gulya,

1988). GBP does not seem to have any pharmacokinetic interaction with PHT; however, co-administration with VGB and PHT results in marked reduction in clearance of PHT (Matar *et al.*, 2000).

It has been found that AEDs increase fenantyl requirement during anesthesia for craniostomy (Tempelhoff *et al.*, 1990). However, this is a dose-effect relationship between the number of AEDs received and the maintenance dose of fentanyl required for balanced anesthesia. AEDs have a similar dose-effect relationship with pipercuronium neuromuscular blockade (myorelaxants), also resulting in induction of a significant effect of AEDs (Jellish *et al.*, 1993).

A case of retroperitoneal hematoma due to interaction between PHT and acenocoumarol, possibly potentiated by concomitant administration of paroxetine, has been reported (Abad-Santos *et al.*, 1995).

The fact that over-the-counter drugs and nutritional supplements are increasingly being self-administered by patients creates the risk of drug interactions. Internet self-diagnosed and self-treated cases can also contribute to drug–drug interactions.

Interactions with folk medicine

In many countries folk medicine is frequently used for various reasons. Knowledge of active ingredients and possible interactions with AEDs is usually poor. Widely used ginkgo preparations are a good example. Co-medication of ginkgo and AEDs may result in decreased effectiveness of AEDs due to the presence of seizure provoking contaminants in some ginkgo preparations. Ginkgo products may contain neurotoxin 4′-O-methylpyridoxine, which is a B_6 antivitamin (Wada *et al.*, 1985). When seizures occur in patients for the first time, particularly in children, it is recommended that subjects be asked whether they have been taking ginkgo seeds or leaf extracts (Arenz *et al.*, 1996; Yagi *et al.*, 1993). In the probable mechanism of seizures, 4′-O-methylpyridoxine appears to inhibit pyridoxal kinase and when taken in a sufficient amount may result in convulsions. The amount of this neurotoxin in gingko leaves or seeds depends on the growing seasons during which the product was harvested (Arenz *et al.*, 1996).

Another example is primrose oil. Concurrent use of evening primrose oil and AEDs may result in seizures (Holman and Bell, 1983). Combination of phenothiazines (for presumed schizophrenia) and evening primrose oil resulted in epileptic seizures. Withdrawal of primrose oil and CBZ administration resulted in seizure control. Evening primrose oil activated temporal lobe epilepsy in two patients with schizophrenia (Vaddadi, 1981). For the same reason, evening primrose oil is contraindicated in patients with mania and epilepsy (Barber, 1998; Newall *et al.*, 1996).

AEDs in non-epileptic disorders

Carbamazepine

CBZ is one of the most commonly used AEDs in epilepsy and other neurological and psychiatric disorders. CBZ mechanisms involve inhibitory action on sodium and on calcium (L- and N-type) channels, inhibitory effect on the release of somatostatin, increase of 5-HT release, effect on synaptic transmission and receptors, purine, monoamine, acetylcholine, adenosine and NMDA receptors (Crowder and Bradford, 1987; Lampe and Bigalke, 1990; Worley and Baraban, 1987). Its broad spectrum of pharmacological actions may explain the potent effect of CBZ in disorders other than epilepsy.

The analgesic effect is most comprehensively documented in neuralgias (Cambell *et al.*, 1966; Nicol, 1969; Rockliff and Davis, 1966). However, it is also used in diabetic polyneuropathy (Rull *et al.*, 1969), phantom limb pain syndrome, thalamic pain, cerebellar tremors and migraine (Leijon and Boivie, 1989; McQuay *et al.*, 1995; Rompel and Bauermeister, 1970; Sechi *et al.*, 1989).

There are reports that CBZ is also effective in hemifacial spasm, myotonia, restless legs syndrome (Montagna, 1992; Telstad *et al.*, 1984) and hyperactivity disorders in children (Silva *et al.*, 1996). In patients with dementia, CBZ is given to alleviate agitation, aggressiveness or other behavioral abnormalities. There are many reports and a long history of CBZ use in alcoholism, psychiatric disorders such as acute mania, bipolar disorders and mood stabilizing in affective and aggressive disorders (Dunn *et al.*, 1998; Kishimoto *et al.*, 1983; Mayo-Smith, 1997; Post *et al.*, 1997; Post, 1988).

Gabapentin

GBP is widely and more frequently used in fields other than epilepsy. This may be due to its multiple mechanisms of action and to the fact that it is not associated with any significant pharmacokinetic interaction with other drugs. Most frequently, GBP is indicated for various pain syndromes and bipolar disorders. In these health conditions GBP efficacy is well documented in clinical controlled trials.

In pain-resistant conditions, combination of GBP with other analgesics is frequently used. In these cases GBP is the optional drug in elderly patients because in this population polytherapy is frequently used and GBP, usually, does not interact with other drugs. However, antacids (Maalox (R)) given concurrently with GBP reduced GBP bioavailability by 20% and when given 2 h after GBP, reduction was by 5% only (Product Information: Neurontin (R), Pfizer, New York, 2002).

GBP in combination with antiretroviral medication showed some effects in neuropathic pain due to immunodeficiency syndrome (Nevill, 2000). Amitriptyline or GBP are alternatives for postherpetic neuralgia, and other AEDs (GBP, LTG, TGB and TPM) are alternatives for seizures since indinavir interaction with CBZ causes antiretroviral therapy failure (Hugen *et al.*, 2000). Adding GBP to stable opioid medication in neuropathic cancer pain resulted in significant pain reduction without new adverse events (Caraceni *et al.*, 1999). However, concurrent use of GBP and morphine may result in an increase of GBP plasma concentration (Product Information: Neurontin (R), Pfizer, New York, NY, 2002), requiring GBP dosage reduction in the elderly.

GBP administration resulted in significant reduction of spontaneous or evoked pain (brush-induced allodynia, cold-induced allodynia and hyperalgesia) (Attal *et al.*, 1998). Good effects of GBP were reported in newly diagnosed trigeminal neuralgia (Magnus, 1999), in diabetic neuropathy in randomized studies (Backonja *et al.*, 1998) and in postherpetic neuropathy (Rowbotham *et al.*, 1998).

GBP (1800–2400 mg/day) administered in patients with migraine resulted in significant prophylactic migraine attack reduction: in 36% of the patients, 50% reduction of migraine attacks was observed (in comparison with 14% in the placebo group) (Mathew *et al.*, 1999).

In patients with bipolar or monopolar disorders and mild depression, moderate to marked response was reported using GBP (Ghaemi *et al.*, 1998; Harden *et al.*, 1999; Ryback *et al.*, 1997). Good effect was also observed in the treatment of acute mania using GBP alone or in combination with other antimanic drugs (Grunze *et al.*, 1999; Hatzimanolis *et al.*, 1999). These positive effects were observed in open-label study, on rather small number of patients and short-treatment duration. However, placebo-controlled studies showed that GBP does not have such beneficial effects in bipolar psychosis (Frye *et al.*, 2000).

Other neurological disorders: GBP administration resulted in significant beneficial effects in spasticity and paroxysmal symptoms associated with multiple sclerosis (Cutter *et al.*, 2000). In Parkinson's disease GBP in addition to dopaminergics showed a significant improvement in favour of GBP over a short period of co-medication (Olson *et al.*, 1997). In amyotrophic lateral sclerosis controversial results were reported during GBP administration (Miller *et al.*, 1996; Mazzini *et al.*, 1998).

GBP was administered in Huntington's disease and other movement paroxysmal disorders (Cosentino *et al.*, 1996; Hardoy *et al.*, 1999; Kothare *et al.*, 2000). In open studies, long-term GBP administration of 900 mg showed moderate to good beneficial effects, without adverse events in tardive diskinesia, facial diskinesia, blepharospasm, hemichorea or hemibalismus. On the other hand, various movement disorders appeared when GBP was initiated; these disappeared when GBP was withdrawn. In 48% of the patients with restless legs syndrome clinical improvement was observed during GBP administration (Alder, 1997).

Paroxysmal dystonic movement, in both hands, occurred during combination of 900 mg GBP with propranolol in the elderly. After reduction of propranolol to

40 mg/day the paroxysmal dystonia subsided immediately. A pharmacodynamic interaction effect was suggested (Palomeras *et al.*, 2000).

Combination of GBP with propranolol led to significant tremor improvement (Gironell *et al.*, 1999). Orthostatic tremor was reduced in the majority of patients with GBP treatment (Onofrj *et al.*, 1998). In another study, however, GBP 1800 mg/day was added for 2 weeks to baseline anti-tremor treatment without any significant tremor reduction compared to the placebo (Pahwa *et al.*, 1998). No drug interactions were reported.

Various rare neurological conditions: GBP was administered in reflex sympathetic dystrophy, central pain, myokymia, cramp syndrome, idiopathic chronic hiccup and usually with clinical improvement (Merren, 1998).

Since GBP is eliminated predominantly by renal excretion, it may be influenced or may affect pharmacokinetics of other drugs showing the same pattern of elimination at the renal site (McLean, 1994). In patients with renal dysfunction or in the elderly, the daily dose of GBP should be downwardly adjusted according to creatinine clearance decrease.

Lamotrigine

LTG has multiple mechanisms of action including decrease of glutamate release in addition to inhibition of sodium and calcium (L- and N-type) currents, and increase of GABA.

It has been suggested that LTG possesses distinct psychotropic effects in addition to its antiepileptic action (Brodie, 1992; Uvebrant and Bauziene, 1994). Placebo-controlled trials in epilepsy treatment show some mood improvement (greater well-being) (Jawad *et al.*, 1989; Smith *et al.*, 1993) and there are theoretical reasons to suggest that LTG, like other AEDs, may possess mood-stabilizing properties. Polytherapy is usually used in bipolar psychoses, since there is no single mood stabilizer (Frye *et al.*, 2000; Shelton and Calabrese, 2000). LTG monotherapy administered in two groups of patients with bipolar-I depression showed that 250 mg of LTG was significantly better than the placebo. LTG was effective in patients with rapid-cycling bipolar disorder and was useful in the treatment of bipolar-II disorder. LTG has not been shown to have clear efficacy in the treatment of mania or unipolar depression (Calabrese *et al.*, 1999, 2000). Based on efficacy, adverse events and costs, it has been suggested that the use of LTG in mood disorders should probably be on the basis of a second-line agent for bipolar depression (Hurley, 2002).

Levetiracetam

LEV is an AED with unique profile of activity with potent broad-spectrum efficacy including effect on the high voltage N-type calcium channel, and at GABA and glycine-gated channels.

Information concerning LEV usage in non-epileptic disorders is too limited to allow any firm conclusions to be made. However, a number of preliminary reports show that LEV is well tolerated and effective in a wide variety of pain states (cervical and lumbar radiculopathy, traumatic peripheral nerve injury, neuropathic component in neoplastic pain, postherpetic neuralgia, allodynia, myelopathic pain and paresthesis in multiple sclerosis). LEV is presently undergoing extensive evaluation for the treatment of various neuropathic pains and migraines; however, it is only registered for the treatment of epilepsy (Mealy *et al.*, 2002; Pakalnis, 2002).

Migraine and various headaches are other disorders in which LEV has been used with positive effects in reducing severity and frequency with modest side effects (Drake *et al.*, 2001; Krusz, 2001). In refractory migraines LEV was given intravenously (i.v.) with good effect and was well tolerated (Krusz and Daniel, 2002).

There is also a suggestion that LEV may by used as a mood stabilizer (Bowden, 2001).

LEV is not associated with any pharmacokinetic interactions.

Oxcarbazepine

There are few publications concerning the use of O-CBZ in non-epilepsy conditions, although it has been used to treat acute mania (Emrich, 1990). However, since O-CBZ is better-tolerated than CBZ (with the exception of more common hyponatremia), and has similar mechanisms of action, it may be used in indications similar to those for CBZ (Asconape, 2002). O-CBZ is associated with far fewer pharmacokinetic interactions than CBZ.

Phenobarbital

Phenobarbital is the oldest AED in use and is still extensively used in developing countries. The mechanism of action of PB involves antagonism of AMPA receptor subtype and includes enhancement of GABAergic inhibition, enhancement of ionic currents by interactions with $GABA_A$ receptor, decrease of excitatory amino acid release and post-synaptic response due to blocking of the excitatory glutamate response (Smith and Riskin, 1991). A broad spectrum of pharmacological actions may contribute to potential therapeutic activity in neurological conditions other than epilepsy. However, cognitive impairment, morning sedation, potential for abuse, severe toxicity and withdrawal syndrome are contraindications for routine use of PB (strong inducer) in such disorders.

In the past, i.v. injections of PB were frequently used to prevent cerebral hemorrhage in preterm neonates. However, a critical review of the literature suggests that PB has no beneficial effect (Crowther and Henderson-Smart, 2000) and in fact increased the incidence of intraventricular hemorrhage in infants with respiratory disease (Porter *et al.*, 1985).

PB has also been used in increased intracranial pressure to reduce the effect of cerebral blood flow and metabolism (Trauner, 1986). However, it may impair cerebral perfusion pressure by inducing hypotension (Roberts, 2000) and therefore the benefit to risk ratio is low.

Neonatal hyperbilirubinemia can be controlled with a high single dose of PB (12 mg/kg) after birth (Wallin and Boreus, 1984). However, such a dose results in a prolonged sleep-state. In this condition, infants spend more time sleeping than they do with smaller doses.

Combination of chenodeoxycholic acid (750 mg/day) with PB (90–180 mg/day) was effective on the rate-limiting enzymes of liver cholesterol and bile acid synthesis. In patients with gallstones this effect was more pronounced than when each drug was used alone. Thus, an advantageous interaction was observed (Coyne *et al.*, 1975; 1976).

When asthmatic children were treated with PB, theophylline clearance increased by 42%, resulting in a 30% decrease in steady-state serum theophylline concentration (Saccar *et al.*, 1985). This drug combination requires theophylline dosage upward adjustment.

Reversible toxic encephalopathy was reported in a girl, possibly due to the toxic effect of ifosamide (cytostaticum) in combination with PB (Ghosn *et al.*, 1988).

The rapidly fatal outcome of fulminant hepatitis caused by nilutamide, a non-steroidal antiandrogen derivative, was enhanced by co-administration with PB (Pescatore *et al.*, 1993).

Phenytoin

PHT seems to be used much more frequently in the USA and the UK than in other European countries. In Poland, PHT constitutes 6.7% of the pharmaceutical market. PHT is a strong inducer of hepatic enzymes and is involved in numerous drug interactions with AEDs and non-AEDs. Moreover, due to non-linear pharmacokinetics and side effects, PHT is less frequently used today in non-epileptic disorders than it was before the introduction of the new generation of AEDs.

PHT has a broad spectrum of pharmacological action on neurotransmitter receptors and ion channels and this may explain why PHT is so effective in conditions other than epilepsy, such as: neuropathic pain, various pain syndromes, spasticity, myotonia and other disorders. However, evidence on the efficacy of PHT from randomized clinical trials in these and other non-epileptic conditions is rather scant.

Neuropathic pain: It has been reported that PHT may have a beneficial effect in trigeminal neuralgia, glossopharyngeal and superior laryngeal neuralgias, postherpetic and diabetic neuropathy, thalamic syndrome, phantom limb pain, diabetic pain and cancer pain. The efficacy of PHT in other pain syndromes is at best modest

(Chadda and Mathur, 1978; Saudek *et al.*, 1977). Unlike CBZ, evidence for efficacy of PHT in trigeminal neuralgia and similar conditions is based on an uncontrolled study only. However, PHT was more effective than aspirin in reducing pain in glycolipid lipidosis (Fabry disease) (Lockman *et al.*, 1973).

In myotonic treatment, PHT and CBZ were used interchangeably and their efficacy was comparable to the efficacy of procainamide (Munsat, 1967; Sechi *et al.*, 1983). However, adverse events may be more pronounced. In a double-blind placebo-controlled study PHT had a positive effect on motion sickness (Stern *et al.*, 1994).

Pregabalin

PGB $((S)-(+)-3$ isobutylgaba) is a GABA derivative, but does not interact with $GABA_A$ or $GABA_B$ receptors and does not influence GABA concentrations (Whitworth and Quick, 2001). Instead, PGB binds to sub-units β_2, α_1, $\alpha_2-\delta$ of the Ca^{2+} channel and this reduces the release of glutamate, noradrenaline and substance P (Dooley *et al.*, 2000; Errante and Petroff, 2003). These mechanisms of action seem to be important in the treatment of epileptic seizures, pain and anxiety (Field *et al.*, 2001). PGB is not associated with any pharmacokinetic interactions with CBZ, LTG, PB, PHT, TGB, TPM or VPA.

Primidone

PRM has been used in prospective, randomized clinical trials in essential tremor (Findley *et al.*, 1985; Gorman *et al.*, 1986) and is as effective as propranolol (Gorman *et al.*, 1986; Sasso *et al.*, 1990) and more effective than PB (Baruzzi *et al.*, 1983).

Possible adverse events associated with PRM are similar to those with PB, which limits their use.

Tiagabine

TGB is an inhibitor of GABA uptake. The drug was developed specifically for use as an AED based on the concept of the GABAergic mechanism of epileptic seizures. Since reduction in GABAergic neuronal activity has been proposed not only in epilepsy but also in various neuropsychological disorders, anxiety and pain (Krogsgaard-Larsen, 1988; Meldrum, 1982), TGB may have a beneficial effect in these health conditions.

TGB has been evaluated in various GABAergic mechanism-related disorders e.g. sleep disorders (Meldrum and Chapman, 1999), pain (postherpetic and diabetic neuropathy), movement disorders (related to basal ganglia disorders, e.g. tardive diskinesia) (Gao *et al.*, 1994; Thaker *et al.*, 1987), spasticity (Holden and Titus, 1999), bipolar disorders (Kaufman, 1998), anxiety (Neilson, 1988) and neuroprotection against ischemia-induced cell loss (Johansen and Diemer, 1991). A moderate effect of TGB in migraine has been observed (Drake *et al.*, 1999; Freitag *et al.*, 2000).

In casuistic observation TGB was administered in psychiatric patients (bipolar disorders) as add-on therapy to venlafaxine, lithium, flurazepam, bupropion, methylphenidate and paroxetine (Kaufman, 1998; Schaffer and Schaffer, 1999).

Dosages of TGB should be adjusted in patients with liver dysfunction (Beydoun and Passaro, 2002).

In general, preliminary reports suggest that TGB use in non-epileptic conditions requires longer-term studies based on larger numbers of patients and on evidence-based medical principle. The few reports relating drug interactions between TGB and non-AEDs are discussed in Chapter 8.

Topiramate

The mechanisms of action of TPM involve: sodium channel blockade, inhibition of AMPA glutamate receptors, potentiation of GABA-related neuroinhibition at $GABA_A$ receptors (White, 1999); blocking of excitatory neurotransmission mediated by non-NMDA receptors. TPM is also a weak carbonic anhydrase inhibitor (Dodgson *et al.*, 2000) and may have an inhibitory effect on calcium channels (Zhang *et al.*, 2000).

Preliminary data suggest that TPM, with multiple pharmacological properties, may have therapeutic effects in various chronic pain syndromes, migraine and cluster headache prophylaxis, tremor and certain psychiatric disorders.

Analgesic effect of TPM combination with opioids was reported in neuropathic pain; and these effects were not the result of any drug interaction.

TPM was prophylactically effective in migraine and other headaches (Potter *et al.*, 2000; Wheeler and Carrazana, 1999). TPM and propranolol combination resulted in control of essential tremor, particularly in the hands compared to the head or voice (Connor, 2000; Galvez-Jimenez and Hargreave, 2000). No drug interaction was reported.

In psychiatric disorders TPM was combined with tricyclic antidepressants (Ortho McNeil Pharmacological) or with serotonin reuptake (Edwards *et al.*, 2000). TPM has been used as an alternative treatment for bipolar disorder (Doose *et al.*, 1999a), and was effective in 55% of initially manic patients after a mean of 312 days of treatment. There was no clinically significant effect of TPM on haloperidol serum concentrations (Doose *et al.*, 1999b) but a modest decrease in lithium serum concentration was observed though the interaction was without clinical relevance.

Nightmares and binge-eating responded well to TPM in an open-label trial (Shapira *et al.*, 2000). Two patients with Tourette's syndrome were successfully treated with TPM while previous medications were discontinued (Abuzzahab, 2001). No interaction was reported.

In general, the reports on TPM administration in non-epileptic disorders are based on short preliminary studies and/or small numbers of patients.

Valproic acid

VPA is an AED with broad-spectrum efficacy against various forms of epileptic seizure. This is due to the combination of several neurochemical and neurophysiologic mechanisms (Löscher, 1999; Zeise *et al.*, 1991), which may explain its effects in various neuronal dysfunctions. The mechanisms of VPA action include

1 increase of GABA turnover potentiating GABAergic functions in various specific brain regions,
2 inhibitory effect on voltage-sensitive sodium channels (Löscher, 1999),
3 inhibitory effect on neuronal excitation mediated by the NMDA (Zeise *et al.*, 1991).

Several double-blind controlled trials have demonstrated the efficacy of VPA in migraine treatment and prophylaxis (Hering and Kuritzky, 1992; Jensen *et al.*, 1994; Klapper, 1997). Migraines with paroxysmal discharges in the electroencephalograph (EEG), mainly of the dysrhythmic type, were successfully treated with VPA (Viswanathan *et al.*, 1995). VPA is also effective in chronic headaches, (Mathew and Ali, 1991), and in cluster-form headaches (Hering and Kuritzky, 1989). VPA can occasionally be combined with other groups of medication for migraine treatment, including β-adrenergic channel blockers or anti-inflammatory drugs. In such cases potential drug interaction with VPA may occur (see Chapter 8).

In addition to its analgesic effect (DeFeudis, 1984), VPA also shows efficacy in various psychiatric and neurotic disorders. It was reported that VPA is effective in patients with acute mania and its subtypes (Emrich and Wolf, 1992; Pope *et al.*, 1991), depression (Brown, 1989; Young *et al.*, 2000) and bipolar disorders (Goldberg *et al.*, 1998; Hirschfeld *et al.*, 1999; Schaff *et al.*, 1993). Moreover, VPA has been used in anxiety disorders, stress condition, aggressive behavior and tardive diskinesia.

Evidence-based medicine varies greatly but even so, VPA is widely used in fields other than epilepsy in the majority of countries.

Summary

Many drug interactions can be demonstrated but only a few of them are so clinically significant that they require adjustment of drug dosages. However, some drug combinations may produce unexpected changes of various extents and directions in different subjects and in different health conditions. The reasons for this variability include genetic control of the rate of drug metabolism as well as internal factors, such as serum changes, renal or hepatic disorders, gender and ageing. In this chapter, clinically and/or potentially significant drug interactions between AEDs and non-AEDs in health conditions other than epilepsy are discussed. Case reports of toxic effects due to drug interactions are presented as a warning signal calling for attention when polytherapy has to be used. In such cases, careful drug selection and dosage adjustment based on serum drug monitoring and clinical observation are the main rules for risk minimization. Awareness and knowledge of possible drug interactions is a good starting point before making treatment decisions.

REFERENCES

Abad-Santos F, Carcass AJ, F-Capitan C, *et al.* Retroperitoneal haematoma in a patient treated with acenocoumarol, phenytoin and paroxetine. *Clin Labor Haematol* 1995; **17**: 195–197.

Abuzzahab FS. Control of Tourette's syndrome with topiramate. *Am J Psychiat* 2001; **158**: 968.

Alder CH. Treatment of restless legs syndrome with gabapentin. *Clin Nauropharmacol* 1997; **20**: 148–151.

American Academy of Neurology. Practice parameter: evidence based guidelines for migraine headache (an evidence based review). Report on the Quality Standards Subcommittee of the American Academy of Neurology. *Neurology* 2000; **55**: 754–763.

Arenz A, Klein M, Fiehe K, *et al.* Occurrence of neurotoxic $4'$-O-methylpyridoxine in Ginkgo biloba leaves, Ginkgo medications and Japanese Ginkgo food. *Planta Medica* 1996; **62**: 548–551.

Asconape JJ. Some common issues in the use of antiepileptic drugs. *Semin Neurol* 2002; **22**: 27–39.

Attal N, Brasseur L, Parker F, *et al.* Effect of gabapentin on the different components of peripheral and central neuropathic pain syndromes: a pilot study. *Eur Neurol* 1998; **40**: 191–200.

Backonja M, Beydoun A, Edwards KR, *et al.* Gabapentin for the symptomatic treatment of painful neuropathy in patients with diabetes mellitus. A randomised controlled trial. *J Am Med Assoc* 1998; **280**: 1831–1836.

Barber AJ. Evening primrose oil: a panacea? *Pharm J* 1998; (June 4): 723–725.

Baruzzi A, Procaccianti G, Martinelli P, *et al.* Phenobarbital and propranolol in essential tremor: a double-blind controlled clinical trial. *Neurology* 1983; **33**: 296–300.

Beydoun A, Passaro EA. Appropriate use of medications for seizures. *Postgrad Med* 2002; **111**: 69–70.

Bowden CL. The role of anticonvulsants as mood stabiliser. *J Clin Psychiat* 2001; **62** (Suppl. 14): 3–4.

Brau ME, Dreimann M, Olschewski A, *et al.* Effect of drugs used for neuropathic pain management on tetrodotoxim-resistant Na(+) currents in rat sensory neurons. *Anaesthesiology* 2001; **94**: 137–144.

Brodie MJ. Lamotrigine. *Lancet* 1992; **339**: 1397–1399.

Brown R. US experience with valproate in manic depressive illness: a multicenter trial. *J Clin Psychiat* 1989; **50**: 13–16.

Calabrese J, Bowden C, Sachs D, *et al*. A double-blind placebo-controlled study of lamotrigine monotherapy in out-patients with bipolar I depression. *J Clin Psychiat* 1999; **60**: 79–88.

Calabrese J, Susppes T, Bowden C, *et al*. A double-blind placebo-controlled, prophylaxis study of lamotrigine in rapid cycling bipolar disorders. *J Clin Psychiat* 2000; **61**: 841–850.

Cambell FG, Graham JG, Zilkha KJ. Clinical trial of carbamazepine (Tegretol) in trigeminal neuralgia. *J Neurol Neurosurg Psychiatr* 1966; **29**: 265–267.

Caraceni A, Zecca E, Martini C, *et al*. Gabapentin as an adjuvant to opioid analgesia for neuropathic cancer pain. *J Pain Symp Manage* 1999; **17**: 441–445.

Carter GT, Galer BS. Advances in the management of neuropathic pain. *Phys Med Rehabil Clin North Am* 2001; **12**: 447–459.

Chadda VS, Matthur MS. Double blind study of the effects of diphenylhydantoin sodium on diabetic neuropathy. *J Assoc Physic Ind* 1978; **26**: 403–406.

Chen C, Veronese L, Yin Y. The effects of lamotrigine on the pharmacokinetics of lithium. *Br J Clin Pharmacol* 2000; **50**: 193–195.

Cloyd JC, Lackner TE, Leppik IE. Antiepileptics in the elderly. Pharmacoepidemiology and pharmacokinetics. *Family Med* 1994; **3**: 589–598.

Connor GG. Topiramate as a novel treatment for essential tremor. Poster, abstract presented at *Headache World*, London, 2000.

Cosentino C, Torres L, Cuba JM. Gabapentin for Huntington's disease. *J Neurol* 1996; **243** (Suppl. 2): 75–76.

Coyne MJ, Bonorris GG, Chung A, *et al*. Treatment of gallstones with chenodeoxycholic acid and phenobarbital. *New Engl J Med* 1975; **292**: 604–607.

Coyne MJ, Bonorris GG, Goldstein LI, *et al*. Effect of chenodeoxycholic acid and phenobarbital on the rate-limiting enzymes of hepatic cholesterol and bile acid synthesis in patients with gallstones. *J Lab Clin Med* 1976; **87**: 281–291.

Crowder JM, Bradford HH. Common anticonvulsants inhibit Ca^{2+} uptake and amino acid neurotransmitter release in vitro. *Epilepsia* 1987; **28**: 378–382.

Crowther CA, Henderson-Smart DJ. Phenobarbital prior to preterm birth for preventing neonatal periventricular hemorrhage. *Cochrane Database of Systematic Reviews* 2000: CD000 164.

Cutter NC, Scott DD, Johnson JC, *et al*. Gabapentin effect on spasticity in multiple sclerosis: a placebo-controlled, randomised trial. *Arch Med Rehabil* 2000; **81**: 164–169.

D'Andrea G, Bonavita V, Rigamonti A, *et al*. Treatment of migraine with aura: comments and perspectives. *Neurol Sci* 2003; **23**: 271–278.

Dasgupta A, Emerson L. Interaction of valproic acid with nonsteroidal antiinflammatory drugs mefenamic acid and fenoprofen in normal and uremic sera: lack of interaction in uremic sera due to the presence of endogenous factors. *Ther Drug Monit* 1996; **18**: 654–659.

Dasgupta A, Luke M. Valproic acid–ketoconazole interaction in normal, hypoalbuminemic, and uremic sera: lack of interaction in uremic serum caused by the presence of inhibitor. *Ther Drug Monit* 1997; **19**: 281–285.

Dasgupta A, Thompson WC. Carbamazepine–salicylate interaction in normal and uremic sera: reduced interaction in uremic sera. *Ther Drug Monit* 1995; **17**: 199–202.

Dasgupta A, Volk A. Displacement of valproic acid and carbamazepine from protein binding in normal and uremic sera by tolmetin, ibuprofen, and naproxen: presence of inhibitor in uremic serum that blocks valproic acid–naproxen interactions. *Ther Drug Monit* 1966; **18**: 284–287.

DeFeudis FW. Gamma-aminobutyric acid-ergic analgesia: implication for gamma-aminobutyric acid-ergic therapy for drug addiction. *Drug Alcohol Depend* 1984; **14**: 101–111.

Dodgson SJ, Shank RP, Maryanoff BE. Topiramate as an inhibitor of carbonic anhydrase isozymes. *Epilepsia* 2000; **41**(Suppl. 1): 35–39.

Dooley DJ, Mieske CA, Borosky SA. Inhibition of K^+-evoked glutamate release from rat neocortical and hippocampal slices by gabapentin. *Neurosci Lett* 2000; **280**: 107–110.

Doose DR, Kohl KA, Desai-Krieger D, *et al.* No clinically significant effect of topiramate on haloperidol plasma concentration. *Eur Neuropsychopharmacol* 1999a; **9**(Suppl. 5): 357.

Doose DR, Kohl KA, Desai-Krieger D, *et al.* No significant effect of topiramate on lithium serum concentration. Poster presented at the *1999 World Congress of Psychiatry*, Hamburg, Germany, 1999b.

Drake Jr ME, Kay AM, Knapp MS, *et al.* An open-label trial of tiagabine for migraine prophylaxis. *Headache* 1999; **39**: 352 (abstract).

Drake ME, Greathous NI, Armenbright AD, *et al.* Levetiracetam for preventive treatment of migraine. *Cephalalgia* 2001; **21**: 373 (abstract P-113).

Dunn RT, Frye MS, Kimbrell TA, *et al.* The efficacy and use of anticonvulsants in mood disorders. *Clin Neuropharmacol* 1998; **21**: 215–235.

Edwards KR, Glantz MJ, Button J, *et al.* Efficacy and safety of topiramate in the treatment of painful diabetic neuropathy: a double-blind, placebo-controlled study. *Neurology* 2000; **54**(Suppl. 3): A81 (abstract).

Emrich HM. Studies with oxcarbazepine in acute mania. *Int Clin Psychopharmacol* 1990; **5**(Suppl. 1): 83–88.

Emrich HM, Wolf R. Valproate treatment of mania. *Prog Neuropsychopharmacol Biol Psychiat* 1992; **16**: 691–701.

Errante LD, Petroff OAC. Acute effects of gabapentin and pregabalin on rat forebrain cellular GABA, glutamate, and glutamine concentrations. *Seizure* 2003; **12**: 300–306.

Field MJ, McLeary S, Hughes J, *et al.* Gabapentin and pregabalin, but not morphine and amitriptyline, block both static and dynamic components of mechanical allodynia induced by streptozocin in the rat. *Pain* 1999; **80**: 391–398.

Field MJ, Oles RJ, Singh L. Pregabalin may represent a novel class of anxiolytic agents with a broad spectrum of activity. *Br J Pharmacol* 2001; **132**: 1–4.

Fillastre JP, Taburet AM, Fialaire A, *et al.* Pharmacokinetics of lamotrigine in patients with renal impairment: influence of haemodialysis. *Drug Exp Clin Res* 1993; **19**: 25–32.

Findley LJ, Cleaves L, Calzetti S. Primidone in essential tremor of the hand and head: a double blind controlled clinical study. *J Neurol Neurosurg Psychiat* 1985; **48**: 911–915.

Fleishaker JC, Pearson LK, Peters GR. Gender does not affect the degree of induction of tirilazad clearance by phenobarbital. *Eur J Clin Pharmacol* 1996; **50**: 139–145.

Freitag FG, Diamond S, Diamond ML, *et al.* An open use trial of tiagabine in migraine. *Headache* 2000; **11**: 133–134.

Frye MA, Hetter TA, Kimbrell TA, *et al.* A placebo-controlled study of lamotrigine and gabapentin monotherapy in refractory mood disorders. *J Clin Psychopharmacol* 2000; **20**: 607–614.

Frye M, Ketter K, Leverich G, *et al.* The increasing use of polypharmacotherapy for refractory mood disorders: 22 years of study. *J Clin Psychiat* 2000; **61**: 9–15.

Galvez-Jimenez N, Hargreave M. Topiramate and essential tremor. *Ann Neurol* 2000; **47**: 837–838.

Gao XM, Kakigi T, Friedman MB, *et al.* Tiagabine inhibits haloperidol-induced oral dyskinesias in rats. *J Neurol Transm* 1994; **95**: 63–69.

Ghaemi SN, Katzow JJ, Desai SP, *et al.* Gabapentin treatment of mood disorders: a preliminary study. *J Clin Psychiat* 1998; **59**: 426–429.

Ghosn M, Carde P, Leclerq B, *et al.* Ifosfamide/mesna related encephalopathy: a case report with a possible role of phenobarbital in enhancing neurotoxicity. *Bull Cancer* 1988; **75**: 391–392.

Gironell A, Kulisevsky J, Barbanoj M, *et al.* A randomised placebo-controlled comparative trial of gabapentin and propranolol in essential tremor. *Arch Neurol* 1999; **56**: 475–480.

Glaxo Wellcome Inc. Product information of LAMICTAL (lamotrigine) tablets and LAMICTAL (lamotrigine) chewable dispersible tablets. In: *Physicians' Desk Reference*, 53rd edn. Montvale, NJ: Medical Economics, 1999: A143.

Goldberg JF, Garno, JL, Leon AC, *et al.* Rapid titration of mood stabilisers predicts remission from mixed or pure mania in bipolar patients. *J Clin Psychiat* 1998; **59**: 151–158.

Gorman WP, Cooper R, Pocock P, *et al.* A comparison of primidone, propranolol, and placebo in essential tremor, using quantitative analysis. *J Neurol Neurosurg Psychiat* 1986; **49**: 64–68.

Greendyke RM, Gulya A. Effects of pindolol administration on serum levels of thioridazine, haloperidol, phenytoin, and phenobarbital. *J Clin Psychiat* 1988; **49**: 105–107.

Grunze H, Erfurth A, Amaun B, *et al.* Gabapentin in the treatment of mania. *Fortschr Neurol Psychiat* 1999; **67**: 257–260.

Harden CL, Lazar LM, Pick LH, *et al.* A beneficial effect on mood in partial epilepsy patients treated with gabapentin. *Epilepsia* 1999; **40**: 1129–1134.

Hardoy MC, Hardoy MJ, Carta MG, *et al.* Gabapentin as a promising treatment for antipsychotic-induced movement disorders in schizoaffective and bipolar patients. *J Affect Disord* 1999; **54**: 315–317.

Hatzimanolis J, Lykouraz L, Qulis P, *et al.* Gabapentin as monotherapy in the treatment of acute mania. *Eur Neuropsychopharmacol* 1999; **9**: 257–258.

Hering R, Kuritzky A. Sodium valproate in the treatment of cluster headache: an open clinical trail. *Cephalalgia* 1989; **9**: 195–199.

Hering R, Kuritzky A. Sodium valproate in the prophylactic treatment of migraine: a double-blind study versus placebo. *Cephalalgia* 1992; **12**: 81–84.

Hirschfeld RM, Allen MH, McEvoy JP, *et al.* Safety and tolerability of oral loading divalproex sodium in acutely manic bipolar patients. *J Clin Psychiatr* 1999; **60**: 815–818.

Hoffmann-Trager A, Peiker G, Glockner R, *et al.* The influence of phenobarbital on the pharmacokinetics of propranolol in pregnancy. *Biol Res Preg Perinatol* 1987; **8**: 57–59.

Holden KR, Titus MO. The effect of tiagabine on spasticity in children with intractable epilepsy: a pilot study. *Pediat Neurol* 1999; **21**: 728–730.

Holman CP, Bell AFJ. A trial of evening primrose oil in the treatment of chronic schizophrenia. *J Orthomol Psychiat* 1983; **12**: 302–304.

Hugen PW, Burger DM, Brinkman K, *et al.* Carbamazepine–indavir interaction causes anti-retroviral therapy failure. *Ann Pharmacpther* 2000; **34**: 465–470.

Hurley SC. Lamotrigine update and its use in mood disorders. *Ann Pharmacother* 2002; **36**: 860–873.

IMS, Health Poland, Sanofi-Synthelabo/BUCNSM, 2002.

IMS, PGSM, 2000, 2001, 2002.

Jawad S, Richens A, Goodwin G, *et al.* Controlled trial of lamotrigine (Lamictal) for refractory partial seizures. *Epilepsia* 1989; **30**: 356–363.

Jellish WS, Modica PA, Tempelhoff R. Accelerated recovery from pipecuronium in patients treated with chronic anticonvulsant therapy. *J Clin Anesth* 1993; **5**: 105–108.

Jensen R, Brinck T, Olesen J. Sodium valproate has a prophylactic effect in migraine without aura. *Neurology* 1994; **44**: 647–651.

Johansen FF, Diemer NH. Enhancement of GABA neurotransmission after cerebral ischemia in the rat reduces loss of hippocampal CA I pyramidal cells. *Acta Neurol Scand* 1991; **84**: 1–5.

Kandrotas R, Cranfield T, Gal P, Ransom JL, *et al.* Effect of phenobarbital administration on theophylline clearance in premature neonates. *Ther Drug Monit* 1990; **12**, 139–143.

Kaufman KR. Adjunctive tiagabine treatment of psychiatric disorders: three cases. *Ann Clin Psychiatr* 1998; **10**: 181–184.

Kishimoto A, Ogura C, Hazama H. Long-term prophylactic effects of carbamazepine in affective disorder. *Br J Psychiat* 1983; **143**: 327–331.

Klapper JA. Divalproex sodium in migraine prophylaxis: a dose-controlled study. *Cephalalgia* 1997; **17**: 103–108.

Kothare SV, Pollack P, Kulberg AG, *et al.* Gabapentin treatment in a child with delayed-onset hemichorea/hemibalismus. *Pediatr Neurol* 2000; **22**: 68–71.

Kraepelin E. Manic–depressive insanity and paranoia. R. M. Barelay (trans.), G. M. Robertson eds. Edinburgh: E&S Livingstone, 1921.

Krogsgaard-Larsen P. GABA synaptic mechanisms: stereochemical and conformational requirements. *Med Res Rev* 1988; **8**: 27–56.

Krusz JC. Levetiracetam as prophylaxis for resistant headaches. *Cephalalgia* 2001; **21**: 373 (abstract P-112).

Krusz J, Daniel D. Levetiracetam, given intravenously, for acute intractable migraine. *Eur J Neurol* 2002; **9**(Suppl. 2): 154.

Krychmantowski AU, Bigal ME, Moreira PF. New and emerging prophylactic agents for migraine. *CNS Drug* 2002; **16**: 611–634.

Lackner TE, Cloyd JC, Thomas LW, *et al.* Antiepileptic drug use in nursing home residents: effect of age, gender, and comedication on patterns of use. *Epilepsia* 1998; **39**: 1083–1087.

Lampe H, Bigalke H. Carbamazepine blocks NMDA-activated currents in cultured spinal cord neurons. *NeuroReport* 1990; **1**: 8–10.

Leijon G, Boivie J. Central poststroke pain: a controlled trial of amitriptiline and carbamazepine. *Pain* 1989; **36**: 27–36.

Lockman LA, Hunningghake DB, Krivit W, *et al.* Relief of pain of Fabry's disease by diphenylhydantoin. *Neurology* 1973; **23**: 871–875.

Löscher W. Valproate: a reappraisal of its pharmacodynamic properties and mechanisms of action. *Prog Neurobiol* 1999; **58**: 31–59.

Macdonald RL. Cellular effects of antiepileptic drugs. In *Epilepsy: A Comprehensive Text Book.* J. Engel, T. A. Pedley, eds. Philadelphia: Lippincott-Raven, 1997: 1383–1391.

Macdonald RL, McLean MJ. Anticonvulsant drugs: mechanisms of action. *Adv Neurol* 1986; **44**: 713–736.

Magnus L. Nonepileptic use of gabapentin. *Epilepsia* 1999; **40**(Suppl. 6): 66–74.

Matar KM, Nicholls PJ, Tekle A, *et al.* Effect of vigabatrin and gabapentin on phenytoin pharmacokinetics in the dog. *Eur J Drug Metabol Pharmacokinet* 2000; **25**: 189–193.

Mateu-de Antonio J, Grau S, Gimeno-Bayon JL, *et al.* Ritonavir induced carbamazepine toxicity. *Ann Pharmacother* 2001; **35**: 125–126.

Mathew NT, Ali S. Valproate in the treatment of persistent chronic daily headache: an open label study. *Headache* 1991; **31**: 71–74.

Mathew NT, Magnus-Miller L, Saper J, *et al.* Efficacy and safety of gabapentin in migraine prophylaxis. *Cephalgia* 1999; **19**: 380.

May TW, Rambeck B, Jurgens U. Serum concentration of lamotrigine in epileptic patients: the influence of dose and comedication. *Ther Drug Monit* 1996; **18**: 523–531.

Mayo-Smith MF. Pharmacological management of alcohol withdrawal. *J Am Med Assoc* 1997; **278**: 144–151.

Mazzini L, Mora G, Balzarini C, *et al.* The natural history and the effects of gabapentin in amyotrophic lateral sclerosis. *J Neurol Sci* 1998; **160**(Suppl. 1): 57–63.

McLean MJ. Clinical pharmacokinetics of gabapentin. *Neurology* 1994; **44**(Suppl. 5): 17–22.

McQuay H, Carroll D, Jadad AR, *et al.* Anticonvulsant drugs for management of pain: a systemic review. *Br Med J* 1995; **311**: 1047–1052.

Mealy NE, Martini L, Castaner R, *et al.* Treatment of pain. *Drug Future* 2002; **27**: 403–434.

Meldrum B. Pharmacology of GABA. *Clin Neuropharmacol* 1982; **5**: 293–316.

Meldrum BS, Chapman AG. Basic mechanisms of Gabitril (tiagabine) and future potential developments. *Epilepsia* 1999; **40**(Suppl. 9): 2–6.

Merren MD. Gabapentin for treatment of pain and tremor a large case of series. *South Med J* 1998; **91**: 739–744.

Miller RG, Moore D, Young LA, *et al.* Placebo-controlled trial of gabapentin in patients with amyotrophic lateral sclerosis. *Neurology* 1996; **47**: 1383–1388.

Montagna P. Nocturnal paroxysmal dystonia and nocturnal wandering. *Neurology* 1992; **42**(Suppl. 6): 61–67.

Moshē SL. Mechanisms of action of anticonvulsant agents. *Neurology* 2000; **55**(Suppl. 1): 32–40.

Munsat TL. Therapy of myotonia: a double-blind evaluation of diphenylhydantoin, procainamide and placebo. *Neurology* 1967; **17**: 359–367.

Neilson EB. Anxiolytic effect of NO-328, a GABA-uptake inhibitor. *Psychopharmacology (Berlin)* 1988; **96**: 42 (abstract).

Newall CA, Anderson LA, Phillipson JD, eds. *Herbal Medicines: A Guide for Health-Care Professionals.* London, England: The Pharmaceutical Press, 1996.

Nevill MW. Gabapentin in the management of neuropathic pain. *Am J Pain Manage* 2000; **10**: 6–12.

Nicol CF. A four year double blind study of Tegretol in facial pain. *Headache* 1969; **9**: 54–57.

Nobili A, Tettamanti M, Frattura L, *et al.* Drug use by elderly in Italy. *Ann Pharmacother* 1997; **31**: 416–422.

Olson WL, Gruenthal M, Mueller ME, *et al.* Gabapentin for Parkinsonism: a double-blind, placebo-controlled, crossover trial. *Am J Med* 1997; **102**: 60–66.

Onofrj M, Thomas A, Paci C, *et al.* Gabapentin in orthostatic tremor: results of double-blind crossover with placebo in four patients. *Neurology* 1998; **51**: 880–882.

Ortho-McNeil Pharmaceutical. Data on file. Raritan, NJ.

Pahwa R, Lyons K, Hubble JP, *et al.* Double-blind controlled trial of gabapentin in essential tremor. *Mor Disord* 1998; **13**: 465–467.

Pakalnis A. Current therapies for prophylaxis of pediatric migraine. *Rev Neurotherapeut* 2002; **2**: 555–559.

Palomeras E, Sanz P, Cauo A, *et al.* Dystonia in a patient treated with propranolol and gabapentin. *Arch Neurol* 2000; **57**: 570–571.

Pande AC, Crockatt JG, Janney CA, *et al.* Gabapentin in bipolar disorder: a placebo-controlled trial of adjunctive therapy. *Bipolar Disord* 2000; **2**: 249–255.

Perignon F, Pecquinot MA, Ged C, *et al.* Pharmacokinetics of prednisone after oral administration in children with renal grafts. Changed inducted by phenobarbital and renal insufficiency. *Arch Franc Pediatr* 1985; **42**(Suppl. 1): 639–644.

Pescatore P, Hammel P, Durand F, *et al.* Fatal fulminant hepatitis induced by nilutamide. *Gastroenterol Clin Biol* 1993; **17**: 499–501.

Pope Jr HG, McElroy SL, Keck Jr PE, *et al.* Valproate in the treatment of acute mania: a placebo-controlled study. *Arch Gen Psychiatr* 1991; **48**: 62–68.

Porter FL, R, Marshall RE, Moore JA, *et al.* Effect of phenobarbital on motor activity and intra-venticular hemorrhage in preterm infants with respiratory disease weighting less than 1500 grams. *J Perinatol* 1985; **2**: 63–66.

Posner J, Cohen AF, Land G, *et al.* The pharmacokinetics of (BW 430C) in healthy subjects with unconjugated hyperbilirubinemia (Gilbert's syndrome). *Br J Clin Pharmacol* 1989; **28**: 117–120.

Post RM, Weiss SB. Kindling and manic-depressive illness. In *The Clinical Relevance of Kindling*. T. Bowling, M.R. Trimble, eds. Chichester: John Wiley & Sons, 1998: 209–230.

Post RM. Effectiveness of carbamazepine in the treatment of bipolar affective disorders. In *The Use of Anticonvulsants in Psychiatric Disorders: Recent Advances*. S. McElroy, H. G. Pope, eds. Clifton, NJ: Oxford Health Care, 1988: 1–23.

Post RM, Denicoff D, Frye MA, *et al.* Re-evaluation of carbamazepine prophylaxis in bipolar disorders. *Br J Psychiat* 1997; **170**: 202–204.

Potter DL, Hart DE, Calder CS, *et al.* A double-blind, randomized, placebo-controlled, parallel study to determine the efficacy of topiramate in the prophylactic treatment of migraine. *Neurology*, 2000; **54**(Suppl. 3): A15.

Roberts I. Barbiturates for acute traumatic brain injury. *Cochrane Database of Systemic Review* 2000: CD00033.

Robertson A, Brodersen R. Effect of drug combinations on bilirubin–albumin binding. *Develp Pharmaco Therpaut* 1991; **17**: 95–99.

Rockliff BW, Davis EH. Controlled sequential trials of carbamazepine in trigeminal neuralgia. *Arch Neurol* 1966; **15**: 129–136.

Romanelli F, Ryan M. Seizure in HIV-seropositive individuals: epidemiology and treatment. *CNS Drugs* 2002; **16**: 91–98.

Rompel H, Bauermeister PW. Aetiology of migraine and prevention with carbamazepine (Tegretol): results of a double-blind, cross-over study. *Afr Med J* 1970; **44**: 75–80.

Ross EL. The evolving role of antiepileptic drugs in treating neuropathic pain. *Neurology* 2000; **55**(Suppl. 1): 41–46.

Rowbotham M, Harden N, Stacey B, *et al*. Gabapentin for the treatment of postherpetic neuralgia. A randomised controlled trial. *J Am Med Assoc* 1998; **280**: 1837–1842.

Rull JA, Quibrera R, Gonzales-Millan H *et al*. Symptomatic treatment of peripheral diabetic neuropathy with carbamazepine (Tegretol): double blind crossover trial. *Diabetologia* 1969; **5**: 215–218.

Ryback RS, Brodsky L, Munasifi F. Gabapentin in bipolar disorder (Letter). *J Neuropsychiat Clin Neurosci* 1997; **9**: 301.

Saccar C, Danish M, Ragni M, *et al*. The effect of phenobarbital on theophylline disposition in children with asthma. *J Aller Clin Immunol* 1985; **75**: 716–719.

Sasso E, Perucca E, Fava R, *et al*. Primidone in the long-term treatment of essential tremor: a prospective study with computerised quantitative analysis. *Clin Neuropharmacol* 1990; **13**: 67–76.

Saudek CD, Werns S, Reidenberg MM. Phenytoin in the treatment of diabetic symmetrical polyneuropathy. *Clin Pharmacol Ther* 1977; **22**: 196–199.

Schaff MR, Fawcett J, Zajecka JM. Divalproex sodium in the treatment of refractory affective disorders. *J Clin Psychiat* 1993; **54**: 380–384.

Schaffer LC, Schaffer CB. Tiagabine and the treatment of refractory bipolar disorder (Letter). *Am J Psychiat* 1999; **156**: 2014–2015.

Sechi GP, Traccis S, Durelli L, *et al*. Carbamazepine versus diphenylhydantoin in the treatment of myotonia. *Eur Neurol* 1983; **22**: 113–118.

Sechi PP, Zuddas M, Piredda M, *et al*. Treatment of cerebellar tremors with carbamazepine: a controlled trial with long-term follow-up. *Neurology* 1989; **39**: 1113–1115.

Shapira NA, Goldsmith TD, McElroy SL. Treatment of binge-eating disorder with topiramate: a clinical case series. *J Clin Psychiatr* 2000; **61**: 368–372.

Shelton M, Calabrese J. Current concepts in rapid cycling bipolar disorder. *Curr Psychiatr Rep* 2000; **2**: 310–315.

Silva RR, Munoz DM, Alpert M. Carbamazepine use in children and adolescents with features of attention-deficit hyperactivity disorder: a meta-analysis. *J Am Acad Child Adolesc Psychiatr* 1996; **35**: 352–358.

Smith D, Chadwick D, Baker G, *et al*. Seizure severity and the quality of life. *Epilepsia* 1993; **34**(Suppl. 5): 31–35.

Smith MC, Riskin BJ. The clinical use of barbiturates in neurological disorders. *Drugs* 1991; **42**: 365–378.

Stern RM, Uijtdehaage SH, Muth ER, *et al*. Effects of phenytoin on vection-induced motion sickness and gastric myoelectric activity. *Aviat Space Environ Med* 1994; **65**: 518–521.

Stewart RB, Cooper JW. Polypharmacy in aged. Practical solutions. *Drugs Aging* 1994; **4**: 449–461.

Telstad W, Sorensen O, Larsen S, *et al*. Treatment of the restless legs syndrome with carbamazepine. A double blind study. *Br Med J* 1984; **288**: 444–446.

Tempelhoff R, Modica PA, Spitznagel Jr EL. Anticonvulsant therapy increases fentanyl requirements during anaesthesia for craniotomy. *Canad J Anaesth* 1990; **37**: 327–332.

Thaker GK, Tamminga CA, Alphs LD, *et al*. Brain γ-aminobutyric acid abnormality in tardive dyskinesia. *Arch Gen Psychiatr* 1987; **44**: 522–529.

Tomson T, Ohman I, Vitols S. Lamotrigine in pregnancy and lactation: a case report. *Epilepsia* 1997; **38**: 1039–1041.

Trauner DA. Barbiturate therapy in acute brain injury. *J Pediat* 1986; **113**: 742–746.

Uvebrant P, Bauziene R. Interactible epilepsy in children. The efficacy of lamotrigine treatment, including non-seizure related benefits. *Neuropaediatrics* 1994; **25**: 284–289.

Vaddadi KS. The use of gamma-linolenic acid and linoleic acid to differentiate between temporal lobe epilepsy and schizophrenia. *Prostagl Med* 1981; **6**: 375–379.

Viswanathan KN, Sundraram N, Rajendiran C. Sodium valproate in therapy of intractable headaches with EEG changes. *Cephalalgia* 1995; **11**: 282–283.

Wada K, Ishigaki S, Ueda K, *et al*. An antivitamin B6, 4′-O-methoxypyridoxine, from the seed of Ginkgo biloba. *Chem Pharm Bull* 1985; **33**: 3555–3556.

Wallin A, Boreus LO. Phenobarbital prophylaxis for hyperbilirubinemia in preterm infants: a controlled study of bilirubin disappearance and infant behavior. *Acta Paediat Scand* 1984; **73**: 488–497.

Wheeler SD, Carrazana EJ. Topiramate-treated cluster headache. *Neurology* 1999; **3**: 234–236.

White HS. Comparative anticonvulsant and mechanistic profile of the established and newer antiepileptic drugs. *Epilepsia* 1999; **40**(Suppl. 1): 52–60.

Whitworth TL, Quick MW. Upregulation of γ-aminobutyric acid derivatives. *Biochem Soc Trans*, 2001, **29** (part 6).

Wootton R, Soul-Lawton J, Rolan PE, *et al*. Comparison of the pharmacokinetics of lamotrigine in patients with chronic renal failure and healthy volunteers. *Br J Clin Pharmacol* 1997; **43**: 23–27.

Worley PF, Baraban JM. Site of anticonvulsant action on sodium channels: autoradiographic and electrophysiological studies in rat brain. *Neurobiology* 1987; **84**: 3051–3055.

Yagi M, Wada K, Sakata M, *et al*. Studies on the constituents of edible and medicinal plants. IV. Determination of 4′-O-methylpyridoxine in serum of the patient with Gin-non food poisoning. *Yakugaku Zasshi* 1993; **113**: 596–599.

Young MC, Hughes IA. Loss of therapeutic control in congenital adrenal hyperplasia due to interaction between dexamethasone and primidone. *Acta Paediat Scand* 1991; **80**: 120–124.

Young LT, Joffe RT, Robb JC, *et al*. Double-blind comparison of addition of a second mood stabiliser versus an antidepressant to an initial mood stabiliser for treatment of patients with bipolar depression. *Am J Psychiat* 2000; **157**: 124–126.

Zeise ML, Kasparow S, Zieglgansberger W. Valproate suppresses N-methyl-D-aspartate evoked, transient depolarisations in the rat neocortex in vitro. *Brain Res* 1991; **544**: 345–348.

Zhang X-I, Velumian AA, Jones OT, *et al*. Modulation high-voltage-activated calcium channels in dentate granule cells by topiramate. *Epilepsia* 2000; **4**: 52–60.

21

Drug monitoring in combination therapy

Walter Fröscher

Department of Neurology and Epileptology, Die Weissenau (Department of Psychiatry I, University of Ulm), Ravensburg, Germany

Introduction

In 1978 Penry remarked 'The clinical management of epilepsy has improved dramatically in the past decade through the determination of serum antiepileptic drug (AED) concentrations' (Penry, 1978). The recommendations for undertaking therapeutic drug monitoring of AEDs in serum are based on clinical experience and on a number of studies demonstrating a correlation between serum concentrations of AEDs on the one hand, and seizure frequency and dose-dependent adverse effects on the other hand. Such a correlation, which is more significant for some AEDs than for others, has been found for the majority of the established AEDs. As for new AEDs, with the exception of vigabatrin, analogous data are increasingly becoming available (Johannessen *et al.*, 2003).

The relationship between serum concentration, seizure frequency and side effects gives the therapeutic range or target range (Table 21.1). In this range, an AED can be considered to be associated with no dose-dependent side effects in the majority of the patients in whom it is effective. Thus the range provides guide values which give a more rapid identification of a patient's individual therapeutic range, which reflects the patient's clinical susceptibility to seizures, seizure type, etc. However, despite a good deal of anecdotal testimony, surprisingly little has been published demonstrating the benefits of anticonvulsant therapeutic drug monitoring in epileptic populations (Eadie, 1995). In two randomized controlled trials on the clinical impact of therapeutic drug monitoring in patients with epilepsy, the implementation of serum AED level monitoring did not improve overall therapeutic outcome, and the majority of patients could be satisfactorily treated by adjusting dose on clinical grounds (Fröscher *et al.*, 1981; Jannuzzi *et al.*, 2000). In the study by Camfield *et al.* (1985), 82 newly diagnosed children were started on AED therapy and followed prospectively for 12–36 months. Serum concentrations were not observed to be different between children who had a relapse and children who continued to have seizure control; concentrations were within the therapeutic range in both groups. In a study of AED side effects in 197 patients, Laplane and Carydakis

Table 21.1 AED therapeutic ranges

Drug	Therapeutic range (μg/ml)
Carbamazepine	3–12
Ethosuximide	40–100
Felbamate	20–110
Gabapentin	2–60
Lamotrigine	0.5–15
Levetiracetam	3–60
Oxcarbazepine/MHD[a]	10–50
Phenobarbital	10–40
Phenytoin	3–20
Primidone[b]	5–15
Tiagabine	5–70
Topiramate	2–25
Valproic acid	40–100

[a] During oxcarbazepine treatment it is only necessary to determine the pharmacologically active monohydroxy derivative (MHD) metabolite.
[b] During primidone treatment it is only necessary to determine the phenobarbital concentration.

The ranges are compiled from following publications: Fröscher (1992, 2000), Glauser and Pippenger (2000), Patsalos (1999), Regenthal *et al.* (1999), Tomson and Johannessen (2000) and Johannessen *et al.* (2003).

(1985) concluded that the recording of side effects from a case history and a physical examination is far more useful than the determination of the serum concentration. By these results, on the one hand the value of a routine serum concentration determination is doubtful, on the other hand most epileptologists are convinced that monitoring improves the pharmacotherapy of the epilepsies even if there is a lack of statistically significant results. At present, the determination of AEDs is considered to be indicated in the situations which are listed in Table 21.2. These indications are valid not only for the established drugs but also for the new AEDs, with the exception of vigabatrin, which is associated with a somewhat unusual mechanism of action whereby its pharmacological effect long outlasts its serum concentration.

Indications for drug monitoring in antiepileptic combination therapy

The applicability of therapeutic drug monitoring during combination therapy with different AEDs or during combination of an AED and drugs used for the

Table 21.2 Indications for the determination of AEDs in serum

* Therapeutic unresponsiveness (the determination of AEDs in serum helps to clarify the causes of the resistance to therapy, a frequent cause being irregular intake or underdosage; deliberate overdosage due to fear of seizures can also be detected)
* Suspected non-compliance
* Lack of communication (e.g. infants, foreign-language patients, disturbances of consciousness, dementia, aphasia)
* Suspected intoxication (including overdose)
* Combination therapy
* Unusual pharmacokinetics (e.g. children, the elderly, pregnancy, hepatic or renal failure)
* Adjustment of the serum concentration into the therapeutic range to prevent under- or overdosage in patients with a low seizure frequency
* Status epilepticus

treatment of non-epilepsy-related conditions relates to three main considerations, which are discussed below.

Avoidance of underdosage

One of the most frequent prescription errors relates to treatment with two drugs that are below the effective dose. If it is not possible to tell from the case history as to which drug is effective, the determination of the serum concentration can provide invaluable information as to which of the two drugs should be adjusted in relation to its dosage. Thus if a patient continues to have seizures on drug A and a drug B, one will determine the serum concentration of both drugs. If the serum concentration of A is within the target range and the serum concentration of B is below, then a first therapeutic step would be to increase the dosage of drug B. In contrast, in a seizure-free patient with the same treatment regimen described above, one would reduce the dosage of drug B and keep the dosage of drug A the same. Undertaking such a step-wise approach also serves to take into account the possibility of pharmacokinetic interactions. Owing to the possibility of drug interactions, the addition or withdrawal of a drug to or from a drug combination may result in a considerable shift in serum concentration. The immediate detection and correction of such a shift may help to prevent underdosage with recurrences of seizures or intoxication. If a patient is seizure free with a combination of lamotrigine with a medium serum concentration and a low serum concentration of valproic acid, the withdrawal of valproic acid may induce seizures, not because of the high efficiency of the low dose of valproic acid but because of the drop of the lamotrigine serum concentration (valproic acid is an enzyme inhibitor, capable of reducing the rate of metabolism of the co-administered lamotrigine; Patsalos *et al.*, 2002). Although valproic acid withdrawal may be undertaken without knowledge of lamotrigine serum concentrations, their knowledge would allow for a more gradual and predictive therapeutic response.

Another setting whereby underdosage can occur is when an AED, whose metabolism is susceptible to enzyme induction, is co-prescribed with an enzyme-inducing AED. If, for example, in a patient with focal epilepsy the occurrence of tonic–clonic seizures has been stopped by valproic acid monotherapy but complex focal seizures persist, one could add the enzyme-inducing drug carbamazepine. This might induce an increase of seizure frequency by an acceleration of the elimination of valproic acid (Patsalos *et al.*, 2002). The cause of the deterioration of the seizure frequency will be explained quickly by measuring the serum concentration of valproic acid. In another patient, the same combination might not increase the seizure frequency but induce toxicity by an increase of the serum concentration of the carbamazepine-epoxide metabolite. The clinical significance of this interaction is particularly important in children, where high concentrations of carbamazepine-epoxide have been observed, along with severe side effects such as vomiting and tiredness. This example also demonstrates the value of monitoring a pharmacologically active metabolite such as carbamazepine-epoxide in special situations.

When an enzyme-inducing AED such as phenytoin is withdrawn from a treatment regimen, one needs to take into account the consequent de-induction. If phenytoin is discontinued abruptly rather than gradually, the valproic acid concentration will increase to its new steady-state level at about 1 week later. In contrast, a drug with a longer half-life (e.g. phenobarbital) would take longer to reach its new steady-state concentration (Mattson, 1995). In these complex situations, monitoring of serum concentration provides invaluable information for the optimal management of patients.

AED underdosage may also be induced by the addition of a drug which has been indicated for a non-epilepsy-related condition. If, for example, gabapentin is co-ingested with hydroxides of aluminium or magnesium (antacids), the absorption of gabapentin will be reduced (Patsalos *et al.*, 2002). The extent of the reduced absorption is best ascertained by measuring the serum concentration.

Avoidance of intoxication and identification of suspected side effects

Clinically relevant examples of interactions between AEDs with the consequence of an increase of the serum concentration of one of the drugs (or both drugs, e.g. when phenytoin and phenobarbital are co-prescribed) are the combination of the enzyme-inhibiting valproic acid and phenobarbital (increase of phenobarbital), valproic acid and lamotrigine (increase of lamotrigine), topiramate and phenytoin (increase of phenytoin), sulthiame and phenytoin (increase of phenytoin), and the aforementioned combination of valproic acid and carbamazepine (increase of carbamazepine-epoxide; Patsalos *et al.*, 2002; Rambeck *et al.*, 1987).

When combination therapy is associated with symptoms of intoxication, the clinical features and the electroencephalogram (EEG) are often not the right tools to ascertain which AED is responsible. When non-specific neurological symptoms such as tremor and ataxia appear, it is not always clear whether the symptoms are due to intoxication or to the underlying disease, particularly if the disease is progressive. The same is true for psychic symptoms. The difficulty of distinguishing between the symptoms of an underlying disease and intoxication is illustrated by the following case history of a patient on phenytoin monotherapy. We observed a 55-year old epileptic patient with a psychosyndrome, which had been interpreted as postcontusional by the doctor in attendance. The patient was disoriented and decelerated. He was treated with 300 mg phenytoin per day. The neurological examination was hindered because the patient did not cooperate. AED side effects were not expected by the doctor in attendance. The phenytoin level was 53 μg/ml. In reality the psychosyndrome thought to be postcontusional was a pharmacogenetically associated psychosis which disappeared after the withdrawal of phenytoin (Fröscher, 1992).

In ambiguous cases of intoxication in which the concentration of the administered drug is 'normal' and the drug has a pharmacologically active metabolite, the measurement of the metabolite, for example phenylethylmalonamide (PEMA) during primidone therapy or carbamazepine-epoxide during carbamazepine therapy, may be diagnostically helpful. Indeed it should not be forgotten that with AEDs such as carbamazepine and primidone the alleged monotherapy in fact comprises of two or three components (carbamazepine, carbamazepine-epoxide; phenobarbital, PEMA, primidone). Another consideration in doubtful cases of intoxication is the possibility of the intake of drugs which have not been prescribed including over the counter supplements and herbal remedies. Such drugs can only be detected and quantitated by methodologies that are based on basic analytical principles such as high performance liquid chromatography. The use of reagent-based commercial analysis such as enzyme immunoassay may not be sufficient to identify the drug that is responsible for the clinical presentation as the following case history demonstrates. A 28-year old female patient with focal epilepsy was admitted to the hospital because of gait ataxia. The only prescribed drug was carbamazepine. Therefore, at admittance, only the serum concentration of this drug was determined. The carbamazepine value was in the lower part of the target range. With some delay we detected that the patient had continued to take phenytoin which she should have stopped 18 months before. The subsequently measured phenytoin concentration was 60 μg/ml, which was far above the target range.

When AEDs are co-prescribed with drugs for other indications, intoxication can similarly occur. For example, when carbamazepine and erythromycin are co-prescribed, the measurement of carbamazepine serum concentration is indicated because this combination can be associated with a significant increase in carbamazepine concentrations; the extent of which cannot be predicted reliably (Patsalos *et al.*, 2002; Patsalos and Duncan, 1993).

Monitoring of concomitant medication

Another consideration arising from the combination of AEDs and drugs used for other indications may be an underdosage of the latter drugs. If one combines, for example, cyclosporine with an enzyme-inducing drug such as carbamazepine, phenobarbital, phenytoin or oxcarbazepine (Rösche *et al.*, 2001), careful monitoring of cyclosporine is necessary because serum cyclosporine concentrations can be expected to decrease. Thus in patients that have undergone an organ transplantation, this interaction would quickly result in a rejection of the transplanted organ.

Prerequisites of the determination of AEDs in serum

The essential prerequisite for monitoring serum concentrations, both in monotherapy and in combination therapy, is the reliability (accuracy and precision) of the assay methodology (Wilson *et al.*, 1989; Williams *et al.*, 2003). Another important factor is the consideration of the time interval between drug intake and the collection of blood. Thus if a drug has a short half-life value, the blood sampling of a patient in an outpatients setting often does not result in the determination of a trough concentration. In combination with an enzyme-inducing AED, the half-life value of tiagabine, for example, is reduced from 5–8 h (monotherapy) to 2–5 h. When phenobarbital and valproic acid are administered in combination, the half-life value of valproic acid is reduced while the half-life of phenobarbital is increased and its peak concentration is delayed (Patsalos *et al.*, 2002).

Also, as in the case of monotherapy, one has to take into consideration whether or not the measured serum concentration is reflective of steady state. When the dosage is changed, the new serum concentration should not be determined until steady state has been achieved (typically this can be expected to occur after five half-life values of the affected drug).

Measurement of the free (non-protein bound) concentration of AEDs

Some AEDs are highly protein bound in blood to albumin. These include carbamazepine (80%), phenytoin (90%), tiagabine (96%) and valproic acid (95%). Some AEDs may interact at the albumin protein-binding site and free concentration may increase; for example free carbamazepine-epoxide concentrations are significantly increased in patients taking carbamazepine plus valproic acid (Liu *et al.*, 1995). Since only the free concentration can penetrate the blood–brain barrier, several attempts have been made to improve treatment by using free drug concentration measurements; for example by determining AEDs in saliva or by measuring the free concentration in blood by ultrafiltration (Liu and Delgado, 1999). The clinical relevance of the determination of the free AED concentrations is somewhat controversial, even for highly protein bound drugs (Fröscher *et al.*, 1985). Nevertheless, overall there are clinical settings where patient management would best benefit from measurement of free serum concentrations. Indeed, when phenytoin and valproic acid are co-prescribed, measurement of total phenytoin concentrations would be misleading because of the protein-binding displacement interaction that occurs between these AEDs (Patsalos and Perucca, 2003).

Limits and dangers of the determination of serum concentrations of AEDs

The effectiveness of serum concentration determination depends on the accuracy of the therapeutic ranges of the individual AEDs. Therefore, for phenytoin with its narrow therapeutic range the indication for serum concentration monitoring is much clearer than, for example, phenobarbital, for which the upper limit of the therapeutic range is very blurred.

As for the new AEDs, the clinical relevance of drug monitoring is limited by the fact that the target ranges are derived from the clinical trial data collected during their evaluation as add-on therapy (Johannessen *et al.*, 2003). These studies enrol patients that are highly selected and as such are not reflective of patients seen in general clinical practice. Nevertheless, these ranges are valuable as they provide reference values, which can aid patient management. Serum monitoring of new AEDs is particularly useful when interacting AED combinations are co-prescribed.

The appropriate procedure for adjusting the dosage is essentially the same irrespective of whether or not the serum concentration is determined. In both cases the dose is increased slowly until seizures cease or, if seizures persist, until the intoxication limit is reached. The upper limit of the serum concentration is merely a warning signal, not a barrier. The procedure must be similar because the individual therapeutic ranges are different. The lower limit of the target range or therapeutic range is even more indistinct than the upper limit.

It is imperative that therapeutic ranges are appreciated for what they are, that is statistical ranges whereby if a patient achieves a serum concentration within that range, the probability of achieving a desirable therapeutic response (with minimal side effects) is high. A serum concentration should be used in conjunction with the knowledge of the patient, the clinical information and also the pharmacokinetic characteristics of the drug. The therapeutic range should be used as a guide.

Special laboratory tests

Sometimes when there is an interaction associated with AED treatment, a surrogate physiological marker may be necessary other than the measurement of a serum drug concentration, so as to ascertain the interaction. An example of this is the combination of phenprocoumon or warfarin and an enzyme-inducing AED, whereby the serum concentration of phenprocoumone/warfarin will decrease. In this setting the careful monitoring of the prothrombin time (or internationalized normalized ratio, INR) is indicated. Another example is that of valproic acid-induced encephalopathy. Valproic acid occasionally induces stuporous or comatose states. This encephalopathy is frequently accompanied by hyperammonemia without signs of hepatic failure. Valproic acid encephalopathy may occur after initiation of valproic acid as monotherapy or, more often, in combination with other AEDs (e.g. phenobarbital, phenytoin, topiramate). In this setting monitoring of plasma ammonia concentrations would be a valuable diagnostic tool (Hamer *et al.*, 2000).

Future of monitoring

Therapeutic drug monitoring has greatly enhanced the treatment of epilepsy in that it has allowed the individualization of treatment and thus maximized the desirable anticonvulsant effects of AEDs while keeping to a very minimum the undesirable side effects that are associated with AEDs. Monitoring is essential for drugs with a narrow therapeutic index and for those drugs with unacceptable incidence of toxicity. This is particularly exemplified by phenytoin (Gentry and Rodvold, 1995). With regards to the new AEDs, target ranges are at their infancy and will inevitably require fine tuning as our clinical experience with these drugs increases. The usefulness of drug monitoring during combination polytherapy is dependent on the propensity of the combination to interact and the extent and mechanism of the interaction. For pharmacodynamic interactions, drug monitoring is only of value in that it is used to exclude the possibility that an interaction is pharmacokinetic in nature. For many pharmacokinetic interactions, the direction and extent of the associated change in serum drug concentration cannot be reliably predicted. Furthermore, some interactions may be associated with either an increase or a reduction in serum concentration. The likelihood of an unpredictable interaction is much lower with some of the new AEDs compared with the established drugs. Indeed gabapentin and levetiracetam have a particularly low propensity to interact

(Patsalos, 2003). Therefore, the role of drug monitoring will not be important during combination therapy with these AEDs.

Summary

Combination therapy is an important indication for AED therapeutic drug monitoring as it is an invaluable aid in avoiding underdosage and intoxication and also to confirm drug-related side effects.

If it is not possible to conclude from the case history which component of a combination is probably effective, the determination of the serum concentration helps identify which drug dosage should be increased or lowered. In this setting one has to take into account the possibility of drug interactions. In particular, consequent to a pharmacokinetic interaction, the addition or withdrawal of a drug to or from a combination may result in a considerable shift in serum concentration. The early detection and correction of such a shift may help to prevent, for example, underdosage with recurrences of seizures. With the combination of a medium dose of lamotrigine and a low dose of valproic acid, the withdrawal of valproic acid may induce seizures not because of the low dose of valproic acid but as a consequence of the decrease of the lamotrigine serum concentration. When combination therapy has led to intoxication symptoms the clinical picture and the EEG are often not helpful in recognizing the responsible drug. In sedated patients taking a combination of valproic acid and phenobarbital, drug monitoring can help to differentiate between valproic acid encephalopathy with a 'normal' serum concentration and phenobarbital intoxication as the consequence of an inhibitory interaction between phenobarbital and valproic acid with a consequent elevation of phenobarbital serum concentrations.

REFERENCES

Camfield PR, Camfield CS, Smith EC, *et al.* Newly treated childhood epilepsy: a prospective study of recurrences and side effects. *Neurology* 1985; **35**: 722–725.

Eadie MJ. The role of therapeutic drug monitoring in improving the cost-effectiveness of anticonvulsant therapy. *Clin Pharmacokinet* 1995; **29**: 29–35.

Fröscher W. Clinical relevance of the determination of antiepileptic drugs in serum. *Wiener Klinische Wochenschrift* 1992; **191**(Suppl.): 15–18.

Fröscher W. "Therapeutischer" Bereich der Serumspiegel der Antiepileptika. In *Pharmakotherapie der Epilepsien*. W. Fröscher, V. Blankenhorn, Th. W. May, *et al.* eds. Stuttgart: Schattauer-Verlag, 2000: 43–66.

Fröscher W, Eichelbaum M, Gugler R, *et al.* A prospective randomized trial of the effect of monitoring plasma anticonvulsant levels in epilepsy. *J Neurol* 1981; **224**: 193–201.

Fröscher W, Burr W, Penin H, *et al.* Free level monitoring of carbamazepine and valproic acid: clinical significance. *Clin Neuropharmacol* 1985; **8**: 362–371.

Gentry ChA, Rodvold KA. How important is therapeutic drug monitoring in the prediction and avoidance of adverse reactions? *Drug Safety* 1995; **12**: 359–363.

Glauser TA, Pippenger CE. Controversies in blood-level monitoring: reexamining its role in the treatment of epilepsy. *Epilepsia* 2000; **41**(Suppl. 8): S6–S15.

Hamer HM, Knake S, Schomburg U, *et al.* Valproate-induced hyperammonemic encephalopathy in the presence of topiramate. *Neurology* 2000; **54**: 230–232.

Johannessen SI, Battino D, Berry DJ, *et al.* Therapeutic drug monitoring of the newer antiepileptic drugs. *Ther Drug Monit* 2003; **25**: 347–363.

Jannuzzi G, Cian P, Fattore C, *et al.* A multicenter randomized controlled trial on the clinical impact of therapeutic drug monitoring in patients with newly diagnosed epilepsy. *Epilepsia* 2000; **41**: 222–230.

Laplane D, Carydakis C. Les effets secondaires des traitements antiépileptiques. Etude des 197 cas. *Revue Neurologique (Paris)* 1985; **141**: 447–455.

Liu H, Delgado MR. Therapeutic drug concentration monitoring using saliva samples. Focus on anticonvulsants. *Clin Pharmacokin* 1999; **23**: 365–379.

Liu H, Delgado MP, Browne RH. Interactions of valproic acid with carbamazepine and its metabolites, concentrations, concentration ratios, and level/dose ratios in epileptic patients. *Clin Neuropharmacol* 1995; **18**: 1–12.

Mattson H. Antiepileptic drug monitoring: a reappraisal. *Epilepsia* 1995; **36**(Suppl. 5): S22–S29.

Patsalos PN. New antiepileptic drugs. *Ann Clin Biochem* 1999; **36**: 10–19.

Patsalos PN. The pharmacokinetic characteristics of levetiracetam. *Meth Find Exp Clin Pharmacol* 2003; **25**: 123–129.

Patsalos PN, Duncan JS. Antiepileptic drugs – a review of clinically significant drug interactions. *Drug Safety* 1993; **9**: 156–184.

Patsalos PN, Perucca E. Clinically important drug interactions in epilepsy: general features and interactions between antiepileptic drugs. *Lancet Neurol* 2003; **2**: 347–356.

Patsalos PN, Fröscher W, Pisani F, *et al.* The importance of drug interactions in epilepsy therapy. *Epilepsia* 2002; **43**: 365–385.

Penry JK. Reliability of serum antiepileptic concentrations and patient management. In *Antiepileptic Drugs: Quantitative Analysis and Interpretation.* C. E. Pippenger, J. K. Penry, H. Kutt, eds. New York: Raven Press, 1978: 1–5.

Rambeck B, May ThW, Juergens U. Serum concentrations of carbamazepine and its epoxide and diol metabolites in epileptic patients: the influence of dose and comedication. *Ther Drug Monit* 1987; **9**: 298–303.

Regenthal R, Krüger M, Köppel C, *et al.* Zu Möglichkeiten und Grenzen von Therapeutischen und Klinisch-toxikologischen Referenzwerten für Plasma-/Serum-/Vollblutkonzentrationen von Arzneimitteln bei akuten Vergiftungen – eine Übersicht. *Anästhesie Intensivmedizin* 1999; **3**: 129–144.

Rösche J, Fröscher W, Abendroth D, *et al.* Possible oxcarbazepine interaction with cyclosporine serum levels: a single case study. *Clin Neuropharmacol* 2001; **24**: 113–116.

Tomson T, Johannessen SI. Therapeutic monitoring of the new antiepileptic drugs. *Eur J Clin Pharmacol* 2000; **55**: 697–705.

Williams J, Bialer M, Johannessen SI, *et al.* Interlaboratory variability in the quantification of new generation antiepileptic drugs based on external quality assessment data. *Epilepsia* 2003; **44**: 40–45.

Wilson JF, Tsanaclis LM, Williams J, *et al.* Evaluation of assay techniques for the measurement of antiepileptic drugs in serum: a study based on external quality assurance data. *Ther Drug Monit* 1989; **11**: 185–195.

22

Cognitive side-effects due to antiepileptic drug combinations and interactions

Albert P. Aldenkamp[1,2,3], Mark de Krom[1], Irene Kotsopoulos[1] and Jan Vermeulen[4]

[1] Department of Neurology, University Hospital of Maastricht, The Netherlands
[2] Department of Behavioral Science, Epilepsy Centre Kempenhaeghe, Heeze, The Netherlands
[3] University of Amsterdam, SCI Kohnstamm Research Institute, Amsterdam, The Netherlands
[4] Epilepsy centre SEIN, Heemstede, The Netherlands

Introduction

The possibility that cognitive impairment may develop as a consequence or aftermath of epilepsy was raised as early as 1885 when Gowers described 'epileptic dementia' as an effect of the pathological sequela of seizures. Nonetheless, the topic was not coupled to antiepileptic drug (AED) treatment until the 1970s.

It has now been established that AED treatment may be associated with a variety of side-effects (Aldenkamp, 1995, 1998; Vermeulen and Aldenkamp, 1995, 2001). Some effects appear immediately after the start of drug exposure, such as nystagmus, but are relatively benign because they show habituation (Kulig and Meinardi, 1977), or are reversible when they are dose dependent. Others may be of insidious onset, emerging only after extended periods of treatment (i.e. chronic side-effects). A multitude of such chronic side-effects have been documented (Reynolds, 1975), but the most frequently reported effects concern central nervous system (CNS) effects. This chapter reviews some of our knowledge about a specific subgroup of such CNS-related chronic side-effects of AED treatment, that is, cognitive side effects: the adverse effects of drug treatment on information-processing systems.

Such effects are considered to be much more moderate than for example, some of the idiosyncratic reactions to drugs and normally do not lead to discontinuation of drug treatment. Nonetheless, a number of studies have claimed that the drug-induced cognitive impairments may have a much greater impact on daily life function than had hitherto been suspected (Trimble, 1983, 1987a, b), for example through the impact on critical functions, that is, learning in children (Aldenkamp, 1995) or driving capacities in adults (often requiring milliseconds precision), or on vulnerable functions such as memory function in elderly. Moreover, as the cognitive side-effects represent the long-term outcome of AEDs, the effects may increase with prolonged therapy, which may contribute to the impact on daily life functioning in patients with refractory epilepsies (Committee on Drugs, 1985).

Review of psychometric studies

The interest in the cognitive side-effects of AED treatment is of relatively recent origin and the first studies are from the 1970s (Ideström *et al.*, 1972; Dodrill and Troupin, 1977), probably stimulated by the widening range of possibilities for drug treatment during that period; valproate (VPA) and carbamazepine (CBZ) were clinically introduced in this same period and many studies compare these drugs with phenytoin (PHT). A first paragraph of this chapter reviews the literature in lines of evidence-based medicine, that is, reviewing the empirical data that were published in peer-reviewed journals. Potentially relevant studies were identified through computerized and manual searches of the English-language literature published from January 1970 through December 1994. A computerized search of the DIMDI database was conducted. In addition, the bibliographies of several reviews on the same topic were examined (Trimble and Thompson, 1981, 1983; Trimble, 1983, 1987a; Evans and Gualtieri, 1985; Novelly *et al.*, 1986; Smith, 1991; Dodrill, 1992). Criteria for selection of the papers were:

1 English-language report of original research, published in peer-reviewed journals in the period 1970–1994; studies after 1970 were all done at a time when most of the current AEDs had become available and modern cognitive tests had come into widespread use.
2 Studies that report psychometrically assessed cognitive functions (excluding for example clinical observations).
3 Only current AEDs (excluding experimental drugs that have been removed from study programmes, such as zonisamide (ZNS), felbamate or flunarizine).
4 Only studies on patients with epilepsy (excluding AED studies in for example psychiatric patients). The resulting meta-analysis has been published on the data concerning monotherapy (Vermeulen and Aldenkamp, 1995). Here we focus on the results for combination therapy or polytherapy.

In the meta-analysis, studies were classified into the polytherapy category if subjects were treated with more than one drug at a time and no comparisons between individual drugs, or single drug vs. no AED, were possible. Studies that were identified through the aforementioned procedure and involving polytherapy are listed in Table 22.1 (Reynolds and Travers, 1974; Debakan and Lehman, 1975; Matthews and Harley, 1975; Sommerbeck *et al.*, 1977; Wilensky *et al.*, 1981; Thompson and Trimble, 1980, 1982, 1983; Corbett *et al.*, 1985; Ludgate *et al.*, 1985; Berent *et al.*, 1987; Durwen *et al.*, 1989; Prevey *et al.*, 1989; Duncan *et al.*, 1990; Van

Rijckevorsel–Harmant, 1990; Dodrill and Wilensky, 1992; Durwen *et al.*, 1992; May *et al.*, 1992; McGuire *et al.*, 1992; McKee *et al.*, 1992; Pieters *et al.*, 1992; Chataway *et al.*, 1993; Dodrill *et al.*, 1993; Durwen and Elger, 1993; Gilham *et al.*, 1993; Mitchell *et al.*, 1993; Smith *et al.*, 1993; McKee *et al.*, 1994).

From Table 22.1, the following points can be noted:

1 *Treatments.* This section shows the treatment conditions associated with assessment points. The nomenclature and abbreviations for individual AEDs comply with the recommendations in *Epilepsia*, 1993, 34, 1151. In addition: P, polytherapy; SAD, single additional dose; Mono, monotherapy; plac, placebo; none, no AEDs. Subscripts: AED_{cr}, controlled release formulation; $AED_{Dhi/Dme/Dlo}$, high, medium, low dosage; $AED_{Shi/Slo}$, high vs. low serum (or saliva) levels; $P_{red, mod}$, P reduction [c.q.], other modification; $P_{AED+/-}$, P with vs. without a particular AED; $P_{tox+/-}$, P with toxic vs. non-toxic serum levels. Slashes (/) indicate contrasts under study in a parallel group or post-test-only design. Crosses ($\times$) indicate crossover elements. Arrows ($\rightarrow$) indicate change of one treatment to another. Plus signs ($+$) indicate that medication is added to an existing regimen.

2 *Number of subjects.* The numbers are shown separately for each treatment condition and untreated controls; they indicate the number of subjects who completed the trial and for who test data were available. A range is given for *n* when not all subjects completed all tests. Occasionally, we were unable to determine these numbers for the separate treatments (e.g. when only an overall *n* was provided), or for one or more outcome measures. This is indicated by a question mark.

3 *Drop-out rate.* This gives a rough indication as to whether a selection artefact might have developed during the trial. An overall rate is given separately for subjects on AEDs and untreated controls. About half the studies reviewed mention dropout losses and present sufficient data to compute a drop-out rate for each outcome measure. A range may be given here as well as due to incompletion in various degrees. A few studies explicitly state that no dropout losses occurred (–). In others, dropout losses are mentioned but insufficient data is provided to compute a loss rate (?). Often, dropout losses or their absence are not mentioned (n.m.), which may or may not mean that no such losses occurred. Sometimes a minimum rate is quoted ($\geqslant$), more subjects may have been lost, but the data are unclear or ambiguous in this regard.

4 *Design.* (Table 22.2 gives an overview of the general design types encountered.) The term design as used here refers to the scheduling of treatments (i.e. AEDs, placebo, no treatment) and outcome measurement sessions, and to the way subjects were assigned to treatment groups (i.e. on a random basis or not). Occasionally, we were unable to discover a consistent principle underlying

Table 22.1 Review summary of polytherapy polytherapy studies (1970–1994)

Study	Treatments	Subjects (N) On AEDs	Untreated controls	Drop-out rate	Design	Cognitive variables (N)	Time on AED
Reynolds and Travers (1974)	P	57	–	n.m.	Post-test	3	?
Dekaban and Lehman (1975)	$(P_{Dhi} \rightarrow P_{Dme} \rightarrow P_{Dlo})$/none	8–12	6_{NE}	n.m.	Parallel	6	14–20 days
Matthews and Harley (1975)	P_{tox+} /P_{tox-}	35/28	–	n.m.	Post-test	33	?
Sommerbeck *et al.* (1977)	P + (VPA × plac)	8–20	–	33–73%	X-over (R)	30	12 weeks
Thompson and Trimble (1980, 1982)	P/(P → (P_{red}/P_{red} + CBZ))	10/20/15	–	n.m.	Parallel	6	6 months
Wilensky *et al.* (1981)	PHT + (CLZ × PB)	43	–	22%	X-over (R)	?	4 months
Thompson and Trimble (1983)	P_{Shi} × P_{Slo}	28	–	n.m.	X-over	20	3 months
Corbett *et al.* (1985)	P	312	–	n.m.	?	1	?
Ludgate *et al.* (1985)	P → Mono	12	–	33%	Single	17	1 year
Berent *et al.* (1987)	P → (P_{red} + ZNS)	9	–	18%	Single	16	24 weeks
Brodie *et al.* (1987)	P/CBZ/VPA/PHT	66	25	n.m.	Single	20	?
Durwen *et al.* (1989)	P → P_{mod}	13	–	n.m.	Single	18	?
Prevey *et al.* (1989)	P → VPA	8	–	n.m.	Single	17	5 months
Duncan *et al.* (1990)	P/(P → (P_{PHT-}/P_{CBZ-}/P_{VPA-}))	25/20–21/14	–	16–17%	Parallel	8	4 weeks
Van Rijckevorsel *et al.* (1990)	P → P_{mod}	26	–	28%	?	5	3 months
Durwen *et al.* (1992)	P → P_{mod}	13	–	n.m.	Single	18	5 days
Dodrill and Wilensky (1992)	PHT/P_{PHT+}/P_{PHT-}	11/11/11	–	83%	Parallel	20	5 years

McGuire et al. (1992)	P/(P + VGB)	15/15	–	n.m.	Parallel	7	4 weeks
McKee et al. (1992)	CBZ → (CBZ + VPA)	16	–	33%	Single	7	5 days
May et al. (1992)	P_{PHT+}/(P_{PHT+} → P_{PHT-})	12/17	–	n.m.	Parallel	15	10 weeks
Pieters et al. (1992)	(P_{CBZ} → P_{CBZcr})/none	15	15_{NE}	6%	Parallel	22	4 weeks
Bittencourt et al. (1993)	PB + (PHT/CBZ)	50	–	15%	Parallel	?	6 months
Gilham et al. (1993)	P + (VGB × plac)	24	–	13%	X-over (R)	10	12 weeks
Smith et al. (1993)	P + (LTG × plac)	40–44	–	46–51%	X-over (R)	9	18 weeks
Dodrill et al. (1993)	P → (P + (VGB/plac))	83/85	–	8%	Parallel (R)	19	12 weeks
Chataway et al. (1993)	P/(P_{CZP+} → P_{CZP-})	11/11	–	52%	Parallel	4	2 weeks
Durwen and Elger (1993)	P → P_{mod}	27	–	n.m.	Single	19	5 days
Mitchell et al. (1993)	P_{mod}	?	-	n.m.	?	?	?
McKee et al. (1994)	CBZ + (OCBZ × plac)/VPA + (OCBZ × plac)/ PHT + (OCBZ × plac)/OCBZ	9/9/10/7	–	19%	X-over (R)	8	3 weeks

VGB, vigabatrin; LTG, lamotrigine; OCBZ, oxcarbazepine; CLZ, clorazepate.

Randomized treatment allocation, or treatment sequencing in a crossover and parallel design, is indicated by the suffix (R).

Table 22.2 Design nomenclature and classification

Abbreviated designation	Design name	Definition
Post-test	Post-test-only	One or more groups of subjects are tested *after* (but not before) receiving treatment
Single	Single group pre-test–post-test	A single group is tested both before and after the treatment period
Parallel	Parallel groups	Two or more groups are assigned to different treatment conditions and tested both before and after the treatment period
X-over	Crossover	The same subjects are tested under different treatment conditions, counterbalancing the order of treatments

Randomized treatment allocation, or treatment sequencing in a crossover design, is indicated by the suffix (R).

the scheduling of treatments and assessment points, or different schedules were employed for different subjects. In such cases the design was classified as unclear (?).

5 *Number of cognitive variables.* This gives an indication of the possible scope of the study with respect to cognitive functioning; also, this is a statistically relevant characteristic. Uncertainty as to the number of variables actually employed (?) in analysing the data may occur even if the tests used are mentioned; often multiple outcome variables may be derived from a single test (e.g. response speed, accuracy, subscales in intelligence tests).

6 *Time on AED.* This characteristic is important in judging the relevance of the results to chronic AED use. Its meaning depends on the particular design employed. In a post-test-only design the figures quoted relate to the duration of treatment prior to the assessment point. In repeated measurement designs with one or more groups (i.e. single and parallel) this refers to the duration of the experimentally changed AED-treatment or the continuous medication interval studied. With multiple assessment points during the trial, the maximum interval studied is given. In a crossover design where multiple AEDs or dosages are given, this refers to the time on each AED [c.q.] dosage.

Methodological considerations

Closer inspection of the studies that we identified shows many methodological problems, most of which are inherent to polytherapy as such. These methodological problems must be taken into consideration carefully because they restrict the validity of the information from these studies.

Treatment reproducibility

Polytherapy is by nature a heterogeneous treatment category; thus, one finds treatment descriptions such as 'various combinations of the three major AEDs' (Reynolds and Travers, 1974) or 'PHT and one or more other AEDs' [c.q.], 'drug regimens exclusive of PHT' (Dodrill and Wilensky, 1992), or even 'no attempt was made to standardize drug therapy as part of the study' (Mitchell *et al.*, 1993). Obviously, widely different drug regimes would fit such descriptions, and results established with one regimen may not apply to another. Also, the polytherapy manipulations used in many studies are actually quite complex, making replication problematical. For example, *all* polytherapy reduction studies are done as part of individualized programs of therapy rationalization. That is, patients did not have their medications changed for research purposes, and different types of medication change were not subjected to randomization. Rather, changes were typically made 'according to the individual needs of each patient' (Durwen *et al.*, 1992). The clinical considerations underlying the medication changes are a major ingredient of the treatment package, albeit one that may not be easily reproduced.

Drug interactions

Combinations of AEDs may alter metabolism to produce changes in the level of active and/or toxic metabolites. Examples include the decrease in CBZ levels due to the increased elimination of the drug when given together with PHT and/or phenobarbital (PB). Such interactions can alter seizure control efficacy and may be relevant to cognitive functioning. With multiple drugs, identifying the components of a treatment most responsible for any observed effects presents a difficult problem.

Serum concentration-effect relationships

Cognitive AED effects may be examined through an analysis of the relationship between test scores of subjects and their individual serum drug levels, and this approach seems to offer a way out of the problem mentioned above. In fact, a number of studies report such relationships suggesting that, generally, higher serum levels are associated with lower cognitive scores. However, in patients with epilepsy, higher serum concentrations may be the reflection of higher AED doses prescribed for more severe epilepsy (Reynolds, 1989), perhaps with seizures not fully controlled (Butlin *et al.*, 1984). Also, AEDs may interact on receptor sites (pharmacodynamics), which would not necessarily be reflected in the pharmacokinetics expressed in serum concentrations. Such factors greatly reduce the interpretability of relationships between serum concentrations and cognitive performance.

Seizure confound

Polytherapy is typically given to patients with refractory epilepsy, and separating seizure effects from AED effects may thus be very difficult, particularly in add-on studies, where the cognitive evaluation is usually made in connection with an efficacy trial. That is, adverse cognitive AED effects may be masked by beneficial effects of better seizure control. Also, patients with refractory seizures may not be representative of the general population with epilepsy.

Discussion of cognitive effects

Due to the validity threats described above, acting singly or simultaneously, drawing conclusions about the cognitive effects of polytherapy studies is not without complications. Table 22.1 shows a heterogeneous number of treatments and designs. Moreover, the anecdotal-type of information is best illustrated by the large number of question marks both in the column expressing numbers of patients, for the drop-out rates and even for design, number of cognitive variables, and time on AEDs. Starting from the principles of evidence-based medicine we can therefore only proceed carefully. Conclusions will be drawn on a general level.

Reviewing the literature, five types of studies can be distinguished:

- The first type of study is the single measurement polytherapy study. Corbett *et al.* (1985) is an example of studies that analyze polytherapy in a single measurement design. Patients who received polytherapy are analysed for cognitive impairments. Although, without exception all these studies report severe cognitive impairment the design does not allow the isolation of drug effects from the effects of the epilepsy.
- The second type consists of studies comparing monotherapy with polytherapy. Brodie *et al.* (1987) showed no difference between monotherapy CBZ, VPA, PHT and polytherapy at a single assessment study. Other studies did, however, show serious impairments for polytherapy. Bittencourt *et al.* (1993) used a complex add-on with a polytherapy at baseline (with either PHT or CBZ added to an existing low-dose PB regime) and monotherapy (PHT or CBZ) at endpoint. The study shows statistically significant improvements on measures of memory and attention after withdrawal from polytherapy. As for the former type of study, it is extremely difficult to avoid the seizure confound here as polytherapy is mostly given to different patients.
- A convincing group of studies showed the effect of reduction of polytherapy. Durwen *et al.* (1989) showed that reduction of polytherapy resulted in improvements of verbal memory. Duncan *et al.* (1990) used a rather interesting design in which separate drugs (PHT, CBZ, VPA) were removed from polytherapy regimes showing consistent improvements in cognitive function, irrespective of the type of drug that was discontinued. Thompson and Trimble (1980, 1982) Ludgate *et al.*

(1985) and Van Rijckervorsel *et al.* (1990) are other examples of studies that showed marked improvement after reduction of polytherapy.

- In contrast, the fourth type of study does not show convincing effects of polytherapy. In these add-on studies a new drug is added to either monotherapy or to an existing polytherapy. Berents *et al.* (1987) showed impaired verbal learning when a new drug was added to an already existing polytherapy. Most other studies (Dodrill and Wilensky, 1992; McGuire *et al.*, 1992; Pieters *et al.*, 1992; Dodrill *et al.*, 1993; Gilham *et al.*, 1993), however, showed no effects of newer drugs to an existing polytherapy. These are, however, all studies within the context of drug trials in refractory epilepsy, where the added effects of a new drug are difficult to entangle from the beneficial effects of improved seizure control.
- Finally, the last type of study that we could distinguish analyzed the relationship between cognitive impairment in polytherapy with serum level. Dekaban and Lehman (1975) claim a relationship but the study does not control interfering factors such as dose and seizure confound and, hence, does not guarantee valid interpretation. The same situation occurs for other studies such as Reynolds and Travers (1974), Matthews and Harley (1975) and Thompson and Trimble (1983).

The existing evidence from especially the reduction studies, therefore suggests the possibility of potentiation of tolerability problems in polytherapy and specifically an increase of cognitive problems. It may therefore be hypothesized that drug interactions may be responsible for this potentiation. This seems to be a general effect as it occurs in many combinations of drugs and so far not a specific combination has been identified.

Clinical effects

Although the psychometric studies generally show a tendency of cognitive impairments in polytherapy compared to monotherapy, this merely *suggests* a drug interaction effect. As previously mentioned evidence-based confirmation will be extremely difficult due to the methodological problems that occur when studying polytherapy and especially in the light of the many interfering factors, especially the seizure confound. Any study will have difficulties entangling the interfering factors of seizure effects and the effects of polytherapy, when typically polytherapy is used in the more refractory epilepsies.

Nonetheless, we may look at more anecdotal clinical information. In many drug trials a similar effect has been found as suggested by the psychometric studies: a higher incidence of side-effects in combination therapy when compared to the same drug in monotherapy. This is often observed in post-marketing studies. Many of the new drugs are first tested in add-on designs and monotherapy is only used later. A recent example is topiramate showing not only a higher incidence of

Table 22.3 Percentage of side-effects for topiramate (TPM) in polytherapy vs. monotherapy; potentiation of side-effects due to polytherapy?

Most common AEDs with TPM adjunctive therapy*	% Patients	
	Adjunctive therapy TPM 200–400 ($N = 183$)	Monotherapy (0 AEDs at baseline) TPM 200/500 ($N = 71$)
Somnolence	29	13
Dizziness	25	13
Ataxia	16	6
Nervousness	16	6
Abnormal vision	13	3
Psychomotor slowing	13	6
Speech disorders	13	1
Memory difficulty	12	8
Confusion	11	6
Paresthesia	11	38
Diplopia	10	1
Anorexia	10	15

* Incidence $\geq$10% and $\geq$5% difference in incidence vs. placebo.

side-effects in combination therapy but also different types of dominant complaints when compared to monotherapy (Aldenkamp, 2000; Aldenkamp *et al.*, 2000). Table 22.3 illustrates this.

When inspecting this example we see cognitive impairments are reduced in monotherapy, but other impairments, especially paresthesia, are increased. This may lead to the hypothesis of potentiation of some tolerability problems and especially cognitive side-effects.

Of course, it is imperative to emphasize that the monotherapy studies typically include patients with other epilepsies compared to the initial add-on studies, which are done in refractory partial epilepsies with an associated risk of epilepsy-induced cognitive impairments. Moreover, in contrast with the former paragraph of this chapter, these side effects have not been established with formal psychometric or other objective measurements, but are based on clinician ratings of subjective patient complaints.

Subjective patient complaints

We can take this one step further and use the subjective patient complaints as primary outcome measure. This has not been done systematically. We have, however, recently

Table 22.4 Subjective reported side effects in 346 patients in a community-based study

Area and type of side effect[a]	% patients[b]
General CNS	*68.2 (overall CNS complaints)*
Fatigue	20.3
Tiredness	18.8
General slowing	12.1
Headache	8.9
Dizziness	8.1
Motor problems	*31.5 (overall motor complaints)*
Tremor	13.3
Ataxia	13.0
Falling	5.2
Gastrointestinal complaints	*33.2 (overall gastrointestinal complaints)*
Weight gain	12.4
Micturition problems	8.4
Loss of appetite	5.2
Nausea	2.9
Diarrhea	2.3
Weight loss	2.0
Cognition	*61.8 (overall cognitive complaints)*
Memory problems	21.4
Concentration difficulties	16.1
Speech problems	8.7
Language difficulties	7.8
Visual	*7.5 (overall visual complaints)*
Double vision	7.5
Mood and behavior	*22.3 (overall mood/behavior complaints)*
Agitation/irritability	14.8
Depression	7.5
Cosmetic	*20.4 (overall cosmetic complaints)*
Hair loss	7.2
Gum problems	7.8
Skin complaints	5.4
Sleep problems	*8.7 (overall complaints about sleep)*
Insomnia	8.7

[a] One patient may be reporting several side effects.

[b] Summary of both moderate and severe complaints.

finished a community-based study, using subjective patient complaints about side effects of their treatment as primary outcome measure (Carpay *et al.*, 2002).

Taking advantage of the reliable databases of AED use in the pharmacies in the Netherlands we were able to establish a non-selected unbiased community-based study group of adult patients with epilepsy from a suburban area (100 000 inhabitants) with a prevalence equivalent of 0.4% (i.e. 346 patients). All patients finished a rating scale on side-effects of their treatment. Almost half the patients reached a 2-year seizure remission; about one-third considers the seizures unacceptable. About 80% of the patients are on monotherapy. Nonetheless, almost 60% of the patients report side-effects in at least three areas.

Table 22.4 shows that the two areas with clearly most reports are: (a) general CNS-related complaints (such as fatigue and dizziness) with 68% complaints; and (b) cognitive complaints (61.8%). If we combine cognitive and mood areas, then behavioural complaints are, with 84.1% complaints, the dominant complaint in our study group. Within the areas, two types of complaint have been reported by >20% of the patients: memory problems (21.4%) and fatigue (20.3%). Two other complaints are reported by between 15% and 20% of the patients: tiredness (18.8%) and concentration difficulties (16.1%). It is thus clear that cognitive complaints are a dominant complaint even in a group of patients with a well-controlled epilepsy, mainly using monotherapy.

Subsequently, differences in side-effect profile were tested per AED. This was only possible for four groups with >50 patients, that is, patients on monotherapy of VPA, CBZ or PHT and patients on polytherapy (28.7%, 24.7%, 15.7% and 19.1% of the study group respectively). All remaining groups were too small to achieve sufficient statistical power. Table 22.5 shows exclusively the 7 areas with statistical differences between the four groups. On all areas the differences were caused by the higher percentage of complaints in patients using polytherapy. The remaining differences show more concentration difficulties for PHT compared to VPA, more weight gain for both VPA and PHT compared to CBZ.

Conclusion

Systematic analysis of subjective patients complaints about side-effects of AEDs show that the impact of side-effects may be larger than hitherto suspected both in number of patients involved (our community-based sample suggests that almost 60% of the patients with AED have complaints) and the frequency of the complaints. Especially the behavioral (and within this class the cognitive) side-effects occur frequently and require careful monitoring and possible interventions.

Still using subjective patient complaints it is clear that a switch from monotherapy to polytherapy entails a serious risk of increasing side-effects. This has been

Table 22.5 Differences per area of complaint between the four groups: VPA, CBZ, PHT and polytherapy. Results from a community-based study in 346 patients

Complaint	Overall difference: Chi Square based on the Kruskall–Wallis test	Differences between the four groups based on the Mann–Whitney U-test
Tiredness	9.276; df 3; $P = 0.03$	Polytherapy $>$ CBZ ($U = 1834$; $P = 0.02$) Polytherapy $>$ PHT ($U = 1041$; $P = 0.005$)
Ataxia	11.073; df 3; $P = 0.01$	Polytherapy $>$ VPA ($U = 2226.5$; $P = 0.007$) Polytherapy $>$ CBZ ($U = 1952.5$; $P = 0.02$) Polytherapy $>$ PHT ($U = 1170$; $P = 0.03$)
Nausea	8.389; df 3; $P = 0.04$	Polytherapy $>$ VPA ($U = 2334$; $P = 0.03$) Polytherapy $>$ PHT ($U = 1184$; $P = 0.02$)
Tiredness	10.047; df 3; $P = 0.02$	Polytherapy $>$ VPA ($U = 2089$; $P = 0.02$) Polytherapy $>$ CBZ ($U = 1724.5$; $P = 0.003$)
General slowing	9.830; df 3; $P = 0.02$	Polytherapy $>$ VPA ($U = 1995.5$; $P = 0.005$) Polytherapy $>$ CBZ ($U = 1789$; $P = 0.009$)
Concentration difficulties	8.253; df 3; $P = 0.04$	PHT $>$ VPA ($U = 1799$; $P \leqslant 0.05$) Polytherapy $>$ VPA ($U = 2084.5$; $P = 0.01$)
Weight gain	8.040; df 3; $P \leqslant 0.05$	VPA $>$ CBZ ($U = 3234$; $P = 0.05$) PHT $>$ CBZ ($U = 1617$; $P = 0.004$) Polytherapy $>$ CBZ ($U = 2117.5$; $P = 0.02$)

The sign $>$ indicates a high percentage of patients reporting problem for that specific area.

reported from clinical groups, in patients with refractory epilepsy and within the context of many drug trials (most recently for topiramate: Tatum *et al.*, 2001), but is now also confirmed in a community-based sample (Carpay *et al.*, 2005). On the other hand, Bourgeois reports reduction of side effects when reducing polytherapy; this is considered proof for a partially cumulative toxic effect (Bourgeois, 1988). When in clinical decision-making the option of polytherapy arises, the serious risk of an increase in side-effects should be taken into consideration carefully. This is especially important in the light of recent revivals of polytherapy, for example, within the context of rational polytherapy.

A similar effect is often observed when new drugs proceed from initial add-on studies to studies in monotherapy. Although the efficacy profile often remains unchanged, the tolerability profiles often have to be adjusted with much more moderate profiles in monotherapy.

Formal psychometric studies are much more difficult to interpret, especially when formal scientific standards in line with evidence-based medicine are applied.

Nonetheless, we may claim that a systematic review supports these conclusions. It may be considered conceivable that polytherapy increases the risk of behavioral and specifically cognitive impairments. We may therefore hypothesize a potentiation of tolerability problems leading to cognitive impairments due to interactions between AEDs. This seems to be a general effect as it occurs in many combinations of drugs and so far no specific combination has been identified.

REFERENCES

Aldenkamp AP. Cognitive side-effects of antiepileptic drugs. In *Epilepsy in Children and Adolescents.* A. P. Aldenkamp, F. E. Dreifuss, W. O. Renier, eds. New York: CRC-Press Publishers, Boca Raton, 1995: 161–183.

Cognitive side-effects of newer antiepileptic drugs relative to the established AEDs. In *Challenge Epilepsy – New antiepileptic drugs.* H. Stefan, G. Krämer, B. Mamoli, eds. Berlin: Blackwell Science, 1998: 135–151.

Cognitive effects of topiramate, gabapentin and lamotrigine in healthy young adults. *Neurology* 2000; **54**: 270–272.

Aldenkamp AP, Vermeulen J. Cognitive side-effects of antiepileptic drugs. In *Pediatric Epilepsy; Diagnosis and Therapy,* 2nd edn. J. M. Pellock, W. E. Dodson, B. F. D. Bourgeois, eds. 2001: 629–636.

Aldenkamp AP, Baker G, Mulder OG, *et al.* A multicentre randomized clinical study to evaluate the effect on cognitive function of topiramate compared with valproate as add-on therapy to carbamazepine in patients with partial-onset seizures. *Epilepsia* 2000; **41**(9): 1167–1178.

Berent S, Sackellares JC, Giordani B, *et al.* Zonisamide (CI-912) and cognition: results from preliminary study. *Epilepsia* 1987; **28**(1): 61–67.

Bittencourt PRM, Antoniuk SA, Bigarella MM, *et al.* Carabamazepine and phenytoin in epilepsies refractory to barbiturates: efficacy, toxicity and mental function. *Epilepsy Res* 1993; **16**: 147–155.

Bourgeois BFD. Problems of combination drug therapy in children. *Epilepsia* 1988; **29**(Suppl. 3): S20–S24.

Butlin AT, Danta G, Cook ML. Anticonvulsants, folic acid and memory dysfunction in epileptics. *Clin Exp Neur* 1984; **20**: 57–62.

Carpay JA, Aldenkamp AP, Van Donselaar C. Subjective complaints about side-effects of antiepileptic drugs; results from a community-based study. *Epilepsia* 2005 (in press).

Chataway J, Fowler A, Thompson PJ, *et al.* Discontinuation of clonazepam in patients with active epilepsy. *Seizure* 1993; **2**: 295–300.

Committee on Drugs. Behavioral and cognitive effects of anticonvulsant therapy. *Pediatrics* 1985; **76**: 644–647.

Corbett JA, Trimble MR, Nichol TC. Behavioral and cognitive impairments in children with epilepsy: the long-term effects of anticonvulsant therapy. *J Am Acad Child Psychiatr* 1985; **24**: 17–23.

Dekaban AS, Lehman EJB. Effects of different dosages of anticonvulsant drugs on mental performance in patients with chronic epilepsy. *Acta Neurol Scand* 1975; **52**: 319–330.

Dodrill CB. Problems in the assessment of cognitive effects of antiepileptic drugs. *Epilepsia* 1992; **33**(Suppl. 6): S29–S32.

Dodrill CB, Troupin AS. Psychotropic effects of carbamazepine in epilepsy: a double-blind comparison with phenytoin. *Neurology* 1977; **27**: 1023–1028.

Dodrill CB, Wilensky AJ. Neuropsychological abilities before and after 5 years of stable antiepileptic drug therapy. *Epilepsia* 1992; **33**(2): 327–334.

Dodrill CB, Arnett JL, Sommerville KW, *et al.* Evaluation of the effects of vigabatrin on cognitive abilities and quality of life in epilepsy. *Neurology* 1993; **43**: 2501–2507.

Duncan JS, Shorvon SD, Trimble MR. Effects of removal of phenytoin, carbamazepine, and valproate on cognitive function. *Epilepsia* 1990; **31**(5): 584–591.

Durwen HF, Elger CE. Verbal learning differences in epileptic patients with left and right temporal lobe foci – a pharmacologically induced phenomenon? *Acta Neurol Scand* 1993; **87**: 1–8.

Durwen HF, Elger CE, Helmstaedter C, *et al.* Circumscribed improvement of cognitive performance in temporal lobe epilepsy patients with intractable seizures following reduction of anticonvulsant medication. *J. Epilepsy* 1989; **2**: 147–153.

Durwen HF, Hufnagel A, Elger CE. Anticonvulsant drugs affect particular steps of verbal memory processing – an evaluation of 13 patients with intractable complex partial seizures of left temporal lobe origin. *Neuropsychologia* 1992; **30**(7): 623–631.

Evans RW, Gualtieri CT. Carbamazepine: a neuropsychological and psychiatric profile. *Clin Neuropharmacol* 1985; **8**(3): 221–241.

Gilham RA, Blacklaw J, Mckee PJW, *et al.* Effects of vigabatrin on sedation and cognitive function in patients with refractory epilepsy. *J Neurol Neurosur Psychiatr* 1993; **56**: 1271–1275.

Ideström CM, Schalling D, Carlquist U, *et al.* Behavioral and psychological studies: acute effects of diphenylhydantoin in relation to plasma levels. *Psychiat Med* 1972; **2**: 111–120.

Kulig B, Meinardi H. Effects of antiepileptic drugs on motor activity and learned behavior in the rat. In *Advances in Epileptology*. H. Meinardi, A. J. Rowan, eds. Amsterdam: Swets & Zeitlinger, 1977: 98–104.

Ludgate J, Keating J, O'Dwyer R, *et al.* An improvement in cognitive function following polypharmacy reduction in a group of epileptic patients. *Acta Neur Scand* 1985; **71**: 448–452.

Matthews CG, Harley JP. Cognitive and motor-sensory performances in toxic and nontoxic epileptic subjects. *Neurology* 1975; **25**: 184–188.

May TW, Bulmahn A, Wohlhueter M, *et al.* Effects of withdrawal of phenytoin on cognitive and psychomotor functions in hospitalized epileptic patients on polytherapy. *Acta Neur Scand* 1992; **86**(2): 165–170.

McGuire AM, Duncan JS, Trimble MR. Effects of vigabatrin on cognitive function and mood when used as add-on therapy in patients with intractable epilepsy. *Epilepsia* 1992; **33**(1): 128–134.

McKee PJW, Blacklaw J, Butler E, *et al.* Variability and clinical relevance of the interaction between sodium valproate and carbamazepine in epileptic patients. *Epilepsy Res* 1992; **11**: 193–198.

McKee PJW, Blacklaw J, Forrest G, *et al.* A double-blind placebo-controlled interaction study between oxcarbazepine and carbamazepine, sodium valproate and phenytoin in epileptic patients. *Br J clin Pharmac* 1994; **37**: 27–32.

Mitchell WG, Zhou Y, Chavez JM, *et al.* Effects of antiepileptic drugs on reaction time, attention, and impulsivity in children. *Pediatrics* 1993; **91**(1): 101–105.

Novelly RA, Schwartz MM, Mattson RH, *et al.* Behavioral toxicity associated with antiepileptic drugs: concepts and methods of assessment. *Epilepsia* 1986; **27**(4): 331–340.

Pieters MSM, Jennekens-Schinkel A, Stijnen Th, *et al.* Carbamazepine (CBZ) controlled release compared with conventional CBZ: a controlled study of attention and vigilance in children with epilepsy. *Epilepsia* 1992; **33**: 1137–1144.

Prevey ML, Mattson RH, Cramer JA. Improvement in cognitive functioning and mood state after conversion to valproate monotherapy. *Neurology* 1989; **39**: 1640–1641.

Reynolds EH. Chronic antiepileptic toxicity: a review. *Epilepsia* 1975; **16**: 319–352.

Phenytoin: toxicity. In *Antiepileptic Drugs.* R. H. Levy, F. E. Dreifuss, R. H. Mattson *et al.*, eds. New York: Raven Press, 1989: 241–256.

Reynolds EH, Travers RD. Serum anticonvulsant concentrations in epileptic patients with mental symptoms: a preliminary report. *Br J Psychiatr* 1974; **124**: 440–445.

Smith DB. Cognitive effects of antiepileptic drugs. In *Advances in Neurology*, vol. 55. D. Smith, D. Treiman, M. Trimble, eds. New York: Raven Press, 1991: 197–212.

Smith D, Baker G, Davies G, *et al.* Outcomes of add-on treatment with lamotrigine in partial epilepsy. *Epilepsia* 1993; **34**(2): 312–322.

Sommerbeck KW, Theilgaard A, Rasmussen KE. Valproate sodium: evaluation of so-called psychotropic effect. A controlled study. *Epilepsia* 1977; **18**: 159–162.

Tatum WO, French JA, Faught E, *et al.* Postmarketing experience with topiramate and cognition. *Epilepsia* 2001; **42**(9): 1134–1140.

Thompson PJ, Trimble MR. Further studies on anticonvulsant drugs and seizures. *Acta Neurol Scand* 1980; **60**: 51–58.

Anticonvulsant drugs and cognitive functions. *Epilepsia* 1982; **33**: 531–534.

Anticonvulsant serum levels; relationship to impairments of cognitive functioning. *J Neurol Neurosur Psychiatr* 1983; **46**: 227–233.

Trimble MR. Anticonvulsant drugs and psychosocial development: phenobarbitone, sodium valproate, and benzodiazepines. In *Antiepileptic Drug Therapy in Pediatrics.* P. L. Morselli, C. E. Pippenger, J. K. Penry, eds. New York: Raven Press, 1983: 201–217.

Anticonvulsant drugs and cognitive function: a review of the literature. *Epilepsia* 1987a; **28**(S3): 37–45.

Anticonvulsant drugs: mood and cognitive function. In *Epilepsy, Behaviour and Cognitive Function.* M. R. Trimble, E. H. Reynolds, eds. Chichester: John Wiley & Sons, 1987b: 135–145.

Trimble MR, Thompson PJ. Memory, anticonvulsant drugs and seizures. *Acta Neur Scand* 1981; **64**: 31–41.

Anticonvulsant drugs, cognitive function and behaviour. *Epilepsia* 1983; **24**(Suppl. 1): S55–S63.

van Rijckevorsel–Harmant K, Flahaut D, Harman J, *et al.* Event-related potentials and cognitive functions in epileptic treated patients. *Clin Electroencephalog* 1990; **21**(2): 67–73.

Vermeulen J, Aldenkamp AP. Cognitive side-effects of chronic antiepileptic drug treatment: a review of 25 years of research. *Epilepsy Res* 1995; **22**: 65–95.

Wilensky AJ, Ojemann LM, Temkin NR, *et al.* Clorazepate and phenobarbital as antiepileptic drugs: a double-blind study. *Neurology* 1981; **31**(10): 1271–1276.

Part V

Conclusions and future perspectives

23

Selection of drug combinations in clinical practice: current and future perspectives

Jerzy Majkowski

Center for Epilepsy Diagnosis and Treatment, Foundation of Epileptology, Warsaw, Poland

Introduction

Polytherapy has flourished in the long history of epilepsy. In recent decades, it has waxed and waned depending on our current knowledge and availability of antiepileptic drugs (AEDs). Introduction of effective AEDs in the first half of the twentieth century shifted treatment strategy towards monotherapy in the 1950s and 1960s. However, in the 1960s and 1970s, when carbamazepine (CBZ), valproic acid (VPA), benzodiazepines and other AEDs made their appearance, treatment reverted towards polytherapy once again. The concept of treatment was based on the erroneous assumption that polypragmasy improves the effectiveness of AEDs without increasing their toxicity. Besides, clinical trials of AEDs were biased and methodologically dubious (Coatsworth, 1971).

Introduction of double-blind trials and other rules for drug evaluation protocols was an important step in comparative and more objective AED clinical evaluation (Delgado-Escueta *et al.*, 1983; Mattson *et al.*, 1983). Moreover, when the negative aspects of polytherapy were reported in the 1970s and 1980s (Shorvon and Reynolds, 1979; Reynolds and Shorvon, 1981), there was a return to monotherapy in the majority of patients. Tests of AED concentration in the blood serum and credibility of the measurements substantially contributed to this shift in treatment strategy (Pippenger *et al.*, 1976; Richens, 1980).

In the late 1980s and in the 1990s several new AEDs were introduced to the pharmaceutic market and used as add-on therapies. This led to yet another shift towards polytherapy in difficult-to-treat patients. At this time the concept of 'evidence-based medicine' provided more objective quantified drug effect evaluation and the principle of 'good clinical practice' was coined to emphasize the need to individualize the choice of drug(s) and dose.

Rational AED selection and combination is a relatively recent event in the history of treatment of epilepsy based on animal models (Masuda *et al.*, 1981; Löscher and Ebert, 1996; Czuczwar, 1998). However, clinical trials of phenobarbital (PB)

and phenytoin (PHT) monotherapies vs. combination of both drugs were performed many years ago, emphasizing the beneficial effect of this combination (Yahr *et al.*, 1952). Consequently, there is not much clinical experience in this field and there is very little knowledge of how to combine drugs most efficiently. The concept has been developed over the last 10–15 years and a number of new AEDs have been approved for epilepsy treatment in the majority of countries. At present, 15 AEDs are available in all. They have different mechanisms of action, tolerability, pharmacokinetic and pharmacodynamic profiles and possible interactions. The availability of such a variety of AEDs has widened the choice of combinations and made the choice much more complex for clinicians than 15 years ago. But on the other hand, it provides better opportunity for the treatment of patients with fewer adverse events.

Selection of the best AED combination for a given patient is no easy task since there is no simple rule. Moreover, it is good to remember that populations of patients with epilepsy are heterogeneous and therefore it is hard to compare the efficacy of drug combinations in such populations. However, a broad knowledge of the characteristics of old and new AEDs and consideration for the distinctive profile of the patient make it easier to make the most reasonable and knowledgeable decision, and to select the best and optimal patient care for those who are resistant to pharmacotherapy. These patients present the greatest problem and are the biggest challenge for epileptology today. For clinicians, the challenge is to identify patients early and to select the most appropriate AED combinations. For researchers, the challenge is to discover the cause of drug resistance and to synthesize new and more efficient AEDs.

In this chapter, polytherapy with old and new AEDs, current clinical experience with drug combinations and future treatment strategies in pharmacoresistant epilepsies will be discussed.

Pharmacotherapy-resistant seizures

The majority of patients (60–70%) with newly diagnosed epilepsy can apparently be controlled with a single AED. The remaining group with recurrent seizures – so-called refractory epilepsy – requires two or (in a small percentage of patients) even three AEDs to improve seizure control – providing that AED selection is based on currently available knowledge of their pharmacologic profile and drugs are appropriately matched to the unique characteristics of the epileptic patient (type(s) and severity of seizure, age, sex, health condition, medical history, concomitant medications, profession, level of acceptance of seizures and/or adverse events, etc.).

The concept of pharmacotherapy resistance is justified and useful (Table 23.1), even if there is no generally accepted definition (Ohtsuka *et al.*, 1988; Lüders, 1990;

Table 23.1 Justification for concept of pharmacotherapy resistant patients

- Consideration for neurosurgery treatment.
- Requirements to conduct a certain life style.
- Higher risk of sudden unexpected death, memory difficulties, academic difficulties, depression, and impaired psycho-social adjustment and activity.
- Possibility of comparing results of multicenter studies, e.g. new AED evaluation.
- Necessity to search for more efficient drugs.
- Searching for causes of drug resistance.

Camfield and Camfield, 1996; Majkowski, 1996). The need to use more than one drug for seizure control may be called drug resistance. For combination therapy this definition is useful enough for the time being. But when should combination therapy be started? How many monotherapies should be tried when about 15 AEDs are available? Different neurologists answer this question differently. In 14 Mediterranean countries, 23–67% of neurologists chose combination therapy when monotherapy with one drug failed to control seizures, rather than trying a second, alternative monotherapy (Baldy-Moulinier *et al.*, 1998). It seems that in newly diagnosed patients at least two (or even three) drugs with different mechanisms of action should be used in monotherapy before combination therapy is started.

Patients with refractory epilepsy have always been in polytherapy with more or less effective drugs. At present, selection of AED combinations is mainly based on personal experience and on a few clinically documented studies. On the other hand, there are a number of promising studies based on animal seizure and epilepsy models showing that certain combinations of two AEDs are more or less effective than others and have better or worse tolerability (Bourgeois, 1986, 1988; Czuczwar, 1998; Deckers *et al.*, 2000). These results require critical clinical verification, however, for example the beneficial effect of CBZ with calcium channel blockers combination, reported in many experimental animal studies (Czuczwar *et al.*, 1992), has not been confirmed at the clinical level (Chaisewikul *et al.*, 2001a). The authors, in an overview of corresponding literature, do not recommend this comedication because of significant withdrawal rate probably due to side-effects (flunarizine) or not convincing evidence of effectiveness (nifedipine or nimodipine). There is also the question not only of drug combinations but also of dose and side-effect differences in animal models and human beings. It was also shown in experimental studies that synergism of two drugs may be evident at only some drug ratios (Czuczwar and Borowicz, 2002).

Scale of the problem

Mattson (1992) estimates that success of a monotherapy in newly diagnosed partial epilepsies may be observed in 65% of patients. In the remaining 35%, less than

Table 23.2 Mono- and polytherapy in 6117 patients with chronic epilepsy

Number of AEDs	% and (number) of patients
Monotherapy	57.7 (3530)
Duotherapy	31.7 (1940)
Three drugs	8.8 (541)
More than three	1.7 (106)

one-third (10%) may be markedly improved by two-drug combinations and a further 5% by more than two AEDs. Thus, about 35% of newly diagnosed patients are left with partially controlled or uncontrolled seizures and are subject to various drug combinations of two or more AEDs. Taking into consideration incidence, high prevalence, chronic characteristics of epilepsy and possible remissions, it seems that the ratio of patients with chronic epilepsy to newly diagnosed and controlled patients is rather increasing, even if newly diagnosed patients are being successfully treated at the expected level. Thus, the number of patients requiring long-term combination therapy is at least 30–40% of the general epileptic patient population.

This figure is also derived from successive monotherapies with three different AEDs in previously untreated patients (Kwan and Brodie, 2000). Out of 470 previously untreated patients, seizures were successfully controlled by monotherapy in 61% of patients. In our multicentre studies performed on 6204 patients in 13 epilepsy-oriented centres in Poland in 2001, the use of monotherapy and polytherapy was compared (Table 23.2) (Majkowski *et al.*, 2005). The study shows that 42.2% of patients ($n = 2588$) are on polytherapy. The five most frequent combinations of two AEDs, i.e. CBZ + valproate (VPA), VPA + lamotrigine (LTG), CBZ + LTG, CBZ + vigabatrin (VGB), and CBZ + topiramate (TPM), were used in 47% of the patients, 22 combinations were used in 43% and 10% of combinations in the remaining 203 patients with localization-related seizures, thus showing great variability of AED combinations. Deckers *et al.* (2000) reviewed 33 animal and human studies on AED combinations and found that several combinations offered improved effectiveness, but no uniform approach was used in the studies.

Rational polytherapy

The concept of so-called rational polytherapy – broadly discussed in previous chapters – was introduced in the 1990s. This concept is based on a better understanding of pharmacokinetic and pharmacodynamic drug interactions and allows, to some extent, the prediction of their clinical effects. A review of the literature on the possible impact of AED interactions on therapeutic outcome when bitherapy had to be used has recently been published (Patsalos *et al.*, 2002; Patsalos and Perucca, 2003).

The aim of rational polytherapy is to improve the effectiveness to toxicity ratio: effectiveness should be supra-additive or at least additive and toxicity should be lower than additive. Effectiveness of drug combination is measured by frequency and/or severity reduction of seizures. It may also have some economic benefits if combination therapy is cheaper than therapy with either of the drugs or when seizure and/or toxic effects are more successfully controlled, just decreasing indirect costs. Improved well-being of the patients is difficult to calculate.

A good understanding of AED pharmacologic mechanisms of action should help the therapist to choose the best two-AED combination (Czuczwar, 1998; Deckers *et al.*, 2000). It has been proposed that combination of AEDs with different mechanisms of action may have a better clinical effect than drugs with the same mechanisms. It seems logical, for the majority of patients, that combination of drugs with different mechanisms of action is more effective than two drugs with a similar mode of action. Combining a drug facilitating gamma amino butyric acid (GABA)-ergic transmission with a drug reducing the excitatory effects of aminoacids (LTG) or a Na^+ channel blocker (CBZ) with a drug increasing GABA levels (VGB) is probably more advisable than combining two Na^+ channel blockers (e.g. CBZ + PHT). This idea is based on experimental data and theoretical speculations. However, knowledge about various and usually complex or unknown mechanisms of action of the majority of AEDs is incomplete. Tiagabine (TGB) and VGB are the only two drugs which have been developed on the basis of the seizure mechanism concept and both have a single mechanism of action, i.e. both increase GABA-mediated inhibition, but their modes of operation are different. Ethosuximide (ESM) is the third drug with a single mechanism of action (calcium channel blocker). The remaining AEDs have multiple mechanisms of action and therefore act like combination therapy.

Moreover, at the clinical casuistic and experimental level, there are exceptions to this idea, e.g. treatment with two GABA-ergic agents (VGB and TGB) resulted in substantial improvement of seizure control in two patients with refractory epilepsy (Leach and Brodie, 1994). At the experimental level, combination of TGB and gabapentin (GBP) – two drugs affecting the GABA-ergic system – has shown supra-additive interaction without adverse events in mice models of seizures (Luszczki *et al.*, 2003). The authors suggest that this very promising experimental result should be verified clinically.

Combination therapy with old AEDs

The general principles of AED combination are shown in Table 23.3. Additive or supra-additive efficacy was claimed in a number of reports when two drugs were

Table 23.3 General principles of AED combination

1 Failure of monotherapy with two (or even three) successive drugs.
2 Knowledge of pharmacokinetic and pharmacodynamic profiles of the AED.
3 To select drugs considering their interactions.
4 To select drugs which have low probability of adverse events and high therapeutic index.
5 Combining AEDs which have different mechanism of action seems to be more beneficial than using two drugs with similar mechanism.
6 Combination therapy is more effective in two or more different seizure types.
7 Adding or withdrawing AEDs should be carefully monitored clinically (and blood level concentration if appropriate) during first days or weeks of modified treatment because of possible drug interactions.

combined and compared to monotherapy. Many studies, however, are based on small numbers of patients, with possibly some essential methodological pitfalls which are discussed in Chapters 10 and 12. There are also casuistic reports showing exceptions from the rules.

One of the earliest beneficial effects of combination therapy of CBZ with PHT was observed in 15% of patients (5 of 33) in comparison with successful cross-over monotherapy with either drug in 67 of 100 patients (Hakkarainen, 1980).

An additive or even supra-additive effect was observed in refractory absence seizures in five patients following combination of VPA and ESM (Rowan *et al.*, 1983); neither of the drugs used in monotherapy was effective. A pharmaco-dynamic interaction was suggested. In one study of VPA and ESM comedication, serum levels of VPA were significantly ($P < 0.01$) lower in this combination than in VPA monotherapy (Sälke-Kellermann, 1997). The mechanism of this interaction is unknown.

Good efficacy with minor side-effects was obtained with CBZ and VPA comedication (Fröscher *et al.*, 1984). At least 50% seizure reduction was reported in 50% of patients. The best results were observed in patients with generalized seizures as opposed to partial complex ones. In such comedication, the additive anticonvulsant effect seemed to be more significant than the additive effect of neurotoxicity (Bourgeois, 1988). However, it was also reported that combination of CBZ with VPA may result in additive effectiveness and in supra-additive neurotoxicity due to increased CBZ-epoxide levels resulting from inhibition of expoxide hydrolase by VPA (Warner *et al.*, 1992).

Deckers *et al.* (2001) used a different methodological approach to evaluate drug combination. In newly diagnosed patients, CBZ and VPA monotherapy were compared to a half drug load of both. The authors did not find any difference in neurotoxicity or efficacy.

Combination of CBZ with VPA or with PHT resulted in a decrease of generalized tonic–clonic seizures in half of the patients (Mattson and Cramer, 1988). A similar effect of at least 50% seizure frequency reduction and complete seizure control was obtained in one-half of 100 patients with uncontrolled partial and secondarily generalized seizures by switching from CBZ monotherapy to bitherapy combining VPA with CBZ (Dean and Penry, 1988).

Beneficial effects of combination of CBZ and VPA in patients with complex partial seizures and secondarily generalized seizures were observed in 14 of 17 patients who failed to respond to VPA or CBZ monotherapy (Walker and Koon, 1988).

In a double-blind prospective study of patients with complex partial seizures receiving CBZ or PHT in monotherapy, divalproex sodium (an oligomeric complex composed of sodium valproate and VPA in a 1:1 molar ratio) or placebo was randomly added (Willmore *et al.*, 1996). Significant seizure frequency reduction (by 43%) was obtained in patients on drug combination with divalproex compared with the placebo group.

Thus, in localization-related seizures, combination of CBZ with VPA seems to be more effective than monotherapy with CBZ or VPA in some patients resistant to these drugs. The same is true for combination therapy of VPA with ESM in absence seizures.

These favorable effects in various two-drug combination therapies (PHT, PB, CBZ and VPA) were not confirmed by other authors (Schmidt, 1982; Schmidt and Gram, 1995).

Negative drug combinations have also been reported. In clinical practice, combination of benzodiazepines with PB, resulting in additive efficacy and adverse events at the pharmacodynamic level, is not recommended in long-term therapy (Leppik and Wolff, 1993).

Combinations with new AEDs

Lamotrigine plus

Combination of LTG with VPA in refractory localization seizures has been reported in a number of publications (Panayiotopoulos *et al.*, 1993; Pisani *et al.*, 1993, 1999a; Brodie *et al.*, 1997). In a European multicentre study (Brodie *et al.*, 1997), adding LTG to VPA, CBZ or PHT monotherapies produced significantly better efficacy ($P < 0.001$) than combination of CBZ or PHT with LTG. The proportion of responders were 64%, 41% and 38%, respectively. The authors suggest that the lower efficacy of the last two combinations compared with LTG alone may be due to the induction effect of PHT and CBZ on LTG and lower serum concentration.

A pharmacodynamic supra-additive effect of efficacy and infra-additive toxicity of LTG with VPA combination was suggested (Brodie *et al.*, 1997; Frey and Kanner,

1999; Pisani *et al.*, 1999a). However, the contribution of pharmacokinetic interaction cannot be excluded. Serum level of LTG was measured in add-on therapy with VPA or CBZ in 60 patients with resistant partial seizures (Benetello *et al.*, 2002). In 70% of the patients there was complete seizure control or at least 50% seizure reduction. Mean LTG serum level was significantly higher in responders than in non-responders. The best results were in VPA-cotreated patients with the highest LTG serum level. Central nervous system (CNS) toxicity developed in patients with the highest LTG concentrations, whereas CNS toxicity seemed to be unrelated to CBZ or CBZ-epoxide serum concentrations.

In casuistic reports seizure control was achieved with LTG plus VPA combination in unusual refractory myoclonic epilepsy (Ferrie and Panayiotopoulos, 1999) and in very resistant absence seizures (Besag *et al.*, 1995).

The beneficial effect of combination of LTG with CBZ seems to be controversial due to the marked increase in serum CBZ-epoxide concentration: the toxic effect is supra-additive whereas the antiepileptic affect is additive, possibly at the pharmacodynamic level (Warner *et al.*, 1992; Besag *et al.*, 1998; De Romanis and Sopranzi, 1999).

In randomly double-blind add-on therapy, LTG or placebo was added to previous AED medications in 30 therapy-resistant children with generalized epilepsy and Lennox–Gastaut syndrome (Eriksson *et al.*, 1998). There was a statistically significant reduction (>50%) in seizure frequency in the LTG group compared with the placebo group.

In an open-label prospective study LTG was added to previous AED medications in partial epilepsy with drop attacks and secondary bilateral synchrony on electro-cardiogram (EEG) (Bisulli *et al.*, 2001). Good efficacy (seizure reduction >50%) was observed, including EEG improvement in all types of seizures in 12 of 14 patients.

Gabapentin plus

In a casuistic report, five patients with a long history of resistant partial complex seizures and unsuccessful treatment, with various new and conventional drug combinations, became seizure-free when GBP was added to LTG (two patients), to LTG and VPA (two patients) or to LTG and CBZ (one patient) (Pisani *et al.*, 1999). Any attempt to discontinue LTG or GBP resulted in loss of seizure control.

Topiramate plus

In a double-blind, placebo-controlled study, combination of TPM (200 mg/day) added to CBZ in 263 patients with partial-onset seizures was studied (Guberman *et al.*, 2002). Median seizure frequency reduction was 44% in the TPM group and 20% in the placebo group ($P < 0.001$).

It has been reported that the combination of TPM with LTG significantly reduces the frequency of tonic and myoclonic seizures in children (mainly in Lennox–Gastaut syndrome) (Kugler *et al.*, 1997; Delanty *et al.*, 1998). Casuistic observations of this beneficial combination have also been reported (Stephen *et al.*, 1998).

Vigabatrin plus

The combination of VGB with GBP, VGB with LTG or VGB and TGB does not show pharmacokinetic interactions and may be particularly useful in pharmaco-therapy-resistant partial complex seizures (Leach and Brodie, 1994; Ferrendelli, 1995). Indeed, a number of authors reported good efficacy of VGB with LTG combination in localization-related seizures compared with monotherapy with one of the drugs (Fröscher *et al.*, 1992; Stewart *et al.*, 1992; Arzimanoglou *et al.*, 1993; Robinson *et al.*, 1993; Stolarek *et al.*, 1993; Schapel *et al.*, 1996). However, the studies are based on rather small numbers of patients with localization-related seizures, and on casuistic reports. In another study the synergistic effect of LTG and VGB was not confirmed (Sills *et al.*, 1993).

In 215 CBZ-resistant patients with partial seizures, VGB or VPA were randomly added to CBZ treatment (Brodie and Mumford, 1999). Combination therapy of VGB with CBZ or CBZ with VPA had similar effects: 50% of seizure frequency reduction was observed in 53% and 51% of patients, respectively. The authors conclude that VGB and VPA which increase neuronal inhibition mediated by GABA, can be added to or substituted for CBZ when it fails to control seizures.

In newly diagnosed epilepsy, combination therapy of VGB with CBZ was compared to VGB or CBZ monotherapy in 51 of 58 patients. Among 14 patients who had seizures on VGB or CBZ cross-over monotherapy, combination of both drug resulted in seizure control in five patients (Tanganelli and Regesta, 1996). Good efficacy of this combination was also obtained by adding VGB to CBZ in therapy-resistant patients (Muri and Judice, 1995). In both studies VGB with CBZ combination resulted also in toxic side-effects. These effects, which were also observed in our study in localization-related seizures, may be partly due to a pharmacokinetic interaction resulting in an increase of CBZ serum level concentration when VGB is added (Jêdrzejczak *et al.*, 2000).

Tiagabine plus

Combination of CBZ + TGB or PHT + TGB did not result in better seizure control than treatment with TGB alone. However, adverse events were the reason for withdrawal of CBZ or PHT (Biton *et al.*, 1998). This may be an example of pharmacodynamic antagonism of drug combination.

Combination therapy of three or more AEDs

There is no convincing evidence that three or more AEDs are better than a combination of two at the maximally tolerated dose. However, everyday clinical practice suggests that in some pharmacotherapy-resistant patients, combination of three AEDs has a better effect than two drugs. Duncan (1996) noted that refractory patients occasionally achieve better seizure control with three drugs than with two. Cereghino *et al.* (1975) observed that in patients with poorly controlled seizures (generalized and/or partial) the combination of CBZ plus PB plus PHT was more effective than each drug alone or combination of two drugs. A similar casuistic observation has also been reported (Fröscher, 2000).

Favorable combination of three drugs (GBP + LTG + VPA and GBP + LTG + CBZ) resulting in complete seizure control in three patients was already mentioned (Pisani *et al.*, 1999b).

Clinical controlled trials of new AEDs show beneficial effects when a third new AED is added to two previous drugs. As a matter of fact, it is not the study design which is the target for evaluation of combination therapy. The emphasis of the study is put on efficacy of a new AED, regardless of its combination with other drugs. Moreover, the studies are based on a very heterogeneous group with a high proportion of patients with poor prognosis. Despite these limitations, meta-analysis of the controlled clinical trials of oxcarbazepine (O-CBZ) (Castillo *et al.*, 2000), LTG (Ramaratnam *et al.*, 2003), TPM (Jette *et al.*, 2002; Ribacoba Montero and Salas Puig, 2002), TGB (Pereira *et al.*, 2002), levetiracetam (LEV) (Marson *et al.*, 2001; Chaisewikul *et al.*, 2001b), zonisamide (ZNS) (Chadwick and Marson, 2003) in combination with other AEDs showed that 50% of the reduction of localization-related seizure frequency varies between 20% and 50% with about 10% of seizure-free patients.

In our studies, already quoted (Table 23.2), three AEDs were used in 9% (541 patients) and more than three AEDs in 1.7% (106 patients). In 541 patients about 250 different AED combinations were used; the most frequent combinations were: CBZ + VPA + LTG, CBZ + VPA + CZP (clonazepam), CBZ + VPA + VGB, CBZ + VPA + TGB, VPA + LTG + TPM, CBZ + VPA + TPM. These six combinations encompassed 28% of the patients; 25 different three-drug combinations were used in 20% of the patients; in the remaining 52% AED combinations were not repeatable. This reflects dramatic trial and error, and helplessness to improve seizure control rather than knowledge of AEDs – in otherwise therapy-resistant patients with mixed types of seizures and a long history of various drug administrations with unknown sequence of effects of preceding drug on the successive one.

A strategy for temporary administration of three AEDs is proposed by Elger and Fernandez (1999) and in Chapter 10.

Combination of four AEDs which is used in clinical practice, in a rather small percentage of patients, is unlikely to be beneficial – even if concepts of subtherapeutic doses of polytherapy are used.

Combination therapy of AED and non-AED

Such combinations have been used in a more or less controlled way for many years but have not often been subject to systematic study. In catamenial seizures, an intermittent combination of acetazolamide is rather widely used in those phases of the menstrual cycle when the risk of seizures is higher. A beneficial effect was reported for uncontrolled seizures in catamenial epilepsy by adding medroxyprogesterone (Mattson *et al.*, 1982). Clobazam administered paramenstrually had similar effects (Feely and Gibson, 1984). Diazepam given per rectum in cluster seizures or prophylactically in children with febrile convulsions diminished AED requirement (Majkowski *et al.*, 1995).

Combination of 25 mg of PB with 10 mg of procyclidine (anticholinergic agent), known as Didepil, was introduced by Doychinov in the 1960s. This combination in adults (in doses of 75–150 mg of PB + 30–60 mg of procyclidine per day) showed a better effect than monotherapy with PB, PRM, VPA or CBZ (Doychinov, 1980; Łysakowska *et al.*, 1980). Anticholinergic adverse events were observed in a majority of patients, in 23% of them the dose of this combination was decreased. It was suggested that the effect of this combination is synergistic (Doychinov, 1980) but we found increased serum blood level of PB due to procyclidine interaction.

Drug interactions may produce increases in desired metabolites or decreases in the formation of undesired metabolites. For example, danazol inhibits the metabolic epoxide-trans-diol pathway of CBZ, resulting in doubled half-life (Krämer *et al.*, 1986). The relatively low CBZ-epoxide level is possibly responsible for the good tolerability of high CBZ levels, exceeding $20\,\mu g/ml$ (Fröscher, 1998). Propranolol has been used to control tremor induced by VPA; propranolol is just as effective as PRM (Gorman *et al.*, 1986).

New perspectives on resistance to pharmacotherapy

Resistance to pharmacotherapy occurs in a significant number of patients with chronic epilepsy; its pathogenesis and mechanism(s) of development are not fully understood. It is not clear whether the drug resistance already existed before AED therapy began or whether it developed in relation to the number of seizures, AED administration, underlying brain pathology of epilepsy or genetic factors. It is also possible that a combination of various factors contributes to its occurrence (Sisodiya, 2003). Drug resistance seems to be associated with the progressive course of epilepsy. The progressive nature of epilepsy has been observed in the majority of untreated patients with generalized tonic–clonic seizures (Elwes *et al.*, 1988) and with partial seizures (Majkowski, 1998, 2000; Jêdrzejczak *et al.*, 2002); it has also been observed in treated patients despite treatment (Arroyo *et al.*, 2002; Elices and Arroyo, 2002). The currently available AEDs prevent neither primary epileptogenesis nor, in some patients, secondary brain epileptization with its biologic and psycho-social consequences which may be irreversible, particularly, in the developing brain.

The fact that some patients with chronic epilepsy do not respond to various AED therapies may not necessary be due to pharmacologic properties of AEDs but to an intrinsic drug resistance. Three main, and not necessarily mutually exclusive, mechanisms may play a role in drug resistance:

1 loss of pharmacologic target, e.g. GABA receptor;
2 cellular mechanism of drug pharmacologic action is blocked;
3 poor penetration of drug into the CNS (Marroni *et al.*, 2003), which may depend on a number of impaired mechanisms of blood–brain barrier (BBB) drug-crossing or drug transporters.

In experimental models of epilepsy, as in epileptic patients, there are good and bad responders to different AEDs. In recent years a number of studies have shown some reasons for such differences.

Using patch-clamp recordings from resected hippocampal tissue from patients with temporal lobe epilepsy, the mechanism of CBZ action was studied in responders and non-responders to CBZ (Remy *et al.*, 2003). It was found that the mechanism of CBZ action – blocking of voltage-dependent $Na^{(+)}$ channels – was completely lost in CBZ-resistant patients: seizure activity, elicited in human hippocampal slices, was insensitive to CBZ. In contrast, CBZ was effective in blocking $Na^{(+)}$ channels and seizure activity, in vitro, in patients who were responsive to CBZ. Using the same method, the authors demonstrated the ineffectiveness of CBZ on the $Na^{(+)}$ channel in chronic experimental epilepsy. The study suggests that loss of $Na^{(+)}$ channel drug resistance may constitute a novel mechanism underlying the development of drug resistance in epilepsy.

Along this line of experimental research it has been suggested that the PHT effect on after-discharges in the kindling model in rats may be different (Ebert *et al.*, 1999). The authors suggest that the difference between PHT responders and non-responders may be genetically determined rather than due to experimental factors.

In another line of recent studies the role of drug transporters has been emphasized in the disposition of some drugs – not only in epilepsy. Immunohisto-chemical and molecular genetic data have shown an over-expression of a number of genes and proteins that may be responsible for pharmacoresistance (Seegers *et al.*, 2002; Sisodiya *et al.*, 2002; Sisodiya, 2003; Marroni *et al.*, 2003; Potschka *et al.*, 2003a). Because the AED(s) is (are) not reaching the epileptic neurons, secondary epileptization with its progressive symptomatology is taking place, as in untreated patients. In such cases the kindling mechanism is a good candidate for the explanation of the progressive nature of the process in humans (Majkowski, 1999).

One of the mechanisms of resistance which has recently been identified is over-expression of drug-resistance proteins: such as multidrug-resistance gene – 1 P-glycoprotein (MDR 1, ABCB 1) and multidrug-resistance-associated proteins (MRP 1–5). Transporters, particularly MDR 1 and MRP 2, may play an important role in pharmacotherapy-resistant patients with epilepsy. They are crucial in mediating the efflux of some AEDs, such as CBZ, PHT, PB, LTG, and FBM across the BBB (see reviews of the literature by Patsalos and Perucca, 2003; Potschka *et al.*, 2003a). Over-expression of MRD 1 or MRP 2 and possibly other proteins may limit penetration of AEDs to their brain target sites. Over-expression of multidrug-resistance proteins 2 (MRP 2; ABCC 2) was found in the apical membranes of brain capillary endothelial cells of epileptic tissue from drug-resistant patients (Potschka *et al.*, 2003b). A complementary study shows that, in the kindled animal epilepsy model, deficiency of e.g. MRP 2 in mutant rats is associated with increased anticonvulsant response to CBZ (Potschka *et al.*, 2003a).

The role of MRP 2 in drug disposition into the brain is poorly defined. Potschka *et al.* (2003b) used an interesting strategy to determine the contribution of MRP 2 to BBB function. They showed that MRP inhibitor probenecid increases the extra-cellular brain level of PHT in rats, thus indicating that PHT is a substrate of MRP 2 in the BBB. It has also been demonstrated that in MRP 2-deficient rats extra-cellular PHT brain levels were significantly higher compared with a normal strain. In the kindling model, coadministration of probenecid significantly increased the anticonvulsant effect of PHT. The same effect was observed in kindled MRP 2-deficient rats (Potschka *et al.*, 2003b).

It was shown that the proteins may be over-expressed in the brain tissue (neurons and glia) in patients with refractory epilepsy associated with dysembryoplastic tumors, focal cortical dysplasia and hippocampal sclerosis (HS) (Sisodiya *et al.*, 2002). The authors conclude that the over-expressed resistance proteins lower the interstitial concentration of AED in the area of the epileptogenic pathology, resulting in pharmacotherapy-resistant epilepsy. In normal brain tissue MDR 1 is expressed almost exclusively by endothelial cells whereas in epileptic cortex it is expressed by endothelial cells and perivascular astrocytes. The tissue differences may be caused by genomic factors (e.g. DNA level) (Marroni *et al.*, 2003).

However, there is still limited proof that the candidates for mediators of drug resistance are functionally important in human drug resistance (Sisodiya, 2003). Since amygdala kindling does not induce any lasting over-expression of P-glycoprotein in areas involved in the kindling process, the process underlying epilepsy seems to be responsible for the seizures, not for over-expression of the protein (Seegers *et al.*, 2002). Since there are many pathophysiologic and pharmacologic similarities between the kindling model and temporal lobe epilepsy, the authors suggest that drug resistance in patients is the result of uncontrolled seizures, not the underlying pathology of epilepsy.

Siddiqui *et al.* (2003) tested the hypothesis that CC genotype at the ABCB 1 C3435T polymorphism, which is associated with increased protein expression, influences the response to AED. ABCB 1 3435 was genotyped in therapy-resistant and drug-responsive epileptic patients, and in control subjects without epilepsy. These pharmacogenomic results identified a genetic factor (CC genotype at ABCB 1 3435) associated with resistance to AEDs in a majority of epileptic patients.

The role of transporters in the distribution of glutamate may be just as important as AEDs. Increased extra-cellular glutamate levels in the epileptogenic hippocampus have been reported in temporal lobe epilepsy. These increased levels of glutamate transporters may be the result of malfunctioning and/or downregulation of glutamate transporters (Proper *et al.*, 2002). The authors have shown differences in mRNA and protein levels of glutamate transporter subtype in specific hippocampal regions; in the HS subgroup excitatory amino acid transporters were reduced (parallel to severe neuronal cell loss) whereas in epileptic patients without HS there was an increase in number of glutamate transporter subtypes. The functional consequence of these findings is not determined.

These new lines of recent research show, on the one hand, how complex the pathogenesis of drug resistance is, and on the other hand, they show how necessary it is to revise the current preclinical strategy for the development of new AEDs with better penetration across the BBB than presently available drugs. All AEDs have been tested on normal animal models of seizures and epilepsies, assuming that the drugs reach the brain epileptic neurons. However, differences in kindling and AED response in normal animals and animals with developmental brain defects have been found (Majkowski, 1983; Majkowski *et al.*, 1984; Majkowski *et al.*, 1986). Moreover, it has been postulated that animal models of drug-resistant kindled seizures are more promising (Löscher, 2002; Löscher and Leppik, 2002). Current limitations of AED therapy and methodological problems of mono- vs. combination therapy have been recently reviewed by Deckers *et al.* (2003). Indeed, a new approach is needed to prevent undesirable consequences of uncontrolled seizures.

This type of future research in no way limits the concept of more rational therapy based on knowledge of pharmacokinetic and pharmacodynamic drug interactions. Clinical verification of experimental data on combination therapy, in a more homogeneous subgroup of early identified drug-resistant patients, performed in multicentre studies on a sufficient number of subjects, seems to be the best therapeutic strategy for today.

REFERENCES

Arroyo S, Brodie MJ, Avanzini G, *et al*. Is refractory epilepsy preventable? *Epilepsia* 2002; **43**: 437–444.

Arzimanoglou A, Gerardin V, Moszkowski J, *et al*. Lamotrigine in patients with childhood onset intractable epilepsy. *Epilepsia* 1993; **34**(Suppl. 6): 113.

Baldy-Moulinier M, Civanis A, D'Urso S, *et al*. Therapeutic strategies against epilepsy in Mediterranean countries: a report from an international collaborative surgery. *Seizure* 1998; **7**: 513–520.

Benetello P, Furlanut M, Baraldo M, *et al*. Therapeutic drug monitoring of lamotrigine in patients suffering from resistant partial seizures. *Eur Neurol* 2002; **48**: 200–203.

Besag FMC, Panayiotopoulos C, Chivers F, *et al*. Therapeutic interaction of lamotrigine with valproate and suximides. *Epilepsia* 1995; **36**(Suppl. 3): 116.

Besag FMC, Berry DJ, Pool F, *et al*. Carbamazepine toxicity with lamotrigine: pharmacokinetic or pharmacodynamic interactions? *Epilepsia* 1998; **39**: 183–187.

Bisulli F, Baruzzi A, Rosati A, *et al*. Efficacy of lamotrigine add-on therapy in severe partial epilepsy in adults with drop seizures and secondary bilateral synchrony on EEG. *Epileptic Disord* 2001; **3**: 151–156.

Biton V, Vasquez B, Sachedo RC, *et al*. Adjunctive tiagabine compared with phenytoin and carbamazepine in multicenter, double-blind trial of complex partial seizures. *Epilepsia* 1998; **39**(Suppl. 6): 125–126.

Bourgeois BFD. Antiepileptic drug combinations and experimental background: the case of phenobarbital and phenytoin. *Naunyn Schmiedebergs Arch Pharmacol* 1986; **333**: 406–411.

Bourgeois BFD. Combination of valproate and ethosuximide: Antiepileptic and neurotoxic interactions. *J Pharmacol Ther* 1988; **247**: 1128–1132.

Brodie MJ, Yuen AC, 105 Study Group. Lamotrigine substitution study: evidence for synergism with sodium valproate. *Epilepsy Res* 1997; **26**: 423–432.

Brodie MJ, Mumford JP for the 012 Study Group. Double blind substitution of vigabatrin and valproate in carbamazepine-resistant partial epilepsy. *Epilepsy Res* 1999; **40**: 199–205.

Camfield PR, Camfield CS. Antiepileptic drug therapy: when is epilepsy truly intractable? *Epilepsia* 1996; **37**(Suppl. 1): 60–65.

Castillo S, Schmidt DB, White S. Oxcarbazepine add-on for drug-resistant partial epilepsy. *Cochrane Database Syst Rev* 2000; CD002028.

Cereghino JJ, Brock JT, van Meter JC, *et al*. The efficacy of carbamazepine combinations in epilepsy. *Clin Pharmacol Ther* 1975; **18**: 733–741.

Chadwick DW, Marson AG. Zonisamide add-on for drug-resistant partial epilepsy *Cochrane Rev. The Cochrane Library* 2003; Issue, 2. Oxford: Update Software.

Chaisewikul R, Baillie N, Marson AG. Calcium antagonists as an add-on therapy for drug-resistant epilepsy. *Cochrane Rev. Cochrane Library* 2001a; Issue 4, Oxford: Update Software.

Chaisewikul R, Privitera MD, Hutton JL, *et al*. Levetiracetam add-on for drug-resistant localization related (partial) epilepsy. *Cochrane Database Syst Rev* 2001b; CD001901.

Coatsworth JJ. Studies on the clinical efficacy of marketed antiepileptic drugs. NIH PHS USDHEW Bethesda Md 1971; **5**: 393.

Czuczwar SJ. Experimental background for synergistic and additive effects of antiepileptic drugs. *Epileptologia* 1998; **6**(Suppl. 2): 21–29.

Czuczwar SJ, Borowicz KK. Polytherapy in epilepsy: the experimental evidence. *Epilepsy Res* 2002; **52**: 15–23.

Czuczwar SJ, Gasior M, Janusz W, *et al.* Influence of flunarizine, nicardipine and nimodipine on the anticonvulsant activity of different antiepileptic drugs in mice. *Neuropharmacology* 1992; **31**: 1179–1183.

Dean JC, Penry JK. Carbamazepine/valproate therapy in 100 patients with partial seizures failing carbamazepine monotherapy: long-term follow-up. *Epilepsia* 1988; **29**: 687.

Deckers CLP, Czuczwar SJ, Hekster YA, *et al.* Selection of antiepileptic drug polytherapy based on mechanism of action: the evidence reviewed. *Epilepsia* 2000; **41**: 1364–1374.

Deckers CLP, Hekster YA, Keyser A, *et al.* Monotherapy versus polytherapy for epilepsy: A multi-center double-blind randomised study. *Epilepsia* 2001; **42**: 1387–1394.

Deckers CLP, Genton P, Sills GJ, *et al.* Current limitations of antiepileptic drug therapy; a conference review. *Epilepsy Res* 2003; **53**: 1–17.

Delanty N, French JA, Williams SF. Lamotrigine and topiramate combination therapy: experience from postmarking surveillance. *Epilepsia* 1998; **39**(Suppl. 6): 131.

Delgado-Escueta AV, Mattson RH, Smith DB, *et al.* Principles in designing clinical trials for antiepileptic drugs. *Neurology* 1983; **33**(Suppl. 1): 8–13.

De Romanis F, Sopranzi N. Lamotrigine in the therapy of resistant epilepsy. *Clin Therapeutica* 1999; **150**: 279–282.

Doychinov D. Didepil for the treatment of epilepsy. In *Epilepsy: A Clinical and Experimental Research*. J. Majkowski, ed. *Monogr Neural Sci*. Basel: S. Karger, 1980: 112–118.

Duncan JS. Principles of treatment of patients with chronic active epilepsy. In *The Treatment of Epilepsies*. S. Shorvon, F. Dreifuss, D. Fish, D. Thomas, eds. Oxford: Blackwell Science, 1996: 177–190.

Ebert U, Rundfeldt C, Lehmann H, *et al.* Characterization of phenytoin-resistant kindled rats, a new model of drug-resistant partial epilepsy: influence of experimental and environmental factors. *Epilepsy Res* 1999, **33**: 199–215.

Elger CE, Fernandez, G. Options after the first antiepileptic drug has failed. *Epilepsia* 1999; **40**(Suppl. 6): 9–12.

Elices E, Arroyo S. Is drug resistant partial epilepsy progressive? *Rev Neurol* 2002; **34**: 505–510.

Elwes RDC, Johnson AL, Reynolds EH. The course of untreated epilepsy. *Br Med J* 1988; **29**: 948–950.

Eriksson AS, Nergardh A, Hoppu K. The efficacy of lamotrigine in children and adolescent with refractory generalized epilepsy: a randomized, double-blind, crossover study. *Epilepsia* 1998; **39**: 495–501.

Feely M, Gibson J. Intermittent clobazam for catamenial epilepsy: tolerance avoided. *J Neurol Neurosurg Psychiatr* 1984; **47**: 1279–1282.

Ferrie CD, Panayiotopoulos CP. Therapeutic interactions of lamotrigine and sodium valproate in intractable myoclonic epilepsy. Seizure 1999; **3**: 1375–1376.

Ferrendelli JA. Rational polypharmacy. *Epilepsia* 1995; **36**(Suppl. 2): 115–118.

Frey M, Kanner AM. Do lamotrigine and valproic acid have an additive anticonvulsant effect. *Epilepsia* 1999; **40**(Suppl. 7): 144.

Fröscher W. Synergistic and additive effects of antiepileptic drugs in epileptic patients. *Epileptologia* 1998; **6**(Suppl. 2): 31–42.

Fröscher W. Clinical experience with synergistic and additive effects of antiepileptic drugs in epileptic patients – new developments. *Epileptologia* 2000; **8**: 221–227.

Fröscher W, Stodl K-D, Hoffmann F. Kombinationsbehandlung mit Carbamazepin und Valproinsäure bei Problemfällen einer Epilepsie-Ambulanz. *Arzneim Forsch* 1984; **34**: 910–914.

Fröscher W, Rauber A, Rothmeier J, *et al.* Vigabatrin bei pharmakoresistenten Epilepsien. *Akt Neurol* 1992; **19**: 48–49.

Gorman WP, Cooper R, Pocock P, *et al.* A comparison of primidone, propranolol, and placebo in essential tremor, using quantitative analysis. *J Neurol Neurosurg Psychiatr* 1986; **49**: 64–68.

Guberman A, Neto W, Gassmann-Mayer C, EPAJ-119 Study Group. Low-dose topiramate in adults with treatment-resistant partial-onset seizures. *Acta Neurol Scand* 2002; **106**: 183–189.

Hakkarainen H. Carbamazepine vs diphenylhydatoin vs their combination in adult epilepsy. *Neurology* 1980; **30**: 354.

Jette NJ, Marson AG, Hutton JL. Topiramate add-on for drug-resistant partial epilepsy. *Cochrane Database Syst Rev* 2002; CD001417.

Jêdrzejczak J, Dlawichowska E, Owczarek K, *et al.* Effect of vigabatrin addition on carbamazepine blood serum levels in patients with epilepsy. *Epilepsy Res* 2000; **39**: 115–120.

Jêdrzejczak J, Leñska-Mieciek M, Tomik BJ. The dynamics of natural, undiagnosed epilepsy of many years' duration – diagnostic difficulties. Three case studies. *Epileptologia* 2002; **10**: 163–174.

Krämer G, Theisohn M, von Unruh GE, *et al.* Carbamazepine-danazol drug interaction: its metabolism examined by a stable isotope technique. *Ther Drug Monit* 1986; **8**: 387–392.

Kugler St. L, Sachedo RC, Wenger EC, *et al.* Efficacy of combination topiramate and lamotrigine in refractory epilepsy in children. *Epilepsia* 1997; **38**(Suppl. 8): 192–193.

Kwan P, Brodie MJ. Early identification of refractory epilepsy. *Engl J Med* 2000; **342**: 314–319.

Leach JP, Brodie MJ. Synergism with GABA-ergic drugs in refractory epilepsy (letter). *Lancet* 1994; **343**: 1650.

Leppik LE, Wolff DL. Antiepileptic medication interactions. *Neurologic Clinics* 1993; **11**: 905–921.

Löscher W. Animal models of drug-resistant epilepsy. *Novartis Found Symp* 2002; **243**: 149–159.

Löscher W, Ebert U. Basic mechanisms of seizure propagation: targets for rational drug design and rational polypharmacy. *Epilepsy Res Suppl* 1996; **11**: 3–7.

Löscher W, Leppik IE. Critical re-evaluation of previous preclinical strategies for the discovery and the development of new antiepileptic drugs. *Epilepsy Res* 2002; **50**: 17–20.

Luszczki JJ, Swiader M, Parada-Turska J, *et al.* Tiagabine synergistically interacts with gabapentin in the electroconvulsive threshold test in mice. *Neuropsychopharmacology* 2003; **28**: 1817–1830.

Lüders HO. National Institutes of Health Consensus Conference. Surgery for epilepsy. *J Am Med Assoc* 1990; **264**: 729–733.

Łysakowska-Sernicka K, Majkowski J, Biliñska-Nigot B. Antiepileptic and side effects of Didepil. In *Epilepsy: A Clinical and Experimental Research*. J. Majkowski, ed. *Monogr Neural Sci*. Basel: S. Karger, 1980: 119–123.

Majkowski J. Drug effects on after discharge and seizure threshold in lissencephalic ferrets: an epilepsy model for drug evaluation. *Epilepsia* 1983; **24**: 678–685.

Majkowski J. Drug resistant epilepsy and rational polytherapy in the era of new antiepileptic drug. *Epileptologia* 1996; **4**: 281–293.

Majkowski J. Natural course of epileptogenesis: from partial simple to partial complex seizures. A case report. *Epileptologia* 1998; **6**: 99–112.

Majkowski J. Kindling: clinical relevance for epileptogenicity in humans. In *Advances in Neurology*. H. Stefan, F. Andermann, P. Chauvel, S. Shorvon, eds., Philadelphia: Lippincott Williams & Wilkins, 1999; **81**, 105–113.

Majkowski J. The natural progression of epileptogenesis: from partial simple visual seizure to complex and secondary generalised seizures. A case study. *Epileptologia* 2000; **7**: 47–58.

Majkowski J, Lee MH, Kozlowski PB, *et al.* EEG and seizure threshold in normal and lissencephalic ferrets. *Brain Res* 1984; **307**: 29–38.

Majkowski J, Danneberg P, Knappen F. Differences in antiepileptic drug efficacy in hippocampal kindled normal and microcephalic rats. *Brain Res* 1986; **386**: 325–331.

Majkowski J, Sidor K, Wendorff J, *et al.* Prophylaxis and control of febrile convulsion (FC) by rectal administration of diazepam. Prospective study. Preliminary Report. *Epileptologia* 1995; **3**: 111–120.

Majkowski J, Kacinski M, Jedrzejazak J, *et al.* Pharmacological treatment of epilepsy in Poland 2000–2001. Multicenter Prospective Study of 6195 Patients. *Epideplogia* 2005; **13**: In press

Marroni M, Marchi N, Cucullo L, *et al.* Vascular and parenchymal mechanisms in multiple drug resistance: a lesson from human epilepsy. *Curr Drug Targets* 2003; **4**: 297–304.

Marson AG, Hutton JL, Leach JP, *et al.* Levetiracetam, oxcarbazepine and zonisamide for drug resistant localisation related epilepsy: a systemic review. *Epilepsy Res* 2001; **46**: 259–270.

Masuda Y, Utsui Y, Shiraishi Y, *et al.* Evidence for a synergistic interaction between phenytoin and phenobarbital in experimental animals. *J Pharmacol Exp Ther*, 1981; **217**: 805–811.

Mattson RH. Drug treatment of partial epilepsies. *Adv Neurol* 1992; **57**: 643–650.

Mattson RH, Cramer JA. Crossover from polytherapy to monotherapy in primary generalised epilepsy. *Amer J Med* 1988; **84**(Suppl. 1A): 23–38.

Mattson RH, Klein PE, Caldwell BV, *et al.* Medroxyprogesterone treatment of women with uncontrolled seizures. *Epilepsia* 1982; **23**: 436–437.

Mattson RH, Cramer JA, Delgado-Escueta AV, *et al.* A design for the prospective evaluation of the efficacy and toxicity of antiepileptic drugs in adults. *Neurology* 1983; **33**(Suppl. 1): 14–25.

Muri L, Judice A. Vigabatrin as first add-on treatment in carbamazepine-resistant epilepsy patients. *Acta Neurol Scand* 1995; **62**(Suppl. 1): 40–42.

Ohtsuka Y, Ogino T, Amano R, *et al.* Rational treatment of refractory epilepsy in childhood. *Jpn J Psychiatr Neurol* 1988; **42**: 443–447.

Panayiotopoulos CP, Ferrie CD, Knott C, *et al.* Interaction of lamotrigine with sodium valproate (letter). *Lancet* 1993; **341**: 445.

Patsalos PN, Perucca E. Clinically important drug interactions in epilepsy: general features and interactions between antiepileptic drugs. *Lancet Neurol* 2003; **2**: 347–356.

Patsalos PN, Fröscher W, Pisani F, *et al.* The importance of drug interactions in epilepsy therapy. *Epilepsia* 2002; **43**: 365–385.

Pereira J, Marson AG, Hutton JL. Tiagabine add-on for drug-resistant partial epilepsy. *Cochrane Database Syst Pev* 2002; CD001908.

Pippenger CE, Penry JK, White BG, *et al.* Interlaboratory variability in determination of plasma antiepileptic drug concentrations. *Arch Neurol* 1976; **33**: 351–355.

Pisani F, Di Perri R, Perucca E, *et al.* Interaction of lamotrigine with sodium valproate. *Lancet* 1993; **341**: 1224.

Pisani F, Oteri G, Russo MF, *et al.* The efficacy of valproate–lamotrigine comedication in refractory complex partial seizures: evidence for pharmacodynamic interactions. *Epilepsia* 1999a; **40**: 1141–1146.

Pisani F, Oteri G, Antonino F, *et al.* Complete seizure control following gabapentin–lamotrigine comedication. *Epilepsia* 1999b; **40**(Suppl. 2): 253–254.

Potschka H, Fedrowitz M, Löscher W. Brain access and anticonvulsant of carbamazepine, lamotrigine, and felbamate in ARCC2/MRP2 – deficient TR-rats. *Epilepsia* 2003a; **44**: 1479–1486.

Potschka H, Fedrowitz M, Löscher W. Multidrug resistance protein MRP2 contributes to blood–brain barrier function and restricts antiepileptic drug activity. *J Pharmacol Exp Ther* 2003b; **306**: 124–131.

Proper EA, Hoogland G, Kappen SM, *et al.* Distribution of glutamate transporters in the hippocampus of patients with pharmaco-resistant temporal lobe epilepsy. *Brain* 2002; **125**: 32–43.

Ramaratnam S, Marson AG, Baker GA. Lamotrigine add-on for drug-resistant partial epilepsy. *Cochrane Review. Cochrane Library* 2003; Issue 4. Oxford: Update Software.

Remy S, Gabriel S, Urban BW, *et al.* A novel mechanism underlying drug resistance in chronic epilepsy. *Ann. Neurol* 2003; **53**: 469–479.

Reynolds EH, Shorvon SD. Monotherapy or polytherapy for epilepsy? *Epilepsia* 1981; **22**: 1–10.

Ribacoba Montero R, Salas Puig X. Efficacy and tolerability of long term topiramate in drug resistant epilepsy in adults. *Rev Neurol* 2002; **34**: 101–105.

Richens A. Drug level monitoring: the importance of quality control. In *Epilepsy: A Clinical and Experimental Research.* J. Majkowski, ed. *Monogr Neural Sci* 5. Basel: S. Karger, 1980: 176–182.

Robinson MK, Black AB, Schapel GS, *et al.* Combined gamma-vinyl-GABA (vigabatrin) and lamotrigine therapy in management of refractory epilepsy. *Epilepsia* 1993; **34**(Suppl. 2): 109.

Rowan AJ, Meijer JWA, de Beer-Pawlikowski N, *et al.* Valproate–ethosuximide combination therapy for refractory absence seizures. *Arch Neurol* 1983; **40**: 797–802.

Sälke-Kellermann RA, May T, Boenigk HE. Influence of ethosuximide on valproic acid serum concentrations. *Epilepsy Res* 1997; **26**: 345–349.

Schapel GJ, Black AB, Lam EL, *et al.* Combination vigabatrin and lamotrigine therapy for intractable epilepsy. *Seizure* 1996; **5**: 51–56.

Schmidt D. Two antiepileptic drugs for intractable epilepsy with complex partial seizures. *J Neurol Neurosurg Psychiatr* 1982; **45**: 1119–1124.

Schmidt D, Gram L. Monotherapy versus polytherapy in epilepsy. A reappraisal. *CNS Drugs* 1995; **3**: 194–208.

Seegers U, Potschka H, Löscher W. Expression of the multidrug transporter P-glycoprotein in brain parenchyma of amygdala-kindled rats. *Epilepsia* 2002; **43**: 675–684.

Shorvon S, Reynolds EH. Reduction in polypharmacy for epilepsy. *Br Med J* 1979; **2**: 1023–1025.

Siddiqui A, Kerb R, Weale ME, *et al.* Association of multidrug resistance in epilepsy with a polymorphism in the drug-transporter gene ABCB1. *New Engl J Med* 2003; **348**: 1442–1448.

Sills GJ, Thompson GT, Forrest G, *et al.* Lack of experimental interaction between vigabatrin and lamotrigine. *Epilepsia* 1993; **34**(Suppl. 6): 92.

Sisodiya SM. Mechanisms of antiepileptic drug resistance. *Curr Opin Neurol* 2003; **16**: 197–201.

Sisodiya SM, Lin W-R, Harding BN, *et al.* Drug resistance in epilepsy: expression of drug resistance proteins in common causes of refractory epilepsy. *Brain* 2002; **1**: 22–31.

Stephen LJ, Sills GJ, Brodie MJ. Lamotrigine and topiramate may be a useful combination. *Lancet* 1998; **351**: 958–959.

Stewart J, Hughes E, Reynolds EH. Lamotrigine for generalized epilepsies (letter). *Lancet* 1992; **340**: 1223.

Stolarek I, Blacklaw J, Thompson GG, *et al.* Gamma-vinyl-GABA (vigabatrin) and lamotrigine: synergism in a refractory epilepsy? *Epilepsia* 1993; **34**(Suppl. 2): 108–109.

Tanganelli P, Regesta G. Vigabatrin vs carbamazepine monotherapy in newly diagnosed focal epilepsy: a randomised response conditional cross-over study. *Epilepsy Res* 1996; **25**: 257–262.

Walker JE, Koon R. Carbamazepine versus valproate versus combined therapy for refractory partial complex seizures with secondary generalization. *Epilepsia* 1988; **29**: 693.

Warner T, Patsalos PN, Prevett M, *et al.* Lamotrigine-induced carbamazepine toxicity: an interaction with carbamazepine-10, 11-epoxide. *Epilepsy Res* 1992; **11**: 147–150.

Willmore LJ, Shu V, Vallin B, the M 88–194 Study Group. Efficacy and safety of add-on divalproex sodium in the treatment of complex partial seizures. *Neurology* 1996; **46**: 49–53.

Yahr MD, Sciarra D, Carter S. Evaluation of standard anticonvulsant therapy of 319 patients. *J Am Med Assoc* 1952; **150**: 663–667.

24

Future research: an experimental perspective

Rob A. Voskuyl[1,2], Daniel M. Jonker[1,2] and Fernando H. Lopes da Silva[2,3]

[1] LACDR, Division of Pharmacology, Gorlaeus Laboratories, Leiden, The Netherlands
[2] Epilepsy Institute of the Netherlands (SEIN), Achterweg, Heemstede, The Netherlands
[3] Swammerdom Institute of Life Sciences (SILS), University of Amsterdam, The Netherlands

Introduction

The previous chapters have amply demonstrated both the need for effective combinations of antiepileptic drugs (AEDs) and the problems associated with the use of such combinations. The first problem is to choose which drugs should be combined and in which dose ratio. To be superior to monotherapy, the drug combination should either act synergistically with respect to the antiepileptic effect or antagonistically with respect to adverse effects, or both. The second major task is assessment of the efficacy of a combination and the experimental demonstration that the efficacy is significantly better than monotherapy.

It is the challenge for basic research:

1 To provide the theoretical basis to design effective combinations for specific epilepsies.
2 To provide new tools to assess whether the effect of a combination is synergistic, additive or antagonistic.

In this chapter, we will focus only on achieving maximal synergy for the antiepileptic effect. Alternatively, aiming at achieving maximal antagonism could be applied to minimize adverse effects.

Ultimately, the advantage of a combination of drugs over a single drug can be demonstrated only in in vivo experiments. In vitro experiments are highly useful for the analysis of interactions at specific targets, but can never take into account all aspects that contribute to the final efficacy in the intact organism. Therefore, studies on combination therapy should include both approaches. When designing in vivo experiments and choosing an experimental animal model to demonstrate synergy (or antagonism) of drug combinations, a number of points should be taken into consideration. Pharmaco-resistance is associated with a few specific types of epilepsy. Drug combinations should therefore be tested in those types of epilepsy, and appropriate experimental animal models should be selected to investigate the efficacy and usefulness of such combinations. Furthermore, the mechanism of epileptogenesis, the possible progressive nature of the epilepsy and the chronic use of AEDs may all cause modification or functional adaptation of the efficacy of a drug.

In this chapter the factors influencing AED responses will be discussed first. Subsequently, the use of computer simulations based on mechanistic interaction models for designing efficient study protocols and data interpretation will be introduced. Finally, the assessment of the efficacy of combinations based on pharmacokinetic–pharmacodynamic (PK/PD) modeling of concentration–effect data will be dealt with.

Factors influencing AED response

Mechanisms of epileptogenesis

Development of new effective AEDs and therapeutic approaches ideally implies elucidation of the basic mechanisms of epileptogenesis and seizure generation and, thereby, identification of the appropriate targets (Löscher and Ebert, 1996). Different epilepsies have different mechanisms of epileptogenesis. Therefore, the choice of the experimental model to study basic mechanisms is critical. Epileptogenesis and seizure generation seldom depend on a single cause but rather on a combination of factors. This can be, for example, reduction of GABAergic inhibition, enhancement of glutamatergic excitation, a change in properties of voltage-regulated Na^+-channels, etc.; but it may also depend critically on specific neuronal loss, synaptic reorganization and gliosis. Furthermore, developmental abnormalities and tumor growth may be associated with generation of 'epileptogenic networks' characterized by enhanced seizure susceptibility. Intuitively, it might be argued that effective pharmacotherapy will depend on correctly targeting a number of properties of neuronal systems simultaneously. The fact that a remarkable number of AEDs appear to have multiple actions indirectly supports this notion. One approach could be to design drugs that incorporate several specified actions in a single molecule (Löscher and Ebert, 1996). This may be possible at some time, but for the near future it is more feasible to attempt to combine drugs with highly selective actions on specific targets. Such combinations would represent truly rational polytherapy. Presently, drug combinations consist only of compounds with putative antiepileptic action. However, it is conceivable that future combinations will also include drugs that are presently not considered antiepileptic.

Experimental animal models

For studies on drug combinations experimental epilepsy models should be used that mimic human epilepsies and seizure types exhibiting a high percentage of resistance to pharmacotherapy Stables *et al* (2002). The subpopulation of refractory epilepsy is not a well-defined group. About 60% of all refractory patients have temporal lobe epilepsy presenting with complex partial seizures (Reynolds *et al.*, 1983). Refractory epilepsy also occurs very often with severe syndromes such as Lennox–Gastaut (Sillanpää, 1995) and in some forms of primary generalized epilepsy (Reutens and Berkovic, 1995). However, seizures do not persist in all patients with any one of these forms of epilepsy. Regesta and Tanganelli (1999) recently discussed a number of factors that may be useful as predictors of refractoriness. Apart from syndromes and types of epilepsy, this list includes other factors such as frequency of seizures, number of seizures before treatment, status epilepticus, brain lesions, brain tumors and genetic factors.

From the discussion above, it is clear that many factors can contribute to the emergence of pharmaco-resistance. However, at present there are only a few models available that faithfully represent types of epilepsy associated with pharmaco-resistance (Coulter *et al.*, 2002; Löscher, 1997).

Löscher and co-workers developed an interesting model. They observed that a subpopulation of amygdala-kindled animals do not respond to phenytoin (Löscher *et al.*, 1993). In this subpopulation other AEDs are not effective either, with the possible exception of levetiracetam. From their studies, evidence is accumulating that this can be considered as a true model for pharmaco-resistance (Cramer *et al.*, 1998; Löscher, 1997; Löscher *et al.*, 1998).

Recently the 6-Hz-psychomotor seizure model of partial epilepsy was evaluated as a potential screening model of therapy-resistant limbic seizures (Barton *et al.*, 2001). Because of the phenytoin insensitivity, this model was originally abandoned, but this very property may indicate its usefulness as a model of pharmaco-resistant epilepsy. In a study on the effect of twelve established and new AEDs in this model, it was found that at low-stimulus intensity, nearly all drugs exhibited full or partial protection. Increasing the stimulus intensity decreased the efficacy of all AEDs and only levetiracetam and valproate remained fully protective, although with a lower potency.

Generalized epilepsies respond well to monotherapy, as do experimental genetic models of absence-like epilepsies such as the Genetic Absence Epilepsy Rat from Strasbourg (GAERS) and the WAG/Rij rats from Nijmegen (The Netherlands). Accordingly, these models appear to be less relevant for sophisticated drug interaction studies. However, recently a model has been described that appears to reflect properties of atypical absences (Cortez *et al.*, 2001), a progressive form of epilepsy that eventually responds poorly to drug treatment. The model is based on inhibition of cholesterol synthesis in a critical postnatal period. Although it has not yet been characterized rigorously (including response to drug treatment), it might prove an interesting model for drug interaction studies. Since the animals exhibit spontaneous seizures, this model more closely resembles true epilepsy.

A number of experimental models have been developed, based on the long-term effects of induction of status epilepticus, which share a number of properties with human temporal lobe epilepsy. Status epilepticus can be induced either by administration of convulsant drugs (Sperk, 1994; Turski *et al.*, 1989) or application of nearly continuous electrical stimulation to selected brain structures (Gorter *et al.*, 2001; Lothman *et al.*, 1989; Nissinen *et al.*, 2000; Shirasaka and Wasterlain, 1994). Although the models differ in details, they have in common that the animals develop spontaneous seizures after a so-called latent period.

Most pharmacologic studies in these models have involved testing efficacy of anticonvulsant drugs in the acute phase or (less frequently) on spontaneous seizures (Glien *et al.*, 2002; Leite and Cavalheiro, 1995; Nissinen *et al.*, 2004). Other studies have focused on mechanisms of epileptogenesis in order to identify new targets and to prevent cell death, development of spontaneous seizures, etc. (Liu *et al.*, 1999; Mazarati *et al.*, 1998b; Pitkänen *et al.*, 1999; Rice and DeLorenzo, 1999). Only few studies have attempted to characterize development of pharmaco-resistance. It has been noted that the efficacy of AEDs rapidly diminishes after induction of status epilepticus (Kapur and Macdonald, 1997; Mazarati *et al.*, 1998a; Morrisett *et al.*, 1987). However, how induction of status epilepticus and the process of epileptogenesis leading to spontaneous seizures affect the time course and nature of reduction in efficacy of AEDs, has not yet been studied systematically and quantitatively.

Studies in the post-status model of spontaneous seizures after hippocampal electrical stimulation have revealed a novel factor that may underlie pharmaco-resistance, namely a change in the molecular structure of the Na^+ channel, characterized by the emergence of the neonatal form, detrimental to the adult form (Aronica *et al.*, 2001). This is associated with a change of the kinetics of Na^+ currents (Ketelaars *et al.*, 2001) and may account for a change in the sensitivity to AEDs such as carbamazepine (Vreugdenhil and Wadman, 1999; Reny *et al.*, 2003). This illustrates the relevance of using proper experimental animal models for the evaluation of AEDs, alone or in combinations.

An unexplored area is the use of animal models developed by controlled mutations. Identification of the genetic mutations in well-defined human epilepsies in principle provides the tools to induce similar syndromes in animals. This provides exciting opportunities that might become available within a few years.

Disease progression

Some types of epilepsy are clearly progressive in nature and the same is observed in a number of experimental models, for example kindling and the post-status models. This aspect is a central issue of these models. It is likely that progression of the epileptogenic process will alter the response to AEDs. A good example is the failure of *N*-methyl-D-aspartate (NMDA) antagonists in clinical studies (Löscher and

Schmidt, 1994), which may be due to profoundly altered properties of NMDA receptors, as has been observed after kindling (Mody, 1999). Few studies on AEDs have been performed from this perspective. Studies by Cleton *et al.* may serve as an indication of the importance of this aspect and as a proof of concept. The efficacy of midazolam to enhance gamma amino butyric acid alpha ($GABA_A$)-mediated inhibition was compared in fully kindled animals and unstimulated controls, using the increase in the β-frequency band in the electroencephalogram (EEG) as a marker for enhanced inhibition. Kindling reduced the maximal effect by about 25% and similar reductions were found in the cortical stimulation model and in WAG/Rij rats, which exhibit spontaneous absence seizures (Cleton *et al.*, 1998; 1999b). This indicates that this phenomenon is not restricted to a specific experimental model. Remarkably, kindling did not affect the efficacy of tiagabine, a drug that enhances GABAergic inhibition to a similar degree, but by a different mechanism (Cleton *et al.*, 2000a). On the contrary, the potency of tiagabine was *increased*. Thus, alterations in efficacy of AEDs may differ for each drug (and drug combination), depending on the mode of action.

Influence of chronic medication

AEDs are always taken chronically. The continuous exposure of a receptor to a drug may cause adaptation of that receptor. This is commonly called tolerance development, of which the benzodiazepines are the classical example. Studies by Cleton *et al.* on midazolam and tiagabine yielded interesting observations. Chronic treatment with midazolam, either by continuous infusion or by administration via implanted slow-release devices, caused a reduction in efficacy of the order of 50% (Cleton *et al.*, 2000c), similar to the reduction in efficacy in different epilepsy models. Investigation of chloride uptake in synaptoneurosomes from amygdala-kindled animals, and animals chronically treated with midazolam suggested that reduction in efficacy of the administration of midazolam was caused by adaptation of the $GABA_A$ receptor in both cases (Cleton *et al.*, 1999b). Thus, similar adaptive (homeostatic) mechanisms may be present in disease progression and drug tolerance. Nevertheless, chronic administration of tiagabine in amounts that enhanced $GABA_A$-mediated inhibition to the same extent as midazolam, did not affect the efficacy at all (Cleton *et al.*, 2000b). Whether chronic treatment alters the efficacy or not, these observations emphasize that the effect of chronic treatment needs to be taken into account when studying drug combinations.

Pharmacokinetic factors and interactions

When considering the efficacy of drug treatment or when comparing the efficacy of a specific regimen under different conditions, it is of course necessary to ensure that the level of target exposure is known. In other words, pharmacokinetic parameters should be determined as well. Chronic medication, the epileptic state of the brain and disease progression may all influence the pharmacokinetics of a drug. In addition, pharmacokinetic interactions often occur when drugs are given in combination. Thus, it is self-evident that determination of pharmacokinetic properties should always be included in studies on drug efficacy, in particular with drug combinations. In the face of these arguments it is surprising that this is the case only in about half of the studies in the literature. The pharmacokinetic processes that may influence the drug effect are absorption, rate of metabolism, formation of active metabolites, distribution (also within the brain), protein binding, passage of the blood–brain barrier and active transport out of the brain.

Development of drug combinations: a modeling approach

The commonly held view is that only combinations of AEDs with different mechanisms will result in a synergistic action. The logic of this is clear, but beyond this statement the development of effective drug combinations largely remains a matter of trial and error. There is no theoretical basis to predict which combinations of mechanisms will yield a synergistic, additive or antagonistic effect, how large a synergistic or antagonistic effect will be, and how this will depend on the efficacy and concentration (or dose) of each drug. Even in oncology, where combination therapy is the rule rather than the exception, design of new combinations is often simply based on overlap of efficacies and lack of overlap of toxicities (Peters *et al.*, 2000). Two scenarios can be envisaged in which combination therapy could be applied. Refractory epilepsy often starts with an initiating event (e.g. head trauma, febrile seizures or stroke), which sets in motion a cascade of irreversible events ultimately leading to pharmaco-resistance. Each step in the cascade is a potential target for intervention (Löscher, 2002). A cocktail of drugs aimed at these targets could prevent this domino effect. This requires of course, knowledge of the involved risk factors, mechanisms of epileptogenesis and seizure generation, disease progression, and of the time course of the cascade at a level that is presently not available, but it could become feasible in the future. The alternative scenario is to design drug combinations based on knowledge about the various mechanisms presently known to be involved in pharmaco-resistant epilepsies. Also this approach is hampered by a lack of understanding of all the involved factors, but the prospects in this direction are considerably better.

Knowledge of the mechanisms that operate in an interaction can be used to simulate the response of a combination at all concentration pairs. This approach is based on the operational model of agonism introduced by Black and Leff (1983). The key feature of this model is the separation of the drug–receptor interaction and the subsequent transduction into the response. Thus, the model incorporates both drug-related properties (e.g. receptor affinity) and system-related properties

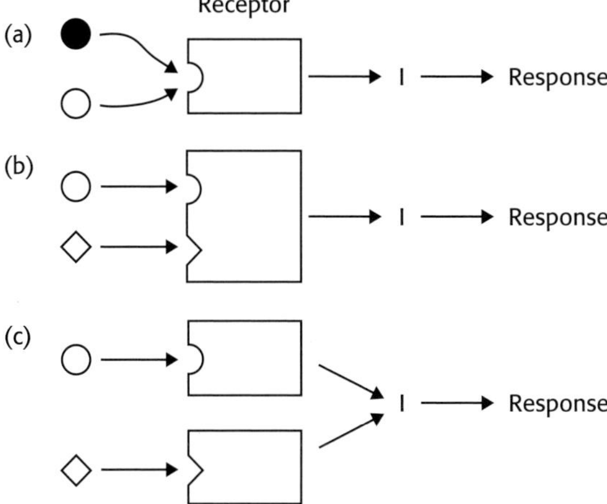

Figure 24.1   In a mechanism-based analysis the pharmacologic effect of a drug is separated into the drug–receptor interaction and the transduction from receptor activation to pharmacologic response. The transduction may take place in one or more steps via intermediate states (indicated as I). In this figure three general types of interaction are displayed. In (a) competition of two agonists for one receptor is shown. In (b) two agonists bind to the same receptor at different sites. A well-known example of this type is allosteric modulation, of $GABA_A$ receptor function by benzodiazepines. In (c) two agonists bind to different receptors and the two transduction pathways converge at some point

(e.g. receptor density). An important system property is the parameter characterizing the transduction efficiency. For a series of analog compounds this parameter indicates the relative efficacy, that is whether a compound is a full or a partial agonist.

The starting point of the study by Jonker and Visser (2005) was the distinction of three general types of interaction (Figure 24.1). The simplest interaction is the competition of two drugs for the same binding site on a receptor (competitive interaction). The second possibility is the binding of two drugs to separate binding sites on the same receptor. In this case the binding of one drug can modulate the binding of the other and the subsequent receptor activation. This so-called allosteric modulation can be in the positive or negative direction. The third type of interaction is the binding of the two drugs to different receptors. In the first two types of interaction the response after receptor activation is generated through a common transduction pathway. In the last case, however, the final response is generated through different transduction pathways that converge after one or more intermediate steps.

To compare the different interaction schemes they developed an elegant method. The classical method used to evaluate drug interactions is the isobolographic analysis (Berenbaum, 1989). In this analysis different concentration pairs of the two drugs needed to elicit an effect of the same magnitude are plotted. If this so-called isobole (or iso-effect line) is linear, the interaction is considered to be additive. Significant deviation of linearity indicates synergy or antagonism. However, this method has several disadvantages. First, the method is purely empirical and therefore does not allow conclusions concerning mechanistic aspects. Second, the shape of the iso-effect line depends on the shape of the concentration–effect relation of each drug. For example, if these relationships are described by a sigmoid E_{max} model with different slope factors for each drug, the iso-effect line will not be linear. Third, if the two drugs differ in maximal response, the isobole is not defined at responses above the lower of the two maxima. Thus, interpretation of such data is not a straightforward matter.

As an alternative, three-dimensional response surfaces were generated to depict the interaction of the drug combinations (Greco *et al.*, 1995; Minto *et al.*, 2000). The response surface predicted by the interaction model is compared to a reference response surface. If an additive interaction is assumed, the reference surface can be constructed according to the concentration–addition method for drug A in the presence of drug B and vice versa (Pöch and Holzmann, 1980). The occurrence of synergy, simple addition or antagonism is then most easily visualized by subtracting the two surfaces. A flat surface of zero effect indicates simple addition, whereas hills and valleys indicate regions of synergy and antagonism, respectively (Figure 24.2). This method is very attractive because it allows recognition of the concentration regions of interest in a single glance and provides insight into the magnitude of the interaction as well. The simulations indicated that the best chances for observing synergism are to be expected with allosteric modulation, and if two different receptors are involved.

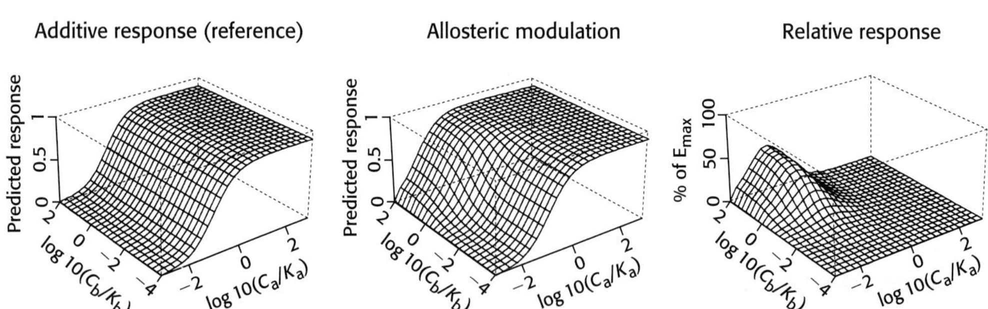

Figure 24.2 Visualization of an allosteric interaction. The concentration–effect relationship for agonist A is characterized by a sigmoid function. The concentration C_a is normalized by dividing C_a by the affinity constant K_a. Drug B binds to the same receptor complex but does not exert an effect of its own. The left panel shows the predicted response surface for simple addition, the middle panel for the allosteric interaction model. The right panel represents the difference between the reference and the allosteric modulation and clearly shows the concentration region of interactions

The interaction models incorporated simple sigmoid functions to describe the drug–receptor interaction and the signal transduction. The translation of receptor activation into effect strongly influences the magnitude of the combined effect. Remarkably, stronger synergism was predicted with moderately efficient than with highly efficient signal transduction. In other words, combinations of partial agonists are more likely to yield synergy than combinations of full agonists. Many other system parameters determine whether synergism will occur. For example, a steep relation between receptor activation and effect increases the maximum degree of synergism. On the other hand, baseline receptor activation can reduce the degree of synergism predicted with allosteric interaction. Simulations have also been carried out for situations where the concentration–effect relationship of a drug cannot be described by a sigmoid function. The interaction was modeled successfully for the case where one of the drugs exerts a biphasic effect. Modeling of drug interactions is therefore not restricted to relatively simple situations. This is important because it is likely that with increasing insight into the mechanisms leading to the final response of a drug, more complex interaction models will be needed.

It should be noted that the interaction models did not only predict synergism, but under certain conditions also antagonism. Thus, in certain concentration ratios, drug combinations can be detrimental to the anticonvulsant effect.

In summary, the computer simulation proposed by Jonker and Visser appears to be a promising tool to predict which drug combinations are likely to be synergistic or antagonistic, based on mechanistic considerations. The simulations have also indicated that synergistic or antagonistic interactions do not occur at all concentration pairs. This offers a considerable advantage for designing experiments to confirm predictions, because the concentration ranges at which combinations need to be tested can be restricted and this will considerably reduce the amount of experimental work required to characterize the efficacy of a drug combination. Finally, it may be applied to establish the mechanism of unknown interactions by comparing the experimentally determined surface plot with theoretical models.

Assessment of efficacy of drug combinations: experimental aspects

When evaluating the efficacy of drug combinations, the objectives are simple. The anticonvulsant effect should be measured in appropriate experimental models of pharmaco-resistant epilepsy, at specified concentrations of each drug. However, in practice this is a formidable task. If we take the post-status model as an example, spontaneous seizures start to appear after a latent period of about 1 week and it takes 8 weeks to reach a steady state of approximately 10 seizures per day (Gorter *et al.*, 2001). If suppression of spontaneous seizures were taken as pharmacodynamic endpoint, it would cost many animals, and months if not years, to characterize the response surfaces of drugs A and B and their combination, to decide whether the combination is synergistic. Furthermore, since seizures occur at unpredictable moments, it would be necessary to maintain drug concentrations at specified levels for appreciable periods of time and to monitor plasma concentrations closely. This is obviously not feasible. Preferably the anticonvulsant efficacy of a drug or a combination should be assessed on seizure activity that can be elicited repeatedly and in a controlled manner. This should be done over a wide range of concentrations and in a reasonably short time. Simultaneously, plasma concentrations of each drug should be determined to account for possible pharmacokinetic interactions and to allow estimation of the concentration at the effect site.

Controlled seizure activity and pharmacologic endpoints

Seizures can be evoked easily by electrical stimulation of various brain areas. However, post-ictal threshold changes and ethical considerations often prevent repeated measurements in the same animal, certainly at short-time intervals. This virtually excludes methods like the maximal electroshock test, but seizures evoked in the kindling model or in the 6-Hz-psychomotor seizure model are useful endpoints. Suppression of seizures is a meaningful endpoint but it is an all-or-nothing event. More accurate information can be obtained by determining the threshold for convulsions, for example by stepwise increase of the stimulus intensity. However, this is a time-consuming procedure, and post-ictal changes may confound threshold values with repeated determination. These disadvantages have been eliminated by stimulation with ramp-shaped pulse trains, which provides a quick and accurate measure for the seizure threshold (Hoogerkamp *et al.*, 1994; Voskuyl *et al.*, 1989, 1992). Moreover, with some restrictions, it may be repeated at very short intervals (minutes) in the same animal. So far, this method has been explored only in cortical motor areas. Seizures can also be elicited by application of convulsant drugs (e.g. pentylenetetrazole) and similarly the threshold can be determined by timed intravenous (i.v.) infusion. The time to the first convulsive event may be used as a measure for the minimal convulsant dose. The plasma concentration of the convulsant at that time point is an even more precise parameter. Unfortunately, this method cannot be repeated at short time intervals, which limits the obtainable information to one data point per animal.

Seizures are usually considered as a single entity, but an interesting possibility is to analyze separate seizure behavioral components and their time sequence in detail (Della Paschoa *et al.*, 1997, 1998b). Seizure semiology plays an important role in clinical diagnosis, but it is seldom used in pharmacologic studies. The effects of AEDs on specific seizure components have been investigated and it has been shown that they can be selectively suppressed (Jonker *et al.*, 2003, 2004).

Methods, which have been developed in ethology for measuring behavior objectively and reproducibly, are utilized for quantification. If drugs can be found that specifically and selectively suppress certain seizure components, and if these components are generated by separate mechanisms, this might provide an interesting approach to develop putatively successful combinations. Moreover, quantitative behavioral analysis can in principle be applied to any seizure type, irrespective of its origin, and in any experimental animal model or even in humans.

It is also possible to use indirect markers for seizure suppression. For example, if a drug combination is expected to modify $GABA_A$ receptor-mediated inhibition, the increase in the EEG in the β-frequency band can be monitored (Mandema *et al.*, 1992)[R.A.3]. Such an approach focuses more on mechanisms of interaction and eventually allows conclusions about the contribution of specific mechanisms to the antiepileptic effect.

The methods described above can be applied initially in naive animals and later in one of the experimental models representative for pharmaco-resistant epilepsy. In the final stage the ultimate test will be the efficacy of a drug combination to suppress spontaneous seizures. The frequency of seizure occurrence, or even better, the distribution of the duration of inter-ictal intervals, is in principle a good measure. A low frequency of seizure occurrence and the inherent unpredictability clearly complicate these measurements, but on the other hand in that stage of development, only a limited range of drug plasma concentrations or dose regimens need to be tested.

Design of experiments

An efficient way to establish the response surface of a drug combination is to give drug A as a continuous i.v. infusion in order to establish a steady-state concentration and to add drug B as an i.v. bolus dose on top of the infusion (Della Paschoa *et al.*, 1998a). By measuring the anticonvulsant effect at regular time intervals after administration of the bolus dose, the effect can be determined over the full concentration range of drug B in the presence of a specified concentration of drug A. Repeating the experiment at different steady-state levels of A, characterizes the complete response surface in a relatively small number of experiments. When necessary, alternative concentration–time profiles can be created. For example, a linearly or stepwise increasing plasma concentration can be achieved easily by programming a computer-controlled infusion pump using the pharmacokinetic parameters of the drug (Cleton *et al.*, 1999a). By using this approach to administer two drugs in a fixed ratio, the response surface can be then determined even more efficiently than by the method described above.

These approaches can be used only under certain conditions. In the first place this is possible only when the anticonvulsant effect can be determined repeatedly.

It is therefore very convenient if cortical stimulation with ramp-shaped pulse trains can be applied or if a continuous measure such as the change in the β-frequency band in the EEG can be used. In the second place, maintaining a steady-state concentration for hours by continuous i.v. infusion is only feasible when the drug is water soluble and available in sufficient amounts. By adding a suitable carrier to the infusion fluid, such as albumin or cyclodextrin, water-solubility might be increased. Alternatively, drugs could be administered by a slow-release device.

Determination of plasma concentrations is of utmost importance when evaluating drug combinations. For the estimation of the concentration of both drugs at the time of effect measurement, it is not sufficient to rely on pharmacokinetic parameters determined for the individual drug in healthy animals. The actual concentrations in combination experiments may be different because of pharmacokinetic interactions, interindividual variability and epilepsy-induced alterations in pharmacokinetics. Furthermore, transport to the brain may be changed as well. Upregulation of transporters in the blood–brain barrier such as P-glycoprotein and multidrug-resistance-associated proteins may lower the brain concentration. Although sophisticated mathematical models may be applied to estimate drug concentrations at the effect site, based on the pharmacokinetics in plasma, this should be confirmed by independent techniques. Methods such as microdialysis, positron emission tomography and magnetic resonance spectroscopy may provide such information.

Integrated PK/PD modeling

Superiority of a combination over a single drug needs to be proven. For this purpose, PK/PD modeling, which describes and characterizes the relationship between drug concentration and pharmacologic response by a mathematical model, is a convenient method. There are many applications of PK/PD modeling, such as optimization of dosage regimens, comparison of drug response under physiologic and pathologic conditions, etc. (Lesko *et al.*, 2001; Sheiner and Steimer, 2000). The particular advantage in this case is that both pharmacokinetic and pharmacodynamic interactions can be identified simultaneously.

Models used to characterize drug action in PK/PD modeling have evolved from simple empirical models such as the sigmoidal E_{max} model to sophisticated mechanistic models that take into account physiologic and pathologic mechanisms, and mechanisms of drug action. Another important development is the application of population modeling (Holford and Peck, 1992; Ouellet *et al.*, 2001), which focuses on characterizing and explaining variability in pharmacokinetics and in pharmacologic response (e.g. inter- and intra-individual variability, influence of covariates such as age, gender, disease, co-medication, etc.). Also the modeling of non-continuous pharmacologic endpoints, such as categorical data, discrete counts or time-to-event is now feasible. This has greatly enhanced the power and applicability of Pk/Pd modeling and will be particularly useful in drug-related epilepsy research.

Summary and conclusions

Despite a long history of research, the science of truly rational polytherapy is still in its infancy. It is generally believed that combining drugs with different mechanisms of action will give the best chance of improving the anticonvulsant efficacy and/or reducing the number and severity of adverse events. This approach appears logical, but sound experimental evidence is still lacking. Assuming that it is true, it is clear that a detailed knowledge of the mechanisms leading to pharmaco-resistant epilepsy, for which combination therapy is primarily intended, is of crucial importance. Present knowledge of experimental animal models proposed for refractory epilepsy indicates that multiple factors contribute to its emergence. This supports the notion that simultaneously aiming drugs at the different targets is likely to be the most successful way to treat refractory epilepsy. Eventually, combinatorial chemistry may provide agents that combine different anticonvulsant properties in a single molecule. For the present, it is more feasible to combine selectively acting drugs. Exploration of mechanism-based mathematical interaction models may help to improve our understanding of drug interactions and to identify the most synergistic (or antagonistic) combinations. Theory predicts that the translation of receptor activation into pharmacologic response is as important as the drug-receptor interaction itself.

Remarkably, drugs with moderate efficacy are predicted to produce more synergism (or antagonism) than drugs with high efficacy. Results of theoretical interaction studies can be elegantly visualized by constructing three-dimensional plots of the concentration–response surface. A plot of the difference between the interaction model and a reference model immediately identifies the concentration regions of synergism and antagonism. These theoretical predictions may be used to design experiments confined to the most interesting concentration regions, which will considerably reduce the amount of experimental work. Combinations need to be tested after acute and chronic dosing in vivo in experimental models faithfully reflecting refractory epilepsy, in order to account for altered drug responses in the epileptic brain. In addition, a careful study of the pharmacokinetics is an indispensable element in studies on drug combinations to account for pharmacokinetic interactions and epilepsy-induced changes in pharmacokinetics. It is advantageous if the anticonvulsant effect can be measured repeatedly in the same animal, because this makes it possible to establish concentration–effect relations in an efficient way. Integrated PK/PD modeling and population modeling provide the best tools to quantify pharmacodynamic interactions.

More and better experimental models of refractory epilepsy are needed. In nearly all the presently available models, epilepsy is induced in essentially healthy animals. The search for combinations should also be applied to minimize side effects and should include complementary studies in vitro. It is believed that a thorough understanding of the mechanisms of epileptogenesis and ictogenesis will pave the way for development of effective drug combinations. Such combinations may contain even more than two agents.

REFERENCES

Aronica E, Yankaya B, Troost D, *et al.* Induction of neonatal sodium channel II and III alpha-isoform mRNAs in neurons and microglia after status epilepticus in the rat hippocampus. *Eur J Neurosci* 2001; **13**: 1261–1266.

Barton ME, Klein BD, Wolf HH, *et al.* Pharmacological characterization of the 6 Hz psychomotor seizure model of partial epilepsy. *Epilepsy Res* 2001; **47**: 217–227.

Berenbaum MC. What is synergy? *Pharmacol Rev* 1989; **41**: 93–141.

Black JW, Leff P. Operational models of pharmacological agonism. *Proc Royal Soc Lond* 1983; **B 220**: 141–162.

Cleton A, Voskuyl RA, Danhof M. Adaptive changes in the pharmacodynamics of midazolam in different experimental models of epilepsy: kindling, cortical stimulation and genetic absence epilepsy. *Br J Pharmacol* 1998; **125**: 615–620.

Cleton A, Mazee D, Voskuyl RA, *et al.* Rate of change of blood concentrations is a major determinant of the pharmacodynamics of midazolam in rats. *Br J Pharmacol* 1999a; **127**: 227–235.

Cleton A, Van der Graaf PH, Ghijsen W, *et al.* Mechanism-based modeling of adaptive changes in the pharmacodynamics of midazolam in the kindling model of epilepsy. *Pharm Res* 1999b; **16**: 1702–1709.

Cleton A, Altorf BA, Voskuyl RA, *et al.* Effect of amygdala kindling on the central nervous system effects of tiagabine: EEG effects *versus* brain GABA levels. *Br J Pharmacol* 2000a; **130**: 1037–1044.

Cleton A, Altorf BA, Voskuyl RA, *et al.* Pharmacokinetic-pharmacodynamic modelling of tiagabine CNS effects upon chronic treatment in rats: lack of change in concentration–EEG effect relationship. *Eur J Pharm Sci* 2000b; **12**: 141–150.

Cleton A, Ödman J, Van der Graaf PH, *et al.* Mechanism-based modeling of functional adaptation upon chronic treatment with midazolam. *Pharm Res* 2000c; **17**: 321–327.

Cortez MA, McKerlie C, Snead III OC. A model of atypical absence seizures. EEG, pharmacology, and developmental characterization. *Neurology* 2001; **56**: 341–349.

Coulter DA, McIntyre DC, Löscher W. Animal models of limbic epilepsies: what can they tell us? *Brain Pathol* 2002; **12**: 240–256.

Cramer S, Ebert U, Löscher W. Characterization of phenytoin-resistant kindled rats, a new model of drug-resistant partial epilepsy: comparison of inbred strains. *Epilepsia* 1998; **39**(10): 1046–1053.

Della Paschoa OE, Kruk MR, Hamstra R, *et al.* Seizure patterns in kindling and cortical stimulation models of experimental epilepsy. *Brain Res* 1997; **770**: 221–227.

Della Paschoa OE, Kruk MR, Hamstra R, *et al.* Pharmacodynamic interaction between phenytoin and sodium valproate changes seizure thresholds and pattern. *Br J Pharmacol* 1998a; **125**: 997–1004.

Della Paschoa OE, Kruk MR, Hamstra R, *et al.* Effects of repeated seizure induction on seizure activity, post-ictal and interictal behavior. *Brain Res* 1998b; **814**: 199–208.

Glien M, Brandt C, Potschka H, *et al.* Effects of the novel antiepileptic drug levetiracetam on spontaneous recurrent seizures in the rat pilocarpine model of temporal lobe epilepsy. *Epilepsia* 2002; **43**: 350–357.

Gorter JA, van Vliet EA, Aronica E, *et al.* Progression of spontaneous seizures after status epilepticus is associated with mossy fibre sprouting and extensive bilateral loss of hilar parvalbumin and somatostatin-immunoreactive neurons. *Eur J Neurosci* 2001; **13**: 657–669.

Greco WR, Bravo G, Parsons JC. The search for synergy: a critical review from a response surface perspective. *Pharmacol Rev* 1995; **47**: 331–385.

Holford NHG, Peck CC. Population pharmacodynamics and drug development. In *The In Vivo Study of Drug Action.* C. J. van Boxtel, N. H. G. Holford, M. Danhof, eds. Amsterdam: Elsevier Science Publishers B.V. 1992: 401–413.

Hoogerkamp A, Vis PW, Danhof M, *et al.* Characterization of the pharmacodynamics of several antiepileptic drugs in a direct cortical stimulation model of anti-convulsant effect in the rat. *J Pharmacol Exp Ther* 1994; **269**: 521–528.

Jonker DM, von de Mheen C, Eilers PH, *et al.* Anticonvulsant drugs differentially suppress individual vital signs: a pharmacokinetic/pharmacodynamic analysis in the cortical stimulation model in the rat. *Beh Neurosis* 2003; **117**: 1075–1085.

Jonker DM, Voskuyl RA, Danhof M. Pharmacodynamic analysis of the anticonvulsant effects of tiagabine and lamotrigine in combination in the rat. Epilepsy 2004; **45**: 424–435.

Jonker DM, Visser SAG, Von der Groof PH, *et al.* Towards a mechanism-based analysis of pharmocodynamic clrug-drug-interventions. Pharm Ther 2005 (In press).

Kapur J, Macdonald RL. Rapid seizure-induced reduction of benzodiazepine and Zn^{2+} sensitivity of hippocampal dentate granule cell $GABA_A$ receptors. *J Neurosci* 1997; **17**: 7532–7540.

Ketelaars SO, Gorter JA, van Vliet EA, *et al.* Sodium currents in isolated rat CA1 pyramidal and dentate granule neurones in the post-status epilepticus model of epilepsy. *Neuroscience* 2001; **105**: 109–120.

Leite JP, Cavalheiro EA. Effects of conventional antiepileptic drugs in a model of spontaneous recurrent seizures in rats. *Epilepsy Res* 1995; **20**: 93–104.

Lesko LJ, Rowland M, Peck CC. Optimizing the science of drug development: opportunities for better candidate selection and accelerated evaluations in humans. *Pharm Res* 2001; **17**: 1335–1344.

Liu H, Mazarati AM, Katsumori H, *et al.* Substance P is expressed in hippocampal principal neurons during status epilepticus and plays a critical role in the maintenance of status epilepticus. *Proc Natl Acad Sci USA* 1999; **96**: 5286–5291.

Löscher W. Animal models of intractable epilepsy. *Prog Neurobiol* 1997; **53**: 239–258.

Löscher W. Current status and future directions in the pharmacotherapy of epilepsy. *Trends Pharmacol Sci* 2002; **23**: 113–118.

Löscher W, Ebert U. Basic mechanisms of seizure propagation: targets for rational drug design and rational polypharmacy. In *Rational Polypharmacy*. Elsevier Science B.V. 1996: 17–43.

Löscher W, Schmidt D. Strategies in antiepileptic drug development: is rational drug design superior to random screening and structural variation? *Epilepsy Res* 1994; **17**: 95–134.

Löscher W, Rundfeldt C, Hönack D. Pharmacological characterization of phenytoin-resistant amygdala-kindled rats, a new model of drug-resistant partial epilepsy. *Epilepsy Res* 1993; **15**: 207–219.

Löscher W, Cramer S, Ebert U. Selection of phenytoin responders and nonresponders in male and female amygdala-kindled Sprague–Dawley rats. *Epilepsia* 1998; **39**: 1138–1147.

Lothman EW, Bertram EH, Bekenstein JW, *et al*. Self-sustaining limbic status epilepticus induced by "continuous" hippocampal stimulation: electrographic and behavioral characteristics. *Epilepsy Res* 1989; **3**: 107–119.

Mandema JW, Kuck MT, Danhof M. Differences in intrinsic efficacy of benzodiazepines are reflected in their concentration–EEG effect relationship. *Br J Pharmacol* 1992; **105**: 164–170.

Mazarati AM, Baldwin RA, Sankar R, *et al*. Time-dependent decrease in the effectiveness of antiepileptic drugs during the course of self-sustaining status epilepticus. *Brain Res* 1998a; **814**: 179–185.

Mazarati AM, Liu H, Soomets U, *et al*. Galanin modulation of seizures and seizure modulation of hippocampal galanin in animal models of status epilepticus. *J Neurosci* 1998b; **18**: 10070–10077.

Minto CF, Schnider TW, Short TG, *et al*. Response surface model for anesthetic drug interactions. *Anesthesiology* 2000; **92**: 1603–1616.

Mody I. Synaptic plasticity in kindling. In *Jasper's Basic Mechanisms of the Epilepsies, Third Edition: Advances in Neurology* A. V. Delgado-Escueta, W. A. Wilson, R. W. Olsen, R. A. Porter, eds. Philadelphia: Lippincott Williams & Wilkins, 1999; **79**: 631–644.

Morrisett RA, Jope RS, Snead III OC. Effects of drugs on the initiation and maintenance of status epilepticus induced by administration of pilocarpine to lithium-pretreated rats. *Exp Neurol* 1987; **97**: 193–200.

Nissinen J, Halonen T, Koivisto E, *et al*. A new model of chronic temporal lobe epilepsy induced by electrical stimulation of the amygdala in rat. *Epilepsy Res* 2000; **38**: 177–205.

Nissinen J, Lange CH, Stratton SC, *et al*. Effect of lamotrigine treatment on epileptogenesis: an experimental study in rat. *Epilepsy Res* 2004; **58**: 119–132.

Ouellet D, Bockbrader HN, Wesche DL, *et al*. Population pharmacokinetics of gabapentin in infants and children. *Epilepsy Res* 2001; **47**: 229–241.

Peters GJ, van der Wilt CL, van Moorsel CJ, *et al*. Basis for effective combination cancer chemotherapy with antimetabolites. *Pharmacol Ther* 2000; **87**: 227–253.

Pitkänen A, Nissinen J, Jolkkonen E, *et al*. Effects of vigabatrin treatment on status epilepticus-induced neuronal damage and mossy fiber sprouting in the rat hippocampus. *Epilepsy Res* 1999; **33**: 67–85.

Pöch G, Holzmann S. Quantitative estimation of overadditive and underadditive drug effects by means of theoretical, additive dose-response curves. *J Pharmacol Meth* 1980; **4**: 179–188.

Regesta G, Tanganelli P. Clinical aspects and biological bases of drug-resistant epilepsies. *Epilepsy Res* 1999; **34**: 109–122.

Remy S, Gabriel S, Urban BW, *et al.* A novel mechanism underlying drug resistance in chronic epilepsy. *Ann Neurol* 2003; **53**: 469–679.

Reutens DC, Berkovic SF. Idiopathic generalized epilepsy of adolescence: are the syndromes clinically distinct? *Neurology* 1995; **45**: 1469–1476.

Reynolds EH, Elwes RDC, Shorvon SD. Why does epilepsy become intractable? *Lancet* 1983; **ii**: 952–954.

Rice AC, DeLorenzo RJ. N-methyl-D-aspartate receptor activation regulates refractoriness of status epilepticus to diazepam. *Neuroscience* 1999; **93**: 117–123.

Sheiner LB, Steimer J-L. Pharmacokinetic/pharmacodynamic modelling in drug development. *Ann Rev Pharmacol Toxicol* 2000; **40**: 67–96.

Shirasaka Y, Wasterlain CG. Chronic epileptogenicity following focal status epilepticus. *Brain Res* 1994; **655**: 33–44.

Sillanpää M. Epidemiology of intractable epilepsy in children. In *Intractable Epilepsy*. S. I. Johannessen, L. Gram, M. Sillanpää, T. Tomson, eds. Petersfield: Wrightson Biomedical Publishing, 1995: 13–25.

Sperk G. Kainic acid seizures in the rat. *Prog Neurobiol* 1994; **42**: 1–32.

Stables JP, Bertram EH, White HJ, *et al.* Models for epilepsy and epileptogenesis: report from the NIH workshop. Bethesda, Maryland. *Epilepsy* 2002; **43**: 1410–1420.

Turski L, Ikonomidou C, Turski WA, *et al.* Review: cholinergic mechanisms and epileptogenesis. The seizures induced by pilocarpine: a novel experimental model of intractable epilepsy. *Synapse* 1989; **3**: 154–171.

Voskuyl RA, Dingemanse J, Danhof M. Determination of the threshold for convulsions by direct cortical stimulation. *Epilepsy Res* 1989; **3**: 120–129.

Voskuyl RA, Hoogerkamp A, Danhof M. Properties of the convulsive threshold determined by direct cortical stimulation in rats. *Epilepsy Res* 1992; **12**: 111–120.

Vreugdenhil M, Wadman WJ. Modulation of sodium currents in rat CA1 neurons by carbamazepine and valproate after kindling epileptogenesis. *Epilepsia* 1999; **40**: 1512–1522.

25

Future research: a clinical perspective

Carlos A. Fontes Ribeiro

Department of Pharmacology, Faculty of Medicine, University of Coimbra, Coimbra, Portugal

Introduction

Although the best standard guideline for the treatment of epilepsy is to treat patients with monotherapy antiepileptic drugs (AEDs) first, the use of AEDs in combination to treat patients with intractable epilepsy is a long-standing clinical practice. The concept of monotherapy is relatively new, having its origin in the mid-1970s (Leppik, 2000). Monotherapy implies the use of a single active entity and its advantages are recognized. These include avoidance of drug–drug interactions, enhancement of compliance and the reduction of adverse effects. But is this true? What is the benefit/risk ratio of polypharmacy compared with monotherapy? Are all the combinations of AEDs useful and/or equally useful? What doses of AEDs in polypharmacy and in monotherapy must be compared?

With our enhanced understanding of the mechanisms of ictal events and mechanisms of action of the traditional and new (second generation) AEDs, as well as the licensing of new AEDs having a variety of mechanisms for antiepileptic action, the concept of 'rational polypharmacy' (RP) has been developed (Homan, 1997). Although it may appear as a paradox, the goals of RP are to minimize total AEDs used, to personalize antiepileptic treatment, to develop more specific targets for therapy and to maximize the therapeutic index. Therefore, the heart of RP is the use of two (and only occasionally more than two) agents to give better seizure control with the lowest dose of each AED and with minimal adverse effects.

Patients with difficult to control epilepsy have traditionally received multiple AEDs in what is essentially random polypharmacy (Homan, 1997). The intent was to develop synergistic therapeutic effects. However, in the majority of cases, although additive efficacy was observed, adverse effects were also significantly potentiated. Consequently, the use of inappropriate drug combinations has long been and remains a problem. RP advocates the use of AEDs with different mechanisms of action and/or appropriate pharmacokinetic properties; however, as to whether this approach is associated with an enhanced risk/benefit ratio compared to monotherapy is unknown.

The inappropriate application of drug combinations has been frequently coupled with inadequate recognition or understanding of epileptic syndromes (Homan, 1997). An individual patient's epilepsy may be treated as a mixed epileptic condition rather than as a single epileptic syndrome with multiple seizure types (Homan, 1997). Is combination of different AEDs necessary to treat different seizure type and epileptic syndromes? With the improvement in the definition of epileptic syndromes, is there stronger indication for RP? What is the timing and target population of RP? What data are needed to develop RP for a specific patient?

Many of the answers to these questions are proposals for future clinical research. Thus, there are two broad lines of research: one is linked to the development of the so-called 'rational antiepileptic polypharmacy', and the other to the study of adverse events induced by drug interactions or combinations.

The development of RP can be supported by an improved definition of epileptic syndromes. Since knowledge about the initiation of the seizure, spread of the ictal activity and arrest of the seizure has been increasing, there are new opportunities to design RP in a single drug (with multiple mechanisms) and/or to design 'curative' antiepileptogenic drugs. Of course, all of these ideas and projects must be tested through clinical studies. Even the accepted combinations of AEDs must be tested through well-designed clinical trials. Another avenue which can be of value in AED combinations is the study of the quality of life and of compliance.

The other past, present and future line of research is related to the risk of drug combinations or interactions. Pharmacovigilance is obligatory and must be improved for the study of drug interactions. Another item related to the safe use of drugs is the development of pharmacogenomics with the possibility of choosing the bespoke AED. Finally, it is important to verify whether or not the serum therapeutic ranges, described for antiepileptic monotherapy, are similar to those necessary during the rational combination of AEDs.

Improved definition of epileptic syndromes: recent and promising tools to study combinations of AEDs

Pharmacological management of epilepsy has targeted only symptoms (i.e. seizures) and not the disease (i.e. epilepsy), and it has been limited to containment of seizure propagation without attention to initiation or rates and routes of the spread of seizure activity (Löscher and Ebert, 1996). There is some evidence indicating that some generalized seizures in children may be exacerbated by carbamazepine (Snead and Hosey, 1985), myoclonic seizures worsened by vigabatrin and juvenile myoclonic epilepsy aggravated by phenytoin, carbamazepine or gabapentin (Leppik, 2000). Therefore, the diagnosis of the epileptic syndrome is useful and when possible must be obtained.

The goal of developing more specific targets for RP includes treatment of the onset of seizures (ictogenesis) and of the onset and maintenance of epilepsy (epileptogenesis) (Lothman, 1996).

Other advances can be obtained through the use of animal models of epilepsy, namely genetic models which are a source that is yet to be optimally used and has the potential to allow evaluation of AEDs, not only for anti-ictal potential but also for antiepileptogenic potential (Homan, 1997). This can be associated with the more classical animal models to study AEDs. Debate over an appropriate model to study polypharmacy continues (Homan, 1997) and must be one of the goals for future research.

Another technique is computer modelling, which may provide the means to develop potential drug combinations. This approach is most relevant to predict rational drug combinations at the pharmacodynamic level (Homan, 1997). Of course, well-designed clinical trials with such suggested drug combinations must always be performed.

In addition to the significant contribution to epilepsy treatment by localizing epileptic foci for surgical excision, functional neuroimaging (e.g. positron emission tomography, PET; single photon emission computed tomography, SPECT) may also contribute by refining the definition of epilepsy (for instance, to demonstrate different epileptic syndromes with the same seizure type).

Probably of still greater potential value are studies designed to define receptor sites. These offer the possibility of refinement diagnosis and, therefore, pharmacological management. Some neurotransmitter systems have been studied, such as the benzodiazepine and the opioid receptors, since there is evidence for their involvement in epilepsy. The opioid receptors appear to be related to seizure termination (Theodore, 1990).

Functional neuroimaging using receptor ligands could give information regarding ictal onset, propagation and containment (Homan, 1997), and could be used to formulate a rational plan for pharmacological management. This would be another area for future research.

Almost all the available drugs have been extensively evaluated for simple and complex partial seizures. Many double blind, placebo-controlled clinical trials are available for the second generation AEDs; initial efficacy studies were done as adjunct therapy with one or two marketed AEDs. The first generation AEDs did not undergo such rigorous testing. The effect of drugs on syndromes of primarily generalized epilepsies have not been studied as extensively, and surely these studies must be developed in the near future.

Initiation of the seizure, spread of the ictal activity and arrest of the seizure

During the past two decades, our knowledge of the mechanisms of seizures has greatly expanded. Distinct events occur during a seizure: initiation of the seizure, spread of the ictal activity and arrest of the seizure. Different mechanisms support these steps (Leppik, 2000), since sodium conductance initiates and maintains the ictal activity, calcium conductance initiates and maintains seizure activity and also contributes to neuronal injury, and potassium conductance is essential in the arrest of a seizure discharge. The principal neurotransmitters involved are the inhibitory gamma amino butyric acid (GABA) neurotransmitter and the excitatory glutamate neurotransmitter.

Since AEDs show distinct profiles regarding these different ion conductances, their combination may be rational. Therefore, it is reasonable that a seizure may be suppressed in its initiation by one drug, another may be more effective in limiting its propagation and a third may enhance the probability of its arrest. In addition, other drugs may need to be developed to shorten the post-ictal state or to limit the neuronal damage caused by the seizures. Thus, sodium conductances are modified by phenytoin, carbamazepine, primidone, valproate, lamotrigine, oxcarbazepine and zonisamide, although some of these drugs have other actions as well; calcium conductance (T-calcium channels) may be modified by ethosuximide and valproate; GABA-mediated chloride conductance may be reinforced by vigabatrin, tiagabine, gabapentin and barbiturates; N-methyl-D-aspartate (NMDA) receptors are affected by topiramate (Table 25.1). Although an AED might have many mechanisms of action, only a few are relevant for the antiepileptic effect. In general, it can concluded that the traditional AEDs act via an action on cation currents, whereas the more recent AEDs reinforce the GABA and/or inhibit the glutamatergic systems.

Based on this knowledge, some AED combinations may be proposed, whereas other might be avoided (Table 25.2). However, this apparent RP must be tested through controlled randomized clinical trials, double blind, and with correct sample size, inclusion and exclusion patient criteria, time of treatment and statistical analysis (including per protocol and intention-to-treat analyses, and characterization of dropouts). This area for research is substantial.

Designing RP in a single drug (with multiple mechanisms)

Many studies suggest that multiple neurotransmitters and subtypes of their receptors are involved in the abnormal neuronal excitability that underlies some models of the epilepsies. For instance, the glutamatergic system (NMDA and non-NMDA mechanisms) may have an important role in excitability, whereas the GABAergic system may play a role in decreasing the epileptiform activity. The RP may use several drugs with a different pharmacodynamic profile or, better, may use a single drug

Table 25.1 AEDs and their mechanisms of action

Blockade of the Na^+ current	Phenytoin, primidone, carbamazepine, valproate, oxcarbazepine, lamotrigine, gabapentin, topiramate, zonisamide
Inhibition of L- and N-Ca^{++} currents	Phenobarbital, phenytoin, gabapentin carbamazepine (weakly), lamotrigine, topiramate
Inhibition of T-Ca^{++} current	Ethosuximide, valproate, zonisamide
Enhancement of GABA-evoked Cl^- current	Phenobarbital, topiramate (all AEDs that increase brain GABA)
Antagonism of AMPA receptor subtype	Phenobarbital, topiramate
Blockade of NMDA responses	Phenytoin, carbamazepine, oxcarbazepine, topiramate
Increase of brain GABA	Phenytoin, valproate, gabapentin, lamotrigine, tiagabine, topiramate, vigabatrin
Decreased glutamate release	Lamotrigine
Antagonism of adenosine receptors	Carbamazepine
Increase of 5-HT release	Carbamazepine, gabapentin

Adapted from Macdonald (1997) and Moshé (2000).
5-HT: 5-hydroxytryptamine.

Table 25.2 Combinations based on the mechanisms of action of AEDs

Most useful (due to widely different mechanisms of action): Carbamazepine or phenytoin with gabapentin, tiagabine and topiramate

Least useful (similar mechanisms of action): Carbamazepine and phenytoin; tiagabine, gabapentin and vigabatrin

with affinity for multiple systems. Therefore, the possibility exists that a drug with affinity for multiple receptors or systems (e.g. inhibiting the glutamatergic system and reinforcing the GABAergic system) may have a considerable efficacy. In addition, if the efficacy for the multiple receptors is low, then the compound may show low toxicity (Sankar and Weaver, 1997) compounds with a high affinity and potency may carry unacceptable toxicity (e.g. sedation when the GABA system is strongly activated). Topiramate, an AED with a broad antiepileptic activity, has at least six mechanisms of action (Table 25.1) and, therefore, may show high efficacy. However, these hypothesis must be confirmed by randomized, controlled clinical trials.

Designing 'curative' antiepileptogenic drugs

The drugs currently available for treating epilepsy are little more than symptomatic agents (Sankar and Weaver, 1997), failing to stop the fundamental pathologic process that initially causes and maintains the susceptibility to seizures. Two important concepts are ictogenesis and epileptogenesis. Ictogenesis is the initiation and propagation of a seizure (in time and space), occurring within seconds or minutes and being a rapid electrical/chemical event, whereas epileptogenesis is the gradual process (occurring through a period of months or years), whereby normal brain is transformed into a state susceptible to spontaneous and recurrent seizures (through the initiation and maturation of an epileptogenic focus) (Sankar and Weaver, 1997).

If the chemistries of these two processes are different, their treatment may also be different, by use of different drugs or a single drug with different mechanisms. To treat ictogenesis, it is necessary to control the opening of Na^+ channels (which underlies brain electrical discharges) and the subsequent involvement of K^+ channels and the Na^+/K^+-ATPase pump, often associated with neurotransmitter systems; since the electrical activity passes from neuron to neuron via the Ca^{++} channel-mediated release of neurotransmitters, these channels represent another process to control. Thus, ictogenesis may be inhibited through the blockade of ion channels involved in depolarization, antagonism of excitatory neurotransmitter and/or activation of inhibitory neurotransmitter systems (Sankar and Weaver, 1997).

The fundamental disturbance that yields epileptogenesis seems to represent a combined, concurrent imbalance of an excessive excitation and a weak inhibition (Sankar and Weaver, 1997). Although glutamatergic and GABAergic processes are leading candidates, some studies (Ernfors *et al.*, 1991) suggest other factors such as the nerve growth factor (NGF), whose production is enhanced in the limbic system of animal models (with the experimental form of epileptogenesis known as kindling). The fact that the intracerebroventricular injection of antibodies to NGF delays the onset of kindled seizures (Fundabashi *et al.*, 1988) seems to confirm the role of this protein. The future design of antiepileptogenic compounds must identify the full range of target molecules (NMDA antagonists, GABA agonists, NGF antagonists and others).

Clinical studies to test combinations of AEDs

Studies designed to test efficacy (and safety) of drug combinations can be observational or experimental (Waning and Montagne, 2001). Investigators in observational studies may plan and identify variables to be measured, but human intervention is not a part of the process. Experimental studies, in contrast, involve intervention in ongoing processes to study any resulting change or difference; they are clinical trials and intervention studies designed to compare outcomes between two or more treatment or intervention groups.

Observational study designs include case reports, cross-sectional studies, case–control studies and cohort studies. A case report is a descriptive study of a single patient, and a case series is a collection of case reports; a cross-sectional study is a prevalence study, examining relationships between a drug use (or interaction) problem and other characteristics of people in a population at one point in time; a case–control study compares people who have the disease or problem or drug interaction (cases) to those who do not have (controls) with respect to characteristics of interest (i.e. potential causes); a cohort study is an incidence study that measures characteristics free of drug problem and relates them to subsequent development of the disease or event in that population as it is followed over time (a longitudinal study).

The majority of studies on AED combinations (random or RP) have been observational, although there are a few cohort studies. These studies are less expensive than the experimental ones and the ethical concerns are less. However, the results obtained are weak and, therefore, there is a need to undertake experimental studies in order to provide sound scientific evidence upon which recommendation of RP can be based.

An experimental study is designed to compare benefits of an intervention with a standard treatment, or no treatment, to show cause and effect. This type of study is performed prospectively. Both study groups (the experimental group receives the drug under investigation; the control group receives the traditional or approved treatment or no treatment or placebo) are studied over the same time period using the same measures of safety and efficacy/effectiveness. The gold standard of an experimental clinical study is the randomized, controlled trial (RCT). RCTs are in general studies of Phase III, performed to submit an application of the AED to the European Agency for the Evaluation of Medicinal Products (EMEA), Food and Drug Administration (FDA) or any national drug agency. It must be emphasized that almost all the studies with new AEDs are add-on studies – all the epileptic patients are treated with a standard AED and then they are randomized to placebo or the new AED (crossover or parallel-group add-on RCT design). The efficacy and the risk of the added active drug or of the placebo can then be calculated and compared. This type of design hardly characterizes the new drug and now study designs are being proposed (Loiseau and Jallon, 2001) (e.g. therapeutic failure design trials, attenuated active-control designs, presurgical withdrawal designs).

A supplemental new drug application is submitted when a drug's sponsor requests approval to promote an existing drug with either a new indication or new labeling (for instance, when two AEDs were used in combination in clinical trials and the sponsor wants the reference to this in the summary product characteristics (SPC), or when there are reports of adverse reactions with some drug combinations and the sponsor is obliged to refer this in the SPC).

Although Phase III clinical trials are the gold standard for demonstrating treatment efficacy, pitfalls can include the selected nature of the subjects, the small number of subjects included, the usually brief follow-up period and the missing intention-to-treat analysis (without characterization of the dropouts). Some of these deficiencies may be addressed by a Phase IV clinical trial, usually called a post-marketing study. This type of trial may establish the effectiveness of the combination of drugs, in the routine setting or in some subgroups of patients. Included in these Phase IV trials are the large, simple trials (LSTs) (Lesko and Mitchell, 2001), which can be designed in order to study AED combinations.

LSTs may be the best solution when it is not possible to completely control confounding by means other than randomization. This approach has also been used successfully to evaluate the risk of adverse drug effects when the more common observational designs have been judged inadequate. These studies are really just very large randomized trials made simple by reducing data collection to the minimum needed to test only a single hypothesis (or at most a few hypotheses). Randomization of treatment assignment is the key feature of the design, which controls for confounding by known and unknown factors. The large study size provides for AED combinations the power needed to evaluate small risks, either absolute or relative, and small differences in effectiveness.

The combination of AEDs will only be considered acceptable if the proposed combination is based on valid therapeutic principles. For this, it can be adopted from the guideline CPMP/EWP/240/95 of the CPMP (Committee for Proprietary Medicinal Products) and of the EMEA, although this guideline had been developed for fixed drug combinations. It is necessary to assess the potential advantages in the clinical situation against possible disadvantages, in order to determine whether the combination meets the requirements with respect to efficacy and safety.

Potential advantages of AED combinations include an improvement of the risk/benefit assessment due to:

(a) addition or potentiation of the therapeutic activities of the two drugs, which results in a level of efficacy similar to the one achievable by each active drug used alone at higher doses than in combination, but associated with a better safety profile, or a level of efficacy above the one achievable by a single drug with an acceptable safety profile;

(b) the counteracting by one drug of an adverse reaction produced by another drug.

Disadvantages of combinations of AEDs include the addition of the different adverse reactions specific to each substance.

Adverse reactions are of two principal types: Type A reactions, which will occur in everyone if adequate amount of the drug is given, because they are due to excess of normal, predicable, dose-related, pharmacodynamic effects. Type B reactions are those that will occur only in some people. They are not dose-related and are due to unusual attributes of the patient interacting with the drug. This class of adverse effects includes unwanted effects due to inherited abnormalities (idiosyncrasy) (differences in pharmacogenetics) and/or immunological processes (drug allergy).

Three subordinate adverse reaction types can also be recognized: Type C reactions due to long-term use (for instance, hyponatremia with carbamazepine or oxcarbazepine, behaviour changes with the majority of the AEDs, weight changes with many AEDs). Type D effects, for example teratogenesis, carcinogenesis (with the majority of AEDs, but particularly with valproic acid and phenytoin – do these adverse effects increase with the combination of drugs, in comparison with monotherapy?). Type E reactions, where discontinuation is too abrupt (increased seizures due to interruption of medication – what happens with polypharmacy when one of the drugs is stopped?). Of course, AED combinations may increase Type B and in certain circumstances Type A reactions. The latter may occur when drugs act through the same mechanism and their sum at the sites of action exceeds the maximal dose of one of them at that site. However, as one of the objectives of RP is to use moderate doses of two or more AEDs, Type A adverse reactions should be avoided but with and increasing efficacy.

Another Type A adverse reaction comprises a failure in increasing efficacy and an increase in the number and severity of seizures. This type of reaction can happen with the prescription of different drug formulations, principally due to the increasing number of generic preparations. The resulting variation in steady-state plasma levels, after substitution of one preparation for another may cause gradual loss of seizure control or the gradual development of drug intoxication. Thus, studies of bioequivalence between generics and reference drugs are necessary and they must be a priority for patients, physicians and national regulatory authorities.

Two main objectives in AED combination therapy that could be researched are as follows:

(a) *Pharmacodynamic objectives*: Frequently, the addition or the potentiation of the pharmacodynamic effects of drugs may constitute the rationale of the AED combination. In this case, several dose combinations for each drug might have to be tested and the concentration–response information can help to select the combination leading to a satisfactory response.

(b) *Pharmacokinetic objectives*: In general, it must be demonstrated that the various drugs do not affect each other's respective pharmacokinetic patterns. These interactions should be studied primarily in healthy volunteers; however, patients should also be studied if the disease modifies the pharmacokinetics of a drug or if high-risk subgroup is to be prescribed the drug combination (elderly, patients with renal failure or hepatic impairment).

Table 25.3 Rational AED combinations

Primary generalized epilepsies	*Localization-related epilepsies*
Valproate and propranolol	Carbamazepine or phenytoin and intermittent clobazam
Valproate and ethosuximide	Carbamazepine or phenytoin and valproate
Valproate and phenytoin or primidone	Carbamazepine or phenytoin and gabapentin
	Carbamazepine or phenytoin and lamotrigine
	Lamotrigine and vigabatrin

Adapted from Homan (1997).

Confirmatory clinical trials are necessary to prove efficacy, preferably by parallel or crossover group comparisons in which the combination is compared to its individual (multilevel factorial design). Inclusion of a placebo group is recommended when feasible, but in patients with epilepsy there are concerns about the use of placebo. However, there are now new trial designs which have been specifically designed to overcome this problem.

In some cases, studies have to be specifically designed to determine the minimal effective dose and usual effective dose of the combination. Multiple dose-effect studies may be required.

Although there are some examples of RP (Table 25.3), these combinations have not been tested in rigorous factorial clinical trials; instead their use is based on anecdotal evidence. In factorial trials the combination of active drugs must be compared with each one. This type of clinical trial has been used to study antihypertensive drugs and could be applied for the studies of AEDs. However, one problem with these studies is that of choosing the dose of each drug to be studied.

Safety aspects

In the case of combinations of AEDs, which are for long-term use, safety data on 300–600 patients for 6 months or longer will be required. Where there are grounds to expect that the combination of AEDs may be substantially more harmful or give rise to much more frequent adverse effects than any individual substances given alone, evidence should be obtained that this does not occur in therapeutic use, or that the advantages of the combination, for example increased efficacy, outweigh such disadvantages.

One of the major problems related to clinical research is the non-publication of trials with negative findings, thus enhancing the risk of bias from omitted research. The communication of these trials must be obligatory, in order to develop potent and useful databases.

Quality of life and RP

Assessing the impact of health care interventions is increasingly shifting from biologic and physician-determined parameters to patient-focused parameters. Although they can be more difficult to quantify, patient-cantered outcomes, such as functional status, life satisfaction and health-related quality of life (HRQOL), are often more clinically relevant.

Fundamental dimensions essential to HRQOL have been proposed and include physical, psychological and social functioning, role activities, overall life satisfaction and perceptions of health status (Berzon *et al.*, 1993; Williams, 2001).

Once the decision to assess patients' HRQOL has been made, an investigator must choose which type of HRQOL assessment is most likely to help for answering the research question. Of course, all the instruments used must show validity and reliability. As no standard measure exists, responsiveness is often measured in several ways; most of the statistics involve dividing change in scores by some indicator of the precision of measurement. General guidelines for interpreting HRQOL data in RCTs have been suggested (Guyatt *et al.*, 1997). Important issues addressed (Williams, 2001) are:

1 how to assess the validity of the HRQOL measures used;
2 whether the HRQOL measures performed as expected;
3 how to evaluate the magnitude of effect on HRQOL outcomes;
4 how to translate HRQOL data from an RCT to daily clinical practice.

Compliance

The process of taking medications as prescribed can be an extremely difficult task during AED polypharmacy, particularly in old age. The complexity of the polypharmacy can be further complicated by cognitive abnormalities, poor vision, motor disturbances and adverse reactions.

The patient's compliance in adhering to drug combinations must be studied and enhanced. Questions that need answering in this regard include: at what time of the day must an AED be ingested? Should AEDs be administered together or should they be separated by a specific time interval? These questions might be best answered by first attaining the optimal dose for each patient and then the best regimen of administration studied and used.

Pharmacovigilance

AEDs, either in monotherapy or in polytherapy, can only be useful if there is scientific evidence of relevant efficacy and a low risk of adverse effects. This risk/benefit ratio is established through pre-marketing and post-marketing drug surveillance. Therefore, drug surveillance or pharmacovigilance is applied to drug interactions or to AED combinations. Regarding AEDs, interactions can happen between each other or between AEDs and other drugs or substances, such as food.

The consequences of these drug interactions can be lower efficacy and/or lower safety, both of concern and a reason for pharmacovigilance. Concerning AEDs, less efficacy resulting from AED interactions must be classified as an adverse drug reaction, and thus it must be subjected to pharmacovigilance.

AEDs can also adversely affect the course of a concomitant medical condition; alternatively, drugs used to treat a medical condition can at times exacerbate epilepsy. Carbamazepine occasionally precipitates arrhythmias in patients with cardiac conduction system disease (Scheuer, 1997). Theophylline can lower seizure threshold in susceptible persons and psychotropic agents also occasionally precipitate seizures (Scheuer, 1997).

Taking into account the pre-clinical studies and clinical trials, either of Phases I, II or III, some drug interactions, at the pharmacokinetic or pharmacodynamic level, are expected. Of course these interactions are fundamental to establish the risk/benefit ratio and they must be specified in the SPC of the respective AED. But there are other adverse events that can occur after licensing of the AED, since the drug is then used in a clinical setting different from that of clinical trials, where restricted inclusion and exclusion criteria are inevitable. Unexpected or serious adverse reactions may happen, which oblige us to re-evaluate the risk/benefit ratio and to add these reactions to the SPC.

During post-marketing pharmacovigilance the majority of adverse events are spontaneously reported by physicians, pharmacists and – in some countries – nurses. They use, for instance, the yellow card to communicate the adverse event to the national pharmacovigilance system. This is the principal way for pharmacovigilance (to follow the drug in the market), since all drugs and health professionals belong to the system. But other studies may be performed during the post-marketing surveillance, such as observational cohort studies, case–control studies, case surveillance and clinical trials.

For any surveillance study, their following phases are essential:

1 report of the adverse event;
2 validation of the report;
3 establishment of causality between drug and event.

Unexpected or serious adverse events must always be reported; the communication of other adverse events is country dependent. The term adverse event or adverse experience intentionally avoids implying a necessary cause-and-effect relationship between the use of the drug and the event. The term includes adverse events that occur during the use of the drug in professional practice or drug study, during a drug overdose, as a result of drug withdrawal and as a result of the failure of the expected pharmacological action (Greenwood, 2000). Regarding AED interactions, namely with the new drugs, the increase of adverse event frequency or the decrease of efficacy must also be reported, whether or not it is clearly considered to be drug-related.

In the European Union each National Pharmacovigilance System is linked to the EMEA. The section of EMEA for pharmacovigilance is the pharmacovigilance working party, which belongs to the CPMP, a part of EMEA. In addition, each member state and EMEA collaborates with the World Health Organization (WHO) (via the Collaborating Centre for International Drug Monitoring, in Uppsala, Sweden). Therefore, each National Pharmacovigilance System is connected to EMEA and both are connected to the WHO Collaborating Centre.

To characterize an adverse event as an adverse reaction due to the AED there must be the establishment of causality. This can be made by different methods of importability that take into account chronological and semeiological criteria and an extrinsic importability (with the classifying of bibliographic data). The majority of the methods of importability take only one drug into account at a time. The other drug may be 'another explanation', decreasing the power of the causal relationship. The relationship between the adverse event and the drug can be definite, probable, possible, conditional or not related. If two drugs are used simultaneously the causal relationship will be rarely identified; however, if the one drug is taken after the other the causality can be more readily established.

Adverse reactions can be characterized as serious and/or unexpected and, as highlighted earlier, they must be reported to the pharmacovigilance system. However, as far as the combination of drugs is concerned, all the aspects of safety must be studied in order to clarify the risk/benefit ratio of the combination (at lower doses of each drug, for instance) compared with the single drug, either used at a high dose or at a mean dose, and in populations of different age, sex or susceptibility. Pre-existing medical conditions must also be known so as to characterize the target population for drug combinations.

The consequences of the adverse drug reaction assessment are as follows:

- To establish the overall risk/benefit ratio.
- To begin a rapid alert for the scientific community.
- To withdraw or to reduce the use of the medicinal product.
- To complete the SPC.
- To develop pharmacoepidemiology and databases.
- To design other studies to confirm or explain the adverse reaction.
- To design rational AED combinations (an example of a possible AED combination whose individual knowledge indicates less adverse effects is the combination of

valproate (or gabapentin, vigabatrin or carbamazepine) with topiramate, since the first ones induce weight gain and the latter weight loss (Greenwood, 2000)).
• To define the non-epileptic drugs which can be associated with an AED.

In addition, each medicinal product must, of course, have periodic safety update reports, which permits the drug to be reanalyzed.

The lack of uniformity of populations, terminology, methods for collecting data, patient experiences and the absence of formal methods for testing for adverse reactions make comparisons of adverse reactions among studies difficult. In spite of these problems, pharmacovigilance is the best way to characterize the safety of drug combinations, since all the epileptic population may be followed (through the spontaneous reporting system) or some specific groups of epileptic patients (case–control or cohort studies or through the prescription monitoring system). Of course, during the Phase III or IV post-marketing clinical trials, important and useful data are collected but the less frequent adverse reactions can only happen during the extensive use of the combination of drugs in the general patient population. Thus, pharmacovigilance is an integral component of all future research of all health systems.

To overcome the problem of terminology to describe patient reports of adverse experiences or events, the terminology used in the United States (Coding Symbols for a Thesaurus of Adverse Reactions Terms: COSTART) and the World Health Organization's Adverse Reaction Terminology (WHO-ART), used in the European Union, will be replaced with the Medical Dictionary for Regulatory Activities (MedDRA). To accomplish this goal, the International Conference on Harmonization (ICH), an organization made up of representatives of industry associations and regulatory authorities in United States, Europe and Japan, has agreed upon the structure and content of the MedDRA. The descriptive terms used for adverse events are expanded and this source has a hierarchical structure to allow greater specificity (Brown *et al.*, 1999). Thus, the international use of MedDRA will make it easier to compare adverse events when characterizing AEDs and their combinations.

In the future prospective, comparative studies of adverse events will be essential. With a better understanding of the circumstances in which each adverse effect occurs, we may be able to know the mechanisms that mediate the adverse reactions and ultimately find ways to prevent them and/or to combine AEDs rationally (or to combine an AED with other non-AEDs). Clearly, more research is needed in this area.

Pharmacogenomics and choice of the personal AED

Genetic factors can contribute in the genesis of unexpected or idiosyncratic adverse reactions, through, for example, the synthesis of variant plasma proteins (which can cause atypical drug–protein binding) or in the existence of abnormal or variant metabolic capacity (e.g. slow phenytoin para-hydroxylators may lead to higher than expected drug levels and unexpected toxicity).

A great part of the interactions of AEDs with other AEDs or with other non-epileptic drugs occur at the metabolic level, principally through the cytochrome P450 system. Practically, only five CYP isoenzymes account for the metabolism of most therapeutic agents studied to date (Levy and Bourgeois, 1997) – CYP1A2, CYP2C9/10, CYP2C19, CYP2D6, CYP3A4. CYP2C19 and CYP2D6 exhibit known genetic polymorphism. The major pathway (60–80%) in phenytoin metabolism is hydroxylation to p-hydroxyphenol-5-phenylhydantoin (p-HPPH) by CYP2C9, whereas the metabolism of carbamazepine to carbamazepine-10,11-epoxide (40–60%) is through the isoenzyme CYP3A4 (Levy and Bourgeois, 1997). Now it is possible to characterize each individual regarding his or her CYP isoenzymes. Thus, if a subject does not have genetic polymorphisms, drug interactions during combination therapy will be minimal. Therefore, a bespoke treatment regimen would be possible in the future.

Validation of therapeutic ranges

For many AEDs, therapeutic serum level ranges are more or less well defined. However, the increasing application of serum AED monitoring led to an awareness that use of multiple AEDs altered the pharmacokinetics of the individual drugs, thereby complicating their use. Drugs with a narrow therapeutic range or low therapeutic index are more likely to be the objects for serious drug interactions. In RP, it is necessary to correlate serum levels with clinical efficacy since the combined drugs may be more active if the serum levels attained by each one in combination therapy are similar to those attained when the drug is used in monotherapy. Moreover, the serum concentrations must be correlated with the type and severity of epilepsy.

REFERENCES

Berzon R, Hays RD, Shumaker SA. International use, application and performance of health-related quality of life instruments. *Qual Life Res* 1993; **2**: 367–368.

Brown EG, Wood L, Wood S. The medical dictionary for regulatory activities (MedDRA). *Drug Safety* 1999; **20**: 109–117.

Committee for Proprietary Medicinal Products (CPMP). Note for guidance on fixed combination medicinal products (CPMP/EWP/240/95) (http://www.eudra.org).

Ernfors P, Bengzon J, Kokaia Z, *et al.* Increased levels of messenger RNAs for neurotrophic factors in the brain during kindling epileptogenesis. *Neuron* 1991; **7**: 165–176.

Fundabashi T, Sasaki H, Kimura F. Intraventricular injection of antiserum to nerve growth factor delays the development of amygdaloid kindling. *Brain Res* 1988; **458**: 132–136.

Greenwood RS. Adverse effects of antiepileptic drugs. *Epilepsia* 2000; **41**(Suppl. 2): s42–s52.

Guyatt GH, Naylor D, Juniper E, *et al.* Users' guides to the medical literature. XII. How to use articles about health-related quality of life. *J Am Med Assoc* 1997; **277**: 1232–1237.

Homan RW. Adjunctive and combination therapy. In *Epilepsy: A Comprehensive Textbook.* J. Engel, T. A. Pedley, eds. Philadelphia: Lippincott-Raven, 1997: 1265–1274.

Leppik IE. Monotherapy and polypharmacy. *Neurology* 2000; **55**(Suppl. 3): s25–s29.

Lesko SM, Mitchell AA. The use of randomized controlled trials for pharmacoepidemiology studies. In *Pharmacoepidemiology.* B. L. Strom, ed. London: Wiley & Sons, 2001: 539–552.

Levy RH, Bourgeois BFD. Drug–drug interactions. In *Epilepsy: A Comprehensive Textbook.* J. Engel, T. A. Pedley, eds. Philadelphia: Lippincott-Raven, 1997: 1175–1179.

Loiseau P, Jallon P. Clinical trials in epilepsy. In *Clinical Trials in Neurologic Practice.* J. Biller, J. Bogousslavsky, eds. Woburn, MA: Butterworth-Heinemann, 2001: 121–145.

Löscher W, Ebert U. Basic mechanisms of seizure propagation: targets for rational drug design and rational polypharmacy. *Epilepsy Res Suppl* 1996; **Suppl. 11**: 17–43.

Lothman EW. Neurobiology as a basis for rational polypharmacy. *Epilepsy Res Suppl* 1996; **Suppl. 11**: 3–7.

Macdonald RL. Cellular effects of antiepileptic drugs. In *Epilepsy: A Comprehensive Textbook.* J. Engel, T. A. Pedley, eds. Philadelphia: Lippincott-Raven, 1997: 1383–1391.

Moshé SL. Mechanisms of action of anticonvulsant agents. *Neurology* 2000; **55**(Suppl. 1): s32–s40.

Sankar R, Weaver DF. Basic principles of medicinal chemistry. In *Epilepsy: A Comprehensive Textbook.* J. Engel, T. A. Pedley, eds. Philadelphia: Lippincott-Raven, 1997: 1393–1403.

Scheuer ML. Drug treatment in the elderly. In *Epilepsy: A Comprehensive Textbook.* J. Engel, T. A. Pedley, eds. Philadelphia: Lippincott-Raven, 1997: 1211–1219.

Snead OC, Hosey LC. Exacerbation of seizures in children by carbamazepine. *New Engl J Med* 1985; **313**: 916–921.

Theodore WH, Blasberg R, Lerdeman D. PET imaging of opiate receptor binding in human epilepsy using 18F-cyclofoxy. *Neurology* 1990; **40**: 257.

Waning B, Montagne M. *Pharmacoepidemiology – Principles and Practice.* New York: McGraw-Hill, 2001.

Williams LS. Randomized controlled trials: methodology, outcomes, and interpretation. In *Clinical Trials in Neurologic Practice.* J. Biller, J. Bogousslavsky, eds. Woburn, MA: Butterworth-Heinemann, 2001: 1–26.

Index

Page numbers in *italic*, e.g. *195*, refer to figures. Page numbers in **bold**, e.g. **183**, signify entries in tables.